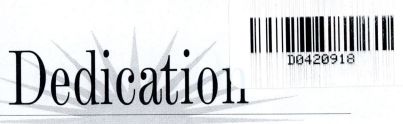

Dedication

This book is dedicated to my mother and father, who always encouraged me to do my best, and to my husband and children, who constantly support me to do so.

Contents

The International Guide to Speech Acquisition

Edited by Sharynne McLeod, PhD

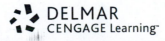

DELMAR
CENGAGE Learning™

Australia • Brazil • Japan • Korea • Mexico • Singapore • Spain • United Kingdom • United States

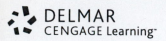
DELMAR
CENGAGE Learning™

**The International Guide to
Speech Acquisition**
Sharynne McLeod

Vice President, Health Care Business Unit:
 William Brottmiller

Director of Learning Solutions: Matthew Kane

Senior Acquisitions Editor: Sherry Dickinson

Managing Editor: Marah Bellegarde

Product Manager: Natalie Pashoukos

Marketing Director: Jennifer McAvey

Marketing Channel Manager:
 Michele McTighe

Production Director: Carolyn Miller

Art Director: Jack Pendleton

Content Project Manager: Stacey Lamodi

For product information and technology assistance, contact us at
Cengage Learning Customer & Sales Support, 1-800-354-9706

For permission to use material from this text or product,
submit all requests online at **www.cengage.com/permissions**
Further permissions questions can be emailed to
permissionrequest@cengage.com

Library of Congress Control Number: 2006038064

ISBN-13: 978-1-4180-5360-4

ISBN-10: 1-4180-5360-0

Delmar
Executive Woods
5 Maxwell Drive
Clifton Park, NY 12065
USA

Cengage Learning is a leading provider of customized learning solutions with office locations around the globe, including Singapore, the United Kingdom, Australia, Mexico, Brazil, and Japan. Locate your local office at **www.cengage.com/global**

Cengage Learning products are represented in Canada by Nelson Education, Ltd.

To learn more about Delmar, visit **www.cengage.com/delmar**

Purchase any of our products at your local bookstore or at our preferred online store **www.cengagebrain.com**

Printed in the United States of America
2 3 4 5 6   19 18 17 16 15

Preface

Learning to speak is one of our most significant achievements. It is remarkable how young children throughout the world decipher the languages they are exposed to and learn to communicate using intelligible speech. *The International Guide to Speech Acquisition* is a comprehensive resource that explores children's speech acquisition.

Typical speech acquisition is used as the framework of the book, as most children accomplish the ability to speak their local language as a natural and effortless part of their daily lives. Some children do not, and require additional input from speech-language pathologists, teachers, and families. Consequently, speech-language pathologists and teachers can use this book as a resource for understanding typical speech acquisition in order to scaffold their assessment, diagnosis, prevention, and intervention plans for children with speech impairment. Linguists, phoneticians, and those interested in children's speech development will also find this book to be relevant to their work.

The International Guide to Speech Acquisition comprehensively addresses *speech* acquisition, including the areas of articulation, phonology, and phonetics. The book does not include information about *language* acquisition. Semantics, morphology, syntax, and discourse are not covered, and readers are directed to other resources to find this information.

Why this book was written

This book could be compared to the *Lonely Planet Guide* or one of the other widely sold travel guides, but this time, specifically written for people who are interested in children's speech from around the world. Instead of containing travel tips, it contains information about children's speech acquisition that is relevant to many languages. This *Lonely Planet Guide* equivalent is timely. In 2005, reciprocity agreements were ratified between the American Speech-Language-Hearing Association (ASHA), the Royal College of Speech-Language Therapists (RCSLT–UK), Speech Pathology Australia, and the Canadian Association of Speech-Language Pathologists and Audiologists (CALSPA). It is likely that other international speech-language pathology associations will also be included in this agreement in future years. Even without this impetus, there is a need for this international resource due to the multicultural composition of schools and speech-language pathology caseloads. Further, professionals such as speech-language pathologists and teachers are educated throughout the world and similarly travel, live, and work with speakers of many different dialects and languages.

Organization of this book

The International Guide to Speech Acquisition is organized in two parts. *Part I, Foundations of Speech Acquisition,* contains an overview of the factors impacting all children's speech acquisition, regardless of the language they speak. Part I is based around the framework of the *International Classification of Functioning, Disability and Health* (ICF; World Health

Organization, 2001), and an explanation of the book's correspondence with the ICF can be found in chapter 1. Using the framework of the ICF has meant an expansion beyond the typical chapters contained in books on children's speech because the ICF embraces a biopsychosocial view of health and wellness. Thus, as well as chapters on genetics, neurology, oromusculature, hearing, articulatory, and linguistic foundations, Part I also includes chapters on historical and international perspectives of childhood, the family, social and educational contexts, activity and participation in society, and personal factors influencing speech acquisition. Learning to speak more than one language is addressed in the chapters on multilingual speech acquisition, children who are internationally adopted, accent modification, and working with interpreters.

Part II, Speech Acquisition Around the World, contains specific information on speech acquisition for English dialects and other languages. The first chapters in Part II outline the unique features of 12 different English dialects. The initial chapter in Part II covers speech acquisition in General American English (GAE). This is then compared with three other American English dialects: African American English, Appalachian English, and Cajun English. English dialects from around the globe are then described: English (from England), Irish English, Scottish English, Australian English, and New Zealand English. Furthermore, English influenced by other major world languages is described in the chapters on Cantonese-influenced English and Spanish-influenced English. It is acknowledged that a number of major American English dialects are not included, specifically the Northern and Southern American English dialects (see Labov, Ash, and Boberg, 2005, for further information). Additionally, South African English and Punjabi-influenced English are major English dialects that are not addressed, and it is anticipated that at least some of these dialects will be included in future editions of the book.

The next chapters in Part II outline the unique features of over 20 different languages. Major language families that are included within Part II are the following:

- Afro-Asiatic languages, represented by the Semitic languages: Arabic, Hebrew, and Maltese
- Altaic languages, represented by Turkish and Korean
- Austro-Asiatic languages, represented by Vietnamese
- Austronesian languages, represented by Filipino and Thai
- Indo-European languages including:
  - Germanic languages, represented by English, German, Dutch, and Norwegian
  - Romance languages, represented by Spanish, Portuguese, and French
  - Celtic languages, represented by Welsh
  - Greek
- Japonic languages, represented by Japanese
- Khoisan langauges, represented by Sesotho
- Sino-Tibetan languages, represented by Cantonese and Putonghua
- Uralic languages, represented by Finnish and Hungarian

This list does not include the following major world language groups: Caucasian, Dravidian, Eskimo-Aleut, Na-Dené, Niger-Congo, Nilo-Saharan, and Pama-Nyungan. In most instances, there is little or no research currently being undertaken on children's acquisition of these languages. Additional language groups should be added in future editions of this book.

Part II Organization

Each chapter in Part II uses exactly the same structure. In this way, readers of the book can flip from one chapter to another, comparing children's speech acquisition. For example, those interested in the acquisition of vowels can find information for each language and dialect under the heading of *Acquired sounds: vowels and diphthongs* and *Percent correct: vowels* in every chapter in Part II. The structure of every chapter is as follows:

1   *General overview of the dialect or language*: provides a general overview of the language, the countries where it is spoken (including a world map), the segmental aspects (consonants, vowels, tones), suprasegmental aspects, and writing system of that language.

2   *Overview of speech acquisition*: contains a comprehensive overview of information available on typical speech acquisition for that English dialect or language. This is supported by the *Summary of Studies Table* found at the end of each chapter.

3   *Overview of typical assessment, intervention, and employment opportunities*: includes professionally oriented information for speech-language pathologists working with children who speak the dialect or language featured in the chapter. This is supported by the *Phonetically Speaking* feature that contains the pronunciation in that language of relevant words such as *tongue, hard palate, sound,* and *sentence* that cannot be found in readily available translation guides.

Features

- Addresses the need for SLPs to have knowledge of dialectal variations in English.
- Chapters consistently organized for ease of locating or comparing information.
- *Phonetically Speaking* feature, appearing at the end of all Part II chapters, demonstrates phonetic pronunciation of certain verses allowing the reader to see the difference one particular verse can have when spoken in different dialects; or contains a table of pronunciations relevant to speech assessment and intervention.
- *Geographic maps* outlining country of focus and areas where the language is spoken is found in each chapter in Part II.
- *Inside front cover* contains a world map indicating areas covered in the book and *inside back cover* contains the International Phonetic Alphabet for easy reference.
- Much of the data presented in Part II has been translated into English for the first time.
  - Scanning the chapters' reference lists will reveal that many studies were written in languages other than English, and many come from doctoral and master's dissertations in those languages. For example, every reference in the chapter on Korean speech acquisition is written in Korean. Similarly, the majority of references in the chapters on Brazilian Portuguese, Israeli Hebrew, Hungarian, Norwegian, Turkish, and Japanese are written in languages other than English.
- Authorship is interdisciplinary and international.
  - The backgrounds of the authors include historians, educators, psychologists, philosophers, geneticists, linguists, phoneticians, audiologists, and speech-language pathologists. Each brings the richness of his or her profession and nationality to a holistic understanding of children's speech acquisition.

Conventions used within this book

The following conventions have been used within the book:

3;6 = 3 years;6 months

C = consonant; V = vowel; G = glide (e.g., /j/)

w = weak stress

S = strong stress (e.g., wwS = weak weak Strong)

$ = syllable boundary

* = not allowable in the language

PCC = percent consonants correct

PVC = percent vowels correct

PCCC = percent consonant clusters correct

IPA = International Phonetic Alphabet

WHO = World Health Organization

'words in single quotation marks' = English translation

italicized word = word in specified language

About the Author

Sharynne McLeod, PhD is an associate professor in speech and language acquisition at Charles Sturt University, Australia, and is a speech-language pathologist. She has published and presented papers internationally on speech acquisition and speech impairment in children. Her research into children's speech development is holistic, encompassing and addressing all aspects of the biopsychosocial framework espoused by the *International Classification of Functioning, Disability and Health* (ICF, World Health Organization [WHO], 2001). Dr. McLeod is a fellow of Speech Pathology Australia and vice president for the International Clinical Linguistics and Phonetics Association. She is editor of *Advances in Speech-Language Pathology* and is on the editorial board of *Clinical Linguistics and Phonetics* (both Taylor and Francis journals). She is an editorial consultant for two journals of the American Speech-Language-Hearing Association: *Language, Speech, and Hearing Services in Schools* and *American Journal of Speech-Language Pathology*. She has been invited to present master classes and seminars at the Speech Pathology Australia National Conference and the American Speech-Language-Hearing Conventions.

Avenue for feedback

Suggestions are welcomed for additional material and chapters to be included in the next edition of this book. Please contact the author at smcleod@csu.edu.au or Delmar, Cengage Learning.

Sharynne McLeod, PhD
Charles Sturt University, Australia

Acknowledgements

This book would not exist without the 72 contributing authors, whom I count as friends as well as colleagues. I thank each of the authors for their generosity of spirit and willingness to work to a template and timelines. There were many respectful discussions among authors to ensure a cohesive book. From reading the chapters it can be seen that the authors have a deep interest in communication and enabling children to realize their potential. This book is a result of more than just their words on paper—it is the result of the collaborative spirit of outstanding professionals within the fields of speech-language pathology, phonetics, linguistics, audiology, philosophy, psychology, history, and education.

Additionally, I am very grateful to the following:

- Ken Bleile, University of Northern Iowa, for his encouragement and nurturing of the idea behind this book.
- The editorial team at Delmar, Cengage Learning, for meeting the challenges of interpreting phonetic symbols, non-English scripts, and the many perspectives presented in this book.
- Steven Gibbs, Spatial Analysis Network, Charles Sturt University, for his ability to listen carefully to authors about the political and linguistic sensitivity of the maps he has drawn.
- David, Brendon, and Jessica, who continually support and encourage my every endeavor.

Contributors

Each contributor is listed along with the pronunciation of his or her name (using International Phonetic Alphabet conventions). This will enable accurate pronunciation when quoting these authors' work. A short biography and each author's e-mail address are also included. This will enable collaborative efforts to increase the knowledge of children's speech acquisition by initiating research to address the gaps identified within each chapter in Part II.

Mousa Amayreh [ˈmuːsa ʔaˈmaːjra] is a native speaker of Arabic with degrees in English, linguistics, and speech-language pathology. His research focuses on normal and disordered Arabic phonology. He is currently director of the Center for Phonetics Research and an associate professor of the Department of Hearing and Speech Sciences at the University of Jordan. e-mail: mamayreh@ju.edu.jo

Jessica Ball [ˌdʒɛsəkə ˈbaɬ] is a professor in child and youth care at the University of Victoria, Canada. She is a clinical-developmental psychologist specializing in Indigenous child and family development. Her recent research and publications focus on assessment and early intervention services for Indigenous children. Along with colleagues, she has done some of the first work in Canada on varieties of English among Aboriginal peoples and implications of cultural differences for the professionals in speech-language pathology, early intervention, and school-based remediation programs. Web site: www.ecdip.org. e-mail: jball@uvic.ca

Martin J. Ball [ˈmɑtɪn ˈbɔl] is Hawthorne Endowed Professor, and Department of Communicative Disorders head, University of Louisiana, Lafayette, USA. He is Honorary Fellow of the Royal College of Speech and Language Therapists, co-editor of *Clinical Linguistics and Phonetics*, and former president of the International Clinical Phonetics and Linguistics Association. He has researched and written widely on clinical phonetics and Welsh linguistics. e-mail: mjball@louisiana.edu

Avivit Ben-David [aviˈvit ben daˈvid] is a practicing speech clinician, with a B.A. and M.A. in communication disorders, and a PhD in linguistics from Tel Aviv University Israel. She is a teaching instructor in phonetics, phonology, and articulation disorders at Tel Aviv University and a lecturer in phonological development and clinical intervention at Hadassah College, Jerusalem. Her research areas include phonological acquisition and phonological disorders in Hebrew. e-mail: bdavid@post.tau.ac.il

Ruth Berman [ʁut ˈbeʁman], née Aronson, is professor emeritus of linguistics and chair in language across the life span at Tel Aviv University, Israel. Her publications include *Modern Hebrew Structure* (Tel Aviv, 1978), *Acquisition of Hebrew* (Erlbaum, 1985), *Relating*

Events in Narrative (with Dan I. Slobin, Erlbaum 1994), and editing of Volume 3 in the *Trends in Language Acquisition Research* series (Benjamins, 2004) and cross-linguistic special issues of *Written Language & Literacy* (2002) and *Journal of Pragmatics* (2005). e-mail: rberman@post.tau.ac.il

Barbara May Handford Bernhardt [ˈbɑɪbɹə ˈmeɪ ˈbɚ-nˌhɑɹt] is an associate professor and speech-language pathologist in the School of Audiology and Speech Sciences, University of British Columbia, Canada. Her research focuses on phonological and phonetic intervention, and early identification of speech and language impairment. A recent study with Drs. Jessica Ball and Jeff Deby has been exploring the topic of First Nations English dialects in Canada. She is a native speaker of western Canadian English. e-mail: bernharb@interchange.ubc.ca

Ken M. Bleile [kɛn blaɪl] is a professor in the Department of Communicative Disorders, University of Northern Iowa, USA. During periods in the last several years he has also served as a visiting scholar in the University of Anatolia, Turkey; in the Ministry of Health, Singapore; in Hertzen University, Saint Petersburg, Russia; and in the University of Canterbury, New Zealand. Dr. Bleile was Speech-Language Pathology chair of the 2003 ASHA conference, and is a recent associate editor for the *American Journal of Speech-Language Pathology*. Dr. Bleile publishes extensively in the areas of phonology, the neurological basis of speech disorders, pediatric head injury, and tracheotomy in children. e-mail: Ken.bleile@uni.edu

Caroline Bowen [ˌkæɹəˈlaɪn ˈbouwən] is an honorary associate in linguistics at Macquarie University, Australia, and operates a solo speech-language pathology practice surrounded by native bushland in Australia's World Heritage-listed Blue Mountains National Park, 100 km from Sydney. Never humdrum, Dr. Bowen's workload combines an enjoyable mix of clinical consulting, research, teaching, and writing. Web site: www.slpsite.com. e-mail: cbowen@ihug.com.au

Li-Rong Lilly Cheng [li ɹɑŋ lɪli tʃɛŋ] is professor in the School of Speech, Language, and Hearing Sciences at San Diego State University, California, USA, and the director of the Chinese Studies Institute. She is a fellow of the American Speech-Language Hearing Association (ASHA) and the recipient of the 1997 ASHA Award for special contributions to Multicultural Affairs. Dr. Cheng is the recipient of the 2002 Diversity Award from the California Speech and Hearing Association. She has numerous publications and has lectured all over the world. Dr. Cheng is the chair of the Education Committee of the International Association of Logopedics and Phoniatrics. She is a consultant for The Children's Workshop, Sesame Street. e-mail: lcheng@mail.sdsu.edu

Barbara L. Davis [baɚbɚɹɑɛldevɪs] is a professor in the Department of Communication Sciences and Disorders at the University of Texas at Austin, USA. Her research centers on understanding the interactive influences of production and perception in speech acquisition and includes studies of typically developing infants in diverse language environments, children receiving cochlear implants, and children diagnosed with developmental speech disorders. e-mail: babs@mail.utexas.edu

Jeff Deby [dʒɛf dəˈbi] is a Vancouver-based freelance sociolinguist. Dr. Deby specializes in the interaction of language with social and cultural identities. A recent study with Drs. Barbara Bernhardt and Jessica Ball has been exploring the topic of First Nations English dialects in Canada. He is a native speaker of western Canadian English. e-mail: jeff.deby@shaw.ca

Katherine Demuth [ˈkæθɚɪn ˈdiməθ] is professor of cognitive and linguistic sciences at Brown University, USA. Her research focuses on teasing apart the biological and environmental contributions to language learning. Much of this research has involved the comparative study of languages with different grammatical structures (English, Spanish, French, Sesotho), exploring children's developing phonological, morphological, and syntactic representations. She is especially known for her research on Sesotho. e-mail: Katherine_Demuth@brown.edu

Alice Dyson [ˈæləs ˈdaɪsən] currently teaches at Ball State University, USA. Her research interests are normal phonological acquisition and cross-linguistic phonology. She is associated with Arabic phonology through her work with Dr. Mousa Amayreh at the University of Jordan over the past 15 years, first as a mentor and later as a colleague. e-mail: adyson@bsu.edu

David J. Ertmer [ˈdeɪvəd ˈɜˑtˈmɚ] is a speech-language pathologist and an associate professor in speech, language, and hearing sciences at Purdue University, USA. He teaches courses in aural rehabilitation and clinical practices in speech-language pathology to undergraduate and graduate students. His current research focuses on early speech development in infants and toddlers who receive cochlear implants. e-mail: dertmer@purdue.edu

Peter Flipsen Jr. [ˈpitɚ ˈflɪpsn̩] is an associate professor of speech-language pathology at the University of Tennessee, Knoxville, USA. Dr. Flipsen teaches classes in phonetics, speech sound disorders, and appraisal of speech and language disorders. His research focuses on long-term outcomes in children with delayed speech and speech development in children with cochlear implants. Dr. Flipsen is originally from Canada and has a long-standing personal interest in the dialects of North American English. e-mail: pflipsen@utk.edu

Annette V. Fox [anɛtə fɔks] has been trained and worked as an SLP in Germany before furthering her education with an M.Sc. in neuropsycholinguistics and a PhD in the acquisition of phonology and the classification of speech disorders in German-speaking children at the Department of Speech at the University of Newcastle upon Tyne in northeast England. In 2003 she became professor of speech and language therapy at the first university for SLT in Germany. e-mail: fox@fh-fresenius.de

Ellen Gerrits [ˈɛlən ˈχɛrɪts] is a licensed speech-language pathologist. In 2001, she received her PhD in phonetic sciences. At present she is affiliated with the Department of Otorhinolaryngology of the University Hospital Maastricht, The Netherlands. Her clinical and research interests include language acquisition of children with hearing loss, children with specific language impairment (SLI), and dyslexia. e-mail: e.gerrits@np.unimaas.nl

Steven Gibbs [stivən gɪbz] is a research support officer for the Spatial Data Analysis Network at Charles Sturt University, Australia. He specializes in using geographic information systems and broader methods in human geography to address issues of policy and social research. In recent years he has worked on and produced maps for road safety reports, pedestrian modeling, rural teacher education, and community surveys. e-mail: stgibbs@csu.edu.au

Gail T. Gillon [gɛeʊ gəˑlən] is an associate professor in the Department of Communication Disorders, University of Canterbury, New Zealand. A native New Zealander, she worked as a speech-language therapist in New Zealand and Australia for several years. Following the completion of her PhD in speech and hearing in 1995, her research has explored the relationship between spoken and written language disorders and the prevention of literacy difficulties for children with speech impairment. e-mail: gail.gillon@canterbury.ac.nz

Brian A. Goldstein [ˈbɹɑɪən ˈɡoldstin] is an associate professor in the Department of Communication Sciences at Temple University, USA. He holds the Certificate of Clinical Competence (CCC) in speech-language pathology. His research interests are phonological development and disorders in Spanish-speaking children. He was also the editor of *Language, Speech, and Hearing Services in Schools* (2004–2006). e-mail: briang@temple.edu

Olga Gordeeva [ˈɔɫɡə ɡɔɹˈdeivə] is a postdoctoral research fellow at Queen Margaret University, Edinburgh, UK. She has a PhD in speech and language sciences, and studied segmental and suprasegmental aspects of typical monolingual acquisition in Scottish English children. e-mail: ogordeeva@gmail.com

Helen Grech [hɛlɛn ɡɹɛk] is a senior lecturer and co-ordinates the Communication Therapy Division within the Institute of Health Care of the University of Malta. Dr. Grech is a native Maltese speaker. Like most of the Maltese, Helen Grech is multilingual. Her doctoral dissertation was related to the phonological acquisition of Maltese-speaking children. e-mail: helen.grech@um.edu.mt

Jacqueline A. Guendouzi [dʒæki ɡɛnduzi] is currently associate professor in communicative disorders at the University of South Alabama, USA, and previously worked at Southeastern Louisiana University and the University of Central England. She has co-authored a book, *Discourse Approaches to Dementia*, and has published in the areas of communication disorders, social interaction, and discourse analysis. e-mail: jguendouzi@usouthal.edu

Linda J. Harrison [ˈlɪndə ˈhæɹəsən] is a senior lecturer in early childhood education at Charles Sturt University, Australia. Dr. Harrison's research addresses child care and family influences on children's development, with a particular focus on the nature of children's relationships with important adults and the ways these relationships impact on adjustment at key periods in development. Linda is involved with a number of longitudinal studies including The Sydney Family Development Project, Child Care Choices, and Growing Up in Australia: The Longitudinal Study of Australian Children (LSAC). e-mail: lharrison@csu.edu.au

Alison Holm [ˈæləsən ˈhɒlm] is a postdoctoral researcher (funded by the National Health and Medical Research Council) in the Perinatal Research Centre at the Royal Brisbane and Women's Hospital in Queensland, Australia. Dr. Holm's research interests are the communication outcomes of preterm children and the phonological development and impairments of monolingual and bilingual children. e-mail: a.holm@uq.edu.au

Sara Howard [ˈsɛəɹə ˈhaʊəd] is a senior lecturer in clinical phonetics and linguistics in the Department of Human Communication Sciences, University of Sheffield, UK. As well as her academic qualifications in phonetics and linguistics, she is professionally qualified as a speech-language therapist/pathologist. Dr. Howard has published and presented widely in the area of clinical phonetics and phonology, with a particular emphasis on the perceptual and instrumental phonetic analysis of developmental speech disorders. e-mail: s.howard@sheffield.ac.uk

Deborah Hwa-Froelich [dɛb wa fɹelɪk], associate professor in the Department of Communication Sciences and Disorders, Saint Louis University, USA, and board-certified child language specialist, has research interests in the assessment and treatment of social-emotional and language-based learning problems in young children and children from culturally and linguistically diverse backgrounds. She is the ASHA Division 14 *Perspectives* editor, a board member for *Word of Mouth*, and coordinator for the SLU International Adoption Clinic. e-mail: hwafroda@slu.edu

Kim M. Isaac [kɪm aɪzæk] completed her PhD studies in 2003 in the area of SLP-interpreter partnerships and has been involved in similar research with colleagues from the University of Newcastle and Macquarie University (Sydney) in Australia. She has also been involved in the education of interpreters through the NSW Health Care Interpreter Service and currently works in private practice. e-mail: kim@headstartforkids.com.au

Raymond D. Kent [ɹeɪ kent] is professor emeritus of Communicative Disorders at the University of Wisconsin-Madison, USA. His primary research interests are neurogenic speech disorders in children and adults, speech development in infants and young children, measurement of speech intelligibility and quality, and the acoustic analysis of speech. e-mail: kent@waisman.wisc.edu

Ghada Khattab [ˈɣaːda χaˈtˤʕːaːb] is a phonetics lecturer in the School of Education, Communication, and Language Sciences at Newcastle University, UK. She is a native speaker of Lebanese Arabic and has a PhD in linguistics from the University of Leeds. Her research interests include monolingual and bilingual phonological development and sociolinguistics. e-mail: ghada.khattab@ncl.ac.uk

Minjung Kim [min tɕʌŋ kim] is a Korean speech-language pathologist and a senior lecturer in the Department of Speech-Language Therapy at Woosong University, Korea. She is interested in Korean children's phonological development and phonological disorders and has written several papers dealing with Korean children's speech acquisition and phonological processes for the identification of phonological disorders of Korean children. e-mail: kimmj@wsu.ac.kr

Kristian Emil Kristoffersen [ˈkʰrɪstjan eˈmɪl kʰrɪˈstofəʃən] is a professor of general linguistics at the University of Oslo, Norway. His main fields of research are clinical linguistics, with focus on phonetic and phonological disorders, and cognitive linguistics, with focus on the semantic structure of spatial particles. Norwegian is his first language. e-mail: k.e.kristoffersen@iln.uio.no

Sari Kunnari [sɑri kunːɑri] is a native Finnish speaker and her research has been primarily in the areas of typical speech and language acquisition of children acquiring Finnish. Dr. Kunnari is a senior lecturer of speech and language pathology at the University of Oulu, Finland. She is currently engaged in several cross-linguistic research projects. e-mail: sari.kunnari@oulu.fi

Felicia Lee [fəˈlɪʃə ˈliː] is affiliated with the University of British Columbia, Canada, and the University of California, Los Angeles, USA. Dr. Lee's research focuses on the syntax and semantics of San Lucas Quiaviní Zapotec (SLQZ), with a special interest in the syntax/semantics interface. Recent publications have addressed issues such as tense, wh-movement, and binding/coreference in SLQZ. She is a co-investigator on the research project on the first language acquisition of Zapotec. e-mail: leefa99@earthlink.net

Clara Levelt [ˈklaːra ˈleːvɛlt] teaches at the Department of Linguistics, Leiden University, The Netherlands, and specializes in child language phonology. She has written a PhD thesis and several articles on the acquisition of Dutch phonology. Together with Paula Fikkert she set up a large database of Dutch developmental data, available (soon) through CHILDES. e-mail: c.c.levelt@let.leidenuniv.nl

Barbara A. Lewis [baɪbaɹə e luɪs] is an associate professor at Case Western Reserve University, USA. Her primary area of expertise is the biological bases of speech and language impairments. She has been conducting research into the genetic basis of speech sound disorders and its comorbidity with language and reading impairment for over 20 years. e-mail: barbara.lewis@case.edu

John L. Locke [dʒɒn lɒk] is professor of speech-language-hearing sciences and director of the interdisciplinary program in linguistics at Lehman College, City University of New York, USA, and a member of the doctoral faculty at the CUNY Graduate Center. He is the author of over 120 publications on the development and evolution of language, including *Phonological Acquisition and Change* (Academic Press, 1983) and *The Child's Path to Spoken Language* (Harvard University Press, 1993). e-mail: john.locke@lehman.cuny.edu

Preeya Lorwatanapongsa [ʔpɹija: lɔ:watʰna: pʰɔ: ŋsa] is a speech-language pathologist and lecturer at the Department of Rehabilitation Medicine, Chulalongkorn University, King Chulalongkorn Memorial Hospital, Bangkok, Thailand. Her specialty is Thai phonology. She has extensive clinical experience with children. She received formal training in Thailand and in the USA. e-mail: preeyalor@hotmail.com

Margaret Maclagan [mäɡɹət məklægən] is a linguist and an associate professor in the Department of Communication Disorders at the University of Canterbury, New Zealand. Her research interests include the study of New Zealand English, especially its overall development and sound changes currently in progress. e-mail: margaret.maclagan@canterbury.ac.nz

Valerie Malabonga [ʋalerie ɱalaboɲa] is a senior research associate at the Center for Applied Linguistics, Washington, DC, USA. Dr. Malabonga's research focus is the assessment of the language and literacy of English language learner children, specifically native speakers of Spanish and Filipino. She is a native speaker of Filipino. e-mail: valerie@cal.org

Stefka H. Marinova-Todd [stefka ɱarinovạtodd] is an assistant professor at the School of Audiology and Speech Sciences at the University of British Columbia in Vancouver, Canada. Her research focus is on oral proficiency and literacy development in the home (Cantonese, Mandarin, and Filipino) and school languages of children who are learning English as a second language. e-mail: stefka@audiospeech.ubc.ca

Sumalai Maroonroge [suma:lai ma:ɹuɲro:ʔt] is an associate professor and the director of audiology in the Department of Communication Disorders at Lamar University, USA. She has provided considerable assistance in the development of educational curricula for clinicians in Thailand and Taiwan. Her research focus is speech perception and electrophysiology measurement. e-mail: Maroonroge@aol.com

Ben Matthews [bɛn ˈmæθjuːz] is a linguist with interests in child speech, cross-linguistic variation, and sign language. His PhD involved a longitudinal study of Scottish English vowel acquisition. He is a lecturer at Queen Margaret University, Scotland. e-mail: bmatthews@qmu.ac.uk

Ineke Mennen [ˈinəkə ˈmɛnən] is a senior lecturer at Queen Margaret University, Scotland. She has worked as a speech-language pathologist in the Netherlands, Greece, and the UK. She also holds a B.Sc. Hons degree in Greek language and literature, and a PhD in linguistics from the University of Edinburgh. She specializes in acquisition of intonation and prosody in monolingual, bilingual, and clinical populations. e-mail: imennen@qmu.ac.uk

Sharynne McLeod [ˈʃæɹən məˈklaʊd] is associate professor in speech and language acquisition at Charles Sturt University, Australia, and has a PhD in speech-language pathology. She has published and presented papers internationally on speech acquisition and speech impairment in children. She is vice president of the International Clinical Linguistics and Phonetics Association, editor of *Advances in Speech-Language Pathology* (Taylor & Francis) and is on the editorial board of *Clinical Linguistics and Phonetics*. e-mail: smcleod@csu.edu.au.

Helena B. Mota [ɛlena mɔta] is associate professor of speech and language pathology and audiology at the Federal University of Santa Maria, Santa Maria-RS, Brazil. She is the coordinator of the research center of speech and language studies. Her areas of interest are clinical phonology, phonological acquisition, and language disorders. e-mail: hbm@viars.net

Nicole Müller [nɪˈkɔl ˈmʏlɐ] is professor in communicative disorders at the University of Louisiana at Lafayette, USA, and also holds a Hawthorne endowed professorship. Particular areas of interest include clinical discourse studies and pragmatics, specifically as applied to dementia; and multilingualism and Welsh linguistics. She is co-editor of *Clinical Linguistics and Phonetics*. e-mail: nmueller@louisiana.edu

Siân M. Munro [ˈʃɑn mʌnˈɹo] is head of the Centre for Speech and Language Therapy Studies at the University of Wales Institute, Cardiff. She is a fellow of the Royal College of Speech and Language Therapists. Her areas of interest include normal and abnormal speech and language development in Welsh-speaking children. e-mail: smunro@uwic.ac.uk

Janna Oetting [dʒæ̃nə ɛɾĩŋ] is a professor at Louisiana State University in Baton Rouge, USA. Her research focuses on child language acquisition and childhood language impairment. In recent years, she has examined both of these topics within the context of dialect diversity and poverty. e-mail: cdjanna@lsu.edu

Areti Okalidou [ɐɾɛˈti okɐˈliðu] is an assistant professor at the University of Macedonia in Greece and has worked as an ASHA-certified speech-language pathologist in the USA and in Greece. She holds a PhD in speech and hearing sciences from the City University of New York, Graduate Center. Her research interests include speech production of normal and developing Greek, but also speech of the hearing-impaired and children with implants. e-mail: okalidou@uom.gr

Mitsuhiko Ota [oːta mitsɯ́çiko] is lecturer in linguistics at the University of Edinburgh, Scotland. His research interests include the acquisition of prosodic structure, the development of pitch phonology, and the phonological lexicon. Much of his work investigates these issues by studying the speech production of 1- to 2-year-old Japanese children. e-mail: mits@ling.ed.ac.uk

Soyeong Pae [so jʌŋ pe] is a professor at Hallym Univeristy, Korea. She is focusing her research on Korean children's speech and language development to develop assessment and intervention materials for Korean children with speech-language and reading impairments. With other Korean speech pathologists she developed several test materials to identify Korean language impairment and has been interested in Korean children's noun and verb acquisition as well as grammatical morphemes. e-mail: spae@hallym.ac.kr

Karen E. Pollock [ˈkɛɹən ˈpɑlək] is a professor and chair of the Department of Speech Pathology and Audiology at the University of Alberta, Canada. Her research interests focus on children's phonological development and disorders. Recent projects have investigated vowel errors in children and speech-language development in children adopted internationally. e-mail: karen.pollock@ualberta.ca

Joan Rahilly [dʒoːn ˈɹahɪli] is senior lecturer in English language and linguistics at the Queen's University of Belfast, Northern Ireland. Dr. Rahilly's research focuses on Irish English and on aspects of speech impairment in English. e-mail: j.rahilly@qub.ac.uk

Leonora Ritter [liənɔɹə ɹɪtɐ] is an associate professor of history and politics and the head of the School of Social Sciences and Liberal Studies, Charles Sturt University, Australia. Her research into childhood includes publications in the areas of the history of juvenile delinquency, and a tentative taxonomy of childhood published in *disClosure, a Journal of Social Theory*. e-mail: lritter@csu.edu.au

Yvan Rose [ivã ʁoz], a native speaker of Québec French, obtained his PhD in linguistics from McGill University (Montréal, Canada) in 2000. His thesis is the first longitudinal study of phonological development in Québec French. His current research focuses on theoretical and developmental aspects of phonology, from a cross-linguistic perspective. e-mail: yrose@mun.ca

Susan Rvachew [ˈsuzən ɹəˈvæʃu] practiced pediatric speech-language pathology for 20 years before taking an academic position in the School of Communication Sciences and Disorders, McGill University, Canada, in order to focus on research full-time. Dr. Rvachew's research is concerned with the relationship between speech perception and speech production skills in infants and children and the development of effective interventions for speech sound disorders. e-mail: susan.rvachew@staff.mcgill.ca

Tuula Savinainen-Makkonen [tuːlɑ sɑʋinɑinenmɑkːonen] is a native Finnish speaker, and her research has been primarily in the areas of typical speech and language acquisition of children acquiring Finnish. Dr. Savinainen-Makkonen is senior research fellow at the Department of Speech Sciences, at the University of Helsinki, Finland. She has conducted research into early phonological development. She is working also as an SLP at Helsinki University Hospital. e-mail: tuula.savinainen-makkonen@helsinki.fi

James M. Scobbie [ˈdʒɪm ˈskɒbe̩] is a native of Glasgow, Scotland. He is a senior research fellow at Queen Margaret University, Scotland. Dr. Scobbie has a PhD in theoretical phonology and has been involved in a variety of research projects on Scottish English and Gaelic sound systems, including a longitudinal acoustic study of consonant cluster acquisition in Scottish children with developmental phonological disorder. e-mail: jscobbie@qmu.ac.uk

Ann Bosma Smit [æn bɒzmə smɪt] earned the master's degree at the University of Iowa and the PhD at the University of Maryland, USA. Currently, she is a professor at Kansas State University, USA. Her areas of study include the development of speech sound production in children who are acquiring General American English, remediation for articulatory and phonological disorders, and fluency disorders. e-mail: asmit@humec.ksu.edu

Lydia K. H. So (So Chau Kan Hoi) 蘇周簡開 [sou₅₅ tsau₅₅ kan₂₅ hɔi₅₅] is currently an associate professor at the University of Hong Kong, and Cantonese is her mother tongue. She qualified as a speech therapist in London and obtained her M.A. and Ph.D in linguistics at Macquarie University, Australia. Her research concentrates in the area of phonological development and disorder in monolingual and bilingual children. e-mail: lydiaso@hkucc.hku.hk

Joseph Paul Stemberger [ˈdʒousəf ˈstɛmˌbɹ̩gɹ̩] is a professor in the Department of Linguistics, University of British Columbia, Canada. His research focuses on mental representations and the processing of phonological and morphological information during language production, addressing implications for psychological models and linguistic theories.

He focuses especially on nonsystematic errors in adult production and on systematic errors in child production. He is currently engaged in a research project on the first language acquisition of Zapotec. e-mail: stemberg@interchange.ubc.ca

Ida J. Stockman [ɑɪdʌ dʒɔnz stɑkmɪn] is a professor in the Department of Communicative Sciences and Disorders at Michigan State University, USA, where she has taught separate courses on phonetics, phonological disorders, speech/language development, and multicultural issues. Her research includes a focus on developmental and clinical assessment issues related to the speech sound articulation of African American children. e-mail: stockma1@msu.edu

Carol Stoel-Gammon [ˈkɛɹəl ˈstol ˌɡæmən] is professor in the Department of Speech and Hearing Sciences at the University of Washington, Seattle, USA, and an adjunct professor in the Department of Linguistics. Her research interests include the study of prelinguistic vocal development, speech and language development in early childhood, and the identification of speech/language disorders in toddlers. e-mail: csg@u.washington.edu

Christie Tilkens [kɹɪstɪ tɪlkənz] received her undergraduate degree in communicative disorders at the University of Wisconsin-Madison, USA, and is currently enrolled in its master's program. She has worked for two years in Professor Lawrence Shriberg's laboratory as a phonetic transcriber and speech acoustics project assistant. e-mail: mctilkens@yahoo.com

Seyhun Topbaş [sɛjhun topbaʃ] trained as a linguist and received her M.A. in applied English language teaching. She furthered her education with an M.Sc. in clinical human communication disorders at the Department of Clinical Communication Studies, City University of London, and a PhD in the phonological analysis and the classification of speech disorders in Turkish-speaking children at Anadolu University in Turkey. In 1999, she pioneered the foundation of the Education, Research and Training Center and first Speech-Language Pathology Department in Turkey by initiating the M.Sc. and PhD programs. She became a professor of SLP in 2005. e-mail: stopbas@anadolu.edu.tr

Isao Ueda [ɯeda isao] is professor at Osaka University of Foreign Studies, Japan, where he obtained his M.A. in linguistics. His research interest lies in phonological acquisition and disorders of children. He serves as an editorial board member for *Journal of Multilingual Communication Disorders*. e-mail: uedais@osaka-gaidai.ac.jp

Nicole Watts Pappas [ˌnəˈkoʊl ˌwɒts ˈpæpəs] is a doctoral student in speech pathology at Charles Sturt University, Australia, researching involvement of families in intervention for speech impairment. She is also actively involved in clinical work in a community clinic in Brisbane, Australia, endeavoring to use family-centered practices in her work with young children and their families. e-mail: nwattspappas@hotmail.com

Sophie Wauquier-Gravelines [sofi vokje ɡʀavəlin] is a professor in the Speech Science Department at the University of Paris 8, France. She teaches linguistics, phonology, morphology, and psycholinguistics. Her current research focuses on the interrelations between adult psycholinguistics, developmental linguistics, and theoretical phonology, in addition to acquisition and speech pathology. She has worked mainly on French. e-mail: wauquiers@wanadoo.fr

Amy L. Weiss [ɛmi waɪs] is a professor at the Department of Communicative Disorders, University of Rhode Island, Kingston, USA. She teaches graduate courses in child language development and disorders, phonological disorders, fluency disorders, and multicultural issues in service delivery, along with maintaining an active research program.

A board-recognized specialist in child language (ASHA), she is the current coordinator of ASHA's Special Interest Division 1: Language Learning and Education. e-mail: weissa@mail.uri.edu

Mehmet Yavaş [mɛhmɛt javaʃ] is professor of linguistics at Florida International University, USA. Besides his numerous articles and chapters on applied phonology, his publications include *Applied English Phonology* (2005), *Phonology: Development and Disorders* (1998), *First and Second Language Phonology* (1994), and *Phonological Disorders in Children: Theory, Research, and Practice* (1991). e-mail: yavasm@fiu.edu

Zhu Hua [tʂuhua] is a senior lecturer School of Language, Linguistics and Culture, Birkbeck, University of London, UK. She is the author of *Phonological Development in Specific Contexts: Studies of Chinese-speaking Children* (Multilingual Matters, 2002), joint editor of *Phonological Acquisition and Disorders: A Multilingual Perspective* (Multilingual Matters, 2006); and joint author of *DEAP: Differential Evaluation of Articulation and Phonology* (The Psychological Corporation, 2002). e-mail: zhu.hua@sllc.bbk.ac.uk

Krisztina Zajdó [ˈkristinɔ ˈzɔjdoː] is an assistant professor of speech-language pathology and a linguist at the Division of Communication Disorders, University of Wyoming, Laramie, USA. Dr. Zajdó's research focuses on the phonetic and phonological aspects of speech acquisition in children from diverse language communities. She has co-edited a book, *Syllable Development: The Frame/content Theory and Beyond*, and has published in the areas of speech timing and phonological development. Recently she and colleagues from Amsterdam and Russia have been exploring the topic of cross-linguistic vowel acquisition in monolingual Hungarian-, Dutch-, and Russian-speaking children. She is a native speaker of Standard Hungarian. e-mail: kzajdo@uwyo.edu; zajdo@hotmail.com.

Introduction

International Perspectives
of Speech Acquisition

Li-Rong Lilly Cheng

This book is long overdue. There are more than 6.5 billion people living on the planet Earth (Xin Hua Net, June, 2005). By 2050, the world population is expected to reach 9.1 billion. The global population speaks more than 6,700 languages and over 399,000 dialects. Most of these languages are mutually unintelligible, and some languages are spoken by only a small number of people. However, some major languages are spoken by millions of people, including Mandarin Chinese (Putonghua), English, Hindi, Bengali, Spanish, French, and Russian. Besides the major languages spoken by large populations, there are also many languages spoken in isolated areas or islands. For example, over 1,200 indigenous languages are spoken among the five million inhabitants of the Pacific Islands; they belong to the Austronesian language family and include Charmorro, Marshallese, Trukese, Carolinian, Papua New Guinean, Korean, Japanese, Ponepean, Samoan, Hawaiian, Fijian, and Tahitian (Cheng, 1991). The five *lingua francas* used by the Pacific Islanders are French, English, Pidgin, Spanish, and Bahasa Indonesian/Malaysian. English is spoken on Guam, American Samoa, Saipan, and many of the Pacific Islands (Cheng, 1995). In the past, most individuals could survive by speaking their mother tongue, and knowledge of another language was not a requirement. At the same time, many groups of people in Africa, Asia, and Europe grew up speaking several languages and acquired fluency and the speech patterns of these various languages as a way of life and a means of survival.

In the early part of the last century, people traveled by boats and ocean liners, trains and cars to reach remote corners of the world. Today, one can travel to most parts of the world by jet within a day's time. The revolution of e-mail and Internet makes it possible to be connected and linked instantly. What used to take months or years to do can be done in a split second. The speed of traveling brings us closer and presents challenges to us as well. In his book entitled *The World Is Flat: A Brief History of the Twenty-first Century*, Thomas Friedman (2005) talks about how the flattening of the world happened at the dawn of the twenty-first century and what it means to countries, companies, communities, and individuals. More recently, the formation of the European Union and the North American Free Trade Agreement (NAFTA) created opportunities for people to travel and work in many corners of Europe and North America. Governments and societies can and must adapt to the flattening of the world.

Today, as the globe is shrinking rapidly, as technology continues to be developed, and as people work and travel all over the world, the need for speech and hearing professionals to have a guide to speech acquisition of the many languages in the world becomes pressing and paramount. In many work settings, speech–language pathologists encounter children who are not able to communicate effectively, and their parents ask for information on the speech acquisition of particular languages. Such information at the current time is not easy to come by, although there have been many research articles and professional papers on the topics of speech acquisition of many languages. The intent of this book is to organize the existing resources so that speech and language professionals can have this timely resource.

A lot of discussion in language diversity deals with the issues surrounding dialects and accents. All the languages and dialects of the world share some common properties, they all have sounds, and yet the specific phonetic features may differ tremendously. These features impact on the ways people speak versions of English. As speech–language pathologists become more involved in providing services to enhance the English communication skill of individuals who are nonnative speakers of English, there is a need to be cognizant about these speech characteristics and the acquisition process.

Our future will bring us more cultural and language diversity, varied experiences, increased insight into the culture of poverty, awareness of challenges for world literacy, and conflicts and unrest. A good example appears in an article entitled "Do boats have eyes?" where Friedman (2003) describes the children in Sikim, a mountain nation in South Asia, and how they learn. How they understand the world and the use of words and language is so different from what our textbooks tell us. These children believe that boats have eyes and can see in the ocean and can go places because they have eyes. The impact of culture is crucial in our understanding of the world around us. Speech–language pathologists need to be prepared to deal with such diverse thoughts and concepts.

Many children experience immigration and uprooting and some are very poor. The following excerpt from an unknown author is fitting here to illustrate the point: "I had seven brothers and when I was five, my dad told me I had to leave… I started to get beaten by my new family. I could not go to school because I had to work to earn money for my new family." The children we encounter may not have gone to school in their homeland and may have experienced poverty, wars, conflicts, and disasters. What effects will this have on their speech-language acquisition and the acquisition of literacy of our world's children? These challenges force professionals in speech and hearing to be more engaged in understanding about speech acquisition around the globe.

The International Guide to Speech Acquisition uses the *International Classification of Functioning, Disability and Health* (World Health Organization, 2001) as its framework in order to address biopsychosocial aspects of speech acquisition. Additionally it contains information on specific languages and English dialects, including the geographical area where the dialect/language is spoken, components of the dialect/language, age of acquisition, speech assessment, and speech intervention. This book is indeed a noteworthy effort from a dedicated group of individuals whose collective wisdom and cumulative knowledge will guide readers along the intricate path toward better understanding the acquisition of speech across the globe. The rich content and hidden treasures of this book need to be savored and cherished.

References

Cheng, L. (1991). *Assessing Asian language performance: Guidelines for evaluating limited-English-proficient students.* Oceanside, CA: Academic Communication Associates.

Cheng, L. (1995). The Pacific Islander populations and the challenges they face. In L. Cheng, (Ed.), *Integrating language and learning for inclusion* (pp. 45–55). San Diego, CA: Singular.

Friedman, T. L. (2003). *Do boats have eyes?* Publisher: unknown.

Friedman, T. L. (2005). *The world is flat: A brief history of the twenty-first century.* New York: Farrar, Straus and Giroux.

Languages of the world. (June 2005). Xin Hua News Bureau, Beijing, China.

World Health Organization. (2001). *ICF : International classification of functioning, disability and health.* Geneva: Author.

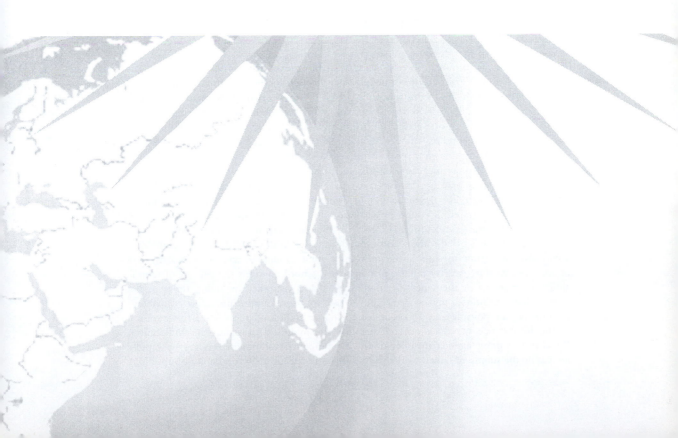

Part 1

Foundations of Speech Acquisition

Chapter 1

The ICF and ICF-CY as a Framework for Children's Speech Acquisition

Sharynne McLeod and Ken M. Bleile

INTRODUCTION

Speech is pivotal to human society as it is the major means of communication throughout the world. Within groups of people, speech often serves to define membership—ours is the group that speaks this way, and yours is the group that speaks that way. Speech and its written equivalents have largely replaced instinct as the means for passing on what is needful to know from one generation to the next (Bleile, 2004).

Reflecting the centrality of speech in human society, negative consequences may ensue when a person does not speak as others do in the community. A child with mild speech impairment may be teased or socially isolated, while persons with more severe speech impairments may be disadvantaged in health, education, and vocation (Lewis, Freebairn, and Taylor, 2000). Challenges encountered by a person with a speech impairment may be aggravated in countries with more limited health and education resources. As the World Bank's Millennium Project (2005) emphasizes, child mortality rates are tied to poverty, lack of education, and limited access to health care. To illustrate, in Mali, a West African nation, the mortality rate in poor, rural families is twice as high as in rich, urban ones. Worldwide, 100 million primary-aged school children remain out of school, almost 60 percent of them girls. To the extent that a disability, including those in the speech domain, limits a person's educational and vocational opportunities, it contributes to poverty and, possibly as a consequence, to higher childhood mortality. In recognition of the importance of education and disability to childhood mortality, the Millennium Project's five-point agenda includes improving human development services by rapidly increasing the supply of skilled workers in health and education (World Bank Group, 2005).

Children's acquisition of speech is a remarkable process, and it is suggested that the acquisition of speech and language is the most impressive feat some people will ever master. The acquisition of speech is unique for each child, yet there are also general trends that guide our understanding of speech acquisition.

A comprehensive understanding of speech acquisition is vital for assessment and intervention for children who are having difficulties with their speech (see Chapter 9). Researchers who study speech impairment have developed frameworks within which to analyze speech production. Concepts such as phonetic inventories, phonological processes, and prosody are useful tools to both researchers and clinicians (summarized in Part II of this book). A framework within which to consider the larger role of speech acquisition in human society may serve a similar heuristic purpose. Consequently the *International Classification of Functioning, Disability and Health* (ICF) (WHO, 2001) has been used as a framework for considering speech acquisition within this book (see Table 1-1).

The ICF and ICF-CY as a framework for considering speech acquisition

The International Classification of Functioning, Disability and Health (ICF)

The ICF is the culmination of over 21 years of development of a classification system of health and wellness. The first version was titled *International Classification of Impairments, Disabilities and Handicaps* (ICIDH) (WHO, 1980). The latest version, the *International Classification of Functioning, Disability and Health* (ICF) (WHO, 2001) draws on biological, psychological, and social aspects of health. Simeonsson (2003, p. S6) indicates that "additional detail is still needed in the ICF to document characteristics and environments unique to children." Consequently the ICF Children and Youth (ICF-CY), released in 2007,

TABLE 1-1   Application of *International Classification of Functioning, Disability and Health* (ICF) to speech acquisition

ICF parts	ICF components	ICF domains identified as relating to speech acquisition	Indicative chapters in this book
Functioning and disability	**Body functions**	• Global mental functions (including temperament and personality functions) • Specific mental functions (including perceptual functions and mental functions of language) • Voice and speech functions (including voice functions, articulation functions, and fluency and rhythm of speech) • Hearing and vestibular functions	• Applications of typical developmental information to understanding of speech impairment • Articulatory foundations • Linguistic foundations • Multilingual speech acquisition • Each chapter in Part II relating to different languages and English dialects • Aural foundations • Perceptual foundations
	Body structures	• Structures of the nervous system (including structure of the brain) • Structure of the eye, ear, and related structures (specifically structure of the external, middle, and inner ear) • Structures involved in voice and speech (including structure of the nose, mouth, pharynx, and larynx) • Structures of the cardiovascular, immunology and respiratory systems (specifically structure of respiratory systems)	• Neurological foundations • Aural foundations • Oromotor foundations

Table 1-1 continued

ICF parts	ICF components	ICF domains identified as relating to speech acquisition	Indicative chapters in this book
	Activities and participation	• Learning and applying knowledge (including listening, learning to read, thinking) • Communication (including communicating – receiving, communicating – producing, conversation and use of communication devices and techniques) • Domestic life • Interpersonal interactions and relationships (including family relationships) • Major life areas (including education) • Community, social, and civic life	• The social and educational context • The family context • Speech acquisition and participation in society
Contextual factors	**Environmental factors**	• Products and technology • Support and relationships (including immediate and extended family, friends, health professionals) • Attitudes (including societal attitudes, social norms, practices, and ideologies) • Services, systems, and policies (including those for communication, health, and education)	• The social and educational context • The family context • Historical and international perspectives of childhood • Cross-cultural sensitivity • Speech acquisition in second first language learners • Working with interpreters • Accent modification
	Personal factors	• Attributes of the person, and the internal influences on functioning and disability	• Personal factors • Variability in speech acquisition

Note. Data from WHO (2001).

provides additional biopsychosocial insight into children's development.

The ICF has two parts, each with two components. Part 1 is titled "Functioning and disability" and includes (a) Body Functions and Structures and (b) Activities and Participation. Part 2 is titled "Contextual factors" and includes (a) Environmental Factors and (b) Personal Factors. Capitalization is used to delineate the difference between the ICF application and other uses of these terms. Within the ICF framework, people's overall functioning is considered. As the result of a health condition or disease, people may have an impairment of Body Function and Structure, a limitation of Activity, and/or a restriction of Participation. The term *disability* "serves as an umbrella term for impairments, Activity limitation and Participation restrictions" (WHO, 2001, p. 3). The extent of a person's impairment, limitation, or restriction is informed by consideration of Personal and Environmental Contextual Factors.

Application of the ICF to speech acquisition

The ICF (and its predecessors) have been applied as a framework for practice for working with children and adults with communication disorders (e.g., American Speech-Language-Hearing Association, 2001; Baylor, Yorkston, and Eadie, 2005; Bourgeois, 1998; Eadie, 2003; Hersh, 1999; Hodge, 1983; Ma and Yiu, 2001; McLeod, 2004, 2006; McLeod and Bleile, 2004; Skeat et al., 2003; Threats, 2000, 2001, 2006; Threats and Worrall, 2004; Worrall, 2001). Simeonsson (2003) is illuminating in his application of the ICF to children with communication disabilities in general. The ICF has been specifically applied to children with speech impairment in a few papers (Hodge, 1983; McLeod, 2004, 2006; McLeod and Bleile, 2004), and its application to children's speech acquisition (for children with either typical or impaired speech) is the focus of this book.

Application of the ICF to the framework of this book

Table 1-1 illustrates the interactions between the parts, components, and domains of the ICF and applies them to children's speech acquisition. This book, titled *The International Guide to Speech Acquisition*, aims to encourage consideration of the whole child and his or her milieu by applying the components engendered within the ICF to its chapters. Table 1-1 indicates the components of the ICF that are relevant to this book. As can be seen, some chapters encompass more than one component and domain of the ICF. Other chapters considered to be important for a holistic understanding of children's speech acquisition are not included in the ICF but are included in this book. For example, genetic foundations of speech acquisition are an essential foundational topic for consideration of speech acquisition but are not included in the ICF.

Functioning and disability

Body Functions describe "the physiological functions of body systems (including psychological functions)" (WHO, 2001, p. 10). Included in the component of Body Functions are the following areas relating to speech acquisition: "speech functions," including articulation, "voice functions" such as production and quality of voice, and "mental functions of language," including expression of spoken language. Body Structures refer to the "anatomic parts of the body such as organs, limbs, and their components" (WHO, 2001, p. 8). Parts of the body such as the brain, lungs, nose, mouth, ears, pharynx, and larynx apply to speech acquisition.

Activities and participation

An activity is the "execution of a task or action by an individual" (WHO, 2001, p. 10) and participation is the "involvement in a life situation" (WHO, 2001, p. 10). Thus, under the heading of Activities and Participation, communication in its many forms is included as an entire chapter within the ICF. Some of the highlighted aspects of communication include "communicating with— receiving— spoken messages," "speaking," and "conversation." Other relevant categories of Activity and Participation include learning and applying knowledge, such as "learning to read" and "learning to write." Within the ICF-CY, additional categories will include "acquiring language." Additionally, Activity and Participation include "interpersonal interactions and relationships," and "major life areas" such as "education" and "community, social and civic life."

Contextual factors

Part 2 of the ICF, titled Contextual factors, includes Environmental and Personal Factors (see Table 1-1). The importance of considering each child as an individual with a unique set of environmental and personal factors cannot be overemphasized. Within some of the speech acquisition literature, individual differences are considered essential companions to general trends in development (see Chapter 10; Vihman and Greenlee, 1987).

Environmental factors "make up the physical, social and attitudinal environment in which people live and conduct their lives" (WHO, 2001, p. 10) and can be facilitators or barriers. Environmental factors relevant to communication include products and technology, support and relationships, attitudes, services, systems, and policies. One of the most important environmental factors relating to children's speech acquisition is "support and relationships," particularly the support of family and friends. For children with speech impairment, the "support of health professionals," including speech–language pathologists, is also important. The impact of moving between different cultures is covered within this book in chapters addressing cross-cultural sensitivity, cross-cultural adoption, multilingual speech acquisition, working with interpreters, and accent modification.

Personal Factors are defined as "the particular background of an individual's life and living, and comprise features of the individual that are not part of a health condition or health states" (WHO, 2001, p. 17). Personal factors include the attributes of the person and the internal influences on functioning and disability. Due to the individuality of this WHO component, personal factors are not specified as chapters within the ICF. A child's unique makeup must be considered within his or her cultural milieu; consequently, the ICF (WHO, 2001, p. 8) recognizes the "large social and cultural variance" and includes race, gender, age, education, past experience, and character style. Research into children's speech acquisition has demonstrated a wide range of individual differences (see Chapter 10).

SUMMARY

- Speech is pivotal to human functioning and underpins access to educational and vocational opportunities.
- Each child is an individual.
- Working with children can be enhanced by considering each child in his or her milieu and placing importance on the child's activity and participation within society.

- The *International Classification of Functioning, Disability and Health* (ICF) (WHO, 2001) is a holistic biopsychosocial framework that can be applied to the consideration of children's speech acquisition.
- The components of the ICF are Body Functions and Structures, Activities and Participation, Environmental Factors, and Personal Factors.

REFERENCES

American Speech-Language-Hearing Association. (2001). *Scope of practice in speech-language pathology.* Rockville, MD: Author.

Baylor, C. R., Yorkston, K. M., and Eadie, T. L. (2005). The consequences of spasmodic dysphonia on communication-related quality of life: A qualitative study of the insider's experiences. *Journal of Communication Disorders, 38*(5), 395–419.

Bleile, K. M. (1991). Individual differences. In K. M. Bleile (Ed.), *Child phonology: A book of exercises for students* (pp. 57–71). San Diego, CA: Singular.

Bleile, K. M. (2004). *Manual of articulation and phonological disorders* (2nd ed.). Clifton Park, NY: Thomson Delmar Learning.

Bourgeois, M. S. (1998). Functional outcome assessment of adults with dementia. *Seminars in Speech and Hearing, 19,* 261–275.

Eadie, T. L. (2003). The ICF: A proposed framework for comprehensive rehabilitation of individuals who use alaryngeal speech. *American Journal of Speech-Language Pathology, 12,* 189–197.

Hersh, D. (1999). Impairment to empowerment: Social model theory and aphasia therapy. In S. McLeod and L. McAllister (Eds.), *Proceedings of the 1999 Speech Pathology Australia National Conference* (pp. 125–130). Melbourne: Speech Pathology Australia.

Hodge, M. (1983). Assessment and treatment of a child with a developmental speech disorder: A biological behavioural perspective. *Seminars in Speech and Language, 14,* 128–141.

Lewis, B. A., Freebairn, L. A., & Taylor, H. G. (2000). Academic outcomes in children with histories of speech sound disorders. *Journal of Communication Disorders, 33,* 11–30.

Ma, E. P.-M. and Yiu E. M.-L. (2001). Voice activity and participation profile: Assessing the impact of voice disorders. *Journal of Speech, Language, and Hearing Research, 44,* 511–524.

McLeod, S. (2003). General trends and individual differences: Perspectives on normal speech development. In S. P. Sohov (Ed.), *Advances in Psychology Research* (Vol. 22, pp. 189–202). New York: Nova Science.

McLeod, S. (2004). Speech pathologists' application of the ICF to children with speech impairment. *Advances in Speech-Language Pathology, 6*(1), 75–81.

McLeod, S. (2006). An holistic view of a child with unintelligible speech: Insights from the ICF and ICF-CY. *Advances in Speech-Language Pathology, 8*(3), 293–315.

McLeod, S., and Bleile, K. (2004). The ICF: A proposed framework for setting goals for children with speech impairment. *Child Language Teaching and Therapy, 20*(3), 199–219.

Skeat, J., Perry, A., Morris, M., Unsworth, C., Duckett, S., Dodd, K., & Taylor, N. (2003). *The use of the ICF framework in an allied health outcome measure: Australian Therapy Outcome Measures (AusTOMs).* In Australian Institute of Health and Welfare (AIHW) ICF Australian User Guide. Version 1.0. Disability Series. AIHW Cat. No. DIS 33. Canberra: AIHW.

Simeonsson, R. J. (2003). Classification of communication disabilities in children: Contribution of the International Classification of Functioning, Disability, and Health. *International Journal of Audiology, 42,* S2–S8.

Threats, T. T. (2000). The World Health Organization's revised classification: What does it mean for speech-language pathology. *Journal of Medical Speech-Language Pathology, 8,* 13–18.

Threats, T. T. (2001). New classifications will aid assessment and intervention. *ASHA Leader, 6,* 12–13.

Threats, T. T. (2006). Towards an international framework for communication disorders: Use of the ICF. *Journal of Communication Disorders, 39,* 251–265.

Threats, T. T. and Worrall, L. (2004). Classifying communication disability using the ICF. *Advances in Speech-Language Pathology, 6,* 53–62.

Vihman, M. M., and Greenlee, M. (1987). Individual differences in phonological development: Ages one and three years. *Journal of Speech & Hearing Research, 30*(4), 503–521.

World Bank Group. (2005). IBRD & IDA: Working for a world free of poverty. Retrieved December 8, 2005, from www.worldbank.org

World Health Organization. (1980). *ICIDH: International classification of impairment, disabilities and handicaps*. Geneva, Switzerland: Author.

World Health Organization. (2001). *ICF: International classification of functioning, disability and health*. Geneva, Switzerland: Author.

Worrall, L. (2001). The social approach: Another new fashion in speech-language pathology? *Advances in Speech-Language Pathology, 3*, 51–54.

Chapter 2

Oromotor Foundations of Speech Acquisition

Raymond D. Kent and Christie Tilkens

INTRODUCTION

The motor foundations for speech are distributed over more than 100 muscles situated in the abdomen, chest, neck, and head. These muscles are recruited for a variety of purposes pertaining to basic life support (e.g., ventilation and nutrition) and for the species-specific task of speech. It is convenient to discuss motor control first in respect to major systems and individual structures, and then to consolidate the information in a larger view that addresses the motor control of speech vis-à-vis more general oral motor functions. The speech systems are the respiratory, laryngeal, and upper airway, but these systems are not in fact anatomically or functionally independent. Rather, they are defined in terms of major roles that commandeer overlapping parts of the anatomy. Each has its own developmental features that are discussed briefly here in respect to structural and functional aspects (for a more detailed discussion and literature citations, see Kent, 1997; Kent and Vorperian, 1995, in press). Table 2-1 presents a summary of anatomical and physiological development. Structure refers to the sizes and shapes of the components, and function refers to actions. It is not known to what degree developmental patterns are influenced by the phonetic properties of a given language. It is assumed that the descriptions given here are universal, but it is certainly possible that certain phonetic properties would affect the development of certain parts of the speech production system.

Oral movements are essential to eating and speech, to oral hygiene, and to patency of the respiratory airway. People normally swallow hundreds of times a day to eat solids, drink liquids, and swallow accumulated saliva and mucus. The swallow is a complicated sequence of movements involving the jaw, lips, tongue, velum, pharynx, larynx, and esophagus. Mastication, essential to the ingestion of most solid foods, is accomplished primarily by

TABLE 2-1 Selected developmental events in the respiratory, laryngeal, and vocal tract systems

	Respiratory	Laryngeal	Vocal tract
Neonate	• Rest breathing rate of 30–80 breaths/minute • Bellows-like action of diaphragm rather than piston-like action in adults • Fetal hemoglobin has high affinity for oxygen; but few alveoli formed	• Larynx is high in neck, making for a shallow laryngopharynx • Vocal folds 2–7 mm long • No lamination of vocal folds	• Vocal tract resembles that of nonhuman primate • Epiglottal-velic approximation • Tongue nearly fills oral cavity • Vocal tract has gentle curvature • Dentition not erupted
2 years	• Rib cage has horizontal orientation, like that in adults		• End of initial growth spurt of most structures
4 years	• Rest breathing rate is about 20–30 breaths/minute • Expiratory work for a given pressure/flow is much greater than in adults	• Vocal ligament formed	• Hypertrophy of nasopharyngeal tonsil (adenoid), prompting velar-adenoidal pattern of closure for many children
6 years	• Nearly adultlike respiratory patterns	• Two layers of vocal ligament begin to develop	• Cranium nearly of adult size • Eruption of permanent dentition
12 years	• Increase in respiratory capacity, especially in boys • Number of alveoli at adult level	• Differentiation of lamina propria nearly complete	• Closure of spheno-occipital synchondrosis (cartilaginous growth center at base of skull) • Eruption of all permanent dentition except wisdom teeth
18 years	• Convergence on adult capacities and volumes	• Adult morphology of vocal folds achieved • Vocal folds about 21 mm long in females and 29 mm in males	• Adult proportions essentially accomplished

the jaw and tongue, although the lips, cheeks, and velopharynx also participate. Speech is the orchestrated action of a multiarticulate system involving the same structures that is unrivaled by any other motor system in terms of its rate of output and the sophistication of its timing control.

Respiratory system

The respiratory system is the complex of organs and tissues needed to exchange blood carbon dioxide (CO_2) with air oxygen (O_2). It is also used as the aerodynamic energy source of speech, by virtue of the airflows and air pressures it generates. This system can be divided into three major functional parts. (1) The conductive portion, consisting of structures that function as ducts, includes the nasal cavity, pharynx, larynx, trachea, bronchi, and bronchioles. The supralaryngeal subportion is known as the upper airway or aerodigestive tract, and it is highly involved with speech, mastication, deglutition, and other oral activities. For basic respiratory purposes, this upper airway must achieve patency. (2) The respiratory portion, consisting of structures in which the exchange of CO_2 and O_2 occurs, refers specifically to the respiratory bronchioles, which terminate in clusters of alveoli called alveolar sacs. (3) The ventilating mechanism, consisting of parts of the thoracic musculoskeletal apparatus and specializations of the lung, provides for the movement of air through the respiratory system.

The neonate's respiratory system has several distinctive features, including a bellows-like displacement of the diaphragm (compared to the pistonlike effect in adults), a paucity of alveoli, a form of hemoglobin that has a high affinity for oxygen, and a rapid rest breathing rate of 30 to 80 breaths/min. By the age of 6 months, the rib cage has assumed a roughly horizontal orientation, and by 1 year, the percentage contribution of rib cage to tidal volume is similar to that in adults. At 1 year, respiratory kinematics for speech differs from that for rest breathing, with less coupling of rib cage and abdomen for speech. It is not until the age of about 7 years that the lung architecture matches the adult form, and at about this same age, there is an essential convergence on an adultlike respiratory pattern. However, children continue to use a greater subglottal air pressure than adults for comparable speaking tasks. This aerodynamic difference can be significant for children with neurologic impairments, such as cerebral palsy.

Laryngeal system

The larynx is both valve and vibrator. As a valve, it regulates the flow of air into or out of the lungs. As a vibrator, it is the source of voicing energy for speech as the result of vibration of the vocal folds. These functions are accomplished through an assembly of cartilage, muscle, and related tissues that are suspended in the neck, with attachments to the hyoid bone, mandible, and thoracic skeleton.

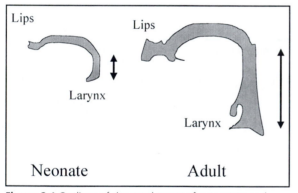

Figure 2-1 Outlines of the vocal tracts of a neonate and adult, as determined from magnetic resonance images of the midsagittal plane. Note that the neonate's vocal tract is not only smaller but has a relatively shorter pharyngeal cavity (double-headed arrow) than is seen in the adult.

The neonatal larynx is located high in the neck between the first and fourth cervical vertebrae (Figure 2-1). This relatively high location gives the advantage of breathing that can be concurrent with vocalization or deglutition. After birth, the larynx descends until, by the age of 6 years, it has reached the adult position between the fourth and seventh cervical vertebrae. The lower position assumed in adulthood represents a functional trade-off, in which a greater range of articulatory possibilities occurs at the expense

of losing the separation of function between deglutition and breathing. The newborn larynx differs from the adult larynx in several aspects of its internal anatomy. The vocal folds are small (about 2–7 mm long), half or more of the vocal fold length is cartilaginous (compared to one-third for adults), and the entire lamina propria is uniform (lacking the laminated structure seen in adults). The vocal ligament develops by about 4 years, but the full differentiation of the lamina propria is not evident until after 12 years. The well-known adolescent voice change in males begins between 12.5 and 14.5 years.

Upper airway system

This system is known by several different names, depending on the perspective that is given to it (e.g., *upper airway system* from an aerodynamic perspective, *vocal tract* from an acoustic perspective, and *pharyngo-oro-nasal system* from a functional-anatomic perspective). It is a complicated system by virtue of its numerous components that differ in biomechanical and neurophysiological properties.

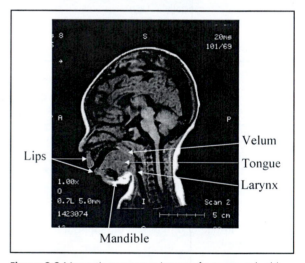

Figure 2-2 Magnetic resonance image of a two-week-old infant, with major speech structures labeled. Note in particular the absence of dentition, the small size of the mandible, and the high position of the larynx. The infant's vocal tract is not smaller than that of the adult, but it differs from the adult's in the relative size and configuration of structures.

A comparison of infant and adult vocal tracts immediately reveals about a threefold difference in size (Figure 2-2). The difference in size is accompanied by differences in relative geometric proportions. The infant vocal tract has been likened to a single tube model, in contrast to the classic two-tube adult model that is evident after the vocal tract is restructured during development. The different vocal tract structures have different growth patterns, so that adult sizes are achieved at different ages, ranging from about 7 to 18 years (Fitch and Giedd, 1999; Kent and Vorperian, 1995; Lieberman, McCarthy, Hiiemae, and Palmer, 2001). The vocal tract of the neonate (Figure 2-1) more closely resembles that of a nonhuman primate than that of an adult human, but it is remodeled in the first few months of life to take on the essential human form. This remodeling includes the descent of the larynx, as noted earlier, which lengthens the pharynx and disengages the epiglottis and soft palate. By 6 months, primary dentition begins to emerge, and the dental arcade eventually serves as an effective boundary for lingual actions in speech. By about 18 months, the jaw has a stable closing pattern, meaning that the first primary molars achieve reliable occlusal contact. At about 3 or 4 years, hypertrophy of the nasopharyngeal tonsil to form adenoidal tissue causes many children to adopt a velar-adenoidal form of velopharyngeal closure. By the age of about 6 years, the nasopharyngeal tonsil typically atrophies, the permanent dentition emerges, and the cranium has reached nearly adult size.

Individual structures are reviewed briefly below, with respect to major structural and functional accomplishments. Although growth patterns are not well established for all structures, an attempt is made to identify periods of growth spurt. Scammon (1930) described three different patterns of growth within the craniofacial complex. The neural calendar, which applies to the cranium and brain, has a relatively rapid growth and approximates adult size at about 6 years. The somatic calendar, observed for skeletal structures including the mandible, has a relatively slow growth during childhood but grows rapidly in adolescence, especially for males, so that adult size is reached at about 16 to18 years. The lymphatic pattern, associated with the tonsils, has a rapid growth in early childhood (3 to 5 years), followed by hypotrophy. Recent observations (Vorperian et al., 2005) indicate that the tongue has a growth calendar that is intermediate between the neural and somatic calendars. It is possible that different parts of the tongue have different growth patterns, with the anterior part reaching adult size by 8 to 10 years, and the posterior part, by 15 to 16 years (Temple, Hutchinson, Laing, and Jinks, 2002).

Mandible

Because the mandible provides skeletal support for the tongue and lower lip, the movements of the latter two structures are predicated on mandibular articulation.

Mandibular muscular activity, in turn, is affected by tongue position (Takahashi, Kuribayashi, Ono, Ishiwata, and Kuroda, 2005). The mandible, the only double-hinged bone in the human body, is carried in a muscular sling that permits movement in three dimensions (Koolstra, 2002). The development of the mandible occurs mainly as increased size without much change in its shape. Growth is accomplished by conversion of growing cartilage at two primary sites, the midline symphysis and the condyles. Another aspect of growth is deposition and resorption of bone. The mandible reaches its adult size at about 18 years in males and somewhat earlier in females (Kent and Vorperian, 1995).

Hyoid bone

The hyoid bone is part of a large tendino-muscular complex, by means of which the hyoid is attached to the base of the skull, mandible, tongue, larynx and scapular belt. It is often described as a "floating bone" (the only such bone in the human body) because it does not articulate with other bones. The hyoid is strategically situated to participate in all functional and nutritional activities of the oro-facial complex (Doual, Leger, Doual, and Hadjiat, 2003). Its position and orientation are adjusted to both mandibular and lingual functions.

Tongue

The tongue is perhaps best modeled as a muscular hydrostat because it is incompressible, maintains a constant volume during position and shape changes, and is capable of localized dimensional adjustments (Kier and Smith, 1985; Hiiemae and Palmer, 2003). The hydrostat model explains the tongue's potential for complex movements and deformations. Specifically, the hydrostat is "a conceptual basis for approaching the morphological and kinematic complexity of the mammal tongue" (Sokoloff, 2004, p. 238). In this model, the tongue is regarded as a constant-volume structure in which movements are produced by changes in shape. The tongue is devoid of an internal skeleton of bone or cartilage, but is tethered by its extrinsic muscles to the cranial base (a fixed skeletal support) and the jaw and hyoid bone (mobile skeletal supports).

Velopharynx

The velopharyngeal opening can be considered as a sphincter-like valve between the oropharynx and the nasopharynx. The lumen of the velopharynx is open for nose breathing and nasal speech sounds but is closed for nonnasal sounds. There are at least four major patterns of velopharyngeal closure; these seem to be determined largely by individual variations in velopharyngeal anatomy, and hence with age and gender (Kent, 1997). A velar-adenoidal pattern predominates in young children, until hypotrophy of the velopharyngeal lymphatic tissue.

Perioral muscles (lips and cheeks)

With respect to soft tissues, the perioral muscles can be considered to act as a "robust muscular hydrostat capable of highly manipulative fine motor movements" (Marshall, Hsu, and Herring, 2005, p. 22). These movements are exploited in speech and in feeding and are coordinated with movements of the jaw and tongue. The newborn's lips are nearly circular and composed of a high percentage of papillae per unit area. The high concentration of papillae makes the labial surface more adhesive, facilitating oral seal during suckle feeding. During development, the lips grow in length, increase in convexity, and change in epithelial composition.

Views of oromotor neural control

Several overarching questions about the motor control for speech can be at least tentatively answered on the basis of recent research. The first question is whether motor control for speech follows the same general pattern as (and perhaps borrows from) motor control for nonspeech behaviors such as mastication and deglutition. A parsimonious view of oromotor development asserts that speech draws on the same motor patterns that are deployed in nonspeech behaviors such as chewing and swallowing.

The frame-then-content theory of MacNeilage and Davis (2001) assumes such a commonality in movement patterning. However, studies have shown task specificity in infants for movements in speech, chewing, and lip protrusion, indicating an early distinction between speechlike movements and movements for nonspeech behaviors (Moore and Ruark, 1996; Ruark and Moore, 1997). Maturation of motor control relates to self-feeding skills in a fairly systematic way. By the age of 12 months, most children can remove food from a spoon with their lips, and by 24 months, they can feed themselves with a spoon without excessive spilling. Both drinking from a sippy cup independently and eating food that requires chewing are accomplished by the age of 18 months (Caruth, Ziegler, Gordon, and Hendricks, 2004).

The second question pertains to the maturational schedule of speech motor control. By the perceptual criterion of phonemic mastery (typically defined statistically as 75% correct production of a given sound), the maturation of speech motor control continues until 7 or 8 years for most children, at least for American English (Sander, 1972). But acoustic and physiologic studies indicate that speech motor control continues to be refined until at least puberty and perhaps as late as 16 years of age in both boys and girls (Smith and Goffman, 2004). Smith and Goffman (2004, p. 204) commented that, "…the late maturation of articulatory motor processes is driven primarily by interaction of speech motor systems with co-developing cognitive-linguistic systems, which are also not adult-like until this late period of development." There is a need for a model of speech development that incorporates macro- and microanatomic changes, motor learning, and neurobehavioral principles.

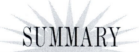

SUMMARY

- Growth and development of the speech production system is a protracted process that continues until about 18 years of age.
- Comparisons of the respiratory, laryngeal, and upper airways in infants and adults reveal a number of striking differences that bear on capabilities for speech sound production.

- The various structures that compose the speech production system have different schedules of maturation, with adultlike size reached anywhere from about 6 to 18 years.
- Although speech and feeding draw on essentially the same anatomic system, there are indications that these behaviors have distinctive modes of neural control and distinctive patterns of development.

REFERENCES

Carruth, B. R., Ziegler, P. J., Gordon, A., and Hendricks, K. (2004). Developmental milestones and self-feeding behaviors in infants and toddlers. *Journal of the American Dietetic Association, 104* (Suppl. 1), S51–S56.

Doual, A., Leger, J. L., Doual, J. M., and Hadjiat, F. (2003). LA DIMENSION VERTICALE (Congrès de Santander). Chapitre 5 : L'os hyoïde et la dimension verticale [The hyoid bone and vertical dimension]. *Orthodontie. Francais., 74,* 333–363.

Fitch, W. T., and Giedd, J. (1999). Morphology and development of the human vocal tract: A study using magnetic resonance imaging. *Journal of the Acoustical Society of America,* 106, 1511–1522.

Hiiemae, K. M., and Palmer, J. B. (2003). Tongue movements in feeding and speech. *Critical Reviews in Oral Biology & Medicine, 14,* 413–439.

Kent, R. D. (1997). *The speech sciences.* San Diego, CA: Singular Publishing.

Kent, R. D., and Vorperian, H. K. (1995). Anatomic development of the craniofacial-oral-laryngeal systems: A review. *Journal of Medical Speech-Language Pathology,* 3, 145–190.

Kent, R. D., and Vorperian, H. K. (in press). In the mouths of babes: Anatomic, motor, and sensory foundations of speech development in children. In R. Paul (Ed.), *Language disorders from a developmental perspective.* Mahwah, NJ: Lawrence Erlbaum.

Kier, W. M., and Smith, K. K. (1985). Tongues, tentacles and trunks: The biomechanics of movement in muscular-hydrostats. *Zoological Journal of the Linnean Society,* 83, 307–324.

Koolstra, J. H. (2002). Dynamics of the human masticatory system. *Critical Reviews in Oral Biology & Medicine,* 13, 366–376.

Lieberman, D. E., McCarthy, R. C., Hiiemae, K. M., and Palmer, J. B. (2001). Ontogeny of postnatal hyoid and larynx descent in humans. *Archives of Oral Biology, 46,* 117–128.

MacNeilage, P. F., and Davis, B. L. (2001). Motor mechanisms in speech ontogeny: Phylogenetic, neurobiological and linguistic implications. *Current Opinion in Neurobiology, 11,* 696–700.

Marshall, C. D., Hsu, R. H., and Herring, S. W. (2005). Somatotropic organization of perioral musculature innervation within the pig facial motor nucleus. *Brain & Behavioral Evolution, 66,* 22–34.

Moore, C. A., and Ruark, J. L. (1996). Does speech emerge from earlier appearing motor behaviors? *Journal of Speech and Hearing Research, 39,* 1034–1047.

Ruark, J. L., and Moore, C. A. (1997). Coordination of lip muscle activity by 2-year-old children during speech and nonspeech tasks. *Journal of Speech, Language, and Hearing Research, 40,* 1373–1385.

Sander, R. K. (1972). When are speech sounds learned? *Journal of Speech and Hearing Research, 37,* 55–63.

Scammon, R. E. (1930). The measurement of the body in childhood. In J. A. Harris, C. M. Jackson, D. G. Patterson, and R. E. Scammon (Eds.), *The measurement of man* (pp. 173–215). Minneapolis: University of Minnesota Press.

Sokoloff, A. J. (2004). Activity of tongue muscles during respiration: It takes a village? *Journal of Applied Physiology, 96,* 438–439.

Smith, A., and Goffman, L. (2004). Interaction of motor and language factors in the development of speech. In B. Maassen, R. Kent, H. Peters, P. van Lieshout, and W. Hulstijn (Eds.), *Speech motor control in normal and disordered speech* (pp. 227–252). Oxford, UK: Oxford University Press.

Takahashi, S., Kuribayashi, G., Ono, T., Ishiwata, Y., and Kuroda, T. (2005). Modulation of masticatory muscle activity by tongue position. *Angle Orthodontist, 75,* 35–39.

Temple, E. C., Hutchinson, I., Laing, D. G., and Jinks, A. L. (2002). Taste development: Differential growth rates of tongue regions in humans. *Brain Research: Developmental Brain Research, 135,* 65–70.

Vorperian, H. K., Kent, R. D., Lindstrom, M. J., Kalina, C. M., Gentry, L. R., and Yandell, B. S. (2005). Development of vocal tract length during early childhood: A magnetic resonance imaging study. *Journal of the Acoustical Society of America, 117,* 338–350.

Chapter 3

Neurological Foundations of Speech Acquisition

Ken M. Bleile

INTRODUCTION

A legacy of humanity's evolutionary past is the fact that extensive brain development occurs after a child is born (Gibson, 1990; Killackey, 1995). Humans, without a genetic inheritance that includes a specialized body and mind fitted to a specific environmental niche, instead have a brain that grows while exposed to the environment. Brain development and the environment interact. A child is born with an ability to grasp complex patterns and learn from a wide number of possible environments. Interaction with the environment shapes a child's brain, narrowing its learning potential to fit the actual community in which the child lives.

The discussion in this chapter summarizes selected recent advances in understanding childhood neurological development related to speech acquisition. Topics include development in connections between cells and development of major brain functions and structures that underlie speech. A major conclusion of the chapter is that central aspects of speech acquisition reflect neurological development during childhood.

Connections between cells

It is well understood that at the neurological level all learning—including speech learning—entails making connections between cells. The human brain contains approximately 100 billion neurons, fed from blood flowing through several major arteries and floating in a chemical bath of neurotransmitters. It is variously estimated that each brain cell connects to between 12,000 and 15,000 other brain cells. Everything a person knows, remembers, plans, thinks of, and learns is a connection between these cells. Two processes underlie how brain cells learn to connect during childhood: selective elimination, and growth and elaboration.

Selective elimination

Between birth and young adulthood a person typically loses approximately one-third of his or her brain cells through a process called selective elimination. Selective elimination is sometimes also called "pruning" and "arborization" by analogy to how gardeners shape and trim a bush (Geschwind and Galaburda, 1987; Neville, 1991). The analogy is apt. The extra brain cells present at birth represent potential to learn from a range of environments; the ones that remain in young adulthood are those actually used. This "use it or lose it" principle shapes a brain to fit the child's environment. An important characteristic of selective elimination is that it appears tied to chronological age, with cells in various areas of the brain being eliminated within specific age ranges. In general, sensory areas of the brain mature earliest and those involved in higher reasoning functions mature later.

Growth and elaboration

Selective elimination is complete by young adulthood, approximately 22 to 25 years of age. Capacity to learn does not stop at that age because cells also interconnect through a second process, called growth and elaboration. Whereas selective elimination appears tied to chronological age and ends in young adulthood, growth and elaboration continue lifelong and are tied to a person's interests, attention, motivation, and exposure to the environment (Buell and Coleman, 1979).

Studies of early intervention for rats illustrate the effects of growth and elaboration (Black, Isaacs, Anderson, Alcantara, and Greenbough, 1990; Chang, Isaacs, and Greenbough, 1991). In these studies, young rats are divided into two groups. Rats in the first group (experimental group) receive a type of early intervention in the form of being reared in an enriched environment with many wheels to run on and objects to climb and move. Rats in the second group (control group) receive a more typical laboratory rat environment—not a deprived environment, only one without the additional stimulation of the environments afforded the experimental group. After the rats reach maturity, those in both groups are killed, their brains are dissected, and synapses in the cerebellum

are counted. Typical of the results of many different studies, Black et al. (1990) found that an enriched environment increased the number of synapses per neuron in the rat cerebellum by 25 percent.

Increases in synaptic connections through growth and elaboration have been demonstrated in many species, including humans. To illustrate, on average, a person with a Ph.D. has more synaptic connections in Wernicke's Area than a person with a B.A., who in turn on average has more synaptic connections in the same area compared to a person with a high school diploma (Jacobs, Schall, and Scheibel, 1993). In our culture, women on average are considered more verbal than men; studies indicate the neurological reflection of this is that women on average have more brain cell connections in Wernicke's Area than males (Jacobs et al., 1993). In old age, as the absolute number of brain cells decreases the number of connections per cell tends to increase, indicating a capacity for lifelong learning (Buell and Coleman, 1979). Last, speech-language pathologists (SLPs) might speculate that growth and elaboration is the process that makes language learning possible as an adult and permits a determined adult to compensate for loss of brain functions after a stroke or head injury.

Major brain areas and functions

Many areas and functions of the brain that support speech acquisition undergo extensive development during childhood.

Brain weight

Brain size gives humans the capacity to grasp complex patterns, including those that underlie speech. The human brain at birth is about 25 percent of its adult weight, it grows maximally to 80 percent of its adult weight during the first 4 years of life, and it reaches its mature size at adulthood (Gibson, 1990; Kretschmann, Kammradt, Krauthausen, Sauer, and Wingert, 1986). A child's play during the first few years of life reflects rapid brain growth. To illustrate, an infant's play with toys typically involves banging, throwing, mouthing, and shaking. Near 12 months, primitive play begins to emerge, perhaps with a child speaking into a pretend telephone. Full representational play begins near 18 to 20 months and is well established by 22 to 24 months (Hedrick, Prather, and Tobin, 1984). In representational play, a child lets one object stand for or symbolize another. For example, a child may introduce absent objects into play by pretending to feed a doll even without having a spoon. Such play is significant because it resembles language, in which words and sentences represent or symbolize events and objects in the real world. It is perhaps not surprising that the neurological growth that permits representational play also makes possible representational language.

Myelin sheaths

Myelin is a white, fatty substance on axons that acts as an insulator and speeds electrical transmission of signals between cells. Myelin is critical for gross and fine motor movements, including speech. Its effect on motor skills is evidenced by multiple sclerosis (MS), a demyelinating disease that may cause profound speech difficulties and other motor problems. Myelination of the brain begins three months before a full-term child is born, achieves its peak growth between birth and the end of the first year, and continues to grow until adulthood (Evans and Hutchins, 2002). Rapid myelination during the first year in conjunction with structural changes in an infant's throat and face may provide one foundation for vocal and speech development.

Hippocampus

The hippocampus is important to working memory and is deeply involved in such important speech activities as memory retention and retrieval (Benes, 1997). The hippocampus, like other memory systems, develops after the child is born, especially during the second year of life (Liston and Kagan, 2002). Increased ability to retain words in memory, along with other neurological and social factors, may contribute to the rapid growth of vocabulary in toddlers.

Prefrontal cortex

The prefrontal lobes are critical to many cognitive activities that underlie speech, including reasoning, planning, judgment, and attention. Cell connections in the prefrontal lobes develop slowly throughout childhood and do not reach maturity until early adulthood (Casey, Gledd, and Thomas, 2000; Sowell, Dells, Stiles, and Jernigan, 2001). Teenagers are famous for lack of planning and judgment, and this has been attributed to lack of maturity of cell connections in the prefrontal lobes. Recognizing the importance of this aspect of brain development, in 2005 the U.S. Supreme Court outlawed the execution of juvenile offenders.

Speech areas

The topics in this section focus on differences in development in brain areas involved in speech perception and speech production.

Speech perception

Visual and auditory areas mature early to provide a child a reliable source of perceptual information to serve as a foundation for learning. Visual and auditory areas peak in number of cell connections during the first half of the first year and achieve a mature number of cell connections during the second half of the first year (Pascallis, de Haan, and Nelson, 2002). Development of speech perception during the first year fine-tunes an infant's speech perception system to fit the ambient language. To illustrate, many languages (called tone languages) use pitch to distinguish between word meanings, and so a child must perceive differences between pitches. Newborns around the world notice pitch differences that in languages such as Mandarin Chinese and Vietnamese signal differences between words (Pascallis et al., 2002). Children born to English-speaking families lose this ability by the end of their first year, while those born to Chinese-speaking families retain it. A "use it or lose it" principle appears operative: children everywhere are born with the same ability to perceive pitch, but those who grow up speaking languages such as Chinese establish and retain these brain cell connections, while those who speak a nontone language such as English lose those potential cell connections.

Speech production

Cortical areas involved in speech production mature at a different rate than those for speech perception. Density of cell connections in Broca's Area does not peak until 15 months and does not reach a mature number of connections until 6 to 8 years (Schade and van Groenigen, 1961; Scheibel, 1993; Simonds and Scheibel, 1989). While a child's perceptual system is well tuned to the ambient language before the first birthday, speech production systems require many years to reach maturity. To illustrate, at 2 years a toddler's speech is largely restricted to sounds made either with articulators touching (stops and nasals) or far apart (vowels and glides). Sounds made between these two extremes (fricatives, affricates, liquids) may not be completely acquired until the early school years. Additionally, a child speaks more slowly than an adult and, consequently, the duration of a child's phrases and sentences is longer (Kent and Forner, 1980), perhaps reflecting that a child is less experienced than an adult in planning and executing speech.

Linking speech perception and speech production

Because speech perception areas develop early and speech production areas develop relatively late, for approximately the first 6 to 8 years a disparity exists between what a child hears and what can be produced. This gap can be enormous early in language development, but it lessens with age. It also varies by individual child. Some can easily leap over the gap between perception and production; for others, it is a chasm wide and deep. The latter type of child may require professional assistance from an SLP to acquire speech.

Imagined as an inverted speech triangle (Figure 3-1), perceptual development begins broadly and ends narrowly. That is, a child starts life with the potential to perceive broad perceptual distinctions needed to acquire any of the world's languages; with development, broad perceptual abilities narrow to fit perceptual distinctions encountered in the language of a child's community. Development of speech production proceeds in the opposite direction: a child begins life producing a narrow range of vegetative sounds; with development, production abilities broaden until a child can pronounce the sounds encountered in the community's language.

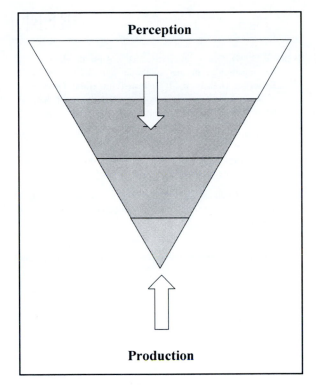

Figure 3-1 Speech triangle

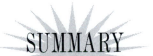

SUMMARY

- Speech development progresses as it does largely because of brain development during childhood.
- Through selective elimination and growth and elaboration, brain cells learn to connect during speech learning.
- A child begins life with barely 25 percent of his or her full brain size, but the brain grows rapidly during the first 4 years of life.
- Meanwhile, myelin is laid down, facilitating speech movements, especially during the first year of life.

- Short-term memory, so important for learning in general and word learning in particular, develops remarkably during the second year of life.
- In the speech domain itself, speech perception systems mature early, affording a child an avenue to learn about the world.
- The speech production system lags, creating a split between what a child perceives and is able to produce.
- Much of phonological development is learning to develop a link between advanced perceptual systems and limited means of production.

REFERENCES

Benes, F. (1997). Corticolimbis circuitry and the development of psychopathology during childhood and adolescence. In N. Krasnegor, G. Lyon, and P. Golman-Rakic (Eds.), *Development of the prefrontal cortex: Evolution, neurobiology, and behavior.* Baltimore, MD: Paul H. Brookes.

Black, J., Isaacs, K., Anderson, B., Alcantara, A., and Greenbough, W. (1990). Learning causes synaptogenesis, whereas motor activity causes angiogenesis, in cerebellar cortex in adult rats. *Proceedings of the National Academy of Sciences, 87,* 5568–5572.

Buell, S., and Coleman, P. (1979). Dendritic growth in the aged human brain and failure of growth in senile dementia. *Science, 206,* 854–856.

Casey, B., Gledd, J., and Thomas, K. (2000). Structural and functional brain development and its relation to cognitive development. *Biological Psychology, 54,* 241–257.

Chang, F., Isaacs, K., and Greenbough, W. (1991). Synapse formation occurs in association with the induction of long-term potentiation in two-year-old rat hippocampus in vitro. *Neurobiology of Aging, 12,* 517–522.

Evans, O. B., and Hutchins, J. B. (2002). Development of the nervous system. In D. E. Haines (Ed.), *Fundamental Neuroscience* (pp. 71–89). New York: Churchhill Livingstone.

Geschwind, N., and Galaburda, A. (1987). *Cerebral lateralization: Biological mechanisms, associations, and pathologies.* Cambridge, MA: MIT Press.

Gibson, K. R. (1990). New perspectives on instincts and intelligence: Brain size and the emergence of hierarchical mental constructional skills. In S. T. Parker and K. R. Gibson (Eds). *"Language" and intelligence in monkeys and apes: Comparative developmental perspectives* (pp. 17–38). New York: Cambridge University Press.

Hedrick, D., Prather, E., and Tobin, A. (1984). *Sequenced inventory of communication development.* Seattle: University of Washington Press.

Jacobs, B., Schall, M, and Scheibel, A. (1993). A quantitative dendritic analysis of Wernicke's area. II. Gender, hemispheric, and environmental factors. *Journal of Comparative Neurology, 237,* 97–111.

Kent, R. D., and Forner, L. L. (1980). Speech segment durations in sentence recitations by children and adults. *Journal of Phonetics, 8,* 157–168.

Killackey, H. (1995). Evolution of the human brain: A neuroanatomical perspective. In M. Gazzaniga (Ed.), *The cognitive neurosciences* (pp. 327–335). Cambridge, MA: MIT Press.

Kretschmann, H., Kammradt, G., Krauthausen, I., Sauer, B., and Wingert, F. (1986). Brain growth in man. *Bibliography of Anatomy, 28,* 1–26.

Liston, C., and Kagan, J. (2002). Memory enhancement in early childhood. *Nature, 419,* 896.

Neville, H. (1991). Neurobiology of cognitive and language processing: Effects of early experience. In K. R. Gibson and A. C. Peterson (Eds.), *Brain maturation and cognitive development* (pp. 47–59). New York: Aladine de Gruyter Press.

Pascallis, O., de Haan, M., and Nelson, C. (2002). Is face processing species specific during the first year of life? *Science, 296,* 1321–1323.

Schade, J. P., and van Groenigen, W. B. (1961). Structural organization of the human cerebral cortex. I. Maturation of the middle frontal gyrus. *Acta Anatomica 47,* 72–111.

Scheibel, A. B. (1993). Dendritic structure and language development. In B. de Boysson-Bardies (Ed.), *Developmental neurocognition: Speech and face processing in the first year of life* (pp. 43–50). New York: Kluwer Academic Publishers.

Simonds, R. J., and Scheibel, A. B. (1989). The postnatal development of the motor speech area: A preliminary study. *Brain and Language 37,* 42–58.

Sowell, E., Dells, D., Stiles, T., and Jernigan, J. (2001). Improved memory functioning and frontal lobe maturation between childhood and adolescence: A structural MRI study. *Journal of the International Neuropsychological Society, 7,* 312–322.

Chapter 4

Auditory Foundations
of Speech Acquisition

David J. Ertmer

INTRODUCTION

The human auditory system is elegant in its ability to perceive and process spoken language. Because this system works so well, children with normal hearing typically learn to produce the speech patterns of their native languages simply by listening to mature speakers and to their own utterances. In contrast, deaf children always require intensive instruction to learn how to produce a full range of speech sounds, words, and sentences. Even with considerable practice and the use of hearing aids, their speech remains, on average, only 20 percent intelligible to unfamiliar listeners (Osberger, 1992). These phenomena illustrate how closely speech development is tied to hearing acuity. In this chapter, six main topics will be considered as this robust relationship is examined. These topics are (1) the anatomy and physiology of the peripheral hearing system, (2) classifications of hearing impairments, (3) the acoustic characteristics of speech sounds, (4) sensory aids for children with hearing impairment, (5) the effects of profound hearing loss on speech development, and (6) speech intervention for children with severe to profound hearing impairments.

Hearing anatomy and physiology

Studying the human auditory system is a bit like reading an intriguing novel for which no ending has yet been written. Although much has been learned about how we hear, many intricacies of the auditory system remain unknown today. The following is a very basic description of the anatomy of the peripheral auditory system and the processes by which acoustic energy (i.e., vibrating air molecules) is changed into a signal that can be passed to the central nervous system. Readers are referred to Gelfand (2001) for a more comprehensive treatment of these subjects.

The peripheral auditory system

The peripheral auditory system consists of the outer, middle, and inner ear or cochlea (Figure 4-1). The outer ear extends from the pinna to the tympanic membrane or "eardrum." The pinna gathers acoustic energy (sound) from the environment and directs it along the external auditory meatus or "ear canal." The pinna also helps listeners to localize sound sources. As sound passes through the ear canal, some frequencies associated with speech receive a boost in intensity; increasing the strength of the speech signal (as well as nonspeech sounds in this range of frequencies) over sounds with lower or higher frequency characteristics. Next, sound reaches the taut and thin tympanic membrane and causes it to vibrate. The vibrations of the tympanic membrane cause the ossicles (three connected bones in the middle ears: the malleus, incus, and stapes) to move very rapidly within the air-filled space known as the middle ear. As Figure 4-1 shows, the ossicular chain is attached to the tympanic membrane at one end and the oval window of the cochlea at the other. The vibrations of the tympanic membrane and the ossicles preserve the frequency (perceived as pitch), timing (durations of sounds and silent periods), and intensity (perceived as loudness and softness) characteristics of the original acoustic signal and transmit this information to the cochlea.

The inner ear consists of the vestibular system, which is responsible for balance and movement sensation, and the cochlea, which is the main organ for hearing. The cochlea is a snail-shaped organ that changes the mechanical vibrations of the ossicles into a signal that can be processed by the central nervous system (Figure 4-1). As shown in a cross-sectional view in Figure 4-2, it has three fluid-filled chambers: the scala vestibuli, scala media, and scala tympani. The basilar membrane winds around the turns of the cochlea from the base to the apex (tip), separating the scala media from the scala tympani. The organ of Corti, which rests on the basilar membrane, has three rows of outer hair cells and one row of inner hair cells as well as their respective supporting bodies. Spiral ganglion are also present throughout the cochlea, connecting it to the auditory nerve (VIII cranial).

How does the cochlea accomplish its complex task? Very basically, the mechanical vibrations conveyed by the stapes to the oval window are converted into fluid waves that displace the basilar membrane at frequency-specific locations within the cochlea; low-frequency sounds cause

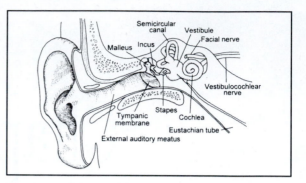

Figure 4-1 Schematic of frontal section revealing outer, middle, and inner ear structures.

displacement near the apex of the cochlea while mid- and high-frequency sounds cause displacement toward the middle and base of the cochlea, respectively. These displacements force hair cells to bend and to release chemical substances, creating action potentials. Auditory nerve fibers synapse on the hair cells, forming the spiral ganglion that relays the electrochemical signal to the auditory nerve and higher levels in the central nervous system. Once again, the frequency, intensity, and timing characteristics of speech are preserved during this conversion. For children with hearing impairments, however, speech and environmental sounds may be less audible or undetected because components of their auditory systems do not function properly.

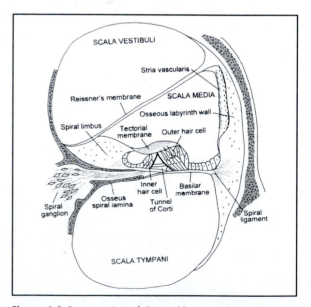

Figure 4-2 Cross-section of the cochlea, revealing scala vestibuli, scala media, and scala tympani.

Classifications of hearing impairments

Hearing impairments are classified by three main characteristics: type of hearing impairment, age at onset, and severity.

Types of hearing impairments

There are three types of hearing impairments: conductive, sensorineural, and mixed hearing.

Conductive impairments

Conductive impairments are characterized by malfunctions in the outer or middle ear with normal functioning in the inner ear. Examples of conductive impairments include occlusions (blockages) of the auditory meatus, otitus media (fluid buildup in the middle ear), ossicular disconnection (separation in the ossicular chain), and otosclerosis (a disease in which bone deteriorates and the movement of the ossicular chain becomes limited). In many cases, conductive hearing impairments are medically correctable, and treatment often results in the restoration of near-normal hearing acuity.

Sensorineural impairments

Sensorineural impairments result from a cochlear or retrocochlear (neurological) malfunction. Causes of sensorineural impairments include ototoxic drugs, genetic factors, and excessive exposure to loud sounds, along with other etiologies. Sensorineural hearing losses are not medically correctable at the present time. Successful application of gene therapy with deaf guinea pigs (Izumikawa et al., 2005) suggests that this approach might one day be effective for overcoming sensorineural hearing impairment in humans.

Mixed hearing impairments

Mixed hearing impairments result from malfunctions in the outer or middle ear and physiological breakdowns in the cochlea or retrocochlear systems.

Age at onset

Four broad classifications are used to classify hearing impairments according to when they begin: congenital (present at birth), prelingual (onset between birth and 3 years), perilingual (onset between 3 years and adolescence), and postlingual (onset during the teens or adulthood). In general, the earlier the onset of a hearing impairment, the greater the impact on speech development.

Severity

Hearing acuity is commonly measured by testing children's ability to detect pure tones of varying intensities across the frequencies 250–8000 Hz (hertz). To do this, audiologists present tones to each ear separately and then plot the lowest-intensity responses to each of the frequencies presented on an audiogram. The completed audiogram reveals the presence or absence of a hearing impairment and the severity of any impairment that is identified. Children's hearing acuity is often described using six levels that are based on hearing thresholds:

1. Normal, 0–20 dB HL (decibels, Hearing Level)
2. Slight-mild hearing impairment, 21–40 dB HL
3. Mild-moderate hearing impairment, 41–55 dB HL
4. Moderate hearing impairment, 56–70 dB HL
5. Severe hearing impairment, 71–90 dB HL
6. Profound hearing impairment, ≥91 dB HL

Figure 4-3 shows an audiogram for a hypothetical child named Sally. The horizontal axis of the audiogram represents frequency levels from "low pitch" tones (e.g., 250 Hz) to "high pitch" tones (e.g., 8000 Hz). The vertical axis represents sound intensity from barely audible (e.g., 0 dB HL) to very loud (e.g., 120 dB HL). The "X" symbols represent the intensity level at which Sally detected pure tones 50% of the time when they were presented to her left ear. This level of performance is called a threshold. The "O" symbols represent thresholds for the right ear. Although additional tests would also be undertaken during a complete hearing evaluation, these thresholds show that Sally has a severe, bilateral hearing impairment with relatively poorer hearing for frequencies above 1000 Hz.

Acoustic characteristics of speech sounds

The "banana-shaped" area in the upper part of Sally's audiogram (Figure 4-3) provides an estimate of the frequency and intensity locations of speech sounds when they produced at conversational intensity levels at a distance of approximately 2 meters. As this area shows, vowels are generally more intense than consonants, and classes of consonants differ from each other in their associated frequencies. For example, the nasals /m/ and /n/ have strong low-frequency characteristics whereas the fricatives /s/ and /f/ are high-frequency sounds. Comparing a child's pure-tone thresholds to the frequency and intensity characteristics of

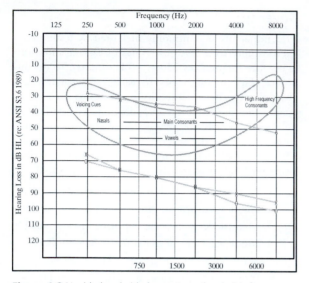

Figure 4-3 Unaided and aided pure-tone thresholds for "Sally," a hypothetical child. The shaded area shows the intensity and frequency ranges of the components of speech when produced at conversational intensity levels.

Sensory aids for children with hearing impairments

Two sensory aids are commonly used to help children with hearing impairments gain access to environmental sounds and speech: hearing aids (HAs) and cochlear implants (CIs).

Hearing aids

Hearing aids are the most commonly used sensory aid for overcoming mild, moderate, and severe hearing impairments. These battery-powered devices amplify speech and environmental sounds so that users can perceive them through their residual hearing. However, HAs typically provide incomplete access to conversational speech for individuals who have profound hearing impairments. In this situation, cochlear implantation may be considered as an alternative to hearing aid use.

Cochlear implants

Cochlear implants are surgically implanted electronic devices that increase hearing sensitivity in individuals who receive little benefit from hearing aids. These devices improve hearing ability by circumventing damaged receptor hair cells in the cochlea and providing electrical stimulation directly to the auditory nerve. CIs typically enable deaf children to make substantial improvements in hearing sensitivity, speech perception, and spoken language abilities (Ertmer, 2005; Niparko, et al., 2000).

Effects of profound hearing impairment on speech acquisition

Speech development is strongly associated with children's residual hearing levels (Monsen, 1978; Smith, 1975). For instance, children with mild and moderate hearing impairments are likely to develop speech at closer-to-typical rates and to achieve higher levels of speech intelligibility than those with severe or profound hearing impairments. Although mild-moderate hearing impairments can interfere with speech development, children with this level of hearing impairment often respond well to hearing aids and traditional speech training methods. Consequently, the remainder of this chapter will focus on children with severe-profound, bilateral, sensorineural hearing impairments because these children typically experience substantial delays in

conversational-intensity speech sounds can give some idea of the audibility of classes of vowels and consonants for a particular child. That is, if the classes of speech sounds are at least 10 dB greater than the child's corresponding threshold, they are likely to be detected by the child (Ling, 1989). It is important to remember, however, that hearing impairment often results in distortion of what is heard. Distortion may affect speech perception, making it difficult for children to decide whether two sounds are the same or different (discrimination), to recognize familiar sounds (identification), and to understand the meaning of spoken messages (comprehension).

The "A" symbols in Figure 4-3 represent Sally's thresholds when using hearing aids to listen to pure tones presented through loudspeakers. Her aided thresholds suggest that she should be able to detect many vowels and consonants, but that high-frequency sounds (e.g., /s/ and /f/) are likely to be inaudible when using amplification. Thus, even though hearing aids will greatly improve Sally's ability to detect conversational speech, she will not hear it as well as children with normal hearing and she may also need auditory training to improve her speech perception abilities (Blamey and Alcantara, 1994).

speech development and require special intervention strategies.

Prelinguistic speech development

Infants and toddlers with profound hearing impairments show extensive deficits in prelinguistic speech development. In general, they begin to babble (i.e., produce consonant-vowel syllable strings with adultlike timing) later than their hearing peers (Oller and Eilers, 1988; Stark, 1983), their vowel-like productions are restricted in their formant frequency locations (Kent, Osberger, Netsell, and Hustedde, 1987), and they have comparatively smaller consonant, vowel, and syllable shape inventories than peers with normal hearing (Stoel-Gammon, 1988). These prelinguistic deficits contribute to delays in the development of meaningful speech.

Phonological development

The production of meaningful speech can be affected in many ways for children who have severe-profound hearing impairments (for reviews see Ling, 1976; Osberger and McGarr, 1982). At a very basic level, speech breathing patterns may be abnormal. That is, children may not learn to inhale rapidly and control exhalation for speech production purposes. Achieving normal phonation can also be problematic. Children's voices may be perceived as too breathy, harsh, loud, or soft. Their fundamental frequencies (perceived as "pitch") may seem inappropriately high or low. The timing of speech is usually much slower than normal due to abnormally long syllable durations and pauses. Atypical intonation and stress patterns are also commonly observed. Last, many phonemes may be misarticulated. The most common phonemic errors for deaf children are vowel omissions, vowel substitutions, consonant substitutions, and consonant distortions (Smith, 1975). In general, phonemes produced at the front of the mouth are more often correct than those produced at the back or in the middle of the mouth because they are visually salient. Special intervention approaches are needed to overcome these problems and to help children optimize their ability to communicate orally.

Speech intervention for children with severe to profound hearing impairments

Short descriptions of speech training approaches for infants, toddlers, and school-age children and related Web sites are provided below. Although the approaches will not be described in detail, several basic principles should be kept in mind when implementing speech training with children who have hearing impairments. First, to be most effective, intervention activities should be appropriate to the age and interests of the child. Although direct instruction and guided practice may be needed to establish some speech targets, meaningful and enjoyable follow-up activities are also important for promoting carryover of new skills and maintaining motivation. Second, families and teachers should be actively involved in the program so that progress toward speech goals can be encouraged and reinforced throughout the day. Third, children with profound hearing impairments often need intensive intervention to improve their speech production skills. Clinicians, parents, and teachers should monitor speech progress to ensure that adequate amounts of service are provided.

Speech training approaches and oral communication resources

Short periods of prelinguistic input (SPPI; Ertmer, et al., 2002) uses speech modeling to stimulate prelinguistic speech development in infants and toddlers.

Baby talk

A practical guide by Kozak and Moog Brooks (2001) provides ideas for stimulating listening, speech, and oral language development in very young children. It is intended for parents but is also a useful resource for speech-language pathologists and aural rehabilitation specialists.

The Ling system

A comprehensive program by Ling (1976, 1989) includes assessment procedures and intervention strategies at the Phonetic (prosodic and segmental) and the Phonological (meaningful speech) levels. Detailed suggestions for eliciting and establishing consonant and vowel production are included in both of Ling's textbooks. The Ling system is the most thorough approach to speech training for deaf children available today.

Guidelines for establishing oral communication

A tutorial by Robbins (1994) discusses six instructional strategies for improving speech and language skills in children with cochlear implants. These techniques are also useful for children with hearing aids.

Cochlear implants for kids

This book (Estabrooks, 1998) offers case studies of oral communication development in young children with cochlear implants. It includes lesson plans for each case and discusses rationales for intervention activities.

The source for children with cochlear implants

A text by Ertmer (2005) provides information about cochlear implant technology, implant candidacy requirements, communication modalities, and intervention approaches for infants and toddlers, preschoolers, and school-age children.

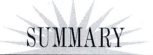

SUMMARY

- Speech development is closely tied to children's hearing acuity levels.
- The human auditory system preserves the frequency, intensity, and timing characteristics of speech as acoustic energy is converted into a signal that the nervous system can process.
- The main types of hearing impairment are conductive, sensorineural, and mixed.

- Hearing aids are the most commonly used technology for treating hearing impairments.
- Cochlear implants are often recommended for children who have profound, bilateral hearing impairments and receive limited benefits from hearing aids.
- Children with severe-profound hearing impairments typically require intensive speech intervention to acquire functional oral communication skills.

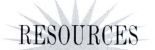

RESOURCES

Web sites relating to auditory foundations of speech acquisition

- *Alexander Graham Bell Association for the Deaf*
  http://www.agbell.org
  The home page of the Alexander Graham Bell Association for the Deaf contains information and resources related to developing oral communication in children with hearing impairments.

- *Beginnings for Parents of Children who are Deaf or Hard of Hearing*
  http://www.beginningssvcs.com
  This parent-centered Web site offers information about childhood deafness and a balanced perspective on oral and signed communication options. It contains Internet links to many related sites.

- *Laurent Clerc National Deaf Education Center*
  http://www.clerccenter.gallaudet.edu
  The Laurent Clerc National Deaf Education Center offers products, training, and resources for families and professionals. Information about oral and manual communication is available.

- *SKI-HI*
  http://www.coe.usu.edu/skihi/index.html
  The SKI-HI (pronounced "sky high") institute Web site provides materials, resources, and training opportunities for professionals and families. Information about deaf-blindness and children with multiple impairments is also presented.

- *John Tracy Clinic*
  http://www.jtc.org
  The John Tracy Clinic offers correspondence courses for parents who wish to optimize their child's listening and speaking skills.

- *Vocal Development.com*
  http://www.vocaldevelopment.com
  This Web site describes three levels of prelinguistic speech development and provides audio-recordings of vocalizations from each level, video examples of language stimulation strategies, and information about Short Periods of Prelinguistic Input (SPPI), an approach to stimulating early speech development in children with hearing impairments.

REFERENCES

Blamey, P. J., and Alcantara, J. I. (1994). Research in auditory training. *Journal of the Academy of Rehabilitative Audiology, 27* (Suppl.), 161–192.

Ertmer, D. J. (2005). *The source for children with cochlear implants.* East Moline, IL: LinguiSystems.

Ertmer, D. J., Young, N., Grohne, K., Mellon, J. A., Johnson, C., Corbett, K., and Saindon, K. (2002). Vocal development in young children with cochlear implants: Profiles and implications for intervention. *Language, Speech, and Hearing Services in Schools, 33,* 184–195.

Estabrooks, W. (1998). *Cochlear implants for kids.* Washington, DC: A. G. Bell Association.

Gelfand, S. A. (2001). *Essentials of audiology* (2nd ed.). New York: Thieme Publishing.

Izumikawa, M., Minoda, R., Kawamoto, K., Abrashkin, K., Swiderski, D., Dolan, D., Brough, D. and Raphael, Y. (2005). Auditory hair cell replacement and hearing improvement by *Atoh1* gene therapy in deaf mammals. *Nature Medicine, 11,* 271–276.

Kent, R., Osberger, M. J., Netsell, R., and Hustedde, C. (1987). Phonetic development in identical twins differing in auditory function. *Journal of Speech and Hearing Disorders, 52,* 64–75.

Kozak, V. J., and Moog Brooks, B. (2001). *Baby talk.* St. Louis: Central Institute for the Deaf.

Ling, D. (1976). *Speech and the hearing-impaired child: Theory and practice.* Washington DC: A. G. Bell Association.

Ling, D. (1989). *Foundations of spoken language for hearing-impaired children.* Washington, DC: A. G. Bell Association.

Monsen, R. B. (1978). Towards measuring how well hearing-impaired children speak. *Journal of Speech and Hearing Research, 21,* 197–219.

Niparko, J., Kirk, K., Mellon, N., Robbins, A., Tucci, D., and Wilson, B. (2000). *Cochlear implants: Principles and practices.* Philadelphia: Lippincott Williams & Wilkins.

Oller, D. K., and Eilers, R. (1988). The role of audition in infant babbling. *Child Development, 59,* 441–449.

Osberger, M. J. (1992). Speech intelligibility in the hearing impaired: Research and clinical implications. In R. D. Kent (Ed.), *Speech intelligibility in speech disorders* (pp. 233–263), Philadelphia: John Benjamins.

Osberger, M. J., and McGarr, N. S. (1982). Speech production characteristics of the hearing impaired: Speech and language. *Advances in Basic Research and Practice, 8,* 221–283.

Robbins, A. M. (1994). Guidelines for establishing oral communication. *Volta Review, 96,* 75–82.

Smith, C. R. (1975). Residual hearing and speech production in deaf children. *Journal of Speech and Hearing Research 18,* 795–811.

Stark, R. E. (1983). Phonatory development in young normally hearing and hearing-impaired children. In I. Hochberg, H. Levitt, and M. J. Osberger (Eds.), *Speech of the hearing-impaired: Research, training, and personnel preparation* (pp. 297–312). Baltimore: University Park.

Stoel-Gammon, C. (1988). Prelinguistic vocalizations of hearing-impaired and normally hearing subjects: A comparison of consonantal inventories. *Journal of Speech and Hearing Disorders, 53,* 302–315.

Chapter 5

Perceptual Foundations
of Speech Acquisition

Susan Rvachew

INTRODUCTION

Popular approaches to speech therapy are based on models of speech processing in which continuously changing acoustic input is transformed directly into discrete linguistic units that form the basis for all further language processing. These influential models have supported the use of intervention practices that have the goal of changing the rules, processes, or constraints that are said to account for the child's production of inaccurate speech output despite presumably adultlike underlying representations (Baker, Croot, McLeod, and Paul, 2001). The purpose of this chapter is to introduce recent theoretical models that, in a significant departure from prior models, emphasise the role of speech perception in phonological acquisition. The clinical implications of these new models for the remediation of speech sound impairment and differences will be briefly discussed.

Theoretical perspectives on speech perception and speech production

Exemplar models of speech perception were developed to account for the finding that the acoustic details of the speech signal are not discarded during the process of perceiving speech. Rather, words are stored as detailed acoustic memories (exemplars). The acoustic details of the listener's set of stored exemplars of a word influence the way in which that particular word is processed during future encounters (Goldinger, 1998; Pierrehumbert, 2003). The acoustic cues that are associated with any given phoneme are word-specific and spread throughout the spoken word (Coleman, 2003). For example, the acoustic characteristics of the vocalic portions of the words *Sue* and *shoe* will be significantly different, as will be the acoustic characteristics of the noise portions of the words *shoe* and *she*. Further acoustic variation in the production of these words is introduced by differences in talker gender, speaking rate, emotional register, and so on. Furthermore, acoustic cues to phoneme identity are language-specific. For example, the vowel /u/ is produced with a much lower second formant frequency by a speaker of Canadian French than by a speaker of Canadian English (Escudero and Polka, 2003). Even though French and English both contain an abstract phonological category for the vowel /u/, English listeners will often misperceive the French /u/ and French listeners will often misperceive the English /u/, depending upon the precise acoustic characteristic of the vowel as produced in different words.

A child must have a great deal of experience with his or her native language in order to develop language-specific perceptual strategies that accurately abstract the appropriate linguistic units from highly variable acoustic input (Nittrouer, 2002). These perceptual strategies, once acquired, resist change; the adult learner of a second language will usually have persistent difficulty with perceiving certain phonemes in the new language. However, perception is influenced by recent experience with speech input throughout the lifespan, as evidenced by the acquisition of a noticeable "accent" after moving from one region to another, arising from changes in the acoustic characteristics of vowel productions to match the local dialect (Munro, Derwing, and Flege, 1999).

A precise knowledge of the acoustic representation of phonological categories is important to the acquisition of speech motor control (Perkell et al., 2000). A talker's goal is to produce an acoustic product that will be perceived as intended, rather than a specific constellation of articulatory gestures. If the talker intends to transmit the phoneme /u/, a number of different acoustic outputs may be produced as long as the acoustic product involves closely spaced first and second formant frequencies. Furthermore, many combinations of jaw, tongue, and lip configurations may be used for producing such a vowel. Auditory feedback is used to develop an internal model of the mapping between the target acoustic space and the articulatory gestures required to achieve the target in different phonetic contexts. Given normal hearing acuity, this internal model can be continuously updated during the lifespan to adjust for changes in the size and shape of the vocal tract and the functional integrity of the articulatory system

(Callan, Kent, Guenther, and Vorperian, 2000; Menard, Schwartz, and Boe, 2002).

Finally, it has been posited that phonological knowledge itself is derived from the process of mapping between acoustic targets and speech motor programs for specific words (Edwards, Fourakis, Beckman, and Fox, 1999). This perspective suggests three potential sources of speech sound errors. The child may have an inaccurate phonological representation for a given word, an imprecise acoustic representation of the word, or an inability to produce the articulatory gestures required for its accurate articulation (Munson, Edwards, and Beckman, 2005). Errors at all three levels of representation may be present for the same phoneme or across phonemes as produced by a single child (Stackhouse and Wells, 1993).

Evidence for the close association of speech perception and speech production

Adults typically produce and perceive speech with a high degree of accuracy, but not all adult speech is equally distinct. For example, different tokens of the words *Sue* and *shoe* will be produced with a variety of peak frequencies in the noise portion of the words; if a talker produces peak frequencies ranging from 6 to 7 kHz for /s/ and from 3 to 4 kHz for /ʃ/, that talker's speech will be perceived to be distinct and intelligible (Newman, Clouse, and Burnham, 2001). If another talker produces these fricatives with peak frequencies between 5 and 8 kHz for /s/ and between 3 and 6 kHz for /ʃ/, this talker's speech will be perceived to be less distinct and intelligible. Adults who produce these phonemes most distinctly show better speech discrimination of these same phonemes (Perkell, Matthies, et al., 2004). A similar finding has been reported for the perception and production of vowels (Perkell, Guenther, et al., 2004).

Relationships between articulation accuracy and speech perception ability have also been reported for normally developing children (Broen, Strange, Doyle, and Heller, 1983) and for children with speech sound disorders (Rvachew and Jamieson, 1989). Furthermore, there is evidence that speech perception development precedes speech production development (Rvachew, 2006), with some knowledge of the acoustic representation for a phoneme being a necessary prerequisite to the acquisition of accurate production of that sound. This has been shown for children with speech disorders (Rvachew,

Nowak, and Cloutier, 2004) and for adult learners of a second language (Bradlow, Pisoni, Akahane-Yamada, and Tohkura, 1997).

Development of speech perception skills

The development of language-specific speech perception begins at birth and is strongly impacted by speech input, which serves to maintain, enhance, or attenuate the infant's ability to perceive certain phonetic contrasts (Polka, Rvachew, and Mattock, in press). The infant identifies the phonetic units that are functionally contrastive in the language by attending to the distributional properties of the input (Maye, Werker, and Gerken, 2002). For example, an infant learning English will hear his or her mother produce voiceless sibilant sounds such as /s/ and /ʃ/ with a broad range of peak frequencies, but these different productions will form a bimodal distribution with many productions having a relatively low peak frequency, many others having a higher peak frequency, and a small proportion falling in between. If the mother's language contains only one sibilant, however, the infant will also hear a large number of sibilant productions representing a broad range of peak frequencies, but the distribution of these productions will be unimodal, with most productions being close to a single value. These differences in the distribution of the different exemplars of words containing these phonemes will lead to the formation of a language-specific set of acoustic and phonological representations.

Descriptions of infant speech perception development often imply that there is very little individual variation in the course of this process. It has not been established, however, that all infants can discriminate all possible phonetic contrasts at birth; nor is it true that all infants lose the ability to perceive all nonnative speech sound contrasts during the first year of life. Infants may retain the ability to discriminate certain contrasts despite the absence of appropriate input (Polka and Bohn, 2003), while others have difficulty perceiving certain contrasts despite receiving appropriate input (Nittrouer, 2001). Individual differences in perceptual performance may be due to variations in acoustic salience of the target phoneme, innate perceptual biases on the part of the infant, and the ability to hear and attend to different aspects of the speech input. Selective attention is emerging as a critical variable, as individual differences in perceptual performance are greater when speech is presented in a noisy or distracting environment (Newman, 2005; Polka, Rvachew, and Molnar, 2006).

Years of experience with language input are required for maturation of speech perception skills. Hazan and Barrett (2000) assessed the ability of children aged 6 to 12 years to identify synthesized words representing contrasts of voice, place, and manner of articulation. While the youngest children were able to identify prototypical versions of the test words with adultlike accuracy, even the oldest children were unable to identify more ambiguous tokens of the words with adultlike consistency and accuracy. Edwards, Fox, and Rogers (2002) found that children aged 3 to 8 years were unable to identify naturally produced words that had undergone minimal acoustic degradation with adultlike accuracy. Children with speech sound disorders demonstrated even poorer perceptual performance than children with typical speech. Speech perception skills were correlated with both receptive vocabulary size and articulation accuracy.

The development of accurate, consistent, and distinct speech production is also a protracted process that follows the development of the child's speech perception abilities. Three stages in the development of adultlike acoustic, phonological, and articulatory representations have been proposed. First, when the child is unaware of a given phonological contrast (e.g., /s/ - /θ/), both members of the contrast will be realized in a phonetically and acoustically similar manner (e.g., [θ]). Then, as the child becomes aware of the phonological contrast, the child will produce target /s/ and target /θ/ with acoustically different realizations that may not, however, be perceptually distinguishable to other listeners. Finally, as the child develops a precise acoustic representation of the contrast, increasing numbers of target /s/ and target /θ/ productions will be acoustically and phonetically accurate (e.g., Velleman, 1988).

Clinical implications

The facts about speech perception development that have been highlighted here show that speech-language pathologists and other clinicians need more sophisticated tools for assessing their clients' speech perception skills. Live-voice presentations of prototypical words for identification or discrimination do not provide sufficient information about the maturity of speech perception development to rule out or establish the presence of a speech perception deficit as an etiological factor. When helping children to acquire accurate and consistent production of speech sounds it is necessary to ensure that the child has a detailed understanding of the acoustic characteristics of misarticulated phonemes. Remediating speech perception deficits is facilitated by presenting the child with many and varied exemplars of words containing the target phoneme, produced with

varying degrees of accuracy and distinctness. Procedures that require the child to make perceptual judgments about this kind of input have been shown to enhance speech production learning and speed the child's progress toward the acquisition of age-appropriate articulation accuracy (Rvachew et al., 2004).

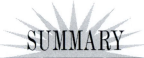

SUMMARY

- Many years of language experience are required in order to develop language-specific perceptual strategies for abstracting linguistic units from highly variable acoustic input.
- A precise knowledge of the acoustic representation of phonological categories is important to the acquisition of speech motor control.
- Distinctness and accuracy of speech production is closely correlated with speech perception performance for specific phonemes in both adults and children.
- Speech perception development begins in infancy and is still not adultlike in late childhood.
- Although children will typically demonstrate good perception of prototypical exemplars of target words presented in ideal listening conditions, they have more difficulty than adults in perceiving less-than-ideal

exemplars of the target words or performing a speech perception task when the words are presented in noisy or distracting conditions.
- Children with speech sound disorders, on average, have significant difficulty with accurate speech perception relative to children with typical speech, especially when the test items involve the speech sounds that they misarticulate.
- Improving children's speech perception skills facilitates the acquisition of accurate speech sound production.
- A speech perception intervention should involve asking the child to make perceptual judgments about many and varied exemplars of words containing the target phoneme, produced with varying degrees of accuracy and distinctness.

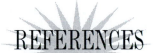

REFERENCES

Baker, E., Croot, K., McLeod, S., and Paul, R. (2001). Psycholinguistic models of speech development and their application to clinical practice. *Journal of Speech, Language, and Hearing Research, 44*, 685–702.

Bradlow, A. R., Pisoni, D., Akahane-Yamada, R., and Tohkura, Y. (1997). Training Japanese listeners to identify English /r/ and /l/: IV. Some effects of perceptual learning on speech production. *Journal of the Acoustical Society of America, 101*, 2299–2310.

Broen, P. A., Strange, W., Doyle, S. S., and Heller, J. H. (1983). Perception and production of approximant consonants by normal and articulation-delayed preschool children. *Journal of Speech and Hearing Research, 26*(4), 601–608.

Callan, D. E., Kent, R. D., Guenther, F. H., and Vorperian, H. K. (2000). An auditory-feedback-based neural network model of

speech production that is robust to developmental changes in the size and shape of the articulatory system. *Journal of Speech, Language, and Hearing Research, 43*, 721–738.

Coleman, J. (2003). Discovering the acoustic correlates of phonological contrasts. *Journal of Phonetics, 31*, 351–372.

Edwards, J., Fourakis, M., Beckman, M. E., and Fox, R. A. (1999). Characterizing knowledge deficits in phonological disorders. *Journal of Speech, Language, and Hearing Research, 42*, 169–186.

Edwards, J., Fox, R. A., and Rogers, C. L. (2002). Final consonant discrimination in children: Effects of phonological disorder, vocabulary size, and articulatory accuracy. *Journal of Speech, Language, and Hearing Research, 45*, 231–242.

Escudero, P., and Polka, L. (2003). *A cross-language study of vowel categorization and vowel acoustics: Canadian English versus*

Canadian French. Paper presented at the 15th International Congress of Phonetic Sciences, Barcelona.

Goldinger, S. D. (1998). Echoes of echoes? An episodic theory of lexical access. *Psychological Review, 105*(2), 251–279.

Hazan, V., and Barrett, S. (2000). The development of phonemic categorization in children aged 6–12. *Journal of Phonetics, 28*, 377–396.

Maye, J., Werker, J. F., and Gerken, L. (2002). Infant sensitivity to distributional information can affect phonetic discrimination. *Cognition, 82*, B101–B111.

Menard, L., Schwartz, J., and Boe, L. (2002). Auditory normalization of French vowels synthesized by an articulatory model simulating growth from birth to adulthood. *Journal of the Acoustical Society of America, 111*(4), 1892–1905.

Munro, M. J., Derwing, T. M., and Flege, J. E. (1999). Canadians in Alabama: A perceptual study of dialect acquisition in adults. *Journal of Phonetics, 27*, 385–403.

Munson, B., Edwards, J., and Beckman, M. E. (2005). Phonological knowledge in typical and atypical speech-sound development. *Topics in Language Disorders: Clinical Perspectives on Speech Sound Disorders, 25*(3), 190–206.

Newman, R. S. (2005). The cocktail party effect revisited: Listening to one's own name in noise. *Developmental Psychology, 41*(2), 352–362.

Newman, R. S., Clouse, S. A., and Burnham, J. L. (2001). The perceptual consequences of within-talker variability in fricative production. *Journal of the Acoustical Society of America, 109*(3), 1181–1196.

Nittrouer, S. (2001). Challenging the notion of innate phonetic boundaries. *Journal of the Acoustical Society of America, 110*(3), 1598–1605.

Nittrouer, S. (2002). From ear to cortex: A perspective on what clinicians need to understand about speech perception and language processing. *Language, Speech, and Hearing Services in Schools, 33*, 237–252.

Perkell, J., Guenther, F. H., Lane, H., Matthies, M. L., Perrier, P., Vick, J., Wilhelms-Tricarico, R., & Zandipour, Z. (2000). A theory of speech motor control and supporting data from speakers with normal hearing and with profound hearing loss. *Journal of Phonetics, 28*, 233–272.

Perkell, J., Guenther, F. H., Lane, H., Matthies, M., Stockmann, E., Tiede, M., Zandipour, M. (2004). The distinctness of speakers' productions of vowel contrasts is related to their discrimination of the contrasts. *Journal of the Acoustical Society of America, 116*(4), 2338–2344.

Perkell, J., Matthies, M. L., Tiede, M., Lane, H., Zandipour, M., Marrone, M., Stockmann, E., & Guenther, F.H. (2004). The distinctness of speakers' /s/–/ʃ/ contrast is related to their auditory discrimination and use of an articulatory saturation effect. *Journal of Speech, Language, and Hearing Research, 47*, 1259–1269.

Pierrehumbert, J. (2003). Probabilistic phonology: Discrimination and robustness. In R. Bod, J. Hay and S. Jannedy (Eds.), *Probability theory in linguistics* (pp. 177–228). Cambridge, MA: MIT Press.

Polka, L., and Bohn, O. (2003). Asymmetries in vowel perception. *Speech Communication, 41*, 221–231.

Polka, L., Rvachew, S., and Mattock, K. (in press). Experiential influences on speech perception and speech production in infancy. In E. Hoff and M. Shatz (Eds.), *Handbook of Language development*. Malden, MA: Blackwell.

Polka, L., Rvachew, S., and Molnar, M. (2005). Infant perception of speech in noise: Direct evidence for nonsensory effects. Manuscript submitted for publication.

Rvachew, S. (2006). Longitudinal prediction of implicit phonological awareness skills. *American Journal of Speech-Language Pathology, 15*, 165–176.

Rvachew, S., and Jamieson, D. G. (1989). Perception of voiceless fricatives by children with a functional articulation disorder. *Journal of Speech and Hearing Disorders, 54*, 193–208.

Rvachew, S., Nowak, M., and Cloutier, G. (2004). Effect of phonemic perception training on the speech production and phonological awareness skills of children with expressive phonological delay. *American Journal of Speech-Language Pathology, 13*, 250–263.

Stackhouse, J., and Wells, B. (1993). Psycholinguistic assessment of developmental speech disorders. *European Journal of Disorders of Communication, 28*, 331–348.

Velleman, S. L. (1988). The role of linguistic perception in later phonological development. *Applied Psycholinguistics, 9*, 221–236.

Chapter 6

Genetic Foundations of Speech Acquisition and Impairment

Barbara A. Lewis

INTRODUCTION

Both environmental and genetic factors contribute to the child's development of the speech sound system. It is likely that many genes contribute to this process as speech acquisition is complex and requires the coordination of respiratory, motor, and neurological systems. A multifactorial model may best explain typical speech acquisition. This model holds that many genes of small effect combine with environmental factors to influence speech acquisition. At present, specific genes for speech acquisition have not been identified. However, genes have been identified that are expressed in the muscles, lungs, and brain and whose products influence development, growth, structure, and function. As genetic studies of typical speech acquisition are not yet available, the following chapter reviews genetic studies of children with speech impairments. These studies may provide a model for genetic studies of speech acquisition and suggest possible candidate chromosome regions for study.

Children with speech impairments represent the largest group of children with communication impairments served by speech-language pathologists. The residual effects of childhood speech impairments may be lifelong, and yet for the majority of individuals the etiological basis of the disorder is unknown. More than half of children with early speech impairments encounter later academic difficulties in language, reading, and spelling (Aram and Hall, 1990; Bishop and Adams, 1990; Felsenfeld, McGue, and Broen, 1995; Menyuk, et al., 1991; Nathan, Stackhouse, Goulandris, and Snowling, 2004; Shriberg and Kwiatkowski, 1988). Recent advances in the identification of genetic mechanisms for speech and language impairment have suggested a possible genetic basis to speech impairment and hold promise in furthering our understanding of causal mechanisms, delineating the biological basis for speech acquisition, and ultimately guiding our clinical practice.

Genetic studies may reveal the biological underpinnings of speech impairment by discovering key genetic pathways (i.e., functional studies of the proteins that the genes code and the resulting metabolic, structure, signaling, transcription regulation, or other cellular pathways), bridging the gap between genetics and the neurobiological basis of these disorders (Fisher and DeFries, 2002). Identification of genetic influences may also result in improved diagnosis and early identification of those at risk, allowing for environmental intervention at a young age (Fisher and DeFries, 2002). Children with family histories of speech impairment may be identified at birth, considered at risk for communication difficulties, screened at a young age, and followed into the school-age years. Understanding the genetic overlap of speech, language, and reading impairments may assist in the development of meaningful diagnostic categories based on shared underlying deficits, such as impaired phonological representational processes (Raitano, Pennington, Tunick, Boada, and Shriberg, 2004; Tunick and Pennington, 2002). The goal of this chapter is to review recent genetic findings in speech impairment, to explore shared genetic influences for speech, language, and reading impairments, and to consider implications for clinical practice. Portions of this chapter are based on a review by Lewis et al. (2005).

Prevalence and comorbidity

Speech-language pathologists often encounter children with combined difficulties in both speech and language in their clinical practice. Examination of the prevalence rates for each disorder and their comorbidity suggests shared genetic influences as well as unique genetic factors. The prevalence of speech impairment in 6-year-old children was reported by Shriberg, Tomblin, and McSweeny (1999) as 3.8 percent with rates of 4.5 percent for boys and 3.1 percent for girls. Rates for younger children are much higher, with some studies reporting rates of 15.6 percent in 3-year-old children (Campbell et al., 2003). The prevalence of language impairment at kindergarten has been reported at 8 percent for boys and 6 percent for girls with an overall rate of 7.4 percent (Tomblin et al., 1997). Shriberg et al. (1999) report rates of comorbidity between speech delay and language

impairment in children with persistent speech delay of 11 percent to 15 percent at 6 years of age, with considerably higher rates of 40 percent to 60 percent reported for preschool children (Shriberg and Austin, 1998). The comorbidity of speech impairment and language impairment was estimated at 6 percent to 21 percent for receptive language impairments and at 38 percent to 62 percent for expressive language impairments. Thus, the risk for comorbid expressive language impairment is two to three times greater than for receptive language impairment (Shriberg and Austin, 1998).

Reading impairment also is often comorbid with speech and language impairment. The prevalence rate of reading impairment in the population is estimated at 5 percent in school-age children (Francks, MacPhie, and Monaco, 2002). In a sample of children at high risk for reading impairment, 28 percent were referred to speech therapy compared with 12.5 percent of children at low risk for reading disability (Pennington and Lefly, 2001). Follow-up studies of children with preschool speech impairment have found later academic difficulties in 50 percent–75 percent of their samples (Aram and Hall, 1990; Bishop and Adams, 1990; Lewis, Ekelman, and Aram, 1989; King, Jones, and Lasky, 1982; Nathan et al., 2004). Our follow-up study of children with preschool speech impairment found that 18 percent of children with speech impairment alone and 75 percent of children with both speech impairment and comorbid language impairment had reading problems in mid-elementary school (Lewis, Freebairn, Hansen, and Taylor, 2002). Rates of comorbidity may vary depending on whether they are derived from children identified with speech, language, or reading impairments.

Genetic heterogeneity of speech impairment

The etiology of speech impairment is most likely heterogeneous with multiple underlying genetic and environmental etiologies. Speech impairment may be due in part to genes that affect processes unique to speech production, such as motor planning, oral motor ability, and some aspects of auditory discrimination. Alternatively, as discussed above, high rates of comorbidities of speech, language, and reading impairments suggest common genetic influences. Plomin and Kovas (2005) recently proposed a theory of generalist genes in which they hypothesize shared genes that exert influence on processes (such as phonological processing) that may be common across disorders. A partly shared genetic etiology may explain shared deficits in phonological awareness, phonological memory, and phonological code retrieval that are common to speech, language, and reading impairment. Thus, speech may be viewed as a complex human trait. The identification of candidate chromosome regions and genes that may be associated with speech impairment has just begun. The study of the genetic bases of spoken and written language began with behavioral genetic methods that utilized statistical techniques and progressed to more sophisticated molecular genetic methods. The findings from these studies are reviewed below.

Family aggregation studies

Early studies of speech, language, and reading impairment sought to establish that the disorder "ran in families" (Pennington, 1997). These familial aggregation studies demonstrated that the prevalence of a disorder within a family of a proband (a child presenting with an impairment) was greater than the prevalence of the disorder in the population as a whole. Most studies of familial aggregation have not distinguished between language impairment and speech impairment. These studies have reported 23 percent to 43 percent of first-degree family members of probands are affected for speech and language impairment (Felsenfeld et al., 1995; Gopnik and Crago, 1991; Lahey and Edwards, 1995; Lewis, 1992; Spitz, Tallal, Flax, and Benasich, 1997; Tallal, Ross, and Curtiss, 1989; Tomblin, 1989). Similarly, studies of familial aggregation of reading impairment have not considered comorbid speech impairment (Decker and DeFries, 1980; DeFries, Singer, Foch, and Lewitter, 1978; Finucci, 1978; Gilger, Pennington, and DeFries, 1991; Hallgren, 1950; Smith, Pennington, Kimberling, and Ing, 1990). However, these studies have reported familial aggregation of specific skills associated with reading, such as phonological short-term memory, phonological decoding, and spelling that may be common to speech impairment (Raskind, Hsu, Berninger, Thompson, and Wijsman, 2000). Of the studies that have specifically examined familial aggregation in families of children with speech impairment, all have reported a higher percentage of family members affected for speech and language impairment than in control families (Felsenfeld et al., 1995; Lewis et al., 1989). Approximately 26 percent of nuclear family members and 13.6 percent of extended family members were affected (Lewis, 1992). Brothers showed higher rates (40 percent) than sisters (19 percent), with mothers 8 percent) and fathers (18 percent) equally affected.

Family studies, however, cannot separate genetic influences from shared family environment. Twin studies are conducted to tease apart environmental and genetic influences.

Twin studies

Twin studies examine the concordance for the impairment in monozygotic twins (MZ) and dizygotic twins (DZ). If concordance rates are higher for MZ than DZ twins, a genetic component to the disorder is implied, as MZ twins are identical genetically whereas DZ twins share on the average 50 percent of segregating genes. Similar to familial aggregation studies, early twin studies of speech and language impairment did not distinguish twins with comorbid disorders. Twin studies of speech impairment report a higher concordance for MZ twins (.95) than DZ twins (.22) (Lewis and Thompson, 1992). Studies of language impairment have also found higher concordant rates for MZ twins than DZ twins, with concordance ranges of .70 to .86 for MZ twins and .38 to .46 for DZ twins (Bishop, North, and Dolan, 1996; Tomblin and Buckwalter, 1998). Thus, a genetic contribution to speech impairment is suggested as MZ twins show higher concordant rates than DZ twins and an environmental component is suggested as MZ twins do not demonstrate complete concordance. Estimates of heritability of speech and language impairment (how much of the variance may be attributed to genetic factors) range from .38 to .76 (Viding Spinath, Price, Dale, and Plomin, 2004).

Molecular genetic studies

Next, molecular genetic studies were conducted to examine the DNA of individual family members. Methods such as linkage analyses were employed to identify regions of chromosomes where potential genes for speech impairment may be located. To date, specific genes for speech impairment have not been identified. However, three research groups provided evidence for their existence.

The first evidence of a gene for speech impairment came from the study of a single large family pedigree known as the K.E. family from the United Kingdom. Fisher, Vargha-Khadem, Watkins, Monaco, and Pembrey (1998) performed a genome-wide linkage study on the K.E. family and identified a region on chromosome 7 that appeared to cosegregate with speech impairment and language disorder. They further localized the gene locus for the family's speech impairment, designated as

SPCH1, to a region at 7q31 and finally identified the causative gene called FOXP2. Individuals who carry the mutant FOXP2 allele present a variety of deficits, including poor speech as well as impairments in reading, writing, comprehension, use of grammar, and IQ. Oral facial apraxia is posited by the authors to be the core deficit in this family. The affected individuals show bilateral atrophy of the caudate nucleus, among an array of other neuroimaging findings. The caudate nucleus is part of the basal ganglia, which has well-described associations with motor control. FOXP2 is widely expressed in both mouse and human tissues including the brain and the lungs (Kaestner et al., 1993; Lai, Fisher, Hurst, Vargha-Khadem, and Monaco, 2001). Recently, a mouse model for the FOXP2 gene was developed (Shu et al., 2005). Mice with disruption in the FOXP2 demonstrated a disruption in vocalization related to social communication.

Several families with other variants of the FOXP2 gene (one with a translocation) have been identified. A recent report found that 1 child out of 49 children with developmental apraxia of speech demonstrated a mutation that resulted in an abnormal protein product (MacDermot et al., 2005). This child's mother and sibling also carried the mutation. The rarity of this mutation suggests that, while the FOXP2 gene may account for the speech impairment in a few isolated families, such mutations do not account for speech impairment in the population as a whole. It is likely that multiple genes contribute to speech impairment in the population, some with general effects and others with specific effects that are modified by the environment.

Other studies have examined chromosome regions previously associated with reading impairment for linkage to speech impairment. A recent study by Smith, Pennington, Boada, and Shriberg (2005) examined 111 probands with speech impairment and their 76 siblings. Smith et al. hypothesized that there is symptom, cognitive, and etiological overlap between speech impairment and reading impairment. They examined linkage of speech impairment to loci on chromosomes 1, 6, and 15 that have been well documented to be associated with reading impairment. Results showed that performance on the Goldman-Fristoe Test of Articulation (Goldman and Fristoe, 1986) linked significantly to a region on chromosome 6 and that both performance on the Goldman-Fristoe Test of Articulation and a nonsense word repetition task linked significantly to a region on chromosome 15. These findings support shared genes for reading and speech impairment that may influence neurologic functions.

A third linkage study (Stein et al., 2004) also supported genetic overlap of speech and reading impairments. The participants in these studies were 674 individuals from 151 families ascertained through a proband with a moderate to severe speech impairment. A region on chromosome 3 that was previously associated with reading impairment demonstrated linkage for speech and language impairment, as well as other spoken and written language impairments. Measures of phonologic coding/decoding demonstrated the strongest linkage. Corresponding performance on tests for single-word decoding also demonstrated linkage as did a test of oral motor skills (Stein et al., 2004). These findings suggest that speech impairment and reading impairment share some common genetic basis.

Conclusions

The genetic foundations for speech have been examined primarily in the context of speech impairment rather than typical or advanced speech acquisition skills. Without exception, these studies have concluded that speech impairment is indeed genetic in part. However, it is likely that there is much genetic heterogeneity that may result in speech impairment. A single major gene such as the FOXP2 gene found in the K.E. family may be responsible for the speech impairment. However, this is the exception rather than the rule. It is likely that for most individuals many genes, with small effects, contribute to speech impairment. These genes may have broader effects and impact cognitive/linguistic processes (such as phonological processing) that underlie both spoken and written language.

Environmental effects may modify the expression of these genes. Risk genes interact with environmental factors as well as protective factors to determine an individual's risk for speech impairment. Thus, the same genetic mutation may have different effects in different individuals due to its interaction with other genes or the environment.

Genetic studies examining speech acquisition or speech impairment in multiple countries or languages have not been conducted. However, cross-linguistic studies of reading impairment suggest that common genetic determinants are responsible for impairments across languages. This seems reasonable, as the biological framework for speech, structures and functions, is universal. Genetic pathways that influence neural development, such as in the case of the FOXP2 gene, would result in similar impairments across languages. What may differ is the frequency of genes in different populations or the effect from environment or motor/cognitive demands of the language.

Clinical implications

Although specific genes for speech impairment have not yet been identified and, consequently, screening for genes is not yet a reality, genetic studies have implications for clinical practice. First, speech-language pathologists should routinely take careful and detailed family histories of the children that they serve. History information should include systematic inquiry regarding skills of all first-, second-, and third-degree relatives. An interview format is more desirable than a questionnaire that the caretaker fills out on his or her own. The informant is first queried regarding whether nuclear family members are affected, followed by maternal and paternal families. The gender, age, and education level of each family member is recorded as well as reported genetic syndromes, hearing loss, developmental delays, or other chronic medical conditions. Construction of a pedigree during the interview serves to verify family relationships and promote consideration of each family member individually. Information on comorbid reading, language, spelling, and learning disabilities should be included. Children identified as demonstrating a family history for a disorder should be screened early and followed routinely into elementary school.

SUMMARY

- A multifactorial model of typical speech acquisition is supported. This model holds that many genes of small effect in conjunction with the environment influence speech acquisition.
- Genetic studies of children with speech impairment support a genetic basis for speech and suggest possible chromosome regions that may be associated with speech, language, and reading skills.

- Genetic heterogeneity of speech acquisition is suggested. In some cases the influence of a single major gene, such as the FOXP2 gene, is involved, and in other cases the combination of many genes results in speech skills. Some genes may have broader effects and influences on both spoken and written language.

REFERENCES

Aram, D. M., and Hall, N. E. (1990). Longitudinal follow-up of children with pre-school communication disorders: Treatment implications. *School of Psychology Review, 19,* 487–501.

Bishop, D. V., and Adams, C. (1990). A prospective study of the relationship between specific language impairment, phonological disorders and reading retardation. *Journal of Child Psychology and Psychiatry, 31,* 1027–1050.

Bishop, D. V., North T., and Donlan, C. (1996). Nonword repetition as a behavioural marker for inherited language impairment: Evidence from a twin study. *Journal of Child Psychology and Psychiatry, 37,* 391–403.

Campbell, T. F., Dollaghan, C. A., Rockette, H. E., Paradise, J. L., Feldman, H. M., Shriberg, L. D., Sabo, D. L., and Kurs-Lasky, M. (2003). Risk factors for speech delay of unknown origin in 3-year-old children. *Child Development, 74,* 346–357.

Decker, S. N., and DeFries, J. C. (1980). Cognitive abilities in families of reading-disabled children. *Journal of Learning Disabilities, 13,* 517–522.

DeFries, J. C., Singer, S. M., Foch, T. T., and Lewitter, F. I. (1978). Familial nature of reading disability. *British Journal of Psychiatry, 132,* 361–367.

Felsenfeld, S., McGue, M., and Broen, P. A. (1995). Familial aggregation of phonological disorders: Results from a 28-year follow-up. *Journal of Speech and Hearing Research, 38,* 1091–1107.

Finucci, J. M. (1978). Genetic considerations in dyslexia. In H. R. Myklebust (Ed.), *Progress in Learning Disabilities* (Vol. 4). New York: Greene and Statten.

Fisher, S. E., and DeFries J. C. (2002). Developmental dyslexia: Genetic dissection of a complex cognitive trait. *Nature Review Neuroscience, 3,* 767–780.

Fisher, S. E., Vargha-Khadem, F., Watkins, K. E., Monaco, A. P., and Pembrey, M. E. (1998). Localisation of a gene implicated in a severe speech and language disorder. *Nature Genetics, 18,* 168–170.

Francks, C., MacPhie, I. L., and Monaco, A. P. (2002). The genetic basis of dyslexia. *Lancet Neurology, 1,* 483–490.

Gilger, J. W., Pennington, B. F., and DeFries, J. C. (1991). Risk of reading disability as a function of parental history in three family studies. *Reading and Writing: An Interdisciplinary Journal, 3*, 299–313.

Goldman, R., and Fristoe, M. (1986). *The Goldman Fristoe Test of Articulation.* Circle Pines, MN: American Guidance Service.

Gopnik, M., and Crago, M. B. (1991). Familial aggregation of a developmental language disorder. *Cognition, 39*, 1–50.

Hallgren, B. (1950). Specific dyslexia (congenital word-blindness): A clinical and genetic study. *Acta Psychiatrica Neurological Scandanavian (Supplement), 65*, 1–287.

Kaestner, K. H., Lee, K. H., Schlondorff, J., Hiemisch, H., Monaghan, A. P., and Schutz, G. (1993). Six members of the mouse fork-head gene family are developmentally regulated. *Proceedings of the National Academy of Science USA, 90*, 7628–7631.

King, R. R., Jones, C., and Laskey, E. (1982). In retrospect: A fifteen-year follow-up report of speech-language disordered children. *Language, Speech, and Hearing Services in Schools, 13*, 24–32.

Lahey, M., and Edwards, J. (1995). Specific language impairment: Preliminary investigation of factors associated with family history and with patterns of language performance. *Journal of Speech and Hearing Research, 38*, 643–657.

Lai, C. S., Fisher, S. E., Hurst, J. A., Vargha-Khadem, F., and Monaco, A. P. (2001). A forkhead-domain gene is mutated in a severe speech and language disorder. *Nature, 413*, 519–523.

Lewis, B. A. (1992). Pedigree analysis of children with phonology disorders. *Journal of Learning Disabilities, 25*, 586–597.

Lewis, B. A., Ekelman, B. L., and Aram, D. M. (1989). A familial study of severe phonological disorders. *Journal of Speech and Hearing Research, 32*, 713–724.

Lewis, B. A., Freebairn, L. A., Hansen, A. J., and Taylor, H. G. (2002, July). *School-age follow-up of children with apraxia of speech.* Paper presented at the IX International Congress for the Study of Child Language and the Symposium on Research in Child Language Disorders.

Lewis, B. A., Shriberg, L. D., Freebairn, L. A., Hansen, A. J., Stein, C. M., Taylor, H. G., and Iyengar, S. K. (2005). *The genetic bases of speech sound disorders: Evidence from spoken and written language.* Unpublished manuscript.

Lewis, B. A., and Thompson, L. A. (1992). A study of developmental speech and language disorders in twins. *Journal of Speech and Hearing Research, 35*, 1086–1094.

MacDermot, K. D., Bonora, E., Sykes, N., Coupe, A., Lai, C. S., Vernes, S. C., Vargha-Khadem, F., McKenzie, F., Smith, R. L., Monaco, A. P. and Fisher, S. E. (2005). Identification of FOXP2 truncation as a novel cause of developmental speech and language deficits. *American Journal of Human Genetics, 76*, 1074–1080.

Menyuk, P., Chesnick, M., Liebergott, J. W., Korngold, B., D'Agostino, R., and Belanger, A. (1991). Predicting reading problems in at-risk children. *Journal of Speech and Hearing Research, 34*, 893–903.

Nathan, L., Stackhouse, J., Goulandris, N., and Snowling, M. J. (2004). Educational consequences of developmental speech disorder: Key stage 1 National Curriculum assessment results in English and mathematics. *British Journal of Educational Psychology, 74*, 173–186.

Pennington, B. F. (1997). Using genetics to dissect cognition. *American Journal of Human Genetics, 60*, 13–16.

Pennington, B. F., and Lefly, D. L. (2001). Early reading development in children at family risk for dyslexia. *Child Development, 72*, 816–833.

Plomin, R., and Kovas, Y. (2005). Generalist genes and learning disabilities. *Psychological Bulletin, 131*, 592–617.

Raitano, N. A., Pennington, B. F., Tunick, R. A., Boada, R., and Shriberg, L. D. (2004). Pre-literacy skills of subgroups of children with speech sound disorders. *Journal of Child Psychology and Psychiatry, 45*, 821–835.

Raskind, W. H., Hsu, L., Berninger, V. W., Thompson, J. B., and Wijsman, E. M. (2000). Familial aggregation of dyslexia phenotypes. *Behavior Genetics, 30*, 385–396.

Shriberg, L. D., and Austin, D. (1998). Comorbidity of speech-language disorder: Implications for a phenotype marker for speech delay. In R. Paul (Ed.), *The speech-language connection* (pp. 73–117). Baltimore, MD: Paul H. Brookes.

Shriberg, L. D., and Kwiatkowski, J. (1988). A follow-up study of children with phonologic disorders of unknown origin. *Journal of Speech and Hearing Disorders, 53*, 144–155.

Shriberg, L. D., Tomblin, J. B., and McSweeny, J. L. (1999). Prevalence of speech delay in 6-year-old children and comorbidity with language impairment. *Journal of Speech, Language, and Hearing Research, 42*, 1461–1481.

Shu, W., Cho, J. Y., Jiang, Y., Zhang, M., Weisz, D., Elder, G. A., Schmeidler, J., De Gasperi, R., Gama Sosa, M., Rabidou, D., Santucci, A. C., Perl, D., Morrisey, E., and Buxbaum, J. D. (2005). Altered ultrasonic vocalization in mice with a disruption in the FOXP2 gene. *Proceedings of the National Academy of Science, 102*, 9643–9648.

Smith, S. D., Pennington, B. F., Boada, R., and Shriberg, L. D. (2005). Linkage of speech sound disorder to reading disability loci. *Journal of Child Psychology and Psychiatry, 46*, 1057–1066.

Smith, S. D., Pennington, B. F., Kimberling, W. J., and Ing, P. S. (1990). Familial dyslexia: Use of genetic linkage data to define subtypes. *Journal of the American Academy of Child and Adolescent Psychiatry, 29*, 204–213.

Spitz, R. V., Tallal, P., Flax, J., and Benasich, A. A. (1997). Look who's talking: A prospective study of familial transmission of language impairments. *Journal of Speech, Language, and Hearing Research, 40,* 990–1001.

Stein, C. M., Schick, J. H., Taylor, H. G., Shriberg, L. D., Millard, C., Kundtz-Kluge, A., Russo, K., Minich, N., Hansen, A., Freebairn, L. A., Elston, R. C., Lewis, B. A. and Iyengar, S. K. (2004). Pleiotropic effects of a chromosome 3 locus on speech-sound disorder and reading. *American Journal of Human Genetics, 74,* 283–297.

Tallal P., Ross R., and Curtiss S. (1989). Familial aggregation in specific language impairment. *Journal of Speech and Hearing Disorders, 54,* 167–173.

Tomblin, J. B. (1989). Familial concentration of developmental language impairment. *Journal of Speech and Hearing Disorders, 54,* 287–295.

Tomblin, J., and Buckwalter, P. (1998). Heritability of poor language achievement among twins. *Journal of Speech, Language, and Hearing Research, 41,* 188–199.

Tomblin, J., Records, N., Buckwalter, P., Zhang, X., Smith E., and O'Brien, M. (1997). Prevalence of specific language impairment in kindergarten children. *Journal of Speech, Language, and Hearing Research, 40,* 1245–1260.

Tunick, R. A., and Pennington, B. F. (2002). The etiological relationship between reading disability and phonological disorder. *Annals of Dyslexia, 52,* 75–95.

Viding, E., Spinath, F. M., Price, T., Dale, P. S., and Plomin, R. (2004). Genetic and environmental influences on language impairment in 4-year-old same-sex and opposite sex twins. *Journal of Child Psychology and Psychiatry, 45*(2), 315–325.

Chapter 7

Articulatory Foundations of Speech Acquisition

Martin J. Ball

INTRODUCTION

The articulation of speech sounds is the organic phase of speech production. This means that the vocal organs are used to create a moving column of air that is shaped into the individual consonants and vowels, and the prosodic features that all go to make spoken communication. It is worth recalling that the vocal organs evolved primarily for nonspeech functions (breathing, eating) but have developed further to be particularly suitable for speech production. The vocal organs compose the vocal tract, which is taken here to extend from the lungs, through the trachea and larynx, to the pharynx and oral and nasal cavities (see Chapter 2).

A wide range of speech sounds are found in natural language (i.e., the 5,000 or so languages spoken around the world), and sounds from outside the repertoire of the target language often occur in the speech-language pathology clinic. Further, clients in the clinic may produce atypical sounds, that is, sounds not found in natural language. Both typical and atypical sounds are surveyed in this chapter, as well as sources where you may find out more information.

This chapter will examine the two main phonetics symbols charts needed by speech-language pathologists: the chart of the International Phonetic Alphabet (Appendix A), and the chart showing the Extensions to the International Phonetic Alphabet for transcribing atypical speech (Appendix B). Further descriptions of articulatory phonetics can be found in such texts as Laver (1994), Ball and Rahilly (1999), Ladefoged (2000a, b), and Ball and Müller (2005). For the importance of accurate clinical transcription see Ball, Rahilly, and Tench (1996), and Ball (2005).

Initiation

As noted above, speech requires a moving column of air, and to create such a column air pressure changes must be initiated somewhere in the vocal tract. If pressure is reduced somewhere in the system, then air from outside the system will flow inwards to equalize the pressures within and without the system. If pressure is increased somewhere in the system, then air will flow outwards—again to equalize the pressure differentials. In speech, an airstream flowing outwards from the lungs is normally used. Therefore, the lungs can be termed the *initiator*. Lung air flows out of the lungs when, at the end of the inhalatory part of the breathing cycle, the full lungs start to collapse under the effects of gravity helped by the contraction of the internal intercostal muscles of the ribcage (causing negative air pressure and so outward flow). For speech, unlike quiet breathing, speakers use the external intercostal muscles as a braking mechanism. This slows the exhalatory part of the cycle, allowing speech for many seconds on a single exhalation. Phoneticians term this airstream *pulmonic egressive*. Speaking on an inhalation (*pulmonic ingressive*) is not found in natural language, but it may be used to disguise the voice or may be found in clients with voice impairment, or stuttering (see Ball and Rahilly, 1996), or other speech impairments (Ingram and Terselic, 1983; Gierut and Champion, 2000; Chin, 2003). Pulmonic egressive speech is found in all languages and, even in those languages that use other initiators, pulmonic egressive is used for the vast majority of sounds. The IPA chart displays pulmonic egressive consonants at the top, with the vowels below to the right.

If the larynx is closed tightly and jerked upwards using the extrinsic laryngeal muscles, negative pressure is caused in the supraglottal vocal tract. This causes the small amount of air above the larynx to flow outwards, and it is possible to make individual speech sounds on this airstream. *Ejective* stops, fricatives, and affricates can be made on this *glottalic egressive* airstream, and are shown on the IPA chart (Appendix A) in a table below and to the left of the main pulmonic consonant table. If the larynx is jerked downwards instead, then negative pressure is caused. Sounds made on this airstream are usually accompanied by a small amount of lung air leaking through the glottis and causing vocal fold vibration (voicing; see below). Sounds made on this *glottal ingressive* airstream are called *implosives*, and again can be found in the nonpulmonic table on the IPA chart.

The final initiator used in natural language is the back of the tongue articulating against the velum. The air trapped above the tongue and some constriction further forward (e.g., the tongue tip against the back of the upper front teeth) is rarefied by lowering the tongue body slightly. When the forward constriction is removed, air flows into the mouth from outside to equalize the negative pressure in the mouth. The *velaric ingressive* airstream is used to make *click* sounds. These are normal consonants in some languages, and some are used extralinguistically in English to show annoyance or encouragement. Clicks are also shown in the nonpulmonic table of the IPA chart. Ejectives, implosives, and clicks, when used in natural language, are embedded in a string of otherwise pulmonic egressive sounds.

In impaired speech, clicks have been reportedly used for pulmonic sounds in several studies (Howard, 1993; Bedore, Leonard, and Gandour, 1994; Heselwood, 1997). Ejectives have also been encountered (Chin, 2002; Nicolaides, 2004), and implosives have been reported used for target pulmonic sounds by Higgins, Carney, McCleary, and Rogers (1996) and Pantelemidou, Hermand, and Thomas (2003), both of which deal with hearing impaired speakers, and by Shahin (2002).

Phonation

Air flowing up from the lungs passes through the larynx. It is here that phonation takes place. There are four main phonation types, two of which are used linguistically in all known languages. *Voiceless* phonation occurs when the vocal folds are between 60 percent and 95 percent of their maximal opening, and air flows through with minimal turbulence for most voiceless sounds, or some turbulence for the sound [h]. On the IPA chart (Appendix A), voiceless consonants are always placed on the left of the relevant box (e.g., [p] in the bilabial plosive box of the pulmonic consonants table).

Voiced phonation occurs when air is metered in short puffs through the vibrating vocal folds. The folds are held together relatively tightly, and the air pressure from the lungs builds up until it forces them apart. As the air squeezes through the narrow gap, the Bernouilli effect causes the folds to close again, until the subglottal pressure forces them apart once more and the cycle continues. This stream of short puffs of air through the folds causes a buzzing noise we term *voice*, or *modal voice*. The frequency of vibrations differs according to the pitch of the voice (intonation, or word tone in tone languages) and depends on whether the speaker is a male, a female or a child, but a range of 80–300 Hz is normal for males (Hz = hertz, or cycles per second). Voice is sufficient to distinguish one consonant from an otherwise identical other consonant; so, for example [b] from [p] and [z] from [s]. On the IPA chart all voiced consonants are placed to the right of their relevant box, whether they have a voiceless pair (e.g., [p] and [b]), or when there is only a voiced consonant shown (e.g., [m]). All vowels are voiced, so these are not shown in boxes.

Whisper is made by opening the posterior end of the vocal folds to about 25 percent maximal opening and is used extralinguistically. *Creak* occurs usually at the anterior end of the folds and has low-frequency vibrations of about 50 Hz. This phonation type is used linguistically in some languages and may be a stylistic variant in English (especially at the end of utterances).

Murmur is a combination of whisper at the posterior part of the folds and normal voicing at the anterior part. It has linguistic use in some languages and stylistic use in others. It may also be termed *whispery voice* or (confusingly) *breathy voice*. Many authorities use *breathy voice* to refer to a pathological voice quality where air is forced past open vocal folds causing them to vibrate to some extent; this voice quality uses a large volume of air, so few syllables can be uttered at any one time. The IPA chart has some diacritics for many of these phonation types in its Diacritics table, and uses the term *breathy voice* for what we term *murmur*.

Other combination phonation types may occur, and some of these are pathological. A full set of phonation types is shown on the VoQS chart (see Appendix C, for a full description of this chart). We should note here the *ventricular* phonation type that uses the false vocal folds (situated above the real ones in the larynx), and *diplophonia* (a combination of modal voice and ventricular voice); both are often found in voice clients in the clinic.

Manner of articulation

Once the airstream passes through the larynx it is modified by the movement of the supralaryngeal articulators (active, such as the tongue; passive, such as the hard palate, etc), and by passing through the resonating chambers of the pharynx, the oral cavity, and sometimes the nasal cavity. Individual sound segments can be divided into a number of manners of articulation, definable by considering the placement of the active and passive articulators. When the articulators are held together, *stop* sounds are made (the air is stopped in the mouth). These consist of oral stops or *plosives* (e.g., [p], [d]); nasal stops or *nasals* (e.g., [m], where the velum is lowered so that the air flows out through the nose albeit it cannot flow through the mouth); *trills*, where the stopping takes the form of several

short stoppages with airflow in between (as in the trilled [r] in Spanish *perro*); and *taps*, where the stopping takes the form of a single short stoppage (as in the tapped [ɾ] in Spanish *pero; see* Chapter 52). These stop sound types are found as the first four rows on the pulmonic consonants table (Appendix A).

The next type of sound is where the articulators are held fairly close together so that as the airflow squeezes through the gap, turbulence is caused. This is why the name *fricative* is used for these sounds. The airflow may be central, as in sounds such [f], [v], [s], [z]; or lateral as in the *ll* found in Welsh placenames, given the IPA symbol [ɬ] (see Chapter 56). The fricatives are found on the two rows below the stops (Appendix A).

The final consonant type has the articulators wider apart so that airflow is smooth, and these sounds are termed *approximants*. Again, there are central ones and lateral ones. The approximants make up the last two rows of the pulmonic table (Appendix A). Some approximants such as [j] and [w] (this last found in the Other symbols section of the IPA chart, as it has a double place of articulation) are called *semivowels* because they are in effect rapid vowel-like beginnings to syllables and cannot be prolonged without turning into a vowel ([j] is like the vowel [i], and [w] like the vowel [u]).

The widest channel between articulators is found with the vowels, and we consider this group of sounds below.

Place of articulation

The pulmonic table on the IPA chart lists the places of consonant articulation across the top, and the names indicate the passive articulator involved. *Bilabial* involves the upper and lower lips (e.g., [m]); *labiodental* has articulation between the lower lip and upper front teeth (e.g., [f]). The tongue tip and/or blade is the active articulator in *dental* (against the inside of the upper front teeth), for example [θ] as *th* in *bath*; *alveolar* (against the tooth ridge), as [d] in English; and *postalveolar* (against the back edge of the alveolar ridge), an example being [ʃ] as *sh* in *shop*. The underside of the tongue tip and blade is the active articulator in *retroflex* consonants, which are found in the languages of India and Indian English among others. The middle part of the tongue body (or *dorsum*) is articulated against or toward the hard palate in *palatal* sounds (as [j] denoting *y* in English *yes*); whereas the back part of the dorsum is used with the velum for *velar* sounds such as [k]. The back of the tongue dorsum is also used against the uvula to make *uvular* sounds, such as the back-r in standard French *rue* [ʁy] (see Chapter 40). *Pharyngeal* sounds are made by pulling the root of the tongue into the pharynx and can be illustrated by the

Arabic fricatives [ħ] and [ʕ] (see Chapter 34). Finally, the *glottal* place involves the articulation of the two vocal folds, as in the sound [h].

Some double articulations are shown in the Other symbols part of the IPA chart. These involve simultaneous articulations of the same manner at two different places; for example bilabial and velar for [w].

English Consonant Symbols

The symbols to transcribe the consonants of English are: /p, b, t, d, k, g, m, n, ŋ {=*ng*} f, v, θ {=*th* in *thin*}, ð {=*th* in *then*}, v, s, z, ʃ {=*sh*}, ʒ {=*s* in *treasure*}, h, tʃ{=*ch*}, dʒ{=*j*}, l, ɹ {=*r*}, w, j {=*y*}/.

Vowels

Phoneticians usually recognize three parameters in the description of vowel articulation: height, anteriority, and lip shape. Four main heights are generally noted for vowels and, as the IPA vowel chart shows, these can be termed *close, close-mid, open-mid,* and *open.* These heights refer to how high the highest point of the arched tongue is when making a particular vowel. Three degrees of anteriority are also usually recognized: front, central, and back. Finally, phoneticians normally distinguish rounded lip shape from unrounded (although unrounded may also be divided into spread and neutral shapes). The IPA chart arranges the vowel symbols around a stylized diagram of the vowel area in the oral cavity (i.e., the area in which vowels, as opposed to consonants, are produced). The left-hand symbol of each pair is unrounded, the right-hand one is rounded. The unpaired central vowels are both unrounded, whereas the unpaired vowel at top right is rounded. Diphthongs are vocalic segments where the tongue glides from one position to another during production; they are transcribed with the symbols for the initial and final positions, often with a tie-bar below them as shown on the IPA chart to mark absence of a break.

English Vowel Symbols

The use of vowel symbols is illustrated in Table 7-1, which shows values for American English.

Prosodic features

Speech consists of prosodic or suprasegmental features as well as consonant and vowel segments. These include pitch (intonation, or word tone in tone languages), stress (contrasting stressed and unstressed syllables), length, voice

TABLE 7-1 Symbols for General American English vowels

Long vowels	Open syllable	Closed syllable
i	bee	bead
ɑ	spa	spot
ɔ	paw*	poured
u	do	doom

Short vowels	Open syllable	Closed syllable
ɪ	–	pit
ɛ	–	pet
æ	–	pat
ʌ	–	putt
ʊ	–	put
ə	b<u>a</u>nana, sof<u>a</u>	<u>a</u>ccept, b<u>e</u>lieve

Rhotic vowels	Open syllables	Closed syllables
ɝ	err	word
ɚ	paper	papered

Diphthongs	Open syllable	Closed syllable
eɪ	pay	paid
aɪ	high	hide
ɔɪ	coy	coin
oʊ	low	load
aʊ	bough	bowed

* May also be /ɑ/

quality (derived from both phonation and articulatory settings), loudness, and tempo. All of these can be transcribed and all can be impaired. Symbols to transcribe stress, length, and pitch are given on the IPA chart in the Suprasegmentals section, while tempo and loudness are covered on the extIPA chart, and voice quality on the VoQS chart (Appendix C). Further advice on transcribing intonation contours is given in Ball, Rahilly, and Tench (1996), and Rahilly (2005).

Diacritics

The Diacritics table on the IPA chart (Appendix A) provides the means to add marks to symbols to denote a different sound than the symbol by itself (sometimes this marks just a slight difference, but not always; see the discussion in Ball, 2001). Many of these diacritics have already been described, and several are self-explanatory. Tongue position can be refined with the following diacritics: raised, lowered, advanced/retracted tongue root, advanced, retracted, mid-centralized. Tongue tip (apical) or blade (laminal) use can be marked, and dental or linguolabial (as opposed to alveolar) placement can be shown. The secondary articulations of labialization, palatalization, velarization, and pharyngealized can be transcribed through the use of superscript diacritics. (Secondary articulation involves an approximation of the articulators to the place note simultaneous to the primary articulation; so [sˠ] denotes a slight raising of the back of the tongue toward the velum during the production of the alveolar fricative.) Finally, we can note that nasalization (air flow through the nose as well as through the mouth) is shown by placing a tilde over the relevant symbol, so a nasalized vowel is shown as [ã].

Atypical speech

The extIPA chart (Appendix B) provides symbols for a range of speech sounds encountered in the speech clinic that are not found in natural language, together with the means of transcribing in detail prosodic features

of speech and aspects of voicing. The consonants table includes some novel manners of articulation: *fricative lateral plus median,* where air flows through a central gap between the articulators simultaneously with a lateral gap; *fricative nareal,* where the friction takes place at the nostrils using air forcibly expelled through the nasal cavity; and *percussive,* where sound results from the striking together of two articulators. There are also several novel places of articulation: *dentolabial* (upper lip to lower front teeth); *labioalveolar* (in overbite cases where the lower lip articulates with the alveolar ridge); *interdental* (where the tongue tip protrudes somewhat between the upper and lower dentition); *bidental* (upper and lower teeth together); and *velopharyngeal* (where air is forced through a narrowed velopharyngeal port into the nasal cavity). *Linguolabial* is also included here as a full place of articulation and denotes a tongue tip to upper lip articulation.

Diacritics are available to transcribe lip shape, place of articulation, strength of articulation (useful in dysarthric and stuttered speech for example), reiterated speech (as in stuttering), and different types of nasal airflow or lack thereof. Unexpected airflow direction (such as pulmonic ingressive) can also be marked.

At the base of the extIPA chart is illustrated the means of noting different degrees of uncertainty in clinical transcription, and silent articulation (or *mouthing*). More details on the extIPA chart are given in Ball (2005), Ball and Müller (2005), and Ball, Rahilly, and Tench (1996).

SUMMARY

- Speech production consists of initiation, phonation, and articulation.
- Speech sounds consist of vowels, consonants, and prosodic features.
- SLPs need to be able to transcribe the entire range of speech sounds found in natural language.

- The symbols and diacritics of the IPA allow this range to be transcribed.
- Atypical speech sounds (i.e., sounds not found in natural language) may also be encountered clinically.
- The extIPA and VoQS charts provide symbols for a wide range of segmental and prosodic features found in clinical speech samples.

RESOURCES

Useful Web Sites

- *The International Phonetic Association*
  http://www.arts.gla.ac.uk/ipa/ipa.html
  The homepage of the IPA

- *Voice and Speech Source*
  http://www.yorku.ca/earmstro/ipa/
  Illustrates the symbols of the IPA in sound
- *UCLA Phonetics Lab Data*
  http://phonetics.ucla.edu/
  Links to Web versions of Ladefoged (2000a, b)

REFERENCES

Ball, M. J. (2001). On diacritics. *Journal of the International Phonetic Association, 31,* 259–264.

Ball, M. J. (2005). Transcribing at the segmental level. In N. Müller (Ed.), *Multilayered transcription* (pp. 49–67). San Diego, CA: Plural.

Ball, M. J., Esling, J., and Dickson, C. (1999). Transcription of voice. In R. D. Kent and M. J. Ball (Eds.), *Voice quality measurement* (pp. 49–58). San Diego, CA: Singular.

Ball, M. J., and Müller, N. (2005). *Phonetics for communication disorders.* Mahwah, NJ: Lawrence Erlbaum.

Ball, M. J., and Rahilly, J. (1999). *Phonetics. The science of speech.* London: Edward Arnold.

Ball, M. J., Rahilly, J., and Tench, P. (1996). *The phonetic transcription of disordered speech.* San Diego, CA: Singular.

Bedore, L., Leonard, L., and Gandour, J. (1994). The substitution of a click for sibilants: A case study. *Clinical Linguistics and Phonetics, 8,* 283–293.

Chin, S. (2002). Aspects of stop consonant product by pediatric users of cochlear implants. *Language, Speech, and Hearing Services in Schools, 33,* 38–51.

Heselwood, B. (1997). A case of nasal clicks for target sonorants: A feature geometry account. *Clinical Linguistics and Phonetics, 11,* 43–61.

IPA. (1999). *Handbook of the International Phonetic Association.* Cambridge: Cambridge University Press.

Ladefoged, P. (2000a). *A course in phonetics* (4th ed.). Florence, KY: Heinle.

Ladefoged, P. (2000b). *Vowels and consonants: An introduction to the sounds of languages.* Oxford: Blackwell.

Laver, J. (1994). *Principles of phonetics.* Cambridge: Cambridge University Press.

Rahilly, J. (2005). Transcribing at the suprasegmental level. In N. Müller (Ed.), *Multilayered transcription* (pp. 69–91). San Diego, CA: Plural.

Shahin, K. (2002). Remarks on the speech of Arabic-speaking children with cleft palate. *California Linguistics Notes, 27.* Retrieved September 1, 2005 from http://hss.fullerton.edu/linguistics/cln/sp02/shahin.pdf

Chapter 8

Linguistic Foundations of Speech Production

Joseph Paul Stemberger

INTRODUCTION

Linguistics, as the scientific study of human language, provides many tools and concepts that make up a useful foundation for any research on language and speech, including speech-language pathology and clinical activities. One crucial aspect of linguistics is that it seeks to develop analytic tools and theories that go beyond any one language, to provide a framework that can be applied to any and all human languages. Part of the approach is descriptive, to provide concepts and categories to describe patterns in a way that highlights the similarities and diffeences between patterns in other languages. Part of the approach seeks explanations for why language in general has the characteristics that it does. It is in the nature of theories that they change in response to new discoveries, sometimes radically altering the way that a given phenomenon is viewed. Nonetheless, most fundamental aspects of a linguistic approach have remained unchanged through the years. In this chapter, I briefly review the relationship between linguistics and the study of speech development, distinguishing between descriptive and explanatory aspects. The general expectation is that child phonological systems will be similar to adult phonological systems; anything possible in an adult system might be possible in a child system, and statistical tendencies across children might be similar to statistical tendencies across adult languages.

Basic fundamentals of the description of language

Representations

Features

Distinctive features are designed to capture similarities between different segments that allow for the description of observed patterns. Traditional phonetic categories are too coarse, and they fail to capture phonetic characteristics that turn out to be important for describing phonological patterns. For example, glides and fricatives share the characteristic of continuous airflow through the oral cavity ([+continuant]), and this explains alternations between glides and fricatives in adult phonological systems, and the Gliding of fricatives in child systems (e.g., *zip* /zɪp/ [jɪp]). There are several competing feature systems in linguistics (including one based on gestures), and all do a more-or-less reasonable job of describing adult and child phonological patterns. However, like traditional phonetic labels, the presupposition that all categories are defined universally may obscure some observed patterns in both adult and child phonological systems, and there are phonological patterns that a particular feature system may do a poor job of describing.

Segments

All of the features (or gestures) that occur at the same time are linked together into a *segment*. Segments define the unit of contrast that differentiates one word from another. At one time segments were discrete (e.g., *generative phonology*): all features began and ended in a single segment. Current thinking (e.g., *nonlinear phonology*) allows a feature to last for different amounts of time, for less than one segment or for many segments. Nonetheless, segments define which features may be combined and allow us to describe impossible combinations such as the impossibility of the velar fricative */x/ in adult English (no [+consonantal, +continuant, Dorsal]). Segments allow the group of features to act as a single unit relative to presence (vs. deletion), acquisition, and frequency effects. Because they define categories, they create a tendency toward greater changes than would otherwise be expected (because changing Feature A would result in an impossible segment in the language, Feature B must also change). Thus gliding [+anterior] /z/ results in [-anterior] [j], because there are no [+anterior] glides. While most linguists accept the existence of segments, they are controversial for early child

language (e.g., Studdert-Kennedy and Goodell, 1995) and for adult language (e.g., Browman and Goldstein, 1986).

Suprasegmental levels of structure

Segments are grouped into syllables, syllables into feet, and feet into prosodic words. Syllables are made up of a prominent segment (a vowel in the nucleus, or less commonly a syllabic consonant), usually preceded by a nonprominent segment in an onset (a consonant or, in some languages, two or more consonants). In some languages the prominent segment may be followed by a nonprominent segment in a coda (a consonant or, in some languages, two or more consonants). Feet contain a prominent syllable and may also have one less-prominent syllable; theories disagree as to whether there can be two weak syllables in a single foot. Feet are grouped into prosodic words (about which far less is known).

Inventories

Linguistic theories examine the particular set of possible elements in each language and develop generalizations across languages.

Consonants and vowels

No language allows the full set of segments that are possible for humans to pronounce (e.g., the list of segments in the IPA; see Chapter 7). Although there is a great deal of variability, there are statistical tendencies across languages (e.g., Maddieson, 1984). All languages have oral stops, and almost all have nasal stops; languages tend to have more oral stops than nasal stops. Nasal stops usually are voiced, and few languages allow voiceless nasals, while oral stops are preferentially voiceless, but many languages additionally allow voiced stops. Most languages have fricatives, but fewer fricatives than stops. Languages have few affricates, liquids, or glides; some languages have none. Typologically, English has a fairly average number of consonant contrasts. Vowel systems usually contain a minimum of three vowels (most often [i], [ɑ], [u], but systems with [i], [ɑ], [o] are not uncommon). Additional vowels may be added via distinctions of vowel length, nasalization, vowel height, vowel backness, tenseness (or ATR/RTR), rounding, or diphthongization, or through some combination of the above. Typologically, English has far more than the average number of vowels.

Suprasegmental levels of structure

Some languages do not allow codas; some allow codas after short vowels but not after long vowels or diphthongs.

No language requires codas (though a few require a coda in word-final position). Some languages require onsets in all syllables, while some allow onsetless syllables only in word-initial position. In all languages, the majority of syllable tokens have onsets. Most phonologists assume that all syllables have a nucleus, but it has been argued that some adult languages allow for nucleus-free syllables (Shaw, 1996). In many languages, onsets, nuclei, and codas are restricted to a single segment, but other languages allow complex onsets, codas, and/or diphthongs. Most languages allow a foot with one syllable, but some require two syllables. The prominent syllable may come first (Sw) or second (wS); in some languages, which syllable is prominent is predictable, while in others (including English) it is not fully predictable or not predictable at all. Some languages allow a prosodic word to have only a single foot, but most allow two (or even more) feet in a single word. The combined effects of constraints on the size of syllables, feet, and prosodic words define a minimum and a maximum size for words.

Constraints

When examining inventories of segments and the way that they may be combined into syllables and so on, patterns are apparent. Some combinations of features are absent; some segments are restricted to particular positions in the syllable or word; some segments may not be combined into a sequence at all or used in a particular position (e.g., in an onset). These patterns are usually stated as constraints on what is possible: velar fricatives are not allowed (*/x, ɣ/); labial fricatives must be labiodental; voiced obstruents are impossible in word-final position; if two consonants are in an onset, the first must be an obstruent and the second must be a liquid or glide; the glide-vowel sequence [ji] is impossible; etc. While the five constraints illustrated here are all common in adult languages, there has never been an attempt to catalog all constraints in all languages, or to determine how frequent each constraint is across languages. Constraints limit the range of surface outputs that are possible in a phonological system. They are used to describe the basic segments, syllables, feet, prosodic words, and sequences of segments that are possible in a language.

Alternations

Constraints also are used to explain changes in the pronunciation of a given morpheme. For example, the English plural suffix −s is pronounced [z] after most voiced segments (e.g., *dogs, gloves, heads*), but [s] after voiceless sounds (e.g., *docks, cuffs, cats*) because English (like most languages) does not allow a voiced obstruent to follow a voiceless one at the end of the word (*[kʰætz]). It is pronounced [əz] after /s/ and /z/ because English does not allow sequences of two strident consonants (e.g., [bɹɪdʒəz], not *[bɹɪdʒz]). Since 1980, most theories of phonology have assumed that constraints underlie most alternations, because in most cases alternations eliminate something that never occurs in any output pronunciation in the language. (However, in a small minority of instances, the eliminated sequence does occur elsewhere in the language, and so some theories still allow for more arbitrary alternations.) In the 1980s, *phonological processes/rules* existed as *repair strategies* to eliminate anything that violated a constraint on output; there is a small set of repair strategies that can resolve violations of a particular constraint, and languages develop one or several processes/rules to eliminate the violations (e.g., Paradis, 1988). Currently in *optimality theory*, alternations are handled fully by constraints (e.g., Bernhardt and Stemberger, 1998); there is a trade-off between a constraint on what can be present in the output and a constraint that requires the output to be faithful to the input. Languages differ as to whether output constraints are more (or less) important than faithfulness, and differ on how faithful they are to a particular input characteristic. In any event, all languages in principle must have constraints (since all have limits on what is possible), and there must be either phonological processes/rules or particular constraint rankings that lead to the particular alternations that are observed.

Explanations

Once we have a full set of descriptive tools and descriptions of many languages, linguists often ask *why* the resulting patterns are as they are. In some instances, the explanations are external to the theory. For example, a constraint may make sense because the affected element is difficult to perceive in the relevant environment or because speakers attempt to be intelligible to listeners, but the phonological theory itself does not explain it. In other instances, an explanation is built directly into the theory; this is especially true when the explanation is that a particular characteristic is innate. Explanations are far more variable than descriptions, and vary far more from theory to theory and across time (as theories change). Innateness is a particularly controversial explanation; many approaches rather assume that elements and constraints emerge from more general properties of human cognition, combined with physical properties of the human vocal tract (see Bernhardt and Stemberger, 1998).

Theories of human cognition, including the psychology of language, add additional explanations: perceptual issues; frequency effects (the amount of practice that a speaker gets) on a feature, a segment, a position in the syllable, a sequence of segments, and so forth; the way that different words interfere with or reinforce each other during processing (e.g., neighborhood effects); issues of learning; the role of memory (long-term memory or the phonological loop in short-term memory); and others. Some approaches to phonology attempt to incorporate cognitive explanations and characteristics (e.g., Bernhardt and Stemberger, 1998; Pierrehumbert, 2003).

Descriptive aspects of linguistic theories tend to be more stable across time than explanatory aspects of the theories. Descriptively, linguistic theory lays out what is possible, or in some cases what is possible but quite uncommon across languages; different theoretical explanations can then be brought in to explain the observed facts.

Applying linguistic notions to speech production in children, including in the clinic

The following represents my views about best practice. They are not shared by everyone.

Be careful about explanations

Explanations are far more bound to particular theories than are descriptions. While it is reasonable practice to make use of the explanations in the currently dominant theories in linguistics, it is not necessarily the case that this will always succeed. It is always necessary to evaluate whether the arguments underlying the explanation are valid, either for adult languages in general or for child language in particular. In many instances, explanations may not be compelling.

Consider an observation that X is never observed in any adult human language. Should we expect that X will never be observed for any child? Stemberger (1996) noted that there are at least four distinct explanations for a gap in adult languages. (1) It is impossible in a grammar, for grammar-internal reasons (including, but not limited to, innateness). It should thus not occur in the speech of any child. (2) It is impossible for performance reasons (concerning speech production, perception, or memory). It should thus not occur in the speech of any child. (3) It is simply

a pattern that cannot be learned (due to characteristics of human learning in general, or of learning grammars in particular), because of difficulty going from observed data to the learning of the appropriate constraint or rule. It will be absent from child language only insofar as the child's output patterns arise from inferring constraints/rules on the basis of patterns in the input. (4) It is impossible for diachronic reasons; given characteristics of sound change over time, but there is just no historical source that could lead to a pattern. Insofar as child language shares the same limitations as historical change, the pattern will be impossible in child language. But if a child's output is not limited in the same way as historical change and does not result from inferring analyses of patterns in the input, then characteristic X may be present in child language. Stemberger (1996) discusses a number of phenomena that have been observed only in child phonology (including Consonant Harmony involving [Labial] and [Dorsal]), and argues that these phenomena may be fully possible in grammar and performance for adults, but are absent in adult speech because of limitations on learning or diachronic change. He also argues that child phonology gives a better view of what is possible in phonological systems than adult phonology does, in some instances. Insofar as explanations are built into the descriptive apparatus, this also means that the descriptive tools of linguistics can run into difficulty when applied to child speech production.

It is also important to be leery of explanations that lead to a prediction that all children should be identical. This includes any explanation of the form: "X should develop later than Y because it is more marked, or less salient, or lower in frequency, or more difficult to perceive, or more complex to produce"; or "X should tend to be pronounced Y because of markedness/frequency/similarity/etc." If taken too literally, the explanation does not account for the range of variability in typically developing children. For example, the lateral [l] may appear at 1;4 before any fricatives are produced, or at 4;6 long after the child has mastered most fricatives, or at any time in between. The extreme variability of developmental pathways in speech production is the primary fact of development that must be accounted for. Explanations originating from linguistics and psychology must play a softer role, at best constituting a pressure in a certain direction that leads to statistical probabilities across children, and not to absolutes.

Last, some explanations may not be relevant to children. Some phenomena in adult language are explained as the result of the speaker taking into account what would be most intelligible for the listener. It is unclear whether children know what is most helpful to the listener or take that into account when producing words. For example, in most dialects of English, the rounding of vowels is not very important, because there are no unrounded counterparts; adult speakers routinely reduce rounding to almost nothing when smiling, with no effects on intelligibility. Yet most children develop rounding early. Occasional children who have no rounded vowels shift labiality off the vowel in ways that impact negatively on intelligibility, such as into the onset in *book* /bʊk/ [bwət] or into the coda in *no* /noː/ [nɤːm]. Indeed, sensitivity to intelligibility would exclude many substitutions and processes that have been observed in child language, and lead to a far lower level of between-child variability than observed.

What the descriptive tools lead to

Features

Features define natural classes and should help make sense of patterns, such as the sets of elements in inventories and the types of substitutions that occur. For example, we expect that nasal and oral stops will share patterns ([-continuant]), and that /f, v, w/ will share patterns ([+continuant, Labial]). We do not expect just fricatives and nasals to share patterns, unless oral stops are also included, because no single set of features can include nasals and fricatives without also including oral stops. Standard feature sets make the right predictions across children statistically, but Bernhardt and Stemberger (1998) note the occasional occurrence of patterns in child language that suggest a different feature system. It is interesting that features describing articulation (rather than acoustics) fare quite well with child data, in general. In addition, we expect that the appearance of a feature or feature combination in one segment (e.g., velar place of articulation in /k/, or nasality in /n/ in codas) may generalize to other segments that contain those features, since features and segments are independent levels in phonological representations.

Segments

Segments allow groups of simultaneously occurring features to act as a group, as well as define the possible output categories in the child's speech. (1) There should be frequency effects, such that the more practiced higher-frequency segments should appear earlier than low-frequency segments *controlling for all other variables*. Pye, Ingram, and List (1987) and Ingram (1988) examined the same segments across languages (thus controlling for phonetic difficulty) and show that this is the case. (2) Since segments that are absent from the adult language have zero frequency in the input, and the child does not try to

learn them, such segments should be (and are) uncommon in child language. (3) Segments define a small number of output states that will tend to attract all impossible segments. Thus, if fricatives are impossible and undergo gliding, /s/ will become [j], with a radically different place of articulation and voicing, because there is no voiceless anterior coronal glide in the child's (or in the adult's) phonological system. (4) If a child has not mastered a particular feature, the child may delete the entire segment rather than partially match it, as with the deletion of coda /d/ even though [t] is in the system (e.g., *bed* /bɛd/ [ba] rather than [bat]), or the replacement of initial /l/ with default [ʔ] even though [d] is in the system (e.g., *lie* /laɪ/ [ʔaɪ] rather than [daɪ]). These and other effects are not predicted by systems in which there are no segments.

Higher-level structure

We expect to see effects of markedness, frequency, and complexity relative to higher structure. Extra feet and syllables may be deleted, depending on word-level and foot-level constraints on complexity and on which foot or syllable is prominent. Extra segments may be deleted, coalesced into a single segment, or shifted to a different position in the syllable or word, if constraints prevent them from being realized in their target position (because no codas or complex onsets are allowed). Since many languages prohibit codas after long vowels and diphthongs, as well as in unstressed syllables, we expect such effects to appear for some children (as they in fact do); for example, coda consonants are deleted only after diphthongs, or only in unstressed syllables, and are possible elsewhere.

Constraints and "alternations"

We expect to see the same sorts of constraints in child language that we see in adult language, along with the same sorts of changes to a target segment (deletion in similar environments, or substitution to similar output segments). In particular, we expect the child to be as faithful as possible to the features of a target segment, while avoiding violation of a constraint that prevents faithful output. Thus, if [p] is a possible output, we expect that /f/ will be changed to [p] rather than to [t] (which is indeed statistically the case). We expect to see phenomena from the phonology (and morphology) of different languages arise spontaneously in the speech of English-learning children, as indeed we do, though any given phenomenon may be rare across children. Last, we expect to see children at a comparable level of development resembling each other more closely in terms of what the constraints are (e.g., no fricatives) than in terms of how they resolve those constraints (Stopping, Gliding,

Deletion, etc.), because different resolutions involve being faithful to different aspects of the target, and the theory says that systems are expected to differ along that dimension.

Practical considerations

When constructing materials for clinical use, including assessment tools, it is important to take into account characteristics of different items. If Item A would quite possibly be subject to several constraints (e.g., Labial Harmony in *thumb*) that would not be relevant to Item B (e.g., *thing*, which lacks a labial consonant), it is important to keep that in mind when interpreting the child's pronunciation. When working on establishing a new segment in the child's system, it is important to avoid words that would be subject to other constraints in the child's system that would delay production of the segment for entirely independent reasons.

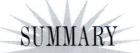

SUMMARY

- Descriptive tools developed for adult languages have proven to be very useful, at least statistically, for analyzing child phonological development, including features, segments, higher-level structure, and constraints.
- Explanations developed for adult languages may be useful, and should be investigated, but they are more theory dependent, change more radically over time, are less reliable tools for dealing with child phonology, and often seem to underestimate the degree to which children differ from each other.
- Structuring materials to reflect the representations, constraints, and even common phenomena of adult human languages is good practice.

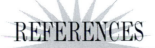

REFERENCES

Bernhardt, B. H., and Stemberger, J. P. (1998). *Handbook of phonological development: From the perspective of constraint-based nonlinear phonology*. San Diego, CA: Academic Press.

Browman, C. P., and Goldstein, L. M. (1986). Towards an articulatory phonology. *Phonology Yearbook, 3*, 219–252.

Ingram, D. (1988). The acquisition of word-initial [v]. *Language and Speech, 31*, 77–85.

Maddieson, I. (1984). *Patterns of sounds*. Cambridge, UK: Cambridge University Press.

Paradis, C. (1988). On constraints and repair strategies. *Linguistic Review, 6*, 71–97.

Pierrehumbert, J. (2003). Probabilistic phonology: Discrimination and robustness. In R. Bod, J. Hay, and S. Jannedy (Eds.), *Probabilistic linguistics* (pp. 177–228). Cambridge, MA: MIT Press.

Pye, C., Ingram, D., and List, H. (1987). A comparison of initial consonant acquisition in English and Quiché. In K. E. Nelson and A. van Kleeck (Eds.), *Children's language* (Vol. 6, pp. 175–190). Hillsdale, NJ: Lawrence Erlbaum.

Shaw, P. A. (1996, January). *Headless and weightless syllables in Salish*. Paper presented at the University of Victoria.

Stemberger, J. P. (1996). The scope of the theory: Where does beyond lie? In L. McNair, K. Singer, L. M. Dobrin, and M. M. Aucoin (Eds.), *Papers from the parasession on theory and data in linguistics, CLS 23* (pp. 139–164). Chicago: Chicago Linguistic Society.

Studdert-Kennedy, M. and Goodell, E. W. (1995). Gestures, features and segments in early child speech. In B. de Gelder and J. Morais (Eds.), *Speech and reading* (pp. 65–88). Hove, UK: Erlbaum, Taylor & Francis.

Chapter 9

Applications of Typical Acquisition Information to Understanding of Speech Impairment

Barbara L. Davis

INTRODUCTION

Knowledge of the typical course of speech and language acquisition constitutes a powerful clinical tool. It provides one essential background for decision making in evaluation and treatment of children diagnosed with speech delay or disorder. Use of typical acquisition information in clinical decision making relies on a *discrepancy model*. The relevant discrepancy is between expected speech and language behaviors at the child's *chronological age* and behaviors observed in clinical evaluation, labeled as the child's *acquisition age* capacities. If behaviors observed during evaluation are not those expected for the child's chronological age, the speech-language pathologist (SLP) determines that a *chronological-acquisition mismatch* is present. Based on this determination regarding core sound system properties, the SLP can decide whether intervention is warranted. This decision is based on a complex of issues including etiology, family expectations, and child motivation (see Chapter 1; Threats and Worrall, 2004, for reviews within the World Health Organization framework).

Considerations in applying typical acquisition information to speech impairment

Chronological-acquisition mismatch

Understanding of speech behaviors expected at a child's chronological age is based on knowledge of typical speech acquisition milestones. Some aspects of typical acquisition may be evaluated relative to comparison with age norms on standardized tests if they are available for the child's native language, for example the *Goldman-Fristoe Test of Articulation-2* for English (Goldman and Fristoe, 2000). If a spontaneous sampling procedure is employed during evaluation, SLP knowledge of typical acquisition milestones at various chronological ages is critical. (See McLeod and Bleile, 2003, for a compilation of normative information on typical speech acquisition for English-speaking children.) In considering chronological-acquisition mismatch, the issue of variability in speech patterns should also be considered (see Chapter 10, for a review of this issue). Until 36 months, variability between children and within the same child in speech production patterns may complicate determining a mismatch between chronological age and acquisition age; after 36 months children are less variable. However, Stoel-Gammon also notes that "in spite of the presence of individual differences, there is clear evidence of common tendencies in patterns of speech acquisition" (see Chapter 10).

The SLP determines a child's acquisition age based on standardized testing and observations of spontaneous communicative behaviors. Acquisition age is determined by comparing the speech behaviors the child exhibits with typical acquisition milestones for his or her chronological age. For example, open CV syllables (e.g., [ba] for [bal]) are expected at 12–18 months chronological age based on studies of young children in this age range across languages as varied as Korean and Equadorean-Quichua (e.g., Gildersleeve-Neumann, 2001; Lee, 2003). When observed in a 6-year-old child, they can indicate a mismatch between chronological age expectations and child acquisition level. The child exhibits an acquisition age of 12–18 months. This chronological-acquisition mismatch forms an important basis for decision making in assessment, choices of goals and targets, and ongoing evaluation of progress.

As SLPs increasingly assess and treat children from varying linguistic backgrounds, knowledge of typical acquisition must expand beyond descriptions of acquisition milestones predominantly derived from studies of English (Davis, 2005). Languages exhibit distinct rules for consonant and vowel phonemes in different word positions, complexity of word and syllable shapes, and prosody (see Maddieson, 1984, for an overview). Spanish has five vowels; Swedish has 22 phonemes. Putonghua and Cantonese are Chinese tone languages; English does not employ tone to contrast word meanings. These divergences occur across the 5,000 or so contemporary spoken languages in varied dimensions of phonology. All dimensions of ambient language phonology must be mastered by children to achieve age-appropriate intelligibility during the preschool and early school age years (e.g., Coplan and Gleason, 1988).

An important challenge to ethical clinical practices is the SLP's ability to use typical speech acquisition milestones using normative data from each child's ambient language. Clearly, ongoing programs of research are needed in a variety of languages to detail the typical course of phonological acquisition. These data are needed to support assessment and intervention with children learning diverse languages. As normative data on diverse phonologies emerge and are included in volumes such as this, information can be employed clinically. Understanding each child's unique language targets will help to avoid making clinical decisions about children from other languages using comparison norms for children learning English.

Delay or disorder

One aspect of clinical assessment is determination of whether a child's speech profile indicates *delay* or *disorder*. Assessment of delay or disorder in the clinical profile of a child impacts selection of intervention goals and targets. This distinction may also impact SLP decisions about prognosis for normalization of speech patterns to expectations for the child's chronological age. Decisions about delay or disorder are founded in part on SLP knowledge of the typical course of speech acquisition in the child's ambient language.

Speech *delay* describes a child who is producing speech or vocalizations expected in a developmentally younger child. An 8-year-old English-speaking child who is producing only /b/ and /d/ in open monosyllabic words, typical behaviors in 8- to 15-month-old children, would provide an example of severe delay in speech acquisition. Children may also present with disordered speech patterns. Speech *disorder* is indicated when a child produces patterns that are not observed during the course of typical speech acquisition. A 5-year-old English-speaking child who produces sequences of glottal closures with /a/ vowels would be diagnosed as having speech disorder based on the expectation that glottal-vowel syllables are not observed in the typical acquisition sequence in English. Related to the issue of variability raised above, it should be noted that the same behavior may simultaneously exhibit patterns indicative of speech delay and patterns of disorder. Typically, developing children are producing rhythmic syllables with oral articulatory labial and alveolar closures by 7–8 months (see Oller, 1980; Vihman, 1996, for reviews). A recent cross-linguistic longitudinal study of 20 Tunisian

Arabic, French, Romanian, Dutch, and Turkish infants (four per language) showed remarkable similarities during the canonical babbling period. The children's speech patterns showed virtually no evidence of ambient language patterns; they produced very similar speech patterns across these diverse languages (Kern and Davis, in press).

Severity level

Assessing the *severity level* of a child's speech delay or disorder is another aspect of clinical practice requiring SLP understanding of typical acquisition milestones (Davis and Bedore, 2003; Shriberg and Kwiatkowski, 1982). Judgments of severity may impact the choice of which children are provided intervention services across intervention settings. Severity level may also be related to length and frequency of intervention in various clinical settings. Determinations of prognosis for improvement to the age-appropriate speech pattern also interface with determination of severity level.

Severity adjectives may help the SLP to communicate effectively with parents to aid in their understanding of the nature of the child's speech impairment. Helping parents to understand that their 4 year old is speaking like an 18-month-old can help to communicate how much difference exists between the child's functional behavior and chronological age expectations. This description is based on comparisons with typical acquisition milestones. Parents often have general knowledge of expected milestones for typical acquisition based on experiences with siblings as well as their child's peers. As a result, communication with parents based on describing a child's acquisition age can support understanding of the severity of speech delay or disorder.

Descriptive terms frequently employed by SLPs, based on results of tests and observations related to core speech behavioral expressions, include *mild, moderate,* and *severe*. These terms are descriptive of the chronological-acquisition mismatch between the functional speech production patterns observed and chronologically based expectations for the child's age. For core speech symptoms, these descriptors are based on evaluation of consonant and vowel phonemes by word position, word and syllable complexity, prosody, and age appropriateness of intelligibility.

Based on studies mainly conducted on children learning English, in a 5-year-old child with *mild* speech impairment, for example, phonetic inventory and phoneme accuracy is incomplete relative to chronological expectations. Most consonant and vowel phonemes as well as word and syllable shapes are produced correctly. Errors are likely distortions (e.g., /ɹ/ distortion) or substitutions (e.g., d/s) considered slightly immature for the child's chronological age. Prosody and vowels are not usually impaired. Intelligibility might be close to 100 percent. However, the child's speech calls attention to itself in spontaneously produced utterances. Typical acquisition comparison level is with children 3;6 to 4;6 years old.

Another 5-year-old with *moderate* delay shows a much less complete phonetic inventory of consonants and syllable/word shapes (i.e., dorsals could be missing or final consonants deleted). Vowel inventory is complete. Even if the child's inventory of consonants, vowels, and syllable/word shapes is complete, it may not be used accurately. Intelligibility is reduced by inconsistent accuracy for the complexity of word targets attempted (i.e., cluster reduction or final consonant deletion). Prosodic aspects of speech production are possibly mildly impaired, reducing intelligibility. This moderately impaired child also shows some atypical patterns indicative of speech disorder. Typical acquisition comparison level is to a typically developing 20- to 30-month-old child using many phonemes of the ambient language (even if complexity of individual words is reduced) and beginning to achieve intelligible speech with most listeners.

The 5-year-old with *severe* delay or disorder demonstrates an incomplete phonetic inventory of consonants, vowels, and syllable/word shapes (i.e., only front vowels and labial consonants as singletons or a few open CV syllables). Accuracy using the available production inventory is poor. Prosody is more likely to be impaired as well. Intelligibility is severely compromised in all communicative contexts. This child probably uses communicative gestures and eye contact to supplement oral communication. Disordered or atypical patterns also occur with more frequency. Typical acquisition comparison behaviors are with the *prespeech* period, consistent with vocal acquisition between 8 and 14 months. This is roughly the period from the onset of speechlike and syllable-based vocalization of canonical babbling until the appearance of the first meaningful words.

Intervention

Continuing analysis of the chronological-acquisition mismatch for core speech-phonological behaviors also enables an ongoing interaction between assessment and intervention. Using available standardized instruments as well as clinical observations of spontaneous communication behaviors, the SLP can compare the child's progress at consistent intervals to the expected acquisition behaviors for his or her chronological age. Changes in speech patterns toward chronological age expectations can serve as one continuing metric of progress in aspects of intervention focused on the core speech sound disorder or delay. This ongoing assessment-intervention interaction is a necessary aspect of establishing the need for continuation of intervention. In addition, periodic assessment of the child's progress relative to the chronological-acquisition mismatch can support the SLP's communication with parents regarding the child's progress in intervention.

SLP selection of goals and targets for intervention is also based partly on knowledge of typical acquisition milestones. Knowledge and use of typical acquisition milestones provides one metric in planning and conducting intervention at the child's present level of function. As an example, knowledge of prelinguistic acquisition milestones allows the SLP to consider earliest behaviors in the typical acquisition sequence in intervention with young clients or those with severe to profound levels of speech delay or disorder. While not based on large normative databases, these milestones have a history in studies of English-learning children (e.g., Davis and MacNeilage, 1995; Mitchell and Kent, 1990; Oller, 1980; Vihman, 1996) and are beginning to be based on a growing body of research on children in other language environments (Kern and Davis, in press).

Typical acquisition behaviors characteristic of the early word period provide another example of the use of typical acquisition milestones in conducting clinical intervention. Sounds include stops, nasals, and glides at labial and alveolar places of articulation and vowels mostly in the lower left quadrant. CV and CVCV word shapes predominate, followed by CVCs, and often at very low frequencies in English (Davis, MacNeilage, and Matyear, 2002) and across languages studied to date (e.g., Gildersleeve-Neumann, 2001). Words are mostly monosyllables in English. Studies of languages in which multisyllables predominate show early use of di- and multisyllables. Reduplication (e.g., [baba]) is most frequent, followed by variegation (e.g., [dædi] or [bada]) (Mitchell and Kent, 1990). When syllables are variegated, consonant manner and vowel height changes predominate, related to lack of independence of articulators from the jaw cycle in earliest vocal sequences in this period (Davis et al., 2002). Children may also utilize idiosyncratic "word recipes," that is, a few restricted ways to fit word targets into favored template(s) (Vihman, 1993). In English, prosodic regularities include first-syllable stress and falling intonation (Pollock, Brammer, and Hageman, 1993; Snow and Stoel-Gammon, 1994). Children learning other languages may show differences related to ambient language in this profile (e.g., Lee, 2003; Teixeira and Davis, 2003). Expressive jargon, intonation contours that are language-like without meaning attached, may be used. Prosodic "sentences" may also occur (e.g., "All gone.").

The discrepancy model, based on comparisons with milestones for typical acquisition in a child's ambient language, represents one perspective on clinical service provision. Multiple approaches to understanding the nature of early developmental speech disorders are in current use in assessment and treatment (see Baker, 2006, for an overview of contemporary approaches). In particular, core vocabulary approaches (e. g., Dodd and Bradford, 2000) and maximal oppositions contrast (Gierut, 2001) present two alternatives that rely far less onchronological-acquisition mismatch. Clinicians will need to continue to stay abreast of this emerging literature to make valid assessment and treatment choices for each individual child's needs. A discrepancy model construct provides one avenue for planning.

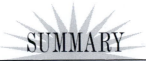

SUMMARY

- Comparisons with milestones for typical acquisition in a child's ambient language represent one aspect of decision making for intervention goals and targets.
- SLP understanding of typical speech acquisition contributes to assessment of delay versus disorder and assignment of severity level, and supports prognostic expectations for clinical outcomes.

- Knowledge of typical speech acquisition milestones also enables ongoing assessment of client improvement during the process of intervention as well as supporting communication with parents about their child's progress.

REFERENCES

Baker, E. (2006). Management of speech impairment in children: The journey so far and the road ahead. *Advances in Speech-Language Pathology, 8*(3), 156–163.

Coplan, J., and Gleason, J. (1988). Unclear speech: Recognition and significance of unintelligible speech in preschool children. *Pediatrics, 82,* 447–452.

Davis, B. L. (2005). Clinical diagnosis of developmental speech disorders. In A.G. Kamhi and K. E. Pollock (Eds.), *Phonological disorders in children: Assessment and intervention* (pp. 3–23). Baltimore, MD: Paul H. Brooks.

Davis, B. L., and Bedore, L. (2003). *Speech disorders clinical archive.* Unpublished multimedia CD-Rom, The University of Texas at Austin, Austin, TX.

Davis, B. L., and MacNeilage, P. F. (1995). The articulatory basis of babbling. *Journal of Speech and Hearing Research, 38,* 1199–1211.

Davis, B. L., MacNeilage, P. F., and Matyear, C. L. (2002). Acquisition of serial complexity in speech production: A comparison of phonetic and phonological approaches to first word production. *Phonetica, 59,* 75–107.

Dodd, B., and Bradford, A. (2000). A comparison of three therapy methods for children with different types of developmental phonological disorder. *International Journal of Language and Communication Disorders, 35,* 189–209.

Gierut, J. A. (2001). Complexity in phonological treatment: Clinical factors. *Language, Speech, and Hearing Services in Schools, 32,* 229–241.

Gildersleeve-Neumann, C. (2001). *Constraints on infant speech production: A cross-linguistic perspective,* Unpublished doctoral dissertation, The University of Texas at Austin, Austin, TX.

Goldman, R., and Fristoe, M. (2000). *Goldman-Fristoe test of articulation-2.* Circle Pines, MN: American Guidance Service.

Kern, S., and Davis, B.L. (in press). *Emergent complexity in early vocal acquisition: Cross-linguistic comparisons of canonical babbling. In* I. Chirotan, C. Coupé, E. Marsico, and F. Pellegrino (Eds), Approaches to phonological complexity. Berlin: Mouton de Gruyter.

Lee, S. (2003). *The phonetic basis of early speech acquisition in Korean.* Unpublished doctoral dissertation, The University of Texas at Austin, Austin, TX.

Maddieson, I. (1984). *Patterns of sounds.* Cambridge, UK: Cambridge University Press.

McLeod, S., and Bleile, K. (2003, November). *Neurological and developmental foundations of speech acquisition* (Invited seminar). Paper presented at the American Speech-Language-Hearing Association Convention, Chicago.

McLeod, S. and Bleile, K. (2004). The ICF: A proposed framework for setting goals for children with speech impairment. *Child Language Teaching and Therapy, 20*(3), 199–219.

Mitchell, P., and Kent, R. (1990). Phonetic variation in multisyllabic babbling. *Journal of Child Language, 17,* 247–265.

Oller, D. K. (1980). The emergence of the sounds of speech in infancy. In G.Yeni-Komshian, J. F. Kavanagh, & C. A. Ferguson (Eds.), *Child phonology, Vol.1: Production* (pp. 93–112). New York: Academic Press.

Pollock, K., Brammer, D. M., and Hageman, C. F. (1993). An acoustic analysis of young children's productions of word stress. *Journal of Phonetics, 21,* 183–203.

Shriberg, L. D., and Kwiatkowski, J. (1982). Phonological disorders III: A procedure for assessing severity of involvement. *Journal of Speech and Hearing Disorders, 47*(3), 256–270.

Snow, D., and Stoel-Gammon, C. (1994). Phrase final lengthening and intonation in early child speech. *Journal of Speech and Hearing Research, 37,* 831–840.

Threats, T. T., and Worrall, L. (2004) Classifying communication disability using the ICF. *Advances in Speech-Language Pathology, 6*(1), 53–62.

Teixeira, E. R., and Davis, B. L. (2003). Early sound patterns in the speech of two Brazilian Portuguese speakers. *Language & Speech, 45*(2), 179–204.

Vihman, M. M. (1993). Variable paths to early word production. *Journal of Phonetics, 21,* 61–82.

Vihman, M. M. (1996). *Phonological acquisition: The origins of language in the child.* Cambridge, MA: Blackwell.

Chapter 10

Variability in Speech Acquisition

Carol Stoel-Gammon

INTRODUCTION

Although the term *variability* often appears in studies of phonological development and disorders, authors are often unclear as to what they are discussing when using this term. Two basic types of variability have been described: variability *between* children, often referred to as "individual differences," and variability *within* the speech patterns of a particular child, usually referring to instances in which words or phonemes are produced differently.

Types of variability

Variability between children

There is a good deal of interchild variability in the early period of speech acquisition, particularly in the transition from babble to words (e.g., Stoel-Gammon and Cooper, 1984; Vihman, Ferguson, and Elbert, 1986) and in word productions of children with vocabularies of 50–100 words (e.g., Ferguson and Farwell, 1975; Vihman, 1993; Vihman and Greenlee, 1987). During this period, typically developing children will differ considerably in the size of their phonetic inventory (i.e., number of different consonants and vowels they can produce), in the accuracy of their productions and in the types of errors that occur, and in levels of intelligibility. The bases for individual differences in acquisition are not known, although investigations of genetic and environmental influences (e.g., differences in input) on speech and language development in children indicate that both factors play a role (Kent and Bauer, 1985; Kovas et al., 2005; Locke, 1989).

In spite of the presence of individual differences, there is clear evidence of common tendencies in patterns of speech acquisition. For example, it is well documented that, regardless of the language community in which a child is raised, prelinguistic vocalizations and early word productions include a greater proportion of consonant-vowel (CV) syllables than CVC syllables and that stop, nasal, and glide consonants occur more frequently than other manner classes (e.g., fricative, liquid). In American English, for example, guidelines for the expected ages of emergence and mastery of phonemes and syllable structures have been established. In the field of communication disorders, it is essential to document patterns of typical development and to determine the range of development that is considered typical. Without this information it is not possible to identify children who fall outside that range. Thus, normative studies of large groups of children serve as the basis for the clinical assessment of speech development.

Variability within a child

Variability of word productions is a hallmark of early child speech. In an oft-cited example from Ferguson and Farwell (1975), a 15-month-old girl produced the word *pen* in 10 different ways within a 30-minute period. Variations occurred in syllable shape, in segments produced, and in the order of segments within productions. None of the productions was accurate, yet each included one or more features of the target form, for example, a nasal consonant, a CVC sequence, a bilabial stop. While this example may be somewhat extreme, variability is clearly a common feature of children's early word productions. As children grow older, their word productions become more consistent; the productions may not be entirely correct, but they are pronounced in the same way each time.

There are at several types of variability in the productions of typically developing children, each with it own characteristics. One common type of variability is based on the position of the phoneme in the word; for example, /b/ may be produced accurately in the word *ball* (word initial) but as a [p] in the word *tub* (word final), or /v/ may be produced as [b] in the word *very* but as [f] in *give*. In both examples, the variable pronunciations are associated with positional differences of the phoneme, specifically word-initial vs. word-final position.

Another type of variability in young children's speech is variable use of a phoneme across lexical targets; thus initial /m/ may be correct in *mommy* but not in *milk*. Variability of this sort cannot be attributed to word position, but it may be affected by phonetic context, most commonly the following vowel. It is common for

initial /k/ to be "fronted" to [t] when /k/ precedes a front vowel, but as [k] preceding back vowels; this means [t] will occur more frequently in words like *key* or *cape* than in *cook* or *call*. A third type of variability is found in multiple productions of the same word as with the child described above (Ferguson and Farwell, 1975), who produced 10 different forms of the word *pen* within a single data collection session. In this case, variability of a particular phoneme is not due to the position of the phoneme within the word or to phonetic context. Given that normal phonological development entails moving from simple, relatively undifferentiated forms (e.g., [da] for *doggie*; [babu] for *bottle*) to adultlike pronunciations, the occurrence of variable productions in early speech is part of the developmental process.

Measuring variability

Two basic types of measures have been used to describe variability in word productions: those that focus on variability of a target phoneme across words (interword variability) and those that focus on variability within multiple productions of the same word (whole-word variability). An example of an interword measure comes from Tyler and colleagues (Tyler and Lewis, 2005; Tyler, Lewis, and Welch, 2003) who analyzed target phonemes to create an "error consistency index." This measure is based on the total number of different sound substitutions/omissions across words produced by a child. To compute the error consistency index (ECI), the total number of substitutions/omissions (i.e., phoneme errors) for each phoneme is summed across all 23 consonantal phonemes of English. If a child makes few errors, the ECI is 0; conversely, a large number of different substitutions across a large number of phoneme targets would yield a high ECI.

Several researchers (Betz and Stoel-Gammon, 2005; Ingram, 2002; Marquardt, Jacks, and Davis, 2004; Shriberg, Aram, and Kwiatkowski, 1997; Stoel-Gammon, 2004; Vogel Sosa and Stoel-Gammon, 2006) have proposed measures of whole-word variability. At the word level, these measures are based on a ratio of the number of phonetic forms of a word (numerator) and the number of productions of that word (denominator). The ratio is then multiplied by 100 to provide the percentage of variability for each word; variability may range from 0 to 100 percent.

An alternative measure, referred to as the "variability ratio," is obtained by dividing the number of different phonetic forms (types) in a sample by the number of different words (types) in the sample (Schwartz, Leonard, Folger, and Wilcox, 1980). For example, if a child produces 60 different words during a recording session and uses 60 different phonetic forms for those words, the *ratio* would be 1.0, indicating no variability. If another child uses 120 different phonetic forms for production of 60 words, the ratio is 2.0 (120/60). In this case, on average, each word had two different pronunciations; it should be noted that this is an *average* and that individual words may be entirely consistent or much more variable.

Finally, Dodd (1995) developed a measure of "whole-word inconsistency" with the goal of designing a set of procedures that would allow her to categorize different types of speech disorders. The measure was based on three productions of a set of 25 words; if a word was produced differently on two of the three trials, the word was said to be variable. Children who exhibited variable production on 10 of the 25 words (a 40 percent level of variability) were classified as exhibiting an inconsistent disorder.

Variability in child speech: Summary of research findings

Variability in children with typically developing speech

This section provides a brief summary of the findings regarding variability in productions of English-speaking children with typically developing speech.

Ages 12–24 months

Regardless of the measure used, studies show that productions of children 12–24 months are quite variable. Vogel Sosa and Stoel-Gammon (2006) analyzed productions of four children followed longitudinally from 12 to 24 months. Percentage of overall intraword variability was calculated for each child at 12, 15, 18, 21, and 24 months based on changes in consonants only; findings revealed high rates of variability (17–59 percent) with a peak corresponding to the onset of combinatorial speech. Schwartz and colleagues (1980), using a slightly different measure, also showed high rates of variability in three children aged 19–21 months; the variability ratio (number of different phonetic forms divided by number of different words in the sample) ranged from 1.23 to 1.65.

Ages 21–33 months

In a longitudinal study of five children producing multiple exemplars of a small set of CVC words, Stoel-Gammon (2004) reported mean variability rates (based on analysis of consonants and vowels) of 60 percent at 21 months, 40 percent at 24 months, 34 percent at 27 months, 42 percent at 30 months, declining to 19 percent at 33 months. During this period, average rates of accurate production for the target words increased from 7 percent at 21 months to 59 percent at 33 months. Thus, even relatively simple CVC words exhibit high rates of variability until 30–33 months. These findings need to be considered in efforts to use variability as an indicator of phonological and/or articulation disorder; however, caution should be applied due to the small numbers of children studied.

Variability in children with speech impairment

Extensive variability may be associated with speech impairment and has been identified as one of the key diagnostic markers of a particular type of disorder: childhood apraxia of speech (Davis, Jakielski, and Marquardt, 1998; Dodd, 1995; Forrest, 2003; Shriberg et al., 1997). Understanding the relationship between variability and speech disorders is important for both assessment and treatment of children with speech impairment.

To date, findings regarding variability and childhood apraxia of speech are ambiguous. Shriberg and colleagues (1997) compared variability in connected speech in children with "suspected" childhood apraxia of speech (CAS) and children with other types of speech disorders and did not find differences between the two groups. Betz and Stoel-Gammon (2005) found high rates of variability in children with severe phonological disorders, not just children with CAS. In a longitudinal study of three children with CAS, Marquardt et al. (2004) reported whole-word variability of 20–60 percent across three age periods. Only one of the children exhibited a consistent decrease in variability with age. Other researchers have noted extensive variability in children with speech disorders but have not reported measures allowing for quantification of this phenomenon.

Variability has also been identified as a possible prognostic marker in children with speech impairment. Tyler et al. (2003; see also Tyler and Lewis, 2005) applied the "error consistency index" (ECI), which is described above, in analyzing speech productions of young children with speech and language disorders. The authors reported that a child's index was a major predictor of phonological change in percentage of consonants correct (PCC) over a 24-week period of intervention, accounting for 31 percent of the variance in PCC. The relationship between the ECI and phonological change was unexpected: children with higher ECI scores (i.e., higher levels of variability) exhibited greater change in PCC than children with lower ECI scores.

Forrest, Elbert, and Dinnsen (2000; see also Forrest, Dinnsen, and Elbert, 1997) found a different association between variability and phonological change. Specifically, children with consistent substitutions for a particular target (e.g., target /k/ is always produced at [t]) acquired the target sound in treatment and generalized the newly acquired sound to other word positions; in contrast, the children with inconsistent substitutions within and across word positions learned the treated sound in the treated position but did not generalize the new production to other word positions. The differences between these two studies are due, at least in part, to different measures, different types of phonological intervention, and different groups of participants. It is clear that further research is needed to determine the relationships between variability and phonological change in children with speech impairment.

Causes of variability

Children with typical development

Explanations for inconsistent productions in children with typical speech and language development tend to fall into two general categories. *Psycholinguistic* explanations attribute variability to incomplete (or underspecified) underlying representations, or to instability of phonological rules that apply to underlying representations to produce the output. *Motor-based* explanations posit that variability stems from immature neuromotor skills that prevent a child from producing a stable form of a target word. In support of this view, it is well documented that young children exhibit variability in many different aspects of motor control, and motor development is characterized as a process of increasing accuracy and decreasing variability (Kent, 1992; Smith and Goffman, 1998).

Specific phonetic features of the target word may also influence phonological variability. For example, it is likely that words with features that are more difficult for a child to pronounce (e.g., certain phonemes; syllable shapes; stress patterns) will exhibit higher levels of variability than words with "easier" phonetic patterns. In this case, variability can be viewed as a trade-off between accuracy of one aspect of a word at the expense of another (Leonard, Rowan, Morris, and Fey, 1982).

Children with speech impairment

It is likely that there are multiple causes of variability in word and phoneme productions of children with speech impairment, and different types of variability may be associated with different types of impairment. Again, most explanations are associated with one of two basic causes: psycholinguistic or motor. Forrest and colleagues (1997) state that positionally based substitutions for a target consonant indicate lack of categorical representation (psycholinguistic cause) of the phoneme. Dodd (1995) also interprets variability as having a psycholinguistic basis, arguing that it stems from a deficit in "phonological planning" (i.e., an incomplete or degraded phonological plan) that results in productions in which the "articulatory parameters" are too broad. Bradford and Dodd (1996) hypothesize that children with phonological planning deficits may have to create a new plan each time they produce a particular word, giving rise to variable productions.

Other investigators believe that variability in the phoneme and/or whole-word productions stems primarily from deficits in the oral-motor system or from a combination of psycholinguistic and motor problems (Crary, 1993; Hall, Jordan, and Robin, 1993).

Clinical implications

Phonological assessment

Given that variability is a key feature of the speech of some children with speech impairment, assessment of variability should be one component of phonological assessment (Hooper and McLeod, 1999; Grunwell, 1992). Unfortunately, traditional single-word articulation tests do not provide the opportunity for obtaining multiple exemplars of the same word and thus cannot serve as a basis for determining levels of variability. Although conversational samples may contain repetitions of some words, these repetitions are often ignored in the analysis. As shown by Hooper and McLeod (1999), analyses that include multiple productions of target words provide a more complete picture of a child's phonological system, particularly with regard to determining phonological inventory.

Phonological intervention

A thorough understanding of a child's phonological system is essential for the design and implementation of an appropriate intervention plan, and part of this understanding derives from assessment of variability. Selection of treatment targets/approaches may differ depending upon level of variability. For example, minimal pair treatment based on contrasting the child's error with the target phoneme may not be appropriate for children with various errors for a target phoneme. Finally, for children with suspected childhood apraxia of speech, treatment will vary depending on beliefs about psycholinguistic vs. motor causes of variability.

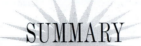

SUMMARY

- Young children with typical speech development may exhibit high levels of variability.
- Extensive variability beyond the age of 36 months may be associated with speech impairment.
- Clinical assessment of speech should include assessment of variability.
- The nature and extent of variability should be considered in designing an intervention plan.

REFERENCES

Betz, S., and Stoel-Gammon, C. (2005). Measuring articulatory error consistency in children with developmental apraxia of speech. *Clinical Linguistics and Phonetics, 19,* 53–66.

Bradford, A., and Dodd, B. (1996). Do all speech-disordered children have motor deficits? *Clinical Linguistics and Phonetics, 10,* 77–101.

Crary, M. (1993). *Developmental motor speech disorders.* San Diego, CA: Singular Press.

Davis, B. L., Jakielski, K. J., and Marquardt, T. P. (1998). Developmental apraxia of speech: Determiners of differential diagnosis. *Clinical Linguistics and Phonetics, 12,* 25–45.

Dodd, B. (Ed.) (1995). *Differential diagnosis and treatment of children with speech disorder.* London: Whurr.

Ferguson, C. A., and Farwell, C. B. (1975). Words and sounds in early language acquisition. *Language, 51,* 419–439.

Forrest, K. (2003). Diagnostic criteria of developmental apraxia of speech used by clinical speech–language pathologists. *American Journal of Speech-Language Pathology, 12,* 376–380.

Forrest, K., Dinnsen, D., and Elbert, M. (1997). Impact of substitution patterns on phonological learning by misarticulating children. *Clinical Linguistics and Phonetics, 11,* 63–76.

Forrest, K., Elbert, M., and Dinnsen, D. (2000). The effect of substitution patterns on phonological treatment outcomes. *Clinical Linguistics and Phonetics, 14,* 519–531.

Grunwell, P. (1992). Assessment of child phonology in the clinical context. In C. A. Ferguson, L. Menn, and C. Stoel-Gammon (Eds.), *Phonological development: Models, research, implications* (pp. 457–483). Timonium, MD: York Press.

Hall, P. K., Jordan, L. S., and Robin, D. A. (1993). *Developmental apraxia of speech: Theory and clinical practice.* Austin, TX: Pro-Ed.

Hooper, S., and McLeod, S. (1999). The impact of speech production variability on phonological analysis. In S. McLeod and L. McAllister (Eds.), *Proceedings of the 1999 Speech Pathology Australia National Conference* (pp. 66–73). Melbourne: Speech Pathology Australia.

Ingram, D. (2002). The measurement of whole-word productions. *Journal of Child Language, 29,* 713–733.

Kent, R. D. (1992). The biology of phonological development. In C. A. Ferguson, L. Menn, and C. Stoel-Gammon (Eds), *Phonological development: Models, research, implications* (pp. 65–90). Timonium, MD: York Press.

Kent, R. D., and Bauer, H. (1985). Vocalizations of one-year-olds. *Journal of Child Language, 12,* 491–526.

Kovas, Y., Hayiou-Thomas, M., Oliver, B., Bishop, D., Dale, P., and Plomin, R. (2005). Genetic influences in different aspects of language development: The etiology of language skills in 4.5-year-old twins. *Child Development, 76,* 632–651.

Leonard, L. B., Rowan, L. E., Morris, B., and Fey, M. E. (1982). Intra-word phon

ological variability in young children. *Journal of Child Language, 9,* 55–69.

Locke, J. (1989). Babbling and early speech: Continuity and individual differences. *First Language, 9,* 191–206.

Marquardt, T., Jacks, A., and Davis, B. (2004). Token-to-token variability in developmental apraxia of speech: Three longitudinal case studies. *Clinical Linguistics and Phonetics, 18,* 127–144.

Schwartz, R. G., Leonard, L. B., Folger, M. K., and Wilcox, M. J. (1980). Early phonological behavior in normal-speaking and language disordered children: Evidence for a synergistic view of language disorders. *Journal of Speech and Hearing Disorders, 45,* 355–377.

Shriberg, L. D., Aram, D., and Kwiatkowski, J. (1997). Developmental apraxia of speech: II. Toward a diagnostic marker. *Journal of Speech, Language, and Hearing Research, 40,* 286–312.

Smith, A., and Goffman, L. (1998). Stability and patterning of speech movement sequences in children and adults. *Journal of Speech, Language, and Hearing Research, 44,* 18–30.

Stoel-Gammon, C. (2004, February). *Variability in the productions of young typically developing children.* Paper presented at the meeting of the International Clinical Phonetics and Linguistics Association, Lafayette, LA.

Stoel-Gammon, C., and Cooper, J. A. (1984). Patterns of early lexical and phonological development. *Journal of Child Language, 11,* 247–271.

Tyler, A., and Lewis, K. (2005). Relationships among consistency/variability and other phonological measures over time. *Topics in Language Disorders, 25,* 243–253.

Tyler, A., Lewis, K., and Welch, C. (2003). Predictors of phonological change following intervention. *American Journal of Speech-Language Pathology, 12,* 289–298.

Vihman, M. M. (1993). Variable paths to early word production. *Journal of Phonetics, 21,* 61–82.

Vihman, M. M., Ferguson, C. A., and Elbert, M. (1986). Phonological development from babbling to early speech: Common tendencies and individual differences. *Applied Psycholinguistics, 7,* 3–40.

Vihman, M. M., and Greenlee, M. (1987). Individual differences in phonological development: Ages one and three years. *Journal of Speech and Hearing Research, 30,* 503–521.

Vogel Sosa, A., and Stoel-Gammon, C. (2006). Patterns of intra-word phonological variability during the second year of life. *Journal of Child Language; 33,* 31–50.

Chapter 11

Speech Acquisition and Participation in Society

Sharynne McLeod

INTRODUCTION

Throughout the world, children and adults participate in society in many different ways. Most will be a member of a family or community and have friends. Most will learn at least one language. Most will participate in education. Many will work and play. Most will participate in organized activities and groups. Many will practice religion. In order to fully participate in society, people should be provided the opportunity to develop to their fullest potential, both in the childhood years and during adulthood. However, it is important that childhood is not seen only as preparation for participation in society as adults. Living a fulfilled life is important in childhood, not just for the future.

Participation from the perspective of the United Nations

An emphasis on participation for children has been fostered by application of The United Nations Convention on the Rights of the Child (UNCRC), which was ratified in 1989 and came into effect in 1990. The UNCRC "sets out rights for the survival, development, protection and participation of children." (UNICEF UK, n.d.). Children's right to participate is a guiding principle of the UNCRC: "The right to participation is relevant to the exercise of all other rights, within the family, the school and the larger community context." As of 2005, the UNCRC has been ratified by every country in the world except the USA and Somalia. Throughout the world many children are now seen as active citizens with their own rights.

The *International Classification of Functioning Disability and Health* (ICF) defines Participation as the "involvement in a life situation" and Activity as "the execution of a task or action by an individual." (World Health Organization, 2001, p. 10). See Chapter 1 for further discussion of the ICF. Within the ICF, Activity and Participation include learning and applying knowledge (e.g., reading), general tasks and demands (e.g., carrying out daily routine), communication (e.g., conversation), mobility (e.g., walking and moving), self-care (e.g., eating and drinking), domestic life (e.g., household tasks), interpersonal interactions and relationships (e.g., family relationships), major life areas (e.g., education), and community, social, and civic life (e.g., recreation and leisure). Participation within each of these areas is enhanced by the ability to communicate effectively (see Eadie et al., 2006). Effective communication is achieved, in part, through effective acquisition of speech and language.

The interrelationship between speech acquisition and realization of life potential

Studies of the long- and short-term outcomes of children with speech impairment provide evidence of the importance of typical speech acquisition in a person's life. The impact of speech impairment may include loss of potential in educational, occupational, and/or social domains. Studies of children with speech impairment will be presented in this review; however, in many instances the participants have co-occurring language or other communication impairments (Blood, Ridenour, Qualls, and Hammer, 2003). In some cases there are better long-term outcomes for those with speech impairments alone than for those with concomitant language impairments (Johnson et al., 1999). Finally, it is important to remember that everyone is unique, and the unique combination of personal and environmental factors, together with the degree of impairment, will result in the extent to which each person can participate in society.

Educational impact

Having a speech impairment as a child can impact on educational outcomes in both the short and long term (Felsenfeld, Broen, and McGue, 1994; Gregory, Shanahan, and Walberg, 1985; Hall and Tomblin, 1978; Harasty and Reed, 1994; Lewis and Freebairn, 1992; Lewis, Freebairn, and Taylor, 2000; Nathan, Stackhouse, Goulandris, and Snowling, 2004; Olson Wagner, Gray, and Potter, 1983). Children with speech impairment can have difficulty with mathematics (Nathan et al.). Children with speech

impairment can also have ongoing difficulties with literacy, including difficulty with phonological awareness, spelling, reading comprehension, and reading accuracy (Bernhardt and Major, 2005; Hesketh, 2004; Larrivee and Catts, 1999; Leitão and Fletcher, 2004; Lewis and Freebairn, 1992; Lewis et al. 2000; Nathan et al.). Severity of speech impairment is indicative of poorer literacy (Larrivee and Catts).

Recent studies in literacy outcomes have attempted to isolate the impact of speech impairment from concomitant speech and language impairment. Lewis et al. (2000) indicated that children with speech impairment alone were more likely to have poor spelling skills relative to their reading and language abilities. Hesketh (2004) indicated that for children with speech impairment alone, phonological awareness at 3;6 to 5;0 years was the best indicator of literacy skills at 6;6 to 7;6 years. Leitão and Fletcher (2004) indicated that children with a nondevelopmental speech impairment at age 5 to 6 years had more significant difficulties with literacy at age 12 to 13 years than children with a developmental speech impairment. However, Lewis et al. (2000) also indicated that children with speech impairment were less likely than children with speech and language impairment to have difficulties with phoneme awareness, language, reading decoding, reading comprehension, and spelling.

Children with speech and/or language impairment require more school-based remedial assistance than their typically developing peers, achieve lower grades (Felsenfeld et al., 1994), and are unlikely to be identified by their teachers as high achievers (McLeod and McKinnon, in press). Adults who had a speech impairment as a child have been reported as completing fewer years of education than their typically developing peers (Felsenfeld et al.).

Occupational impact

A speech impairment may affect one's future economic potential. To illustrate, Felsenfeld et al. (1994) reported that adults with histories of speech impairments were more likely to occupy semiskilled and unskilled jobs than their peers. Many jobs are based on the ability to speak well (Ruben, 2000; Silverman and Paulus, 1989; Weiner, 1974) as opportunities for work that does not require high levels of communication (e.g., in manual labor) become less common in the developed world. Considering the current Western economic climate and the need to present well when seeking placement in a highly competitive job market, a young person with a speech impairment may be at a disadvantage compared with typically developing peers.

Social impact

A communication impairment can also impact children socially (e.g., Fujiki, Brinton, Isaacson, and Summers, 2001; Hart, Fujiki, Brinton, and Hart, 2004; Horowitz, Jansson, Ljungberg, and Hedenbro, 2006; Knox and Conti-Ramsden, 2003). Children with a language impairment have been reported to be withdrawn on the playground and spend less time interacting with their peers when compared with typically developing children (Fujiki et al.). Knox and Conti-Ramsden reported that children with language impairment were more likely to be bullied.

To date, no studies have *directly* examined the social impact of a speech impairment on children; however, indirect studies suggest that this impact may be similar for children with speech impairment. Indirect studies have asked children and adults about their impressions of people with speech impairment. They indicate that children, adolescents, and adults with speech impairment may be perceived negatively by their peers (e.g., Anderson and Antonak, 1972; Crowe Hall 1991; Mowrer, Wahl, and Doolan, 1978; Silverman, 1976; Silverman and Falk, 1992; Silverman and Paulus, 1989). For example, Silverman and Paulus asked high school students to rate a videotape of a hypothetical classmate who substituted /w/ for /r/ along an 81-adjective semantic differential scale. Another group of students rated a "typical" classmate with no speech sound errors on the same scale. The students also said that the speech-impaired person was more tense, nervous, afraid, handicapped, isolated, and uncomfortable, and less employable, friendly, sane, educated, and confident than a typical peer. Silverman and Falk replicated the study of Silverman and Paulus. These negative perceptions and their emotional consequences may be detrimental for adolescents, as this population is strongly influenced by what is fashionable in society and by peer pressure.

Not only do people with typical speech perceive speech-impaired people negatively, but studies have reported that people of all ages with a speech impairment may have a lower self-concept than their non-speech-impaired counterparts (Felsenfeld et al., 1992; Gregory et al., 1985; Silverman and Paulus, 1989).

Behavioral outcomes

Additional studies have compared the communication skills of differing populations with the broader population. Emotionally disturbed adolescents have a higher prevalence of communication impairment. Indeed, Rosenthal (1991) reported that "communication deficits

constituted a central feature of emotional disturbance in adolescence" (Rosenthal, p. 191). Incarcerated people are also reported to have a higher prevalence of communication impairment (Belenchia and Crowe, 1983; Johnson and Hamilton, 1997), including young offenders (Bryan, 2004), and adult female prisoners (Olson Wagner et al., 1983). In most instances, specific studies of speech versus language impairment were not undertaken; however, given the high comorbidity of speech and language impairments, it is likely that many of these people also have speech impairment.

Quality of life

The effect of a communication impairment on quality of life has been studied in adults with a variety of communication impairments, including spasmodic dysphonia (Baylor, Yorkston, and Eadie, 2005). However, there has been limited research on the quality of life of children with speech impairment or their families. One exception is the work by Rudolph, Kummer, Eysholdt, and Rosanowski (2005) who found that mothers of children with speech impairment achieved lower health-related quality of life scores of all subscales except for "bodily pain" and "mental health." The study was unable to identify whether there was a causal link between having a child with a speech impairment and mothers' quality of life.

Health

Children with speech impairment have been reported to have a higher prevalence of health and developmental needs compared with the general population (Keating, Turrell, and Ozanne, 2001). One reason for this could be the high number of health and syndromic conditions resulting in poor speech outcomes (White, 2006), including cleft palate, hearing impairment, Angelman's syndrome (Jolleff, Emmerson, Ryan, and McConachie, 2006), Treacher Collins and Nager's syndromes (Vallino, Peterson-Falzone, and Napoli, 2006), 22q11.2 microdeletion syndrome (Mills, Gosling, and Sell, 2006), congenital nemaline myopathy (Bagnall, Al-Muhaizea, and Manzur, 2006), and Beckwith-Wiedemann syndrome (Shipster, Oliver, and Morgan, 2006).

Listening to children to enable full participation

In order to facilitate full participation for children with speech impairments, it is important to listen to them, to understand their needs, and to consider their rights. There are challenges in respectfully listening to and understanding any child. However, children with speech impairment, particularly those who have unintelligible speech, require careful listening according to specific strategies. Most speech-language pathology assessments and interventions do not specifically target participation in society (McLeod, 2004; McLeod and Bleile, 2004), nor do they focus on listening to children and their families and paying attention to their life aspirations.

Acknowledging children as people with the right to be heard has been condoned during different historical periods and in different cultures (see Chapter 13). However, in recent times there is a growing interest in listening to children (Clark, McQuail, and Moss, 2003; Greene and Hogan, 2005). Children's right to be visible and heard is expressed in Article 12 of the United Nations Convention on the Rights of the Child (UNICEF): "*Article 12* States Parties shall assure to the child who is capable of forming his or her own views the right to express those views freely in all matters affecting the child, the views of the child being given due weight in accordance with the age and maturity of the child."

The Mosaic approach (Clark and Moss, 2001) provides a multimethod framework for creatively listening to children. It involves the use of multimethod techniques for data collection, respectful documentation, and interpretation (Moss, 2001; Smith, 2005). In the Mosaic approach, methods for listening to children can include interviewing, drawing, photography, child conferencing, tours, map making, role play, and observation (Clark, 2001). There are two stages to using the Mosaic approach: first to build up a

"living picture" (Clark, 2001, p. 18), then to draw together all the material or pieces of the Mosaic to "gain a greater understanding of children's priorities" (Clark, 2001, p. 19). Additionally, in stage two, the adult consults with the child about the meaning that has been created, a process called "visible listening."

The Mosaic approach has been adapted for use with children with communication impairments (McLeod and Daniel, 2005). This adaptation includes use of the *Speech Participation and Activity in Children* (SPAA-C) (McLeod, 2004). The SPAA-C was developed by considering the Activity and Participation construct of the *International Classification of Functioning Disability and Health* (ICF) (World Health Organization, 2001). Indicative questions can be used in interviews with any or all of the following: the child with a speech impairment and his or her siblings, parents, friends, teachers, and significant others such as grandparents or neighbors. One component of the SPAA-C is the inclusion of a Likert scale where children indicate how they feel about different scenarios relating to speaking. The 10-question Likert scale has been tested with 95 preschool children who did not have a communication impairment and was found to be appropriate for use with young children (Elliott and McLeod, 2005). The SPAA-C has been extended to include drawings by the interviewed children to further illustrate who they are and the impact of speech impairment on their worlds (Daniel and McLeod, 2006; McLeod, Daniel, and Barr, 2006). Research using the SPAA-C has documented the impact of speech impairment on the lives and families of children with speech impairment (Boase, 2006; McLeod and Daniel, 2006), and specifically siblings of children with speech impairment (Barr, McLeod and Daniel, 2006).

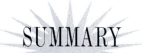

SUMMARY

- Participation in society is a right for both children and adults.
- Having a speech impairment may impact on participation in society in the following domains: educational, occupational, social, behavioral, health, and quality of life.
- The extent of impact of the impairment is influenced by personal and environmental factors.

- In order to fully understand children's potential for participation, it is important to listen to them.
- The Mosaic approach and the SPAA-C are two techniques to allow children, their families, teachers, speech-language pathologists, and others in their world to discuss their activity and participation in society and to consequently form strategies to enable full and effective participation.

REFERENCES

Anderson, R. J., and Antonak, R. F. (1992). The influence of attitudes and contact on reactions to persons with physical and speech disabilities. *Rehabilitation Counselling Bulletin, 35*, 240–247.

Bagnall, A. K., Al-Muhaizea, M. A., and Manzur, A. Y. (2006). Feeding and speech difficulties in typical congenital Nemaline Myopathy. *Advances in Speech-Language Pathology, 8*(1), 7–16.

Barr, J., McLeod, S. and Daniel, G. (2006 in press). Siblings with speech impairments: Cavalry on the hill. Language, Speech, and Hearing Services in Schools.

Baylor, C. R., Yorkston, K. M., and Eadie, T. L. (2005). The consequences of spasmodic dysphonia on communication-related quality of life: A qualitative study of the insider's experiences. *Journal of Communication Disorders, 38*(5), 395–419.

Belenchia, T. A., and Crowe, T. A. (1983). Prevalence of speech and hearing disorders in a state penitentiary population. *Journal of Communication Disorders, 16*, 279–285.

Bernhardt, B., and Major, E. (2005). Speech, language and literacy skills 3 years later: A follow-up study of early phonological and metaphonological intervention. *International Journal of Language & Communication Disorders, 40*, 1–27.

Blood, G. W., Ridenour, V. J., Qualls, C. D., and Hammer, C. S. (2003). Co-occurring disorders in children who stutter. *Journal of Communication Disorders, 36*(6) 427–448.

Boase, A. (2006). *Talking about talking: Children's views on speech.* Unpublished Masters of Medical Science thesis, University of Sheffield, Sheffield, UK.

Bryan, K. (2004). Preliminary study of the prevalence of speech and language difficulties in young offenders. *International Journal of Language & Communication Disorders, 39*, 391–400.

Clark, A. (2001). Say your piece: The Mosaic approach to consulting with children. *Nursery World, 5 July*, 18–19.

Clark, A., and Moss, P. (2001). *Listening to young children: The mosaic approach.* London: National Children's Bureau.

Clark, A., McQuail, S., and Moss, P. (2003). *Exploring the field of listening to and consulting with young children.* Research Report 445. London: Department for Education and Skills.

Crowe Hall, B. J. (1991). Attitudes of fourth and sixth graders towards peers with mild articulation disorders. *Language, Speech, and Hearing Services in Schools, 22*, 334–340.

Daniel, G., and McLeod, S. (2006). Listening to the voice of children with a communication impairment. In G. Whiteford (Ed), *Voice, identity & reflexivity: 2nd qualitative research as interpretive practice conference* (pp. 187–200). Albury, NSW: Charles Sturt University.

Eadie, T. L., Yorkston, K. M., Klasner, E. R., Dudgeon, B. J., Deitz, J. C., Baylor, C. R., Miller, R. M., & Amtmann, D. (2006). Measuring communicative participation: A review of self-report instruments in speech-language pathology. *American Journal of Speech-Language Pathology, 15*, 307–320.

Elliott, A., and McLeod, S. (2005). Children's perceptions of their speech. In C. Heine and L. Brown (Eds.), *Proceedings of the 2005 Speech Pathology Australia National Conference* (pp. 135–142). Melbourne: Speech Pathology Australia.

Felsenfeld, S., Broen, P. A., and McGue, M. (1992). A 28-year follow-up of adults with a history of moderate phonological disorder: Linguistic and personality results. *Journal of Speech and Hearing Research, 35*(5), 1114–1125.

Felsenfeld, S., Broen, P. A., and McGue, M. (1994). A 28-year follow up of adults with a history of moderate phonological disorder: Educational and occupational results. *Journal of Speech and Hearing Research, 37*, 1341–1353.

Fujiki, M., Brinton, B., Isaacson, T., and Summers, C. (2001). Social behaviors of children with language impairment on the playground: A pilot study. *Language, Speech, and Hearing Services in Schools, 32*, 101–113.

Greene, S., and Hogan, D. (2005). *Researching children's experience: Approaches and methods.* London: Sage.

Gregory, A. J. F., Shanahan, T., and Walberg, H. (1985). A descriptive analysis of high school seniors with speech disabilities. *Journal of Communication Disorders, 18*, 295–304.

Hall, P. K., and Tomblin, J. B. (1978). A follow-up study of children with articulation and language disorders. *Journal of Speech and Hearing Disorders, 43*, 227–241.

Harasty, J., and Reed, V. A. (1994). The prevalence of speech and language impairment in two Sydney metropolitan schools. *Australian Journal of Human Communication Disorders, 22*, 1–23.

Hart, K. I., Fujiki, M., Brinton, B., and Hart, C. H. (2004). The relationship between social behaviour and severity of language impairment. *Journal of Speech, Language, and Hearing Research, 47*, 647–662.

Hesketh, A. (2004). Early literacy achievement of children with a history of speech problems. *International Journal of Language and Communication Disorders, 39*, 453–468.

Horowitz, L., Jansson, L., Ljungberg, T., and Hedenbro, M. (2006). Interaction before conflict and conflict resolution in pre-school boys with language impairment. *International Journal of Language & Communication Disorders, 41*(4), 441–466.

Johnson, C. J., Beitchman, J. H., Young, A., Escobar, M., Atkinson, L., Wilson, B., Brownlie, E., Douglas, L., Taback, N., Lam, I., and Wang, M. (1999). Fourteen-year follow-up of children with and without speech/language impairments: Speech/language stability and outcomes. *Journal of Speech, Language, and Hearing Research, 42*(3), 744–760.

Johnson, S., & Hamilton, J. (1997). The causes of crime? *Royal College of Speech Language Therapists, May*, 8–9.

Jolleff, N., Emmerson, F., Ryan, M., and McConachie, H. (2006). Communication skills in Angelman Syndrome: Matching phenotype to genotype. *Advances in Speech-Language Pathology, 8*(1), 28–33.

Keating, D., Turrell, G., and Ozanne, A. (2001). Childhood speech disorders: Reported prevalence, comorbidity and socioeconomic profile. *Journal of Paediatrics & Child Health, 37*(5), 431–436.

Knox, E., and Conti-Ramsden, G. (2003). Bullying risks of 11-year-old children with specific language impairment (SLI): Does school placement matter? *International Journal of Language and Communication Disorders, 38*(1), 1–12.

Larrivee, L. S., and Catts, H. W. (1999). Early reading achievement in children with expressive phonological disorders. *American Journal of Speech-Language Pathology, 8*, 118–128.

Leitão, S., and Fletcher, J. (2004). Literacy outcomes for students with speech impairment: Long-term follow-up. *International Journal of Language and Communication Disorders, 39*, 245–256.

Lewis, B. A., and Freebairn, L. (1992). Residual effects of preschool phonology disorders in grade school, adolescence, and adulthood. *Journal of Speech and Hearing Research, 35*, 819–831.

Lewis, B. A., Freebairn, L. A., and Taylor, H. G. (2000). Academic outcomes in children with histories of speech sound disorders. *Journal of Communication Disorders, 33*, 11–30.

McLeod, S. (2004). Speech pathologists' application of the ICF to children with speech impairment. *Advances in Speech-Language Pathology, 6*(1), 75–81.

McLeod, S., and Bleile, K. (2004). The ICF: A framework for setting goals for children with speech impairment. *Child Language, Teaching, and Therapy, 20* (3), 199–219.

McLeod, S., and Daniel, G. (2005, June). *Application of the Mosaic approach for developing respectful relationships with children with communication impairments.* Presented at the Centre for Equity and Innovation in Early Childhood (CEIEC), Honouring the child honouring equity 5: Reconsidering rights and relationships, Melbourne, Australia.

McLeod, S., and Daniel, G. (2006). *This is my life: Insights from children with speech impairment.* Manuscript in preparation.

McLeod, S., Daniel, G. & Barr, J. (2006). Using children's drawings to listen to how children feel about their speech. Inc. Heine & L. Brown (Eds) *Proceedings of the 2006 Speech Pathology Australia National Conference* (pp. 38–45). Melbourne: Speech Pathology Australia.

McLeod, S., & McKinnon, D. H. (in press). The prevalence of communication disorders compared with other learning needs in 14,500 primary and secondary school students. *International Journal of Language and Communication Disorders.*

Mills, L., Gosling, A., and Sell, D. (2006). Extending the communication phenotype associated with 22q11.2 microdeletion syndrome. *Advances in Speech-Language Pathology, 8*(1), 17–27.

Moss, P. (2001). Listen in: The importance of consulting with children. *Nursery World, 5 July*, 16–17.

Mowrer, D. E., Wahl, P., and Doolan, S. J. (1978). Effect of lisping on audience evaluation of male speakers. *Journal of Speech and Hearing Disorders, 43*, 140–148.

Nathan, L., Stackhouse, J., Goulandris, N., and Snowling, M. J. (2004). The development of early literacy skills among children with speech difficulties: A test of the 'critical age hypothesis.' *Journal of Speech, Language, and Hearing Research, 47*(2), 377–391.

Olson Wagner, C., Gray, L. L., and Potter, R. E. (1983). Communicative disorders in a group of adult female offenders. *Journal of Communication Disorders, 16*, 269–277.

Rosenthal, S. L. (1991). Communication skills in emotionally disturbed and nondisturbed adolescents. *Behavioral Disorders, 16*(3), 192–199.

Ruben, R. J. (2000). Redefining the survival of the fittest: Communication disorders in the 21st century. *Laryngoscope, 110*, 241–245.

Rudolph, M., Kummer, P., Eysholdt, U., and Rosanowski, F. (2005). Quality of life in mothers of speech impaired children. *Logopedics Phoniatrics Vocology, 30*, 3–8.

Shipster, C., Oliver, B., and Morgan, A. (2006). Speech and oral motor skills in children with Beckwith Wiedemann Syndrome: Pre- and post-tongue reduction surgery. *Advances in Speech-Language Pathology, 8*(1), 45–55.

Silverman, E. (1976). Listeners' impressions of speakers with lateral lisps. *Journal of Speech and Hearing Disorders, 41*, 547–552.

Silverman, F. H., and Falk, S. N. (1992). Attitudes of teenagers toward peers who have a single articulation error. *Language, Speech, and Hearing Services in Schools, 23*, 187–188.

Silverman, F. H., and Paulus, P. G. (1989). Peer reactions to teenagers who substitute /w/ for /r/. *Language, Speech, and Hearing Services in Schools, 20*, 219–221.

Smith, K. (2005, June) *Introduction*. Presented at the Centre for Equity and Innovation in Early Childhood (CEIEC), Honouring the child honouring equity 5: Reconsidering rights and relationships, Melbourne, Australia.

UNICEF (n.d.). *The United Nations Convention on the Rights of the Child* (UNCRC). Retrieved August 10, 2005 from http://www.unicef.org/crc/crc.htm

UNICEF UK (n.d.). *UNICEF Youth voice jargon buster.* Retrieved February 10, 2006 from http://www.unicef.org.uk/youth-voice/jargonbuster.asp

Vallino, L. D., Peterson-Falzone, S. J., and Napoli, J. A. (2006). The Syndromes of Treacher Collins and Nager. *Advances in Speech-Language Pathology, 8*(1), 34–44.

Weiner, P. S. (1974). A language delayed child at adolescence. *Journal of Speech and Hearing Disorders, 39*, 202–212.

White, S. (2006). Talking genes. *Advances in Speech-Language Pathology, 8*(1), 2–6.

World Health Organization. (2001). *ICF: International classification of functioning, disability and health.* Geneva: Author.

Chapter 12

The Evolution and Development of Spoken Language

John L. Locke

INTRODUCTION

In 1930, a prospector named Michael Leahy was searching for gold in the highlands of New Guinea when he happened upon the *kanakas*, a reputedly "wild and blood-thirsty" tribe. As Leahy nervously approached, the natives—appearing less fearsome than advertised—could be heard excitedly "jabbering." Sixty-five years later, a prominent psycholinguist thought it noteworthy that the tribesmen, though cut off from the rest of the world, had "language" (Pinker, 1994). But it is also significant that the natives' language was manifested as "jabber" and not erratic gesticulation. We begin by addressing a relationship implicitly identified in the title, that of speech and language. Later we will take up the association between evolution and development. As we will see, the stories of these two relationships are, themselves, intertwined.

Speech and language

In recent years, scholars generally have come to believe that human language is bound by no specific modality, a cognitive capability that responds indifferently to linguistic information that enters the brain by way of the eyes as well as the ears. This conception is due to the fact that signed and spoken languages appear equally easy to learn and use, and they owe much of their processing to common brain mechanisms. Still, except for the signed languages used by the deaf, all four to six thousand of the world's languages are spoken, suggesting that there must be some advantage to the vocal and auditory systems (Locke, 1998; Locke and Hauser, 1999).

In the last few years, research—without any particular fanfare—has been exposing surprisingly intimate relationships between speech and other levels of language, suggesting that speech may not be just one of several ways to express linguistic knowledge. For example, it has been found that the frequency and complexity of vocalization by infants predicts later success in various areas of language, including comprehension (Oller, 2000; see review of volubility literature in Locke and Hauser, 1999). In longitudinal studies carried out in three different countries it has been found that "language" problems in infancy may persist as speech, or even purely articulatory, problems in adolescence and adulthood (Felsenfeld, Broen, and McGue, 1992; Nauclér and Magnusson, 2002; Stothard, Snowling, Bishop, Chipchase, and Kaplan, 1998). Findings in behavioral genetics also support links between language and speech. In studies of monozygotic and dizygotic twins, for example, the highest rates of concordance have come from twins in whom the disorder was primarily expressive—some had disorders that were purely of the articulatory type (Bishop, North, and Donlan, 1995; Lewis, 1990; Lewis and Thompson, 1992). The role played by production factors has also been highlighted by studies of the KE family, about half of whom had morphological problems (Gopnik and Crago, 1991) and verbal and nonverbal dyspraxia (Vargha-Khadem, Watkins, Alcock, Fletcher, and Passingham, 1995). Noting this conjunction, several theorists have toyed with the idea that the family's oral-motor difficulties *caused* their grammatical and comprehension difficulties. "One possibility," wrote Watkins, Dronkers, and Vargha-Khadem (2002), "is that the deviant articulation results in poor phonology, rendering morphological production difficult" (p. 461) "It might be the case," Marcus and Fisher (2003) speculated, "that a deficit restricted to the motor system is fully responsible for the wide-ranging profile of impairment" (p. 261). There could have been a "flow-on effect from articulation to syntax to comprehension," wrote Corballis (2004, p. 548).

Evolution and development

If speech and language are intimately intertwined, their development and evolution are no less so. Young humans are able to acquire a native language because evolution provided them with the genes that build specialized linguistic mechanisms, and the social systems that dispose infants to observe and interact. Evolution also provided

appropriately structured intervals for development and learning: ontogenetic stages. Humans have four—two more stages than the other primates—and all four are needed for the young to reach the proficiency in linguistic communication that characterizes mature members of our species. The first stage, infancy, runs from the prenatal period until 30 to 36 months, when typically developing infants have a lexicon and phonological system, regularly apply morphological and syntactic rules to create novel forms and utterances, and use this material with a basal level of pragmatic force (Locke, 1997).

In humans, the infant stage is no longer than that of other primates—actually, it's shorter—but where social learning is concerned the quality is higher. The reason relates to the fact that our infants are unusually helpless, necessitating round-the-clock handling and care. To be sure, human mothers usually expect to provide the necessary services, but there is still some amount of "parent-offspring conflict" (Trivers, 1972). This is because mothers have other progeny to care for, and other things to do with their time. When they begin to withdraw their attention, as eventually they must, infants begin to "negotiate" continued care. Thus, helplessness, ostensibly a "deficiency," may be responsible for unusually strategic signaling by human infants, including clever ways of using the voice to secure and maintain maternal proximity. Later in development, when able to walk, climb, and manipulate objects, infants need a different form of care ("instruction" about hazardous aspects of their environment), but in evolutionary history the requisite learning would have been unlikely unless infants signaled their interest in dangerous things. Elsewhere, I have suggested that the infants who were able to deal with these new signaling situations were more likely to receive the care and information needed, to engage with potentially helpful others, and therefore to live on to reproductive age themselves (Locke, 2001; in press; 2006). This was a distinct contribution of vocal development to linguistic evolution, since new levels of vocal ability would be carried into later ontogenetic stages where they would be reinforced and elaborated into something that sounded even more like speech (Locke and Bogin, in press).

There may also have been semantic pressures in infancy. According to a proposal by Fitch (2004), hominid parents benefited by exchanging accurate information with their offspring, and with other kin who shared their genes. The better-informed young were more likely to survive into adulthood, passing on to their own offspring genes associated with the improved system of communication. Later, according to Fitch, the new communication system would have been used with genetically unrelated individuals and further elaborated to meet the requirements associated with information transmission.

Early in human development, accomplishments begin to shift from linguistic content and structure to pragmatics and performance. I propose that this shift was of premier importance evolutionarily and was responsible for the interconnectivity of linguistic systems that are sometimes considered autonomous and independent. This is initially seen in childhood, which extends from the end of infancy to 7 years, and has a constellation of traits that is peculiar to humans, including a slowing and stabilization of the rate of growth as well as immature dentition and motor control, dependence on others for food, and extrafamilial friendships. During childhood, there are continuing improvements in phonology, vocabulary, and sentence length as well as syntax. These are invariably credited on the school-oriented language tests that are given by clinicians and teachers, but some of the most important developments in childhood include discourse, narration, and advances in the area of verbal competition and performance, such as joking and the use of preassembled verbal routines. In many cultures, children play verbal games with peers using material learned from family members earlier in infancy, or from unrelated children. These games mark the beginning of various sorts of verbal competition that continue to develop in the next stage, juvenility. Juvenility begins at 8 and ends at 10 years (in girls) or 12 years (in boys) (Bogin, 1999).

The decline of juvenility marks the onset of adolescence, the other ontogenetic stage that is uniquely human (Bogin, 1999). In modern humans, adolescence is marked by a distinct skeletal growth spurt, co-timed with puberty, an intensification of preexisting friendships, and the development of new relationships (Bogin, 1999). I have speculated elsewhere that selection operated throughout ontogeny, but that in adolescence performative behaviors—including socially attractive aspects of articulate vocalization—exerted unusual effects on fitness (Locke and Bogin, in press). In modern human adolescents, there is an increase in a number of verbal functions, several of which fall outside the area of pragmatics as usually defined. These include gossiping, joking, deceiving, mollifying, negotiating, and persuading. Such skills facilitate the achievement and maintenance of social relationships, something that matters a great deal in adolescence, and anthropological reports indicate that in oral societies—which bear a closer relationship to evolutionary contexts than our own—fluent, rhythmic, and elegant speech also facilitates the acquisition of status. It seems likely that vocal and verbal performance played a role in courtship and intrasexual competition

in evolutionary history, and there is evidence that they still do (Locke, 2000).

Were evolutionary ancestors with conspicuous vocal and verbal talent reproductively advantaged? Men who speak in a way that secures attention are also likely to be high in dominance. There are likely to be several vocal and articulatory variables that attract favorable attention, and adaptively so. For example, women prefer voices that are low in frequency (Collins, 2000; Collins and Missing, 2003; Feinberg, Jones, Little, Burt, and Perrett, 2005). This attribute is associated with several indices of fitness—including testosterone and testis volume—that predict coital frequency, social expressivity, and social dominance. Adaptively, female listeners associate a low fundamental frequency and related acoustic variables with greater masculinity, better health, and older age (Feinberg et al., 2005), attributes that women look for in a mate (cf. Buss, 2003). Recently, it was reported that in both men and women, opposite-sex ratings of vocal attractiveness predicted age of first sexual intercourse, number of sexual partners, number of competing sexual relationships, and number of partners that were involved in other sexual relationships (Hughes, Dispenza, and Gallup, 2004).

Conclusion

I have suggested that important aspects of language cannot develop until sexual maturity because functions that emerge at that stage play a key role in its construction. Selection for verbal performance in adolescence reinforces previous developments, sweeping specializations associated with speech and voice, linguistic content and structure, and rules of usage into one large specialization, or network of specialized subsystems. Thus it seems likely that the faculty of language includes a number of disparate capabilities—capabilities that were drawn together in evolution, as they are in modern development, by the whole of human ontogeny.

We are now in a position to see that the two pairs of threads identified in the title—speech and language; development and evolution—must indeed be woven together. For the evolutionary proposals examined here suggest that vocal signals and meanings emerged from the infant period, and were reinforced and elaborated under pressures that applied later in ontogeny. In the weaving, various changes in the form and function of vocalization in early developmental stages led to the expansion of vocal and phonetic capacity, a series of events that must surely have facilitated the evolution of languages that are expressed in "jabber" and not gesticulation.

SUMMARY

- Several different types of evidence suggest that speech is linked to grammar and pragmatics, and therefore must be regarded as something more than the "mouthpiece" for language. As a result, attempts to explain why languages are universally spoken may provide a partial account of the evolution of language itself.
- The evolution of childhood and adolescence, and the remodeling of infancy and juvenility, paved the way for language, which presupposes the appearance of novel behaviors in one or more of these stages. This means that evolution influenced development, which circled back to produce a process that may be thought of, in contemporary shorthand, as "evo-devo-evo."
- The trait of language is the behaviors that evolved, and develop. Some form of the behaviors now considered "precursors" in the development of language may have contributed to its evolution. Integration of these behaviors into a single broad specialization may explain their present-day predictive value.

REFERENCES

Bishop, D. V. M., North, T., and Donlan, C. (1995). Genetic basis for specific language impairment: Evidence from a twin study. *Developmental Medicine and Child Neurology, 37*, 56–71.

Bogin, B. (1999). *Patterns of human growth* (2nd ed.). New York: Cambridge University Press.

Buss, D. M. (2003). *The evolution of desire: Strategies of human mating.* New York: Basic Books.

Collins, S. A. (2000). Men's voices and women's choices. *Animal Behaviour, 60*, 773–780.

Collins, S. A., and Missing, C. (2003). Vocal and visual attractiveness are related in women. *Animal Behaviour, 65*, 997–1004.

Corballis, M. C. (2004). The origins of modernity: Was autonomous speech the critical factor? *Psychological Review, 111*, 543–552.

Feinberg, D. R., Jones, B. C., Little, A. C., Burt, M. D., and Perrett, D. I. (2005). Manipulations of fundamental frequency and formant frequencies influence the attractiveness of human male voices. *Animal Behaviour, 69*, 561–568.

Felsenfeld, S., Broen, P. A., and McGue, M. (1992). A 28-year follow-up of adults with a history of moderate phonological disorder: Linguistic and personality results. *Journal of Speech and Hearing Research, 35*, 1114–1125.

Fitch, W. T. (2004). Kin selection and "mother tongues": A neglected component in language evolution. In D. K. Oller and U. Griebel, (Eds.), *The evolution of communication systems: A comparative approach.* Cambridge, MA: MIT Press.

Gopnik, M., and Crago, M. B. (1991). Familial aggregation of a developmental language disorder. *Cognition, 39*, 1–50.

Hughes, S. M., Dispenza, F., and Gallup, G. G. (2004). Ratings of voice attractiveness predict sexual behavior and body configuration. *Evolution and Human Behavior, 25*, 295–304.

Lewis, B. A. (1990). Familial phonological disorders: Four pedigrees. *Journal of Speech and Hearing Disorders, 55*, 160–170.

Lewis, B. A., and Thompson, L. A. (1992). A study of developmental speech and language disorders in twins. *Journal of Speech and Hearing Research, 35*, 1086–1094.

Locke, J. L. (1997). A theory of neurolinguistic development. *Brain and Language, 58*, 265–326.

Locke, J. L. (1998). Social sound-making as a precursor to spoken language. In J. R. Hurford, M. Studdert-Kennedy, and C. Knight (Eds.), *Approaches to the evolution of language: Social and cognitive bases.* Cambridge, UK: Cambridge University Press.

Locke, J. L. (2000). Rank and relationships in the evolution of spoken language. *Journal of the Royal Anthropological Institute, 7*, 37–50.

Locke, J. L. (2001). First communion: The emergence of vocal relationships. *Social Development, 10*, 294–308.

Locke, J. L. (in press). Parental selection of vocal behavior: Crying, cooing, babbling and the evolution of spoken language. *Human Nature.*

Locke, J. L. (2006). Bimodal signaling in infancy: Motor behavior, reference, and the evolution of spoken language. Manuscript submitted for publication.

Locke, J. L., and Bogin, B. (in press). Language and life history: A new perspective on the evolution and development of linguistic communication. *Behavioral and Brain Science.*

Locke, J. L., and Hauser, M. D. (1999). Sex and status effects on primate volubility: Clues to the origin of vocal languages? *Evolution and Human Behavior, 20*, 151–158.

Marcus, G. F., and Fisher, S. E. (2003). *FOXP2* in focus: What can genes tell us about speech and language? *Trends in Cognitive Sciences, 7*, 257–262.

Nauclér, K., and Magnusson, E. (2002). How do preschool language problems affect language abilities in adolescence? In F. Windsor, M. L. Kelly, and N. Hewlett (Eds.), *Investigations in clinical phonetics and linguistics* (pp. 99–114). Mahwah, NJ: Erlbaum.

Oller, D. K. (2000). *The emergence of the speech capacity.* Mahwah, NJ: Erlbaum.

Pinker, S. (1994). *The language instinct: The new science of language and mind.* London: Allen Lane.

Stothard, S. E., Snowling, M. J., Bishop, D. V. M., Chipchase, B. B., and Kaplan, C. A. (1998). Language-impaired preschoolers: A follow-up into adolescence. *Journal of Speech, Language, and Hearing Research, 41,* 407–418.

Trivers, R. L. (1972). Parental investment and sexual selection. In B. Campbell (Ed.), *Sexual selection and the descent of man, 1871–1971.* Chicago, IL: Aldine.

Vargha-Khadem, F., Watkins, K., Alcock, K., Fletcher, P., and Passingham, R. (1995). Praxic and nonverbal cognitive deficits in a large family with a genetically transmitted speech and language disorder. *Proceedings of the National Academy of Science USA, 92,* 930–933.

Watkins, K. E., Dronkers, N. F., and Vargha-Khadem, F. (2002). Behavioural analysis of an inherited speech and language disorder: Comparison with acquired aphasia. *Brain, 125,* 452–464.

Chapter 13

Historical and International Perspectives of Childhood

Leonora Ritter

INTRODUCTION

We all see children in different ways. Our ideas are shaped by our culture, by tradition, philosophical invention, religious innovation, scientific discovery, and/or cultural colonization. Our views affect the way we treat children, and the way in which children are treated shapes the way children behave, so our views are self-reinforcing. They also tend to be reinforced as we are surrounded by people with similar views, so we tend not to analyze, reflect about, or question them.

This chapter is intended as an aid to reflecting on how you and your clients view children. The most basic variables are whether people see children as the agents and inheritors of their own development or as objects to be shaped for defined purposes, and whether children are trusted or mistrusted as the agents of their destiny.

The child as a social being

A view that trusts the child as a social being is as old as human society and pockets of it can still be found. Documented examples include the Anbarra people of North Arnhem Land (Hamilton, 1981) and the Yequana Indians of Venezuela (Liedloff, 1975). These cultures allow the child to regulate itself within safe boundaries, which are socially maintained because children are seen as belonging to the community. They share in daily activities, learning by observing and by doing. Childhood is lived in the present rather than for the future, ending with a rite of passage around puberty. Discipline is functional and minimal. The Mohave Amerindians, for example, have no word for punishment, and delinquent children are "treated with only a slightly exasperated tolerance" (Zeldin, 1994, p. 382).

In the modern Western world these ideas come to us via Rousseau's idealizing of the primitive savage. They underpin the approaches identified by de Mause (1974, p. 54) as the "helping mode," characterized by the intention to "let the child develop in his own way and time" (Neill, 1966, p. 12). For people who think this way, speech acquisition is expected: "Between two and three most children learn to use the right words in the right order and the right form surprisingly quickly … it seems they are genetically programmed to do this, it is crucial for them to have an adult model to provide them with the speech patterns of language" (Barker, 2001, p. 27). Where a speech impairment develops that does not have a physiological basis and is not the result of poor adult modeling, this approach seeks underlying emotional reasons and psychologically therapeutic solutions (Ritter and Ritter, 1959).

The child as mistrusted agent

There is another view that sees children as agents in their lives, but it is future oriented and does not trust them. It originated with sixteenth-century Puritanism and focuses on salvation of the soul. Within this moralistic view people can see children either as little angels, pure yet vulnerable and therefore to be protected from evil influences and corrected as soon as signs of evil appear, or as little devils, vessels for original sin, which makes it imperative to break their will at all costs. Childhood is a time of strict behavioral codes, moral trial, and earnest endeavor. Right and wrong are absolute; obedience is an end in itself. Parents see themselves as God's agents, teaching their children through authoritarian instruction, reward, and punishment. Discipline is intended both to make the child pay for sin and to ensure that the child will decide to sin no more. Suffering is necessary because of the atonement value of pain. Repentance (saying "sorry") is important and can ameliorate the severity of punishment.

This view is evident in the modern Western emphasis on saying "sorry," the persistence of "obedience" as the measure of a good child, and the use of the word "naughty" (meaning morally worthless) to describe a misbehaving child. Whenever the media tugs our heart strings with stories of lost innocence, it is invoking angel children. Whenever the media whips up paranoia about the evils of uncontrolled youth, it is invoking devil children.

Mistrust of children in the modern world is evident in their being specifically exempted from liberal-democratic laws protecting adult rights. Thus they may be legally assaulted (smacked), deprived of liberty (grounded or placed in time-out), and robbed (toys confiscated) without recourse to law, provided the deed is carried out by a person *in loco parentis*. At the same time they are legally "protected" from living independently or working to earn a living.

Within this view speech impairments are seen more as a sign of the child's "wilfulness" than as something that requires therapy. A graphic nineteenth-century example in Butler's *Way of All Flesh* (1903) involves a father trying to teach a child to say "come" instead of "tum;" try as he might, the child only says "tum." Eventually the father says, "I will give you one more chance, and if you don't say 'come,' I shall know that you are self-willed and naughty." The frightened child says "tum" once more and is beaten and sent to bed (Butler, 1947, p. 92).

The child as object

A number of different views see the child not as a potential agent, but as an object to be shaped for defined purposes; they vary according to the defined purpose. The most individual-centred of these approaches sees children as "future adults'" and focuses on developing their individual physical and intellectual potential. It may segregate the child into educational institutions, in order to concentrate on education and training, or it may use structures, such as apprenticeships, specifically designed to ensure the acquisition of skill. Discipline is corrective, designed to ensure that the child is always doing his or her best. Doctor Spock sells his version of this as ensuring that children will grow up to "make full use of what brains, what skills, what physical attractiveness they have" (1968, p. 4).

This view moves children to center stage and makes them responsible for the future well-being of the human race, with the result that, "We live in a time when anxiety about *what children might turn into* couldn't be higher" (Rosen, 1994, p. 1). It encourages us to enhance learning from the earliest years, choose toys for their educational value, and invest vast amounts of money in schooling. It makes childhood a time of earnest endeavor and lots of homework. The role of speech development within this view is epitomized in the heading: "Ways to encourage your toddler's speech and language development" (Barker, 2001, p. 27). Speech-language pathology has a role in early diagnosis and treatment in order to maximize a child's ability to become a clear and fluent adult.

Another view builds on human potential but changes the priority from benefiting the person to benefiting the nation, seeing children as "future citizens.'" This view mistrusts children as "uncivilized" but sees their potential to become "civilized" given the right experience and training. The desired outcomes depend on the needs of the particular society or nation-state. In ancient Sparta the nation demanded stoic soldiers; in Puritan New England, God-fearing toilers. Traditional Asian authoritarianism develops an obligation to achieve and accept consensus. Hitler's Germany required obedient Aryan nationalists. In the Soviet Union a 1961 advice book to parents, *Roditeli i deti* [Parents and Children], aimed to produce citizens who "better, more quickly, and more joyously fulfill [sic] demands and rules" (Bronfenbrenner, 1970 p. 10).

This approach uses childhood as a time of grading and sorting so that the right people gain status and power, with structural and clearly defined steps toward autonomy. Within this view, SLPs have a role in ensuring that children are sorted by class and the superior ones are taught to speak well in order to enhance their civic roles.

Another outcome-oriented view sees children as a means to an economic end, focusing on making them servants of the economy. This view began with the child as a participant in cottage industries, seeing children as a profitable and convenient source of labor (still prevalent in many third-world countries). It changed to accommodate the Industrial Revolution and economic rationalism, seeing children as potential adult workers. More recently, consumerism wants children to be exploitable consumers. This third phase may appear indulgent, but it puts profits ahead of the welfare of the child, leading child care experts to condemn the influx of "too many" possessions that make the child overwhelmed, demanding, and ungrateful (e.g., Dobson, 1977; Jolly, 1977). It also requires children to be emotionally unsatisfied so that they will go shopping and buy things they do not need in order to cheer themselves up.

This view places speech-language pathology as a service for those parents who can afford it and/or an investment by the state in improving the future employability and earning power of the child.

In the Western world since the Enlightenment, another view that has developed sees children as "subjects of science.'" It has led to the conviction that there is a right or healthy way to rear children and that right diagnosis and treatment can cure everything. Childhood has become a focus of endless study and argument, generating a plethora of professional careers, enormous profits for publishers and the media, and general anxiety for parents. This scientific model of childhood uses such value-laden terms as *normal*, *healthy*, or *correct*, in order to control individual and social behavior, whether through Freud's psychoanalysis, Skinner's behaviorism, or medication for ADHD, all of which are intended to "cure" children or "normalize" their behavior.

This belief that all intervention is for the child's own good according to some objective scientific measure has contributed to the rise of "helping" professions and an unprecedented level of state interference, including state-supported and -controlled clinics, schools, reformatories, health visitors, and welfare workers.

SLPs are embedded in this construct. Their education and approaches are scientific, their solutions are medical, behavioral, or psychological. The scientific view is most dominant where their work focuses on standards rather than functions. For example, Barker advises parents to consult them if a "toddler is not using single words by age eighteen months... [or] two-word sentences by two and a half" (2001, pp. 29–30).

The child as optional extra

All the above views focus in some way or another on children. By contrast, in twenty-first-century Western societies, labor-saving technology, contraception, and women's liberation have made it both possible and desirable to avoid parenthood (the DINK [Double Income, No Kids] model). Children have therefore become optional extras for those who wish to perpetuate their name, prove their fertility, or project their ambitions (Ritter, 2001, p. 25). In this model, childhood is seen as a rather unfortunate stage in human growth, to be managed with as little trouble as possible. Parenting advice manuals and videos focus on how to make children behave and meet their needs (eat, sleep, defecate) in the most convenient ways and as quickly as possible, regardless of the cost to the child. Examples of this are time-out and control crying, both of which disrupt the child's connection with the caregiver by using isolation as a behavior management technique.

To minimize the responsibility of parents for the behavior of their children, genetics or peers are seen as a more important determinant of behavior than parenting, and love and support are reconstructed as "quality time" to license part-time parenting. Optional-extra parents outsource the management of their children as far as possible to professional caregivers: nannies, institutional child care, organized after-school activities, or boarding school.

Optional-extra children have to learn by instruction, as their exclusion from the mundane activities of daily life give them little opportunity for watching and doing. Much of their instruction comes from machines as they tend to interact more with computers and televisions than they do with living people. For these children maximum freedom can be achieved through being no trouble, but attention can be achieved only by being trouble.

This view places responsibility on paid experts, including SLPs, to relieve parents of responsibility for the development of their children. Its prevalence has created concern: "In my opinion recommending parents to seek advice for normal stuttering is a little over the top. Many families do not have easy access to SLPs and such advice is likely to cause an undue amount of stress" (Barker, 2001, p. 30).

Models combined

A number of different views have been identified, but humans are rarely rational or consistent. Thus, the views discussed are rarely found in their pure form, and advice about how to treat children often has internal inconsistencies. The future adult view can, for example, incorporate a trusting element proposing self-regulation and finish with a scientific argument that this is the way to rear healthy adults (Ritter, 1959), or encompass an immortal soul argument stressing the developmental value of obedience and finish with a good-citizen conclusion that it is the way to rear law-abiding adults (Isaacs, 1932).

Western "experts" in the field of parenting advice ensure their popularity and acceptance by incorporating several different views. One of the reasons Benjamin Spock was so successful is that, in spite of being designated as the guru of permissiveness (trusting the child and giving it agency), he managed to simultaneously accommodate most views. Penny Leach, who became popular in the 1970s, similarly combines many approaches. She combines the trusting view in rejecting punishment with the human-potential one in seeing the child as a "person-in-the-making" (1977, p. 3). She also, however, includes the moralistic view in places. On the

subject of the night-wandering child, for example, she says: "the best way of teaching her not to get out is probably to make absolutely sure that she gains nothing by her exploits" (1977, p. 304). Although Leach seemingly rejects the scientific approach, writing that "any set of rules or pre-determined ideas can work well if the rules you choose or follow happen to fit the baby you have" (1977, p. 8), she contradictorily lays down her own laws: "don't ever leave her crying alone, but don't ever get her up again either" (1977, p. 218). She appears to acknowledge the optional-extra view that was emerging at the time of her writing by telling parents, "Fun for her is fun for you" (1977, p. 14), but she ultimately rejects it by pointing out that bringing up a child "involves extremely hard work" (1977, p. 15).

Tension arises for children when the views of the people around them differ. This may occur when different parents hold different views, stepparents enter the picture, home and school clash, carers and experts clash, or parents' own childhoods have imbued them with one set of views but they are drawn intellectually toward a different way of thinking. The debates that accompany these tensions usually center on which way is right or natural (Solter, 2001, p. 2), with "smug predictions of life-long problems" (Barker, 2001, p. 469) for those who get it wrong. This is misleading. The differences are usually about differing models of children rather than which method is objectively or generically best.

Conclusion

In working with children and parents it is important to realize that there are many views of a child, each of which seems valid to its holder. Different views about what children are will therefore produce different expectations of how they should behave and different assumptions of how they should be treated. Children will also have learned different views of themselves, which will dictate how they need to behave and how they expect to be treated. Working effectively with parents and children requires being aware of and accommodating their views, which in turn requires reflection on your own.

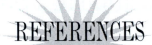

SUMMARY

- There are many different models of childhood.
- One view trusts the child as a social being.
- Another view sees children as agents in their lives, but does not trust them.
- A number of other views see children as objects to be shaped for defined purposes; these include seeing them as future adults, future citizens, means to economic ends, or subjects of science.
- In the twenty-first century, the focus has shifted and children have become optional extras.

- The models discussed are rarely found in their pure form, and advice about how to treat children often has internal inconsistencies.
- Western experts in the field of parenting advice ensure their popularity and acceptance by incorporating several different views.
- Tension arises for children when the people around them hold conflicting models.
- In working with children and parents it is important to realize that there are many views of a child, each of which seems valid to its holder.

REFERENCES

Barker, R. (2001). *The mighty toddler*. Sydney: Macmillan.

Bronfenbrenner, U. (1970). *Two worlds of childhood*. New York: Russell Sage Foundation.

Butler, S. (1947), First published 1903. *The way of all flesh*. Harmondsworth, UK: Penguin Books.

De Mause, L. (1974). *The history of childhood*. London: Souvenir Press.

Dobson, J. (1977). *Dare to discipline*. New York: Bantam Books.

Hamilton, A. (1981). *Nature and nurture*. Canberra: Australian Institute of Aboriginal Studies.

Isaacs, S. (1932). *The nursery years*. London: Routledge & Kegan Paul.

Jolly, H. (1977). *Book of child care*. London: Sphere Books.

Leach, P. (1977). *Baby and child*. Adelaide, Australia: Rigby.

Liedloff, J. (1975). *The continuum concept*. London: Futura.

Neill, A. S. (1966). *Freedom not licence*. New York: Hart Publishing.

Ritter, L. (2001). The many inventions of childhood: A tentative taxonomy. *DisClosure, 10*, 15–34.

Ritter, P., and Ritter, J. (1959). *The free family*. London: Victor Gollancz.

Rosen, M. (Ed.). (1994). *The Penguin book of childhood*. Harmondsworth, UK: Viking.

Solter, A. J. (2001). *The aware baby*. Goelta, CA: Shining Star Press.

Spock, B. (1968). *Baby and child care*. New York: Pocket Books.

Zeldin, T. (1994). *An intimate history of humanity*. London: Sinclair-Stevenson.

Chapter 14

Speech Acquisition in a Social Context

Linda J. Harrison

INTRODUCTION

Children's development, of which speech acquisition is a significant component, is a process that occurs within, and is intricately related to, a social and environmental context. The dynamics of process and context, which are fundamental to understanding children's functioning within their life situation, will be addressed in this chapter.

Bronfenbrenner (1979; 1992/2005) describes the context of development as an ecological system that directly or indirectly influences the person, and development-in-context as an interactive process among the person, the context, and time. His bioecological model of human development has been illustrated by a series of nested circles, each representing direct and indirect systems. The innermost circles, "microsystems," directly influence the child's experiences and include home and out-of-home settings, such as school and child care. The links between microsystems are described as "mesosystems," which describe the interactions, for example, among home and school, school and child care, home and child care. The nature of the home, school, or child care setting is indirectly affected by two outer circles: the "exosystem," which describes external influences on the family such as the workplace and the neighborhood, and the "macrosystem," which comprises the prevailing social, political, economic, and cultural ideologies, conditions, and policies. The social and interpersonal processes that occur within, and are influenced by, these systems are the basis for understanding the unique nature of human development. While all of these levels of influence are relevant to understanding children's development, this chapter will focus primarily at the level of the microsystem. The contexts of home and out-of-home settings, including child care, preschool, and school, will be reviewed in relation to the ways that social and educational environments, and the relationships children form within these environments, affect development.

The process of development is described as reciprocal interaction between the child and his or her immediate environment (microsystems). Interactions at the level of microsystems (proximal processes) are "the primary engines of development" (Bronfenbrenner, 2001/2005, p. 6). Developments in children's speech acquisition, therefore, are produced by proximal processes of verbal and nonverbal interaction between the child and his or her parents, siblings, other adults, and peers. Furthermore, it is through the social, emotional, and intellectual qualities of these interactions and communications that the child develops interpersonal relationships with others and cognitive structures that organize thought. Vygotsky identifies speech—in the form of social dialogue between the child and adults, and spoken or private "inner speech"—as the mechanism by which "the child develops as a thinker and a learner" (cited in Smith, Cowie, and Blades, 2003, pp. 500–501). Accordingly, the organizing and communicative functions of language (and speech) play a key role in the process of development. In this chapter, speech acquisition and functioning are discussed within the context of children's interpersonal relationships and social interactions.

The child's first relationships

Children's earliest relationships are formed within the home environment and familiar out-of-home settings. They develop through the day-to-day communicative interactions that infants have with their parents, siblings, close relatives, and, for a significant proportion of young children, their regular child care providers. Sroufe (1996) describes the early stages of these relationships as being led by the adult caregiver who "reads the infant's signals of distress and other affective communications, imbues them with meaning, and responds to them" (p. 172). In the second half of the first year, however, the baby's contribution to the relationship becomes more active: "the infant specifically and intentionally directs communications to the caregiver, takes purposive action to achieve contact, and flexibly selects and alters behaviors from an expanded repertoire until the goal of interaction or contact is achieved" (p. 172). These child-initiated affective exchanges, such as reaching, crawling, clinging, and directed crying, serve to regulate infant emotion and are evidence that a dyadic attachment relationship has been established.

A further sign of attachment is the baby's use of the caregiver as a "secure base" from which to interact with the immediate environment. The attachment relationship provides the child with the emotional security and confidence needed to venture into novel territory, to explore the world of objects, and to engage socially with others. Communication with the caregiver also broadens once exploration begins, to include "affective sharing" and "joint visual attention" at a distance as well as in close proximity. The mobile infant shares his exploratory successes and interest in objects and activities with the caregiver and engages with her through eye contact, smiles, vocalizations, and gestures.

These three components of the dyadic attachment relationship—emotion regulation, secure base behavior, and affective sharing—lay the foundation for individual development of self-regulation, self-awareness, self-reliance, autonomy, and cognitive growth (Sroufe, 1996), which are important skills for toddlerhood and the preschool years. Further, the nonverbal communicative skills of showing, pointing, offering, and turn taking that infants develop within their attachment relationships have been linked to children's subsequent development of verbal communication (Mundy and Willoughby, 1996). Joint attention, which involves the toddler's nonverbal use of an object to gain the parent or caregiver's attention and share an experience, has also been associated with expressive language and enhanced social behavior (Mundy and Willoughby). Engaging in joint attention is an early indicator of the child's awareness of the inner world of another person, and a precursor to positive social interaction with peers.

Relationships with peers

From a very young age, children are interested in each other. They actively seek social interaction with their siblings (usually children of older or younger ages) and their peers (children of a similar age). Much of this interaction can be described as social play. Table 14-1 summarizes the sequence of behavioral interactions and verbal exchanges that are typical of Western children's play across the toddler, preschool, and school age years. Through play and conversation, children form relationships with their peers that have the potential to become reciprocal and mutual friendships. In toddlers, friendships are seen in children's skillful, primarily nonverbal, complementary interactions and shared intentions in play (Howes, 1996). In preschoolers, friendships are played out in children's verbal and imaginative interactions. Pretend play among friends "opens up a new kind of human relationship for children, a relationship of shared emotion and ideas" (Dunn, 2004, p. 28) and the opportunity for working out fears and imagined experiences. By school age, interactions among friends are characterized by positive affect,

TABLE 14-1 Sequence of childhood social and interpersonal processes

Age period	Social play	Friendship
Toddlerhood (1½–2½ years)	• Nonverbal exchanges: looks, smiles, approaches, offers/takes toy • Child watches and imitates peer's play, makes attempts to join in • Peers show mutual imitation, reinforcement of each other's play • Early turn-taking, complementary actions, shared pretence	• Special relationships shown by preference for particular peers • Stability of friend relations is evident over time
Preschooler (2½–4 years)	• Verbal exchanges: shared plans for play, role-taking in pretend play • Joint pretend with complementary roles, feelings, sequences • Peers negotiate scripts and take on role identities and themes • Causal reasoning is evident in the sequence and emotional content of the narrative • Includes an awareness of the inner world of others, the thoughts, feelings, intentions of the characters	• Children use the term "friend(s)" to identify partner or group special relationships, and to exclude others • Intimacy and trust develops through pretend play and shared feelings/experiences
Early school-age (4–7 years)	• Gender differences evident in pretend play themes: for example, more aggression, rough and tumble, and competitiveness in boys; more social reciprocity, family roles, and cooperation in girls • Social pretend play becomes more complex: for example, children enact scripts from stories, television, videos, and real-life adult scenarios • Evidence of conciliation, negotiation, compromise through verbal exchanges over roles and resources	• Preference for same-sex friendships are evident • Girls' friendships are more intimate, with shared confidences, than boys' • Friendship networks develop, children use "labels" to include or exclude others • Expectation of friend relationships to be trustworthy and loyal and to provide social support
Middle school-age (7–10 years)	• Games with rules: public rules, social expectations, structured game scripts such as video and computer games • Gender differences in outdoor physical play: for example, games requiring large outdoor spaces for boys; more confined areas for girls • Gender "wars" over territory and access to resources are evident	• Same-sex groups differ in size and function; for example, boys' friendships are in large, "extensive" networks of playmates or "gangs;" girls' friendships are in smaller, "intensive" groups of companions or "cliques" • Friends become the child's preferred confidants, over family members • Active efforts are made to please friends and reinforce the relationship

mutually supportive and equitable exchanges, on-task behaviors, and effective ways of managing conflict (Hartup and Abecassis, 2004; Pellegrini and Blatchford, 2000).

At each stage of development, friendships with peers are beneficial for children's social functioning. Research consistently shows that children who have friends are advantaged socially and interpersonally; for example, they are more sociable, more prosocial, more altruistic, more self-confident, less aggressive, and less lonely (reviewed in Hartup and Abecassis, 2004). Furthermore, friendship in middle childhood has been found to decrease the incidence of bullying and to prevent children from having behavior problems (Dunn, 2004).

Social problems associated with childhood speech and language impairment

An understanding of social play and the role of friends is particularly relevant for parents, teachers, and professionals working with children who have speech impairments. Specific language impairment (SLI) has been associated with poor social skills, behavior problems, and difficulty in forming reciprocal friendships (reviewed in Brinton and Fujiki, 2004). These findings hold for both objective (teacher/parent ratings and observed behaviors) and subjective (self-report) measures of social difficulty. For example, in a study of 7 to 8 year old children with specific speech and language difficulties (SSLD) in the United Kingdom, problem behaviors were rated higher than the norm by both teachers and parents (Lindsay and Dockrell, 2001). Similar findings have been noted in the United States (Brinton and Fujiki). Observational data also supports teachers' ratings of peer difficulties. In a two-month study of playground play activities in 6 to 10 year old language-impaired (LI) children enrolled in regular school classrooms and attending speech-language services, and their matched typically developing peers, Fujiki, Brinton, Isaacson, and Summers (2001) observed less peer interaction in the LI children (mean = 54 percent; range = 35–85 percent) compared to typical children (mean = 80 percent; range = 47–100 percent), and more withdrawal/playing alone away from peers (42 percent vs. 17 percent). For the most part, LI children chose play activities that were less demanding of language comprehension or production, and there was little evidence of their being able to compensate for poor verbal abilities by engaging in nonverbal activities such as rough-and-tumble play or games. Interestingly, however, the most successful LI child in the Fujiki et al. study sustained a high level of peer interaction with other girls in a "house" play script by taking the role of "an unruly baby."

Studies have also noted that SLI is associated with problems of bullying by peers. Although Fujiki et al. (2001) found little evidence of aggressive behavior on the playground, when it did occur it tended to be shown by or directed toward the LI children. Subjective measures also note higher levels of bullying in LI children.

In a study of 100 11-year-old children with SLI attending mainstream classes in schools and special education classes, 36 percent reported some experience of bullying; whereas for non-SLI children the figure was 12 percent (Knox and Conti-Ramsden, 2003). The authors offer three interpretations of these findings. First, perceptions of being bullied are higher in SLI children because they are more sensitive to negative interactions or more likely to perceive peers' behavior in a negative light. Second, victimization may be due to SLI children's limited ability to retaliate verbally or a lack of confidence to report bullying. Third, SLI children may provoke others through their own antisocial behavior.

The difficulties that children with speech and/or language impairment have in developing positive peer relationships and friendships are often played out in group settings, such as child care, preschool, and school. Social and interpersonal adjustment and functioning in these settings will be considered in the following sections, which will review contextual feature s of these settings and propose a model for understanding the process of adjustment within the social and educational context.

The child care and early childhood context

When viewed within an ecological model, it is clear that child care and early childhood settings "are embedded within culture and societal organisations" (Howes and James, 2004, p. 140). Child care varies from one country to another in terms of regulatory arrangements, government subsidies, cost to the family, educational provisions, staff ratios and qualifications, and social acceptance/desirability. Within-country variations are similarly diverse (see OECD Early Childhood Education and Care Home Page, online at http://www.oecd.org). A range of options allows parents some opportunity to choose the type of care they prefer or feel is culturally appropriate for their child. Broadly speaking, there are three types of child care in Western contexts: (1) child care centers, in which groups of children of similar ages are cared for by adult caregivers with some level of specialist early childhood or child care qualification, (2) home-based child care, in which a small number of children are cared for by one caregiver who may or may not be supervised by qualified staff, and (3) own-home care for the child and perhaps a sibling or other child, which is provided by a relative, friend, or nanny without external supervision by qualified personnel.

As children move into the preschool years, there is more universal access to early childhood education. Termed "preschool" or "kindergarten," these center-based settings focus primarily on the educational needs of the child in the year(s) prior to entering school, rather than on the child care needs of working parents. In countries where children start school at 5 to 6 years of age, there tends to be a marked increase in attendance in early childhood programs once children reach 4 years: for example, Australia, 96 percent (Harrison and Ungerer, 2005); England, 99 percent (Prior, Courtney, and Charkin, 1999); United States, 65 percent (Kamerman and Gatenio, 2003). Where school entry is later, for example, age 7 years in Finland and Sweden, about two-thirds of 4-year-olds attend preschool: Finland, 66 percent (Valimaki, Ilmonen, Juva, and Hogstrom, 2000); Sweden, 69 percent (Gunnarsson, Korpi, and Nordenstam, 1999). Hours of preschool/kindergarten operation are generally tied to the school term, and working families who choose to use these settings may need to supplement this program with other child care arrangements (Harrison and Ungerer).

In recent years, particular attention has been given to the role that early childhood settings can play in supporting children with developmental difficulties, including speech impairment. A policy of inclusion is common in government-funded schools and services, and teacher training typically includes some provision for working with children with additional needs. The extent to which children's speech and language needs are supported varies between and within countries. In Finland, for example, the law requires that children in need of special care and education have a rehabilitation plan: "day care and rehabilitative early childhood education and care are usually arranged together with other children, (while) ensuring that the child gets the specialist services he or she needs and that the staff have sufficient training (to implement the plan)" (Valimaki et al., 2000, p. 50). In Canada, on the other hand, there are no requirements that services for children under 5 years enroll children with special needs (Doherty, Friendly, and Beach, 2003).

Social and interpersonal relationships in the context of early childhood settings

Child care and early childhood settings provide many children with their first experience of regular contact with adult caregivers/teachers and a group of similar-aged peers. For others, this occurs at school entry. Children's social and interpersonal adjustment to early childhood and school settings is influenced by two interrelated areas: (1) characteristics of the child, including the relationship history he or she has had in the home setting; and (2) the nature of the new relationships the child forms with adults and peers in the care setting. Figure 14-1 illustrates the processes of adjustment and summarizes the key factors and behaviors that impact this process (adapted from Birch and Ladd, 1996, and Howes and James, 2004). Adjustment is described in terms of the child's affective response to the setting, social interaction, and engagement with the learning opportunities that are provided. The dispositions and abilities that are inherent to the child, along with the child's experiences prior to entering a new child care, early childhood, or school setting, contribute directly to the child's adjustment to the new setting. In addition, these characteristics influence the quality of the interpersonal relationships formed in the new setting, which also contributes to adjustment.

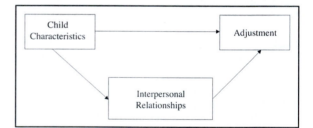

Figure 14-1 Model for understanding the process of adjustment and interpersonal relationships in childcare, early childhood settings, and school.

Friendships are known to have a powerful influence on children's and adolescents' feelings of well-being, classroom behavior, and academic achievement at all levels of schooling (Berndt and Keefe, 1996). Where friendships are characterized by positive features, school adjustment (positive attitudes, better behavior, higher academic achievement) and personal well-being (positive self-esteem, fewer emotional problems, more popularity) are enhanced. In contrast, children whose friendships have more negative features are less well adjusted in school (less classroom involvement, more disruptive behavior). These are important factors to keep in mind when considering the research evidence, presented earlier in this chapter, showing that children with speech and language impairment typically have difficulty interacting with peers and forming friendships. The final section will therefore focus on the ways that early childhood settings and schools can help children to develop supportive and stress-reducing peer relationships.

Educational contexts as supportive social environments

Children as young as 2 years are beginning to construct their own identities and to notice differences between themselves and others, and by age 3 may show stereotyping and bias in their interactions with children with disability (Manning-Morton and Thorp, 2003). Therefore, the types of experiences that children have in their early childhood years are crucial to developing an acceptance of self and of a diverse range of peers. Early childhood services must ensure that all children enjoy an environment that facilitates their development and is free of discrimination. Similarly, teachers and early childhood staff must show that they value everyone and the unique experiences they bring to the group. Fogarty (2003) argues that children who are disenfranchised need extra support and encouragement from teachers. More than that, they need teachers who actively organize peer support for them and challenge children who discriminate or exclude others. She suggests that classrooms can be organized so that children are required to negotiate, cooperate, and resolve problems with their able and less able peers, and are encouraged to focus more on their own behavior and resources rather than on judging or rejecting others.

Similar challenges are evident in schools. Opotow and Deutch (1999) describe the heterogeneous nature of school populations as a "fertile ground for conflict" but also argue that schools provide an environment for learning about conflict and "have immense potential to model and transmit the knowledge, attitudes, and behavior consistent with constructive approaches to conflict" (p. 206). These include cooperative learning, which expects students to work together in a spirit of individual accountability with each member providing appropriate support and assistance to the other; social skills training, which teaches strategies for polite, supportive interaction; conflict resolution training, which teaches students to accept the reality of difference, take the perspective of the other, and be alert to their own tendencies to bias, misperceptions, and stereotyped thinking; anger control; and mediation, which helps partners in conflict negotiate with each other. In these circumstances, learning about managing conflict with peers is by personal involvement or by observation. Bystanders to conflict situations in "conflict-positive" schools, which exemplify constructive conflict resolution in day-to-day functioning, are exposed to the desirability of facing conflict and learn skills for managing it. Constructive approaches to conflict also help victims to recognize that they have a choice in whether to stay in the conflict relationship and to be open and explicit to the other person about what he or she is doing and the effects of his or her actions.

SUMMARY

- Development occurs through a process of reciprocal interaction between the child and his or her immediate social environment, including home and out-of-home settings such as child care, preschool, and school.
- Attachment relationships with family members and nonparental adults are characterized by emotion regulation, secure base behavior, and affective sharing, which lay the foundation for self-regulation, self-awareness, self-reliance, autonomy, and cognitive growth.
- Peer relationships develop through social play, including nonverbal and verbal exchanges, joint pretend, and games.
- Friendships with peers provide social and interpersonal advantages, including greater sociability and more self-confidence, and reduce the incidence of bullying and behavior problems.
- Children with speech and language impairment tend to have poorer social skills, more behavior problems, and more difficulty in forming reciprocal friendships than their nonimpaired peers.
- Early childhood settings and schools must ensure that all children enjoy an environment that facilitates their development and is free of discrimination.
- Teachers can facilitate positive peer relations through active strategies to enhance social interaction, including cooperative learning, social skills training, conflict resolution training, anger control, and mediation.

REFERENCES

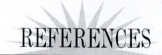

Berndt, T. J., and Keefe, K. (1996). Friends' influence on school adjustment: A motivational analysis. In J. Juvonen and K. R. Wentzel (Eds.), *Social motivation: Understanding children's school adjustment* (pp. 248–278). Cambridge, UK: Cambridge University Press.

Birch, S. H., and Ladd, G. W. (1996). Interpersonal relationships in the school environment and children's early school adjustment: The role of teachers and peers. In J. Juvonen and K. R. Wentzel (Eds.), *Social motivation: Understanding children's school adjustment* (pp. 199–225). Cambridge, UK: Cambridge University Press.

Brinton, B., and Fujiki, M. (2004). Social development in children with specific language impairment and profound hearing loss. In P. K. Smith and C. Hart (Eds.), *Blackwell handbook of childhood social development* (pp. 588–603). Malden, MA: Blackwell Publishing.

Bronfenbrenner, U. (1979) *The ecology of human development.* Cambridge, MA: Harvard University Press.

Bronfenbrenner, U. (1992/2005). Ecological systems theory. In U. Bronfenbrenner, (Ed.), *Making human beings human: Bioecological perspectives on human development* (pp. 106–173). Thousand Oaks, CA: Sage Publications.

Bronfenbrenner, U. (2001/2005). The bioecological theory of human development, In Bronfenbrenner, U. (Ed.) *Making human beings human. Bioecological perspectives on human development* (pp. 3–15). Thousand Oaks, CA: Sage Publications.

Doherty, G., Friendly, M., and Beach, J. (2003). OECD thematic review *early childhood education and care policy: Background report for Canada.* Retrieved November 16, 2006, from http://www.oecd.org/dataoecd/41/36/33852192.pdf

Dunn, J. (2004). *Children's friendships: The beginnings of intimacy.* Malden, MA: Blackwell Publishing.

Fogarty, F. (2003). "I listened carefully to the way children were spoken to"—equality and the under-threes! In L. Abbott and H. Moylett (Eds.), *Working with the under-3s: responding to children's needs* (pp. 142–148). Maidenhead, UK: Oxford University Press.

Fujiki, M., Brinton, B., Isaacson, T., and Summers, C. (2001). Social behaviors of children with language impairment on the playground: A pilot study. *Language, Speech, and Hearing in Schools, 32,* 101–113.

Gunnarsson, L., Korpi, B. M., and Nordenstam, U. (1999). OECD thematic review early childhood education and care. Background report prepared for Sweden. Retrieved November 16, 2006, from http://www.oecd.org/dataoecd/48/17/2479039.pdf

Harrison, L. J., and Ungerer, J. A. (2005). What can the Longitudinal Study of Australian Children tell us about infants' and 4 to 5-year-olds' experiences of education and care? *Family Matters, 72,* 26–35.

Hartup, W., and Abecassis, M. (2004). Friends and enemies. In P. K. Smith and C. Hart (Eds.), *Blackwell handbook of childhood social development* (pp. 285–306). Malden, MA: Blackwell Publishing.

Howes, C. (1996). The earliest friendships. In W. M. Bukowski, A. F. Newcomb, and W. W. Hartup (Eds.), *The company they keep: Friendship in childhood and adolescence* (pp. 66–86). Cambridge, UK: Cambridge University Press.

Howes, C., and James, J. (2004). Children's social development within the socialization context of childcare and early childhood education. In P. K. Smith and C. Hart (Eds.), *Blackwell handbook of childhood social development* (pp. 137–155). Malden, MA: Blackwell Publishing.

Kamerman, S., and Gatenio, S. (2003). Definitions, context, and provision, In U.S. Dept of Education, *OECD thematic review of early childhood education and care. Background report for the United States of America* (pp. 4–22). Available online: http://www.oecd.org/25/55/27856788.pdf

Knox, E., and Conti-Ramsden, G. (2003). Bullying risks of 11-year-old children with a specific language impairment (SLI): Does school placement matter? *International Journal of Language and Communication Disorders, 38,* 1–12.

Lindsay, G., and Dockrell, J. (2000). The behavior and self-esteem of children with specific speech and language difficulties. *British Journal of Educational Psychology, 70,* 583–601.

Manning-Morton, J., and Thorp, M. (2003). *Key times for play: The first three years.* Maidenhead, UK: Open University Press.

Mundy, P., and Willoughby, J. (1996). Nonverbal communication, joint attention, and early socioemotional development. In M. Lewis and M. W. Sullivan (Eds.), *Emotional development in atypical children* (pp. 43–64). Mahwah, NJ: Lawrence Erlbaum.

Opotow, S., and Deutch, M. (1999). Learning to cope with conflict and violence: How schools can help youth. In E. Frydenberg (Ed.), *Learning to cope: Developing as a person in complex societies* (pp. 198–224). Oxford, UK: Oxford University Press.

Pellegrini, A. D., and Blatchford, P. (2000). *The child at school: Interactions with peers and teachers.* London, UK: Arnold.

Prior, G., Courtney, G., and Charkin, E. (1999). *2ⁿᵈ survey of parents of three and four year old children and their use of early years* services, cited in Bertram, T. and Pascal, C. (n.d.). The OECD thematic review of early childhood education and care: Background report for the United Kingdom. Available online: http://www.oecd.org/48/16/2479205.pdf

Smith, P. K., Cowie, H., and Blades, M. (2003). *Understanding children's development* (4ᵗʰ ed.). Malden, MA: Blackwell Publishing.

Sroufe, L. A. (1996). *Emotional development: The organization of emotional life in the early years.* Cambridge, UK: Cambridge University Press.

Valimaki, A-M., Ilmonen, K., Juva, S., and Hogstrom, B. (2000). OECD thematic review of early childhood education and care. Background report for Finland. Available online: http://www.iecd.org/48/55/2476019.pdf

Chapter 15

Speech Acquisition and the Family

Nicole Watts Pappas and Caroline Bowen

INTRODUCTION

In the complex and multilayered ecology of childhood (Bronfenbrenner, 1979), children, families, and communities are interconnected, each influencing the other. Within this context, the astonishing process of speech acquisition is partly innate, and partly the product of observational learning. It cannot unfold without family, no matter what that elusive term implies for a particular child in today's world, where the diversity of family hierarchies and forms, in terms of structure, class, culture, and ethnicity, is emblematic. There is so much diversity that it is doubtful whether any society can still confidently identify its typical family structure. Family may be variously defined in terms of statistical and demographic census categories, in terms of households such as communes and kibbutzim, and in terms of kinship. A family's linguistic environment may be mono- or multicultural, mono- or multilingual, verbal or nonverbal. Family types include nuclear, extended, foster, adoptive, reconstituted, blended, homosexual, and sole parent forms. A remarkable global increase in single-parent families has occurred due to factors such as death, dislocation, lifestyle choice, divorce (where permitted), separation, desertion, and reduced stigmatization and increased social acceptance of single-parent situations. Taking a systemic, cross-cultural view, elders, ancestors, and relatively recently deceased family members influence family functioning and expectations of child rearing, tutelage, and development, even after they are dead, with the family reorganizing around the missing member, as in the case of sudden infant death or the passing of a parent or grandparent.

Human young are unique in their extended period of high reliance on caregivers. Because of this dependency, most of the speech that infants and young children hear comes from their immediate family, or from caregivers and sitters *in loco parentis*, who may or may not be classified by the family as family. These adults and older children exert a pervading influence on children's speech acquisition, even before first words are uttered. Indeed, preverbal children have intonation characteristics that reflect the composition of the ambient language (the language or languages their families speak). But how do prominent caregivers in a child's life listen and talk to them?

Modeling and child-directed speech

A mere 3 days after birth, infants prefer, and selectively attend to, human voices over other acoustic stimuli (Decasper and Fifer, 1980). The ability to imitate sounds is present as young as 4 weeks of age, and by 6 weeks infants engage in both immediate and deferred imitation. When families enjoy and respond positively to infant vocalizations (and who can resist them?), providing models and praising the baby's supposed speech attempts, they actually encourage increased vocalization, thereby fostering speech sound development. Imitation of environmental speech models and the gradual refinement of the syllables of infant babble lead to the production of first words, typically around the time of the baby's first birthday. Throughout this crucial zero to 1 period, and beyond, caregivers and older siblings from many cultures code-switch, altering the prosody of the way they usually speak and using motherese, parentese, or (more familiarly nowadays) child-directed speech (CDS). CDS is characterized by the use of a slower speech rate, shorter utterances, increased mean pitch of utterance, greater pitch range, and more variation in intonation when talking to infants and young children (Papousek and Papousek, 1989). Intriguingly, an infant responds more not only to his or her own mother's voice when she is using CDS but also to the parentese of other people, including siblings. Culturally conditioned, and by no means universal or instinctive, the predilection to use CDS is surmised to reside in a wish to draw children's attention to the speaker, increasing arousal levels, and so facilitating joint attention and speech imitation. Adults vary in their use of CDS, and family composition may affect its frequency. For example, Butler, McMahon and Ungerer (2003) found that twins' mothers use less CDS, possibly due to the time and energy demands of having to allocate care and attention to two babies, and a tendency to let them amuse each other.

Family history

Do typical and advanced speech acquisition run in families? That we do not know. But many studies reveal family aggregation of speech and language impairment. Rates of speech and language impairment in first-degree relatives of children with speech impairment (SI) range from 23 to 41 percent (Lewis, Freebairn, and Taylor, 2000). In a study conducted by Felsenfeld, McGue, and Broen (1995), 33 percent of children whose parent had a history of SI required treatment for that same speech impairment. Speculatively, the tendency for SI to run in families might be because the combined effects of poor speech and language genes, and less-than-favorable communicative environments, provide conditions conducive to the emergence of SI. Plausible though this theory may be, evidence to the contrary shows that the communicative environment provided by a parent with a history of SI does not appear to negatively impact a child's speech sound acquisition. The child whose adoptive parent has a history of SI is not at increased risk of speech difficulty, while an adopted child whose biological parent has an SI history is 1.2–7.5 percent more likely to have SI than a child whose parents have no such history (Felsenfeld and Plomin, 1997).

Socioeconomic status and education

Socioeconomic status (SES) is often invoked as a variable in linguistic and cognitive development, usually in the context of the frequently observed differences in the interpersonal communicative styles of higher and lower SES families. Typifying this body of work, Hart and Risley (1992) compared two groups, finding that higher SES parents spend more time speaking to their children and encourage them to talk more. These high SES parenting practices were positively associated with their children's later IQ scores. Hoff and Tian (2005) found that Chinese high SES mothers used larger vocabularies and longer utterances when speaking to their children than mothers of low SES, with a similar consequence: a positive association with their children's use of vocabulary. Corresponding findings in the area of speech sound acquisition are unavailable so, despite quantitative and qualitative differences between high and low SES parent-child communication patterns, no link has been demonstrated between SES and speech impairment.

Across cultures, parents' education levels influence the way that they interact with their children, while shaping their beliefs about their children's speech and language. Przetacznik-Gierowska, Kielar-Turska, Przetacznik, and Szatko (1992), for instance, found that parents with secondary or higher education were more likely to actively contribute to their children's development of language than parents with primary education only. As well as influencing the way that parents interact with their children and view speech and language, the education levels of parents, especially mothers, are associated with difficulties in speech sound acquisition. Campbell et al. (2003) established that maternal education was positively associated with SI. Importantly, they concluded that if a child was male and had a family history of both speech delay and low maternal education, he was a staggering 7.71 times more likely to have speech delay than a child with none of these features. It is unclear precisely *how* low maternal education might impact on speech sound acquisition, but Campbell and his team suggested that issues such as paucity of nutrition, medical care, and cognitive and language stimulation might combine to increase the risk of speech delay.

The cultural filter

Verbal and nonverbal communication are conditioned by culture, that is, the socially recognized practices, values, and beliefs that inform the way an individual acts and interprets the actions of others. Subject to factors such as age, gender, location, education, and SES, culture influences the communicative style of an individual, subject to factors such as age, gender, location, education, and SES, culture shapes and influences, without dictating responses or prescribing rules, the communicative style of an individual. That is why Hanson (1992, p. 3) preferred to describe culture as a "framework through which actions are filtered or checked as individuals go through daily life." It is important to note at this point that deeply held attitudes and beliefs about child development and adults' interactions with children are often below conscious awareness, differing dramatically between cultures. For example, the information presented here must reflect, to a degree, the authors' inevitable Western cultural bias and a frame of reference, or filter, firmly positioned in the comparatively prosperous industrialized world.

In middle-class Western communities children are considered from birth to be intentional communicators and therefore appropriate conversational partners (Marshall, 2000). By contrast, in some cultures, children are not necessarily regarded in this way until they reach a certain age or stage. For example, Samoan adults do not attribute meaning to infants' vocalizations (Shieffelin and Ochs, 1983), and the infant-parent interactions of Mexican American families (Kayser, 1995) and West African families living in the United Kingdom (Law, 2000) are largely nonverbal.

For the most part in Western culture, children are encouraged to be verbal; they are prompted to initiate conversations with adults, to direct topics, and to ask questions. Beyond the Western frame, there is a wide range of culturally driven rules around how, when, about what, and to whom children should speak. These rules include requiring children to be quietly respectful in the presence of adults and discouraging them from expressing opinions, asking questions, or directing topics. In this regard, Navajo mothers expect children to be quiet in the presence of adults (Marshall, 2000), while the Tamil of Malaysia believe that children should be allowed to speak only when directly addressed by another speaker (van Kleek, 1994). In Mexican American families, where children are not considered equal conversational partners, adults rarely ask children to express their interpretation of events or to say how they feel (Kayser, 1995). Meanwhile, Western Samoan children are obliged to listen and not ask adults questions (Ochs, 1986); and in African American families in the South, adults do not ask children interested questions or rhetorical (known answer) questions in order to engage them in conversation (Heath, 1982).

Beliefs about how children learn to speak also vary, with some caregivers providing explicit articulatory instruction. This happens with West African families living in the United Kingdom who believe talking needs to be specifically taught (Law, 2000), and among Chinese families who trust in nurture rather than nature, employing a directive talking style to teach children language (Johnston and Wong, 2002). But while Kenyan mothers think that children need to be taught in order to acquire motor skills, they do not consider that speech must be taught (Marshall, 2000), and Inuit people hold that speech is learned by observation rather than imitation (Crago, 1990).

Responses to impaired speech acquisition

Cultural and socioeconomic factors may affect a family's attitudes and responses to SI in one of its members, sometimes governing whether they see specialist, outside intervention as a desirable goal, and whether they would want to participate in any treatment regimen, if indeed family involvement were an option in their setting. The age (of a child) at which a family is likely to become concerned about speech difficulties may vary. For instance, Filipino families' understanding is that young children will often outgrow a problem (Roseberry-McKibbin, 1997).

Fatalistic assumptions, superstitions, and spiritual and other beliefs about the nature and causes of impairment are particularly prevalent cross-culturally. For example, some Korean people believe that SI is retribution for sins or parental misdemeanors or foolishness (Erickson, Devlieger, and Sung, 1999). In other cultures SI may be seen as a result of fate, possession by spirits, or a mark of mind-body imbalances (Danesco, 1997; Scheffner Hammer, 1994). In interviews of Mexican American families conducted by Maestas and Erikson (1992), 85 percent of parents understood that a disability was God's punishment for bad behavior, and more than half believed that someone casting evil spells produces disabilities in children. Paradoxically, in many cultures it is accepted that biomedical causes and other causes can co-occur. For example, participants in the study by Maestas and Erikson (1992) said a disability could be caused by God *and* by biomedical antecedents such as the expectant mother having a high fever or ingesting drugs. And of course, a range of cultural factors may deter families from seeking intervention. If SI is regarded as a punishment, a family may be too ashamed to enlist help, or, as in the case of Filipino families, they may fear loss of face for the family (Roseberry-McKibbin, 1997). Others, like those from Chamorro and Carolinian cultures, may see treatment as futile, because disabilities emanate from moral or spiritual sources and are therefore untreatable and incurable (Scheffner Hammer, 1994). In some cultures treatment from a witch doctor or medicine man, rather than intervention from clinicians, may be preferred; or, on the other hand, both interventions may be tried (Danesco, 1997).

There are intense differences and similarities, some subtle and others more overt, between societies, communities, and individuals in adults' expectations of, and relationships with, babies and children. Despite this variety, rates of speech acquisition have been reported to be similar across cultures. Families, it seems, are seeing much the same speech progress in their children, wherever they are.

Part of the expertise of the competent SLP is to be sensitive and open to families' beliefs and practices around development, child rearing, and customary interaction with infants and youngsters growing up, because all of these important factors vary. In a shrinking world, it is also incumbent upon speech and language professionals to recognize, accommodate, and respect the differing roles, expectations, and speech assessment and intervention practices of SLP colleagues, in *their* family, work, and community contexts, internationally. Occurring through a gradual, dynamic, and multifaceted process of genetic endowment, instinct, discovery, and learning, speech acquisition is inevitably the product of elements residing in the child and within the family, shaped by their unique cultural, social, and linguistic milieu.

SUMMARY

- Families are diverse in hierarchy, form, structure, class, culture, and ethnicity.
- Speech acquisition is partly innate and partly learned through observation.
- Families influence speech acquisition even before first words are uttered.
- Across cultures, child-directed speech is used to address children acquiring speech.
- There is a strong tendency for speech impairment (SI) to be inherited.
- Being raised by a parent with SI does not predispose a child to SI.
- Parent-child interactions differ in high and low SES families, but there is no demonstrable link between SES and either speech acquisition or impairment.
- A boy whose family history includes SI, and whose mother is poorly educated, is predisposed to SI.
- Responses to speech impairment differ across cultures.
- A family's culture does not impact the speech acquisition rates of its children.

REFERENCES

brenner, U. (1979). *The ecology of human development.* MA: Harvard University Press.

Butler, S., McMahon, C., and Ungerer, J. A. (2003). Maternal speech style with prelinguistic twin infants. *Infant & Child Development, 12*(2), 129–143.

Campbell, T. F., Dollaghan, C. A., Rockette, H. E., Paradise, J. L., Feldman, H. M., Shriberg, L. D. Sabao, D. L., & Kurs-Lasky, M. (2003). Risk factors for speech delay of unknown origin in 3-year-old children. *Child Development, 74,* 346–357.

Crago, M. (1990). Development of communicative competence, in Inuit children: Implications for speech-language pathology. *Journal of Childhood Communication Disorders, 13,* 73–83.

Danesco, E. R. (1997). Parental beliefs on childhood disability: Insights on culture, child development and intervention. *International Journal of Disability, Development and Education, 44*(1), 41–52.

Decasper, A., and Fifer, W. P. (1980). On human bonding: Newborns prefer their mother's voices. *Science, 208,* 1174–1176.

Erickson, J. G., Devlieger, P. J., and Sung, J. M. (1999). Korean-American female perspectives on disability. *American Journal of Speech-Language Pathology,* 8, 99–108.

Felsenfeld, S., McGue, M., and Broen, P. A. (1995). Familial aggregation of phonological disorders: Results from a 28-year follow-up. *Journal of Speech and Hearing Research, 38*(5), 1091–1107.

Felsenfeld, S., and Plomin, R. (1997). Epidemiological and offspring analyses of developmental speech disorders using data from the Colorado Adoption Project. *Journal of Speech, Language, and Hearing Research, 40*(4), 778–791.

Hanson, M. J. (1992). Ethnic, cultural, and language diversity in intervention settings. In E. W. Lynch and M. J. Hanson (Eds.), *Developing cross-cultural competence: A guide for working with young children and their families* (pp. 3–18). Baltimore: Brookes.

Hart, B., and Risley, T. R. (1992). American parenting of language-learning children: Persisting differences in family-child interactions observed in natural home environments. *Developmental Psychology, 28*(6), 1096–1105.

Heath, S. B. (1982). Questioning at home and at school: A comparative study. In G. Spindler (Ed.), *Doing the ethnography of schooling: Educational anthropology in action* (pp. 102–131). New York: Holt, Rhinehart & Winston.

Hoff, E., and Tian, C. (2005). Socioeconomic status and cultural influences on language. *Journal of Communication Disorders, 38,* 271–278.

Johnston, J. R., and Wong, M. Y. A. (2002). Cultural differences in beliefs and practices concerning talk to children. *Journal of Speech, Language, and Hearing Research, 45,* 916–926.

Kayser, H. (1995). Intervention with children from linguistically and culturally diverse backgrounds. In M. E. Fey, J. Windsor, and S. F. Warren (Eds.), *Language intervention: Preschool through the elementary years* (Vol. 5, pp. 315–331). Baltimore, MA: Paul H. Brookes.

Law, J. (2000). Factors affecting language development in West African children: A pilot study using a qualitative methodology. *Child: Care, Health & Development, 26*(4), 289–308.

Lewis, B. A., Freebairn, L. A., and Taylor, H. G. (2000). Academic outcomes in children with histories of speech sound disorders. *Journal of Communication Disorders, 33*(1), 11–30.

Maestas, A. G., and Erikson, J. G. (1992). Mexican immigrant mothers' beliefs about disabilities. *American Journal of Speech-Language Pathology, 1*(4), 5–10.

Marshall, J. (2000). Critical reflections on the cultural influences in identification and habilitation of children with speech and language difficulties. *International Journal of Disability, Development and Education, 47*(4), 355–369.

Ochs, E. (1986). Introduction. In B. Schieffelin and E. Ochs (Eds.), *Language socialization across cultures* (pp. 1–16). Cambridge, UK: Cambridge University Press.

Papousek, H., and Papousek, M. (1989). Intuitive parenting: Aspects related to educational psychology. *European Journal of Psychology of Education, 4*(2), 201–210.

Przetacznik-Gierwoska, M., Kielar-Turska, M., Przetacznik, J., and Szatko, D. (1992). Parents' beliefs about their children's language development and stimulation. *Polish Psychological Bulletin, 23*(2), 139–152.

Roseberry-McKibbin, C. (1997). Understanding Filipino families: A foundation for effective service delivery. *American Journal of Speech-Language Pathology, 6*(3), 5–14.

Scheffner Hammer, C. (1994). Working with families of Chamorro and Carolinian cultures. *American Journal of Speech-Language Pathology, 3*(3), 5–12.

Schieffelin, B. B., and Ochs, E. (1983). A cultural perspective on the transition from prelinguistic to linguistic communication. In R. M. Golinkoff (Ed.), *The transition from prelinguistic to linguistic communication* (pp. 115–131). Hillsdale, NJ: Lawrence Erlbaum.

van Kleeck, A. (1994). Potential cultural bias in training parents as conversational partners with their children who have delays in language development. *American Journal of Speech-Language Pathology, 3(1),* 67–77.

Chapter 16

Personal Factors and their Influence on Speech Acquisition

Amy L. Weiss

INTRODUCTION

Investigators of child language acquisition have long been interested in describing unified developmental steps and stages. The focus on delineating a uniform path to language competence was probably fueled by the many observed similarities in language development across children and languages (Bates, Dale, and Thal, 1995). At the same time, theories proposed universal principles of speech and language development (Jakobson, 1968; and Stampe, 1973, for speech acquisition). In turn, this belief may have been desirable for clinical practitioners because divergence from a unitary path to language competence would make designation of abnormal development relatively easy.

More recently, however, researchers have reported considerable normal variability in development, both in quality (style) and quantity (rate) of development (Bates, Bretherton, and Snyder, 1988; Bates et al., 1995; Stoel-Gammon, see Chapter 10). Note that the term "normal variability" reflects a stable degree of variation around a core of central developmental tendencies. Leonard, Newhoff, and Mesalem (1980) presented evidence supporting their contention that although young children's early phonological systems may not be identical, the magnitude of their differences does not normally extend beyond specific limits.

One frequently cited example of individual differences in language development focused on vocabulary or lexical acquisition. Nelson (1973) interpreted her study of toddlers' first 50-word vocabulary development as providing evidence for two different lexical styles, one where children acquired a preponderance of nouns and one that was somewhat less noun focused. Additional characteristics appeared to separate the two word-learning groups.

Of particular interest to this chapter was a perceived difference in the articulatory precision observed for members of the two style groupings. The children with larger proportions of nouns in their first vocabularies (referred to as *referential* by Nelson, 1973) tended to be more intelligible than their less noun-focused counterparts (referred to as *expressive* stylists by Nelson) The latter group of vocabulary learners, also referred to as *pronominal* or *holistic* in subsequent studies by other investigators (see Bloom, Lightbown, and Hood, 1975; Nelson, 1981; Peters, 1983), showed a tendency to produce formulae. Although formulae may appear to be multiple words produced as one (e.g., /gɪmidæt/ for *give me that*, or /nowanɪt/ for *no want it*), there is no indication that children recognize that their mega words can be divided further into individual words or sounds. According to Ingram (1976), young children may learn many of their first words in an imitative, nonproductive manner. That is, children are using a top–down or holistic word learning style rather than a bottom–up, analytic style of learning to determine word and phoneme boundaries.

Individual differences have also been observed in specific studies of speech sound acquisition. In a recent analysis of consonant cluster development in Australian English-speaking children, McLeod, van Doorn, and Reed (2001) concluded that although several general trends of development were supported, individual variation was also in evidence. Normal variation manifested itself in the size of cluster repertoire, percentage of consonant clusters correctly produced, and closer approximations to adult phoneme targets. Thus, all of the children were making some gains in consonant cluster development, but McLeod et al. (2001) recognized that capturing evidence of those gains required use of different measurement rubrics.

What explains children's adoption of different pathways to speech acquisition? Are there factors that may be used to explain why some children are slower or more rapid in their rate of developing an adultlike sound system, for example? Further, are these same factors useful in explaining the presence of bona fide disorders of speech acquisition? The answers to these questions can facilitate both better understanding of normal speech and language acquisition and clinical decision making as well. In support of this perspective, Meltzoff (1999) noted that much of the work reported about the language of children diagnosed with autism and Williams syndrome has informed understanding of normal language development in terms of the relationship between cognition and language.

The remainder of this chapter will provide a delineation of proposed personal factors whose role in speech acquisition is only beginning to be understood in most cases. Some of the personal factors that have been investigated more easily lend themselves to study (e.g., age, gender, cognitive ability). Others are more difficult to quantify (e.g., motivation, self-confidence, belief system) but are no less important.

What the child brings to the development table

Age and gender

Age may be the less interesting of the two factors because it is generally accepted that children's speech acquisition will normalize by 9 years (Shriberg, Gruber, and Kwiatkowski, 1994). Age is also easily confounded by maturation in social, physiological, and cognitive realms, making it problematic to study on its own. That is, in the typical child we also assume that development will simultaneously ensue on a number of fronts. For example, it is probable that as children gain more control over their muscle coordination with age and can reliably recognize when their sound productions are not consistent with internalized models, they have attained prerequisite skills for normalizing their speech sound system. Thus, the older the child, the more likely he or she is to have normalized speech, with all other variables held constant.

In one of the largest and most carefully controlled studies of speech acquisition in General American English–speaking children, Smit, Hand, Freilinger, Bernthal, and Bird (1990) documented the speech acquisition patterns of approximately 1,000 children ranging in age from 3;0 (years; months) to 9;0. In this cross-sectional study, the investigators noted that the curves produced by separately plotting the scores (for correct responses) for male and female participants were similar but far from identical. Although the girls' developmental curve could be described as both continuous and steep, the boys' data produced a flatter curve, indicating less rapid development, and a plateau in the middle of the age span tested between 3;6 and 4;6. Ultimately, the gender groups achieved normalization, but the path to that normalization was somewhat different. Based on the Smit et al. data, girls are more likely to acquire speech at a more rapid pace than their male counterparts.

Cognitive ability

It is generally accepted that there is no direct correlation between intelligence and speech acquisition, provided that an individual demonstrates intelligence within the normal range (Bernthal and Bankson, 2004). Persons with IQs below 70, however, are likely to present with some inconsistent articulation errors, most often consonant deletions. The observations by Shriberg and Widder (1990) suggested that the speech patterns of most individuals with mental retardation looked very much like those observed in young children learning their sound system.

Of course cognitive ability is more broadly defined than an intelligence quotient. Developmental psychologists have reported individual differences in infants' abilities to attend to novel stimuli that may have implications for later developmental achievements (Rose and Feldman, 1990). As these researchers noted, differences in attention task performance may be less related to cognitive skill and more influenced by noncognitive factors such as "avoidance of change," a factor that would fit in the category of temperament trait (p. 241). Moreover, Bates and her colleagues (Bates et al., 1988) have suggested that children who adopt a holistic, top-down word-learning strategy, like that observed in *expressive* children, may have more highly developed perceptual competencies than their peers, allowing them to better memorize long strings of sounds for formula production.

Motivation to change speech behavior

There are several anecdotal reports in the speech-language pathology literature reflecting on why and when children with disorders of speech acquisition are motivated to make changes in their speech behavior. Traditionally, motivators for change have been viewed as reinforcement (Shriberg and Kwiatkowski, 1982), but it is also possible that each young child acquiring his or her sound system has an individual, internal "switch" that may enhance or hold back progress.

Weiss (2004) presented the story of a 5 year old boy named Sid with a long-standing speech disorder that rendered his speech mostly unintelligible. Sid had been enrolled in several years of speech therapy that had failed to result in much functional change. After an absence of several weeks due to illness, Sid returned to therapy with a vastly improved speech sound system. The speech-language pathologist (SLP) struggled to determine what had finally precipitated change. She remembered one session shortly before Sid's hiatus when he had asked the SLP whether she understood his much younger sister better than she could understand him. The SLP had answered in the affirmative and noted

Sid's reaction as "a look of sadness" (p. 225). Weiss wondered whether Sid had found himself in an untenable situation where his role as big brother to his sister had been compromised. That is, Sid may have decided to shift his personal construct of identity to be consistent with that of a more intelligible speaker with normalized speech (Hayhow, 1987) as a result of this exchange with his SLP. Accomplishing this feat required him to marshal all of his focus (and prerequisite motor and perceptual skills) to make substantive positive changes to his speech system.

In another example, Kamhi (2000) described the course of speech therapy for his daughter, Franne. Early on in her therapy program, Franne refused to practice her sounds outside of the therapy setting. Her father concluded that Franne was aware, even at her very young age, of "the basic incompatibility between practicing speech sounds and communicating effectively" (p. 183). Kamhi, who characterized his daughter as stubborn, suggested that Franne was able to make the meta-pragmatic distinction between speech as a means for meaningful communication and decontextualized practice. Franne was not interested in her parents' criticisms of how she spoke but instead wanted them to attend to the message she was trying to convey.

It is impossible to do more than speculate about these two children's underlying motivations that facilitated progress, in Sid's case, or threw up a barrier to change, in Franne's case. In light of what we know about children's more precocious cognitive skills (Meltzoff, 1999), however, it may be wise to assume that both children had some control over their progress in therapy. Their differing perspectives provided more or less motivation to work on their speech.

Theory of mind

In Franne's world (see Kamhi, 2000, above), speaking had one important function and that was communicating. Franne recognized that her parents' intentions in their conversations with her were not only for conversation but to use conversation as a therapeutic context. Because Franne was able to perceive the underlying goals her parents had for their interactions with her, we can say that Franne was demonstrating a level of social cognition referred to as *Theory of Mind* (Cutting and Dunn, 1999). In Franne's case, as noted above, her ability to perceive her parents' intentions led to a roadblock in her therapeutic progress due to the mismatch between the child's and parents' perspectives.

In many cases, however, possessing theory of mind may place a young child in line for more success in typical speech acquisition and therapeutic speech habilitation. To understand the underlying beliefs of the conversation partner likely means that actions, such as nodding agreement or quizzical looks, are considered. That is, when a young child is attempting to convey a message, the response of the partner is noted. When misunderstood, the child will be more likely to persist in trying to fix the message so that the intended message is conveyed.

Cutting and Dunn (1999) noted that individual differences were apparent in the social cognition skills of their preschool-age children, including theory of mind. Their findings indicated that parents' occupations and mothers' education levels were positive predictors of the presence of social cognition competencies when language and age were held constant.

Temperament

Temperament has been described as a genetically determined set of traits that can be identified early on in a child's development and may include level of anxiety, degree of stimulus seeking, and orientation on an extroversion-introversion continuum (Strelau, 1998). Others view temperament traits as a subset of personality. Although personality is believed to be a product of social environment, temperament is generally accepted as inherited and left unchallenged by circumstance, persistent in its presence across the life span of an individual.

In terms of speech acquisition, temperament may be associated with perseverance when faced with challenging language-learning tasks. Learning the phonemes of one's language represents only one of several symbol systems involved in language learning. Some children may express frustration in this process while others may embrace the challenge as demonstrated by risk-taking behavior. For example, although they may not have mastered a sound, children do not avoid using words with that sound.

The utility of individual differences

Identifying individual differences in speech acquisition has its practical side as well. When Gierut (1998) summarized the state of treatment efficacy research for children with speech sound disorders, she concluded that a more complete understanding of individual differences in phonological learning was needed. This information would help to determine the facilitating contexts that would enhance change during therapy for individual children. That is, better answers for the "goodness of fit" between child and therapy technique would result.

Similarly, the *Capability-Focus Framework* described by Shriberg (1997) is an attempt to represent the child-centered factors that have been difficult to quantify when analyzing the genesis of success or failure of the therapeutic process. Shriberg noted that children bring to the therapy context varying degrees of "focus" that include both a relative need for external motivational events (reinforcement) as well as the amount of effort exerted by individual children to succeed. The author observed that both retrospective and prospective studies of therapy outcomes have demonstrated "the potential contribution of the focus concept for prediction and treatment decisions" (Shriberg, 1997, p. 126).

Weiss (2004) also proposed that children with speech impairments contribute to the success of their therapy through their willingness to accept responsibility for its outcome. She noted that in the United States, at least, therapy models often neglect the importance of what the child brings to the therapy context in favor of focus on the SLP's techniques. Measures such as the *Child Behavior Checklist* (Achenbach, 1991) and the *Locus of Control Behavior Scale* (Craig, Franklin, and Andrews, 1984) can be used to guide SLPs in understanding the child's view of the speech impairment. That is, is "it" something viewed as outside of his or her control, or is it something viewed as controllable and thus addressable in therapy? Is changing the child's attitude toward the speech impairment a worthy goal in itself for therapy? In this way, the child's temperament is considered as an important factor in determining therapy success or failure. For example, if the child is a risk taker, according to Weiss (2004), he or she will be more willing to attempt tasks that are challenging.

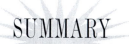

SUMMARY

- There is ample evidence to show that typical children do not acquire speech in exactly the same progression, just as is the case in other areas of language learning.
- Although children's development is not identical, the differences observed fall within "a clearly defined range of possibilities" (Leonard, Newhoff, and Mesalem, 1980, p. 12).

- Personal factors, including age, gender, cognitive ability, motivation, theory of mind, and temperament may be at the heart of why and how children move forward with speech acquisition and why therapy for children with speech impairments succeeds or fails.
- It is important for SLPs to consider individual differences and what each child brings to speech-language therapy.

REFERENCES

Achenbach, T. (1991). *Manual for the child behavior checklist/4-18 and 1991 Profile.* Burlington: University of Vermont Department of Psychiatry.

Bates, E., Bretherton, I., and Snyder, L. (1988). *From first words to grammar: Individual differences and dissociable mechanisms.* New York: Cambridge University Press.

Bates, E., Dale, P., and Thal, D. (1995). Individual differences and their implications for theories of language development. In P. Fletcher and B. MacWhinney (Eds.), *Handbook of child language* (pp. 96–151). Oxford: Basil Blackwell.

Bernthal, J. E., and Bankson, N. W. (2004). *Articulation and phonological disorders* (5th ed.). Boston: Pearson Education.

Bloom, L., Lightbown, L., and Hood, L. (1975). Structure and variation in child language. *Monographs for the Society for Research in Child Development, 40,* Serial #160.

Craig, A., Franklin, J., and Andrews, G. (1984). A scale to measure locus of control of behaviour. *British Journal of Medical Psychology, 57,* 173–180.

Cutting, A., and Dunn, J. (1999). Theory of mind, emotion understanding, language, and family background: Individual differences and interrelations. *Child Development, 70,* 853–865.

Gierut, J. (1998). Treatment efficacy: Functional phonological disorders in children. *Journal of Speech, Language, and Hearing Research, 41(1),* S61–S84.

Hayhow, R. (1987). Personal construct therapy with children who stutter and their families. In C. Levy (Ed.), *Stuttering therapies: Practical approaches* (pp. 1–18). London: Croom Helm.

Ingram, D. (1976). *Phonological disability in children.* London: Edward Arnold.

Jakobson, R. (1968). *Child language, aphasia, and phonological universals.* The Hague: Mouton.

Kamhi, A. (2000). Practice makes perfect: The incompatibility of practicing speech and meaningful communication. *Language, Speech, and Hearing Services in Schools, 31,* 182–185.

Leonard, L., Newhoff, M., and Mesalem, L. (1980). Individual differences in early child phonology. *Applied Psycholinguistics, 1,* 7–30.

McLeod, S., van Doorn, J., and Reed, V. (2001). Consonant cluster development in two-year-olds: General trends and individual difference. *Journal of Speech, Language, and Hearing Research, 44,* 1144–1171.

Meltzoff, A. (1999). Origins of mind, cognition and communication. *Journal of Communication Disorders, 32,* 251–269.

Nelson, K. (1973). Structure and strategy in learning to talk. *Monograph of the Society for Research in Child Development, 38* (1 & 2, Serial #149).

Nelson, K. (1981). Individual differences in language development: Implications for development and language. *Developmental Psychology, 17,* 170–187.

Peters, A. (1983). *The units of language acquisition.* Cambridge, UK: Cambridge University Press.

Rose, S., and Feldman, J. (1990). Infant cognition: Individual differences and developmental continuities. In J. Colombo and J. Fagen (Eds.), *Individual differences in infancy: Reliability, stability, prediction* (pp. 229–246). Hillsdale, NJ: Lawrence Erlbaum.

Shriberg, L. (1997). Developmental phonological disorders: One or many? In B. Hodson and M. Edwards (Eds.), *Perspectives in applied phonology* (pp. 105–131). Gaithersburg, MD: Aspen Publications.

Shriberg, L., Gruber, F., and Kwiatkowski, J. (1994). Developmental phonological disorders III: Long-term speech-sound normalization. *Journal of Speech and Hearing Research, 37,* 1151–1177.

Shriberg, L., and Kwiatkowski, J. (1982). Phonological disorders II: A conceptual framework for management. *Journal of Speech and Hearing Disorders, 47,* 242–256.

Shriberg, L., and Widder, C. (1990). Speech and prosody characteristics of adults with mental retardation. *Journal of Speech and Hearing Research, 33,* 627–653.

Smit, A., Hand, L., Frelinger, J., Bernthal, J., and Bird, A. (1990). The Iowa articulation norms project and its Nebraska replication. *Journal of Speech and Hearing Disorders, 55,* 779–798.

Stampe, D. (1973). *A dissertation on natural phonology.* Unpublished doctoral dissertation, University of Chicago.

Strelau, J. (1998). *Temperament, a psychological perspective.* New York: Plenum Press.

Weiss, A. (2004). The child as agent for change in therapy for phonological disorders. *Child Language Teaching and Therapy, 20(3),* 221–244.

Chapter 17

Multilingual Speech Acquisition

Mehmet Yavaş

INTRODUCTION

The definition of bilingualism (or multilingualism) has been a controversial issue among scholars for a long time, because the concept defies delimitations and is open to a variety of interpretations. While some require nativelike control of two (or more) languages (Bloomfield, 1933), others see the alternate use of two languages as sufficient for bilingualism (Mackey, 1970; Weinreich, 1968). As Beatens-Beardsmore (1982, p. 1) put it elegantly, bilingualism "as a concept has open-ended semantics."

The recognition of the two types of bilingualism is much less controversial. In *simultaneous bilingualism*, languages are acquired simultaneously, while in *successive bilingualism*, the child acquires one language, generally the home language, earlier, and the other language is acquired when he or she enters school.

One system or two

Whether a bilingual (or multilingual) speaker has one or two (or more) systems for the languages he or she uses has also been subject to considerable controversy. This seems to be particularly relevant in the discussion of simultaneous bilingualism. While several researchers (Deuchar and Clark, 1992; Genesee, 1989; Genesee, Nicoladis, and Paradis, 1995; Ingram, 1981) adhere to the idea of separate systems, many others (Burling, 1959; Imedadze, 1967; Leopold, 1949; Major, 1977; Vogel, 1975; Yavaş, 1995) suggest that there is one undifferentiated system. One of the likely reasons for the disagreement is that the researchers studied different stages. The ones who defend one undifferentiated system for two languages have looked at early stages such as the 50-word period, while the proponents of separate systems looked beyond this stage. There is also another view (Vihman, 2002), which argues that the question of whether bilinguals at first have one or two systems is not meaningful, because before the child develops a fairly substantial vocabulary of about 100 words, there is no system at all. This view, however, is different from others, as it is based on phonemic contrasts rather than the phonetic features relevant to the two languages and/or phonological selectivity/avoidance. Thus, we can suggest that, in the beginning, the child is likely to have one undifferentiated system for two languages, and around age 2 the two systems may become differentiated.

Separating one system into two systems does not mean that the individual will have completely independent phonological and phonetic systems, each identical in all ways to those of monolinguals. In other words, as stated by Grosjean (1992, p. 52), the view that "a bilingual has two separate and isolable language competencies and these competencies are similar to those of two corresponding monolinguals" is a myth rather than a fact; the bilingual is not two monolinguals in one person. Watson (1991) argues that while two completely independent systems is a possibility for *perfectly bilingual* bilinguals, a more common occurrence is a bilingual with two systems that differ in some ways from those of monolinguals. The more balanced a bilingual is, the more he or she approximates the nativelike productions in the respective languages. This may manifest itself in productions that are *impressionistically indistinguishable* from monolinguals, but nevertheless not identical when measured instrumentally. Watson interprets this as a sign of economy whereby the speaker does the minimum necessary to be taken as a native speaker of the language without going into the imperceptible details, which are present in the productions of a monolingual.

If the rarely seen *perfectly balanced bilinguals* are not two monolinguals in one person, the typical (not perfectly balanced) ones yield the effects of the dominant language.

Interaction between languages

The interaction between languages (i.e., interference or transfer from one language to the other) has been subject to many studies. Whether a child becomes bilingual simultaneously or successively, it is impossible to rule out interference. This is an important area for speech-language pathologists, because it is crucial to determine if the erroneous patterns with respect to the speech of monolingual speakers are due to the influence of the subject's other language or are indications of a speech-language disorder. The results of interference may manifest themselves because of varying mismatches between the two languages.

Interference in segmental aspects of speech

Missing phoneme

While English has its alveolar fricative phonemes in both voiced and voiceless versions (/s/, /z/), Spanish has only the voiceless one. The target words demanding English /z/ (e.g., *zeal, zip*) may be realized as [sil] and [sip] respectively by a Spanish-English bilingual.

Sounds that are shared by the two languages but have different phonemic status

Two or more sounds may be in contrast in one language, yet they may be allophones of one phoneme in the other language. For example, although sounds [s], [z], and [ʃ] are shared by English and Korean, their phonological status are very different. While these three sounds are in contrast in English, as can be shown in *sip – zip – ship*, they are allophones of the same phoneme in Korean ([ʃ] occurs before /i/, [z] occurs after a nasal, and [s] occurs in other environments). In other words, the three-way phonemic distinction of English is underdifferentiated in Korean. As a result, a sequence such as *sea shells* is likely to be pronounced as [ʃi sɛls] by a Korean-English bilingual.

Salient phonetic differences

Two sounds may have the same phonetic descriptions in two languages but their phonetic realizations may be perceptually very different. A good example of this is the alveolar lateral liquids in English and Arabic. The phonetic realization of American English post-vocalic lateral is a dark /l/, while the realization in Arabic (and many other languages) is a clear /l/. Thus, the practical consequence is that the name *Bill*, which has a dark /l/ in English, would typically be pronounced differently (with a clear /l/) by an Arabic-dominant Arabic-English bilingual.

Different distributional patterns

Two sounds may have the same phonemic status in two languages but may have different distributions. For example, although both English and German contrast voiced and voiceless stops (/p/ – /b/, /t/ – /d/, and /k/ – /g/) in initial and medial positions, only English maintains the contrast in final position; German neutralizes the opposition in favor of the voiceless member of each pair. Consequently, we can find [p, t, k] only in final position in German. The result of this mismatch is the commonly found production of the voiceless member of each pair instead of the voiced English targets (e.g., *cab* realized as [kæp], *bed* realized as [bɛt], *bag* realized as [bæk] by a German-dominant bilingual).

Interference in phonotactic and suprasegmental aspects of speech

Patterns of interference are not restricted to segmental aspects of speech; they are also found in phonotactics as well as suprasegmental aspects. For an example of a mismatch in phonotactic patterns (i.e., sequential patterns) we can compare the syllable structure of English with those of Turkish, Persian, and Korean. While English allows triple onsets (three consonants in syllable-initial position) as in *sprint*, the above-mentioned three languages do not even allow double onsets. Thus, a bilingual person whose dominant language is one of these reveals interferences in attempting double/triple onsets of English (e.g., *spray* realized as [sipire] by a Turkish-English bilingual).

Finally, mismatches in stress and timing are frequent sources of interference. For example, the stress in French falls on the last syllable. In English, by contrast, the placement of stress is variable, and generally not on the last syllable. Thus, the nonnative final stress patterns in English targets are examples commonly found in the speech of French-English bilinguals. Mismatches of timing are rather typical if a bilingual speaks one stress-timed language (i.e., a language in which the stressed syllables tend to occur at roughly equal intervals in time, like English) and one syllable-timed language (i.e., the rhythmic beat by the recurrences of syllables, not stresses; like Spanish). One of the significant differences between the two types of languages lies in the differences of length between stressed and unstressed syllables, and vowel reduction or lack of it. The English word *probability* and its Spanish cognate *probabilidad* reveal the differences nicely. Although the words share the same meaning and the same number of syllables, the similarities end there. In Spanish, the stress is on the last syllable [proßa-iliðăð]. Furthermore, although the remaining syllables are unstressed, they all have full vowels, and the duration of all five syllables is approximately the same. In English [pràbəbíləti] it is the third syllable that receives the main stress and the first syllable has a secondary stress. The first, third, and the last syllables have full vowels, while the second and the fourth have a reduced vowel [ə], which has much less duration than the others. The frequently observed phenomenon in the English of Spanish-dominant bilinguals is the lack of vowel reductions resulting in nonnative productions.

Blurring of interference and developmental processes

While the above examples may have had convincing explanations through interference, the decision may not always be so straightforward in that the nonnative productions may reflect universal developmental simplification processes. This is a situation where we see a cross-linguistically common process occurring in the speech of a child whose dominant language does not provide any evidence of such. For example, if a 5- to 6-year-old Portuguese-dominant Portuguese-English-speaking bilingual reveals a process of final obstruent devoicing (e.g., *bag* realized as [bæk]), we cannot blame the first language, because Portuguese does not allow any stops (voiced or voiceless) in final position. This, however, is a commonly occurring process, which is also experienced by monolingual English-speaking children (typically suppressed before age 3). The reason that a 6-year-old Portuguese-English-speaking child reveals this pattern after the typical age of suppression is the fact that it is not demanded by the structure of Portuguese before then.

There is also another possibility for blurring the distinction between interference and developmental processes. This can occur when a universally motivated developmental process is also part of the dominant language of the bilingual. For example, cross-linguistically the sonorant consonants (liquids, nasals) are preferred over obstruents (stops, fricatives, affricates) as single codas. In other words, if a language permits obstruents as single coda consonants, it automatically allows sonorants in that position, but the reverse does not hold. When a bilingual whose dominant language allows only sonorant codas (e.g., Mandarin Chinese) deals with a language that allows both obstruents (e.g., stops, fricatives, and affricates, /p/, /d/, /s/, /tʃ/) and sonorants (e.g., nasals, liquids, and glides, /n/, /l/ /j/) as single codas (e.g., English), the likelihood of nonnative erroneous productions is on the obstruent codas rather than on the sonorant codas. While this would be in accordance with the patterns of the dominant language, it also is fostered by the cross-linguistically unmarked preference for sonorants in that position.

In all the examples cited above, with respect to interference, the dominant language had the effect on the weaker language. This is not a baseless assumption, especially when there is a very obvious discrepancy in the levels of competence in the two languages involved. Such cases are commonplace in the early stages of the successive bilingual's acquisition of the second language. However, if the imbalance between languages is not that significant, we may end up having a variety of patterns. Gildersleeve, Davis, and Stubbe (1997), while looking at the influence of the vowel systems between two languages (Spanish and English in this case), found that the acoustic characteristics for the majority of vowels produced by their bilingual child subjects were between the values for English monolingual and Spanish monolingual children.

Among the topics studied in contact phonologies, voice onset time (VOT) has been a popular focus of attention. The relevance of studying VOT comes from the fact that its values have been claimed to be closely correlated with overall degree of authentic nativelike speech (Flege and Efting, 1987; Major, 1987).

Kehoe, Lleo, and Rakow (2004) looked at the voice onset time (VOT) patterns in four German-Spanish bilingual children and found a great deal of variability across subjects. While one of the subjects (the most balanced between the two languages) had no cross-language interference, another subject showed transfer of voicing patterns from one system to another. This (German-dominant) subject, at 2;3, produced voiced stops of German with lead voicing (like Spanish voiced stops produced by monolinguals); at 2;6, the same subject showed the transfer of long lag (aspirated) German voiceless stops in the production of Spanish voiceless stops, which are typically short lag (unaspirated). Yavaş (2002), concentrating on voiceless stops, reported instability in the acquisition of VOT by 10 Spanish-English bilingual children (who were aged approximately 7 years but had received consistent exposure to English only since entering school at the age of 5 to 6 years). While two of these subjects showed the expected Spanish influence over English, two others revealed the opposite tendency. The measurements for other subjects all pointed toward mutual influence of the two languages on each other resulting in compromise values. Compromise VOT values were also reported in older populations (Flege, 1987, 1991; Lowie, 1988; Nathan, Anderson, and Budsaba, 1987).

Several studies, however, suggest that early second language (L2) learners may keep their two languages clearly separate and produce stops in an authentic manner in the two languages involved. Williams (1977) reported that children who learned both English and Spanish by age 6 were equal to monolingual English and Spanish speakers in VOT values. Mack (1989) reported similar results for French-English bilinguals at age 7. Conclusions that early bilinguals have nativelike VOT productions can also be found in Flege (1991) and Yavaş (1996).

Besides the information on interference patterns, speech-language pathologists must use information from normal and disordered phonological development in general as well as from the two (or more) languages of the individual. In the bi/multilingual assessment, all languages of the subject should be the focus of attention, and, in order to prevent over- or underdiagnosis, each language should be examined in detail. To this end, all phonemes of the languages should be assessed in different positions, and phonotactic patterns should be carefully evaluated. The unavailability of assessment tools in many languages can make this task difficult, but the assessment tools that are designed for English would be inappropriate for other languages.

Last but not least is the issue of dialect. Since all languages show dialectal variations, to be able to differentiate disorder from differences due to dialectal features, information on the subject's dialectal background is essential. The lack of this information may either result in the misdiagnosis of a phonological disorder or escalate the subject's severity rating.

Acquisition of phonology in speakers who use more than one language is a highly complex phenomenon. In addition to the need to have detailed information on the development of each of the languages separately, we are also in dire need of having bilingual developmental norms, especially with respect to different levels of language dominance.

SUMMARY

- Bilinguals' two language systems constantly interact; they do not have two separate and isolable competencies that are identical to those of two corresponding monolinguals.
- Typically, bilinguals have different degrees of competence in their two languages.
- Even in the most balanced bilinguals, the two phonological systems differ in some ways from those of two corresponding monolinguals.
- In bilinguals where one language is more dominant, interference (or "transfer") is a very important component; this manifests itself in phonetic, phonemic, and prosodic levels.
- Bilingual phonology is also prone to universal tendencies and these may blur the distinction between transfer and developmental processes.
- To fully understand the patterns in the phonology of a bilingual, one also needs to pay close attention to dialectal variations; the lack of such information may result in over/under diagnosis of the productions.

REFERENCES

Beatens-Beardsmore, H. (1982). *Bilingualism: Basic principles.* Clevedon, Avon, UK: Tieto Ltd.

Bloomfield, L. (1933). *Language.* New York: John Wiley.

Burling, R. (1959). Language development of a Garo-speaking child. *Word, 15,* 45–68.

Deuchar, M., and Clark, A. (1992). Bilingual acquisition of the voicing contrasts in word-initial stop consonants in English and in Spanish. *Cognitive Science Research Paper* 213. Brighton, UK: University of Sussex.

Flege, J. E. (1987). The production of new and similar phones in a foreign language: Evidence for the effect of equivalence classification. *Journal of Phonetics, 15,* 47–65.

Flege, J. E. (1991). Age of learning affects the authenticity of voice-onset-time (VOT) in stop consonants produced in second language. *Journal of Acoustical Society of America, 89,* 395–411.

Flege, J. E., and Efting, W. (1987). The production and perception of English stops by Spanish speakers of English. *Journal of Phonetics, 15,* 67–83.

Genesee, F. (1989). Early bilingual development: One language or two? *Journal of Child Language, 16,* 161–179.

Genesee, F., Nicoladis, N., and Paradis, J. (1995). Language differentiation in early bilingual development. *Journal of Child Language, 22,* 611–631.

Gildersleeve, C., Davis, B., and Stubbe, E. (1997). *When monolingual rules don't apply: Speech development in a bilingual environment.* Paper presented at the annual Convention of the American Speech-Language-Hearing Association, Seattle, WA.

Grosjean, F. (1992). Another view of bilingualism. In R. Harris (Ed.), *Cognitive processing in bilinguals* (pp. 51–62). Amsterdam: Elsevier.

Imedadze, N. A. (1967). On the psychological nature of child speech formation under condition of exposure to two languages. *International Journal of Psychology, 2,* 129–132.

Ingram, D. (1981). The emerging phonological system of an Italian-English bilingual child. *Journal of Italian Linguistics, 2,* 95–113.

Kehoe, M., Lleo, C., and Rakow, M. (2004). Voice onset time in bilingual German-Spanish children. *Bilingualism: Language and cognition, 7,* 71–88.

Leopold, W. F. (1949). *Speech development of a bilingual child: A linguist's record. Vocabulary growth in the first two years.* Evanston, IL: Northwestern University.

Lowie, W. (1988). *Age and foreign language pronunciation in the classroom.* Unpublished doctoral dissertation, University of Amsterdam, The Netherlands.

Mack, M. (1989). Consonant and vowel perception and production: Early English-French bilinguals and English monolinguals. *Perception and Psychophysics, 46,* 187–200.

Mackey, W. (1970). Interference, integration and the synchronic fallacy. In J. Alatis (Ed.), *Bilingualism and language contact* (pp. 194–210). Washington, DC: Georgetown University Press.

Major, R. (1977). Phonological differentiation of a bilingual child. *Ohio State University Working Papers in Linguistics, 22,* 88–122.

Major, R. (1987). A model for interlanguage phonology. In G. Ioup and S. Weinberger (Eds.), *Interlanguage phonology: The acquisition of a second language sound system* (pp. 101–124). New York: Newbury House.

Nathan, G. S., Anderson, W., and Budsaba, B. (1987). On the acquisition of aspiration. In G. Ioup and S. Weinberger (Eds.), *Interlanguage phonology: The acquisition of a second language sound system* (pp. 204–212). New York: Newbury House.

Vihman, M. M. (2002). Getting started without a system: From phonetics to phonology in bilingual development. *International Journal of Bilingualism, 6(3),* 239–254.

Vogel, I. (1975). One system or two: An analysis of a two-year old Romanian-English bilingual's phonology, *Papers and Reports on Child Language Development, 9,* 43–62.

Watson, I. (1991). Phonological processing in two languages. In E. Bialystok (Ed.), *Language processing in bilingual children* (pp. 25–48). Cambridge, MA: Cambridge University Press.

Weinreich, U. *Languages in contact.* The Hague: Mouton.

Williams, L. (1977). The perception of stop consonant voicing by Spanish-English bilinguals. *Perception and Psychophysics, 21,* 289–297.

Yavaş, M. (1995). Phonological selectivity in the first fifty words of a bilingual child. *Language and Speech, 38,* 189–202.

Yavaş, M. (1996). Differences in voice onset time in early and later Spanish-English bilinguals. In J. Jensen and A. Roca (Eds.), *Spanish in contact: Issues in bilingualism.* Somerville, MA: Cascadilla Press.

Yavaş, M. (2002). Voice onset time in bilingual phonological development. In F. Windsor, M. L. Kelly, and N. Hewlett (Eds.), *Investigations in clinical phonetics and linguistics* (pp. 341–350). Mahwah, NJ: Lawrence Erlbaum.

Chapter 18

Cross-Cultural Interaction and Children's Speech Acquisition

Barbara May Handford Bernhardt, Jessica Ball, and Jeff Deby

INTRODUCTION

In this chapter, culture is broadly defined as the full range of learned, transmitted human behavior that includes everything one needs to do, know, believe, or have, in order to function in a socially coherent way within a given society (Cole, Gay, Glick, and Sharp, 1971; Ogbu, 1981). In terms of the *International Classification of Functioning, Disability, and Health (ICF)* (World Health Organization, 2001), the issues discussed in this chapter concern the individual's participation in society (see Chapters 1 and 11). The perspectives offered derive from qualitative research (Ball, Bernhardt, and Deby, 2005), an enterprise in which the researcher's life experiences and worldviews are part of the research context (Bateson, 1972; 1987; 1991; Burns and Grove, 2004). The authors of the chapter, a speech-language pathologist, a developmental psychologist, and a sociolinguist, are native English-speaking Canadians of western European cultural heritage. Each of us grew up and currently resides in the culturally diverse area of British Columbia, Canada, although we each lived in other countries at some point in our lives. Our personal life experiences, travel, second-language learning, and academic work have brought each of us into close contact with people of many cultures, languages, and orientations. The perspectives in this chapter derive in part from our life experiences, in part from a recent joint project concerning First Nations (aboriginal) English dialects in British Columbia (Ball, Bernhardt, and Deby, 2006), and in part from the general literature on the topic. The chapter outlines issues in language interaction among people of different groups, the sequelae of such interactions for language acquisition, and the implications for speech and language assessment.

Language interactions among people of different groups

Language is a system of communication composed of elements (e.g., sounds, words, hand movements) and procedures for combining these elements. Any given language comprises a group of different, closely related systems, often called dialects. Dialects are associated with speakers who share various combinations of geography, ethnicity, socioeconomic status, education, first language background, or other social factors. Because different dialects of the same language have slightly different grammars, grammatical "errors" in one dialect might be grammatically correct in another. However, linguists do not view any particular system (dialect) as inherently superior to another. To emphasize this equality linguists often use the term *variety* instead of *dialect*, because to some people, the latter term may imply that dialects are somehow inferior to the "language" itself. Certain varieties are accorded social prestige by being associated with groups that hold power in the social institutions of the dominant cultures, such as royalty, colonizers, and the upper class. Varieties associated with other groups are often stigmatized within these institutions, but they may simultaneously hold *covert prestige* (Trudgill, 1972), that is, status in a social group without formal power in the dominant social groups' institutions, such as a youth-revered street gang, or a rural community. In the broader context of society, a dominant culture's prestige variety is often *standardized*, meaning that one set of grammar and usage "rules" is sanctioned by the groups with political power for use in education, government, and the mass media. Varieties other than the standard tend to be stigmatized (Wardhaugh, 2002). However, as stated above, linguists do not view one language or language variety as inherently better than any other, neither overtly nor covertly. Linguists therefore refer to *standard and nonstandard* varieties, rather than *substandard* varieties. There are many well-known nonstandard varieties of English, for example, African American English (AAE) and Cockney English. Another term, *register,* has been used to refer to varieties such as indigenous Englishes (e.g., Eagleson, 1982). However, linguists define register as referring to a variety that is associated with a specific occupation or activity—for example, legal, air-traffic control, or religious registers (Schiffman, 1997; Wardhaugh). Perhaps the most appropriate term for indigenous varieties is *ethnolect*, that is, a language variety associated with a specific cultural group. An ethnolect is a *social dialect* rather than a regional dialect (Wardhaugh). Another kind of social dialect relates to socioeconomic status (social class). Bernstein (1972) suggested that British working-class and middle-class children may have different ways of using English at home. He suggested that working-class children are socialized into a variety of English that depends heavily on listener inference (*restricted code*), whereas middle-class children are exposed to a variety in which ideas and connections are made more explicit (*elaborated code*). Today, most linguists discount this dichotomous perspective.

Sequelae of cross-cultural interactions for speech and language development

Regardless of the scholarly evidence that languages and varieties of language are equivalent, public beliefs about different languages and language varieties can have social sequelae, which can affect language development and use. Minority languages or nonstandard varieties may be considered low in status and their speakers of lower intelligence, even if they only have an "accent" (Giles and Powesland, 1975; Edwards, 1989; Lippi-Green, 1997). Bernstein (1972), for example, suggested that children whose repertoires were limited to restricted code were hindered in their cognitive and academic development because only elaborated code enabled certain kinds of ideas to occur and flourish. Educational policymakers in some areas adopted the Bernstein perspective, magnifying the institutionalized stigmatization of ethnically different groups, notably the Maori in New Zealand (Hawkins, 1972). Today, developmentalists and linguists discount the perspective that intelligence reflects language variety use. For example, in a review of the literature, Fletcher (1983) notes that nonverbal tests of intelligence show that Native American people have performed as well or better than their non–Native American counterparts (e.g., Havighurst and Hilkevitch, 1944; Levensky, 1970). Nevertheless, if someone speaks a nonstandard variety of the ambient language—whether we call it a dialect, ethnolect, register, or restricted code—Milroy and Milroy (1999) comment that this person may be subject to "linguistic" discrimination, even if public discrimination on the grounds of race, religion, or social class is neither acceptable nor legal.

How do perspectives on languages and language varieties affect a child during speech and language development? This will depend in part on the child's developmental context, that is, the child's family, cultural group, and societal context, and to some extent on the child's age, interest in, and ability to acquire different languages and dialects.

The majority of investigations on the social context of language development have focused on Caucasian, urban, English-learning middle-class children and families who speak the "standard" dialect of the main language of an area. Research on cross-cultural differences in language acquisition is limited, although it is gaining ground. Studies of caregiver-child interactions have revealed strikingly different patterns of interaction across cultures and linguistic groups (see Chapter 15), with different beliefs, values, and expectations observed to be motivating these diverse patterns (e.g., Edwards, Gandini, and Giovaninni, 1996; Heath, 1989; Johnston and Wong, 2002). Parents and communities may have different views on what should happen regarding language or dialect use. Some speakers of a nonstandard dialect may believe that they speak a poor version of the language and encourage their children to speak "better" (Kaldor, Eagleson, and Malcolm, 1982), that is, to adopt the standard pronunciation. However, Kaldor and Malcolm (1991), in their discussion of Aboriginal Australian English, also remark that parents may indirectly value the home language or dialect. Parents may show their valuing of Standard English by wanting their children to learn it in school, but at the same time ascribe Standard English a lower value than the home language or dialect in the home context. Eagleson (1982) observes that using the standard in informal situations among other Aborigines may be condemned as snobbish and self-aggrandizing. This perspective was also expressed in one of our forums on First Nations English dialects, and in ongoing research by Ball (2005) and Ball and Lewis (2005).

Children may consciously or unconsciously select which language or dialect to speak, and which variants of phonemes, words, or grammars to use. These selections may arise out of a desire to fit in or succeed, in their home community, their linguistic or social group, or their educational context. If the child lives in a community where large numbers of speakers use [f] for /θ/, for example, the child may use [f], unless for some reason that child encounters someone or some group that suggests (or taunts) that [f] is "wrong" or "of low prestige" in words such as *think*. The child may start to use [θ] for all words where it is used in the standard variety, or only in those social contexts where use of [θ] avoids discrimination and ensures acceptance; that is, the child may become unidialectal (standard variety) or bidialectal.

Within families, individual children may differ in their degree of bilingualism or bidialectalism.

Implications for speech assessment and intervention

Speech-language pathologists (SLPs) have a challenging task with respect to children who do not use the standard language or language variety of the area. Screening, assessment, and intervention programs embody the cultures and values of researchers and practitioners who designed them, and most of them have been based on the standard varieties of the dominant language or language variety in the area; for example, in English, General American English or the Queen's English (Received Pronunciation). Positive trends are emerging. A recent tool developed by Seymour, Roeper, and De Villiers (*Diagnostic Evaluation of Language Variation, DELV*, 2003) attempts to differentiate language difference from impairment through focusing on the elements that varieties of English have in common. This tool focuses primarily on the differentiation of AAE from General American English, and the stimuli portray many children of African American heritage. The authors admit in their brochure that the tool is not particularly sensitive to Spanish-influenced English in the United States, and it may not yet sufficiently differentiate language difference from impairment for children from other cultural or linguistic backgrounds either. However, it is a strong beginning in this area of test development. More and more standardized tools for speech-language pathology are available in languages other than English.

A speech-language pathologist is unlikely to be fluent in all of the first languages he or she may encounter in practice. However, a number of practices may enable an SLP to evaluate a child's speech development in languages other than the SLP's language(s). The first and crucial step for the SLP is to become proficient in transcription using the entire International Phonetic Alphabet (International Phonetic Association, 1999). The second is for the SLP to find out the phonetic and syllabic inventories of the child's first language or language dialect, through Web and library searches, or through consultation with a native speaker. The third is to have a native speaker compose an audio (and/or video) record of a word list (50–100 words) that includes all or most target phones and structures for that language or language variety, and which (critically) includes the translation for each word into the SLP's native language. The SLP can then create a set of picture or object stimuli that can be presented in a given order. With the help of a native speaker, a speech sample can then be elicited from the child (and recorded on audio and/or video) in that child's native language or dialect in response to the stimuli, the native speaker confirming that the child has indeed uttered the intended words. The IPA-proficient SLP can then transcribe the tape and, by comparison to the targets produced by the native speaker of that language or dialect, proceed to phonological analysis and determination of a management plan (whether that includes dismissal, referral, or treatment). A bilingual or bidialectal child's second language or dialect (presumably the SLP's language) may be elicited by the SLP on a subsequent day, using standard or free conversation procedures. In cases of bilingual or bidialectal speakers, the two phonological analyses may be compared to determine overlap and divergence in phonological development in the two languages (Bernhardt, 2002) or dialects as a basis for a management plan. Through consultation with native speakers of the language or dialect, the SLP will be able to devise a management plan consistent with the child's family's views on impairment and intervention. Although the above practices will be time consuming at first, once a set of stimuli has been developed for a given language or dialect, and the SLP has become more familiar with the views of a particular cultural and linguistic group, clinical efficiencies will follow. Depending on ethical and copyright conditions during development of clinical tools, resources may be shared among SLPs, thereby further increasing efficiency.

In the past few years, several national associations of SLPs have developed position statements and policies promoting sensitivity to cultural differences and recruitment of students from diverse ethnic and linguistic backgrounds into SLP programs (e.g., American Speech-Language-Hearing Association www.asha.org, Canadian Association of Speech-Language Pathology and Audiology, www.caslpa.ca, Speech Pathology Australia www.speechpathologyaustralia.org.au). Position statements and policy papers may not reflect the perspectives of all SLPs of a region, however. Montgomery quotes from a letter to the editor in the *ASHA Leader* (1998) in which the writer, speaking of AAE, states: "there is only one language, one accepted dialect, and that is standard English speech" (Aronson, 1998, cited by Montgomery, 1999, p. 85). The SLP community as a whole may accept the notion of diversity, but individuals may have different perspectives on which language or language variety is best to focus on in language intervention. Furthermore, it remains challenging to distinguish speech impairment from speech difference. Much research remains to be done. Meanwhile, Crago (1992, p. 36) suggests that clinicians and educators "must learn to recognize their own invisible cultural curricula while learning the cultural dimensions of their clients' and students' communication patterns and language use." Crago (1999) suggests that studies of language socialization are helpful starting places to learn about cultural differences and language use; for example, Heath (1986), Schieffelin and Ochs (1986), and Backus (1999). Through development of community-researcher-practitioner partnerships, more will be learned about linguistic and cultural similarities and differences and what practices might work best in a given community (Cheng, 1999). Culturally sensitive practice honors and supports a family's goals for a child's language development, and acknowledges and supports the system of cultural signs and forms of interaction, thus securing a child's attachment and sense of belonging to his or her speech/social community and fostering acquisition of the desired language or language variety.

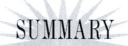

SUMMARY

- Culture can be broadly defined as the full range of learned, transmitted human behavior that includes everything one needs to do, know, believe, or have, in order to function in a socially coherent way within a given society.
- Cross-cultural research often involves qualitative research methodology.

- In qualitative research, the researcher's life experiences are a context of the research and thus are part of the data.
- All languages and language varieties (or dialects) are equally valid.
- Speakers of the standard dialect of a majority language may have greater power, greater educational opportunities, and greater financial success than speakers of minority languages and nonstandard dialects.

- Different families, children, and communities may differ in the degree to which they use their own language or dialect and in which contexts.
- The child's speech acquisition will reflect an interaction of the many factors involved in language or dialect use: opportunity, motivation, family perspective, desire for acceptance.
- Educational and health professionals need to be knowledgeable about the languages and language varieties in their region and respectful of the family's, child's, and communities' wishes regarding language use.

- Policies regarding cross-cultural practice are being defined by some of the national associations of speech-language pathologists, but cross-cultural practices are yet in the infancy stage of development.
- The individual educator or SLP does not have to wait for research to be done before making changes in practice that reflect cross-cultural sensitivity. Because cross-cultural interaction is just that, an interaction, the local SLP can form partnerships with community members from various cultural and linguistic groups in order to develop useful and sensitive assessment and treatment methodologies together.

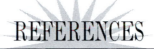

REFERENCES

Backus, A. (1999). Mixed native languages: A challenge to the monolithic view of language. *Topics in Language Disorders, 19*, 11–22.

Ball, J. (2005). Talking points: Exploring needs and concepts for Aboriginal early childhood language facilitation and supports. Technical report prepared for the Public Health Agency of Canada, Aboriginal Head Start in Urban and Northern Communities. Author: University of Victoria.

Ball, J., Bernhardt, B., and Deby, J. (2005, November). *Implications of First Nations English dialects for* supporting First Nations children's language development. Poster presented at the World Indigenous People's Conference on Education, Aotearoa, New Zealand.

Ball, J., Bernhardt, B., and Deby, J. (2006). *First Nations English Dialects: Exploratory Project Proceedings.* Unpublished monograph, University of Victoria and University of British Columbia.

Ball, J., and Lewis, M. M. (2005). First Nations Elders' and parents' views of early language development and goals. Retrieved October 10, 2005, from http://www.ecdip.org/earlylanguage/index/html.

Bateson, G. (1972). *Steps to an ecology of mind: Collected essays in anthropology, psychiatry, evolution, and epistemology.* New York: Ballantine.

Bateson, G. (1987). Conventions of communication: Where validity depends upon belief. In J. Ruesch and G. Bateson (Eds.), *Communication: The social matrix of psychiatry* (pp. 212–227). New York: Norton.

Bateson, G. (1991). The creature and its creations. In R. Donaldson (Ed.),. *A sacred unity: Further steps to an ecology of mind* (pp. 93–110). New York: Harper Collins.

Bernhardt, B. (2002, February). *Phonological disorders in bilingual children: A window into theories of phonology and bilingualism.* Paper presented at the German Linguistics Annual Conference, Mannheim, Germany.

Bernstein, B. (1972). *Class, codes and control, Volume 1: Theoretical studies toward a sociology of language.* London: Routledge and Kegan Paul.

Burns, N., and Grove, S. (2004) *The practice of nursing research: Conduct, critique & utilization* (5th ed.). Philadephia, PA: Saunders.

Cheng, L.-R. L. (1999). Moving beyond accent: Social and cultural realities of living with many tongues. *Topics in Language Disorders, 19*, 1–10.

Cole, M., Gay, J., Glick, J., and Sharp, D. W. (1971). *The cultural context of learning and thinking.* New York: Basic Books.

Crago, M. B. (1990). Development of communicative competence in Inuit children: Implications for speech-language pathology. *Journal of Childhood Communication Disorders, 13*, 73–83.

Crago, M. B. (1992). Ethnography and language socialization: A cross-cultural perspective. *Topics in Language Disorders, 12* (3), 28–39.

Eagleson, R. (1982). Aboriginal English in an urban setting. In R. Eagleson, S. Kaldor, and I. Malcolm (Eds.), *English and the Aboriginal child.* (pp. 113–162). Canberra, Australia: Curriculum Development Centre.

Edwards, C. P., Gandini, L., and Giovaninni, D. (1996). The contrasting developmental timetables of parents and preschool teachers in two cultural communities. In S. Harkness and C. M. Super (Eds.), *Parents' cultural belief systems: Their origins, expressions, and consequences* (pp. 270–288). New York: Guilford Press.

Edwards, J. (1989). *Language and disadvantage.* London: Cole and Whurr.

Fletcher, J. D. (1983). What problems do American Indians have with English? *Journal of American Indian Education, 23*(1), 1–14.

Giles, H., and Powesland, P. (1975). *Speech style and social evaluation.* London: Academic Press.

Havighurst, R., and Hilkevitch, R. (1944). Intelligence of Indian children as measured by a performance scale. *Journal of Social and Abnormal Psychology, 3,* 419–433.

Hawkins, P. R. (1972). Restricted codes and Maori English. *New Zealand Journal of Educational Studies, 7,* 59–68.

Heath, S. B. (1989). The learner as cultural member. In M. Rice and R. Schiefelbusch (Eds.), *The teachability of language* (pp. 333–350). Baltimore, MD: Paul Brookes.

International Phonetic Association. (1999). *Handbook of the International Phonetic Association.* Cambridge, UK: Cambridge University Press.

Johnston, J. R., and Wong, M.-Y. A. (2002). Cultural differences in beliefs and practices concerning talk to children. *Journal of Speech, Language, and Hearing Research, 45,* 1–11.

Kaldor, S., Eagleson, R., and Malcolm, I. (1982). The teacher's task. In R. Eagleson, S. Kaldor, and I. Malcolm (Eds.), *English and the Aboriginal child* (pp. 193–217). Canberra, Australia: Curriculum Development Centre.

Kaldor, S., and Malcolm, I. (1991). Aboriginal English—an overview. In S. Romaine (Ed.), *Language in Australia* (pp. 67–83). Cambridge: Cambridge University Press.

Levensky, K. (1970). *The performance of American Indian children on the Draw-A-Man Test (Paper 111-2).* Washington, DC: National Study of American Indian Education.

Lippi-Green, R. (1997). *English with an accent: Language, ideology, and discrimination in the United States.* New York: Routledge.

Milroy, J., and Milroy, L. (1999). *Authority in language.* New York: Routledge.

Montgomery, J. K. (1999). Accents and dialects: Creating a national professional statement. *Topics in Language Disorders, 19,* 78–86.

Ogbu, J. U. (1981). Origins of human competence: A cultural-ecological perspective. *Child Development, 52,* 413–429.

Schieffelin, B. B., and Ochs, E. (Eds.). (1986). *Language socialization across cultures.* New York: Cambridge University Press.

Schiffman, H. (1997). Linguistic register. author. Retrieved September 4, 2004, from http://ccat.sas.upenn.edu/~haroldfs/messeas/regrep/node2.html.

Seymour, H., Roeper, T., and De Villiers, J. (2003). *Diagnostic evaluation of language variation.* San Antonio, TX: Harcourt.

Trudgill P. (1972). Sex, covert prestige and linguistic change in the urban British English of Norwich. *Language in Society, 1,* 179–195.

van Kleeck, A. (1994). Potential cultural bias in training parents as conversational partners with their children who have delays in language development. *American Journal of Speech-Language Pathology, 3,* 67–78.

Wardhaugh, R. (2002). *An introduction to sociolinguistics.* Malden, MA: Blackwell.

World Health Organization. (2001). *ICF: International classification of functioning, disability and health.* Geneva: Author.

Chapter 19

Speech Acquisition in Second First Language Learners (Children Who Were Adopted Internationally)

Karen E. Pollock

INTRODUCTION

Parents of internationally adopted (IA) children are frequently concerned about speech delays, and the assessment of IA children provides a distinct challenge to speech-language pathologists (SLPs). Although their development may at first glance appear similar to that of bilingual or second language learners, IA children are unique in that (in the majority of cases) exposure to the birth language ceases abruptly at the time of adoption. Without the support of the birth language to build on, IA children are often described as "starting over" with a new first language and are referred to as Second First Language (SFL) learners (Geren, Snedeker, and Ax, 2005; Glennen, 2002b; Roberts et al., 2005). Whereas bilingual children may be assessed in both languages in order to obtain a more complete picture of their development, for SFL learners, assessment in the birth language is often not possible. In addition, because attrition is extremely rapid (e.g., Nicoladis and Grabois, 2002), birth language assessments that are not conducted immediately upon arrival may not be valid (Glennen, 2005). Thus, during the first year or more postadoption, IA children are in limbo—they have no functional language until they learn English, yet they cannot be held to developmental expectations for monolingual English speakers until they have had sufficient exposure to English (Glennen, 2005). Although recent research has begun to establish expectations for SFL learners in the areas of vocabulary and morphosyntax (e.g., Glennen and Masters, 2002; Pollock, 2005), little is known about the acquisition of speech in this unique population.

In addition to experiencing an abrupt switch in language environment, IA children are at risk for speech-language and other developmental delays as a result of early institutional (orphanage) care (e.g., Johnson and Dole, 1999; Miller and Hendrie, 2000). The poorly funded and under-staffed orphanages in which many IA children spend their first months or years do not provide adequate stimulation for speech-language development, with limited language exposure and limited opportunities for interaction with caregivers (Glennen, 2002a).

Facts about international adoption (IA)

Worldwide, the number of IA children has increased dramatically in recent years, but trends vary according to country of birth and country of adoption. For example, in the United States, the total number of international adoptions has increased steadily and rapidly in the past 12 years (from 7,337 in 1993 to 22,884 in 2004) while in Canada the total has remained relatively constant (between 1,738 and 2,222 per year) over the same period of time (Adoption Council of Canada, 2005; U.S. Department of State, 2005). In Australia, the total number of international adoptions fluctuated between 200 and 300 per year from 1993 to 2002, but increased significantly in the next two years to a total of 434 in 2004 (Australian Institute of Health and Welfare, 2005).

The majority of internationally adopted (IA) children are born in non-English-speaking countries in Asia, Eastern Europe, Central and South America, and, more recently, Africa and the Caribbean. They are without caregivers for a variety of reasons, including (but not limited to) the death of both parents, abandonment, or extreme poverty (Child Welfare League of America, 2003). Typically, only countries under severe political or economic stress make their children available for international adoption. For example, recent increases in adoptions from Guatemala are linked to civil wars, repeated national disasters, and widespread poverty. In China, widespread abandonment of infants has been linked to the one-child policy, which was initiated to reduce overpopulation and resultant poverty, and a perceived cultural or family pressure to have sons to carry on the family name and care for the parents in their old age (Johnson, 2004).

In the United States, adoptions from China and Russia predominate, and they have more than tripled in the last 10 years (see Figure 19-1). In Canada, children adopted from China consistently outnumber those from all other countries, accounting for 51 percent of the total IAs in 2004, with the next most frequent country, Haiti, accounting for only 8 percent of the total (Adoption Council of Canada, 2005). In Australia, adoptions from Korea predominated for many years until very recently, when they were outnumbered by a sudden surge in adoptions from China (Australian Institute of Health and Welfare, 2005).

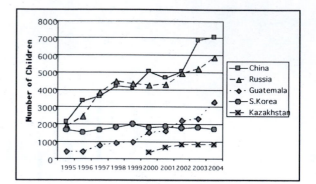

Figure 19-1 Number of international adoptions to the U.S. from 1995–2004 by top five countries of origin (data obtained from http://travel.state.gov/family/adoption/stats/stats_451.html [accessed August 28, 2005])

The largest numbers of IA children have been placed with families in English-speaking countries (e.g., United States, United Kingdom, Canada, Australia, New Zealand), but many have also been adopted into families in Norway, Sweden, the Netherlands, and elsewhere. This review will be limited to children adopted into English-speaking families.

Child characteristics

The children available for adoption vary considerably according to circumstances in the country of origin. In China, 98 percent are healthy infant girls, abandoned soon after birth. In contrast, roughly equal numbers of boys and girls are adopted from other countries. By far the largest numbers of IA children are infants and toddlers. In 2001, 44 percent of IA children were under 1 year of age, and an additional 43 percent were under 4 years of age (Child Welfare League of America, 2003). However, this also varied by country/region of origin. For example, more older children were adopted from Africa (53 percent over 5, 15 percent under 1) and more younger children from Asia (58 percent under 1, 5 percent over 5).

Parent characteristics

Parents who adopt internationally must meet certain eligibility requirements (e.g., age, income, health status, family structure) set by the country of origin, adoption agencies, and immigration laws. For example, to adopt from China, parents must be 30–55 years of age, married at least 6 months, and have no more than 4 children already in the home. Single heterosexual parents are also eligible to adopt from China, but are limited to no more than 8 percent of the total applicants. In contrast, parents adopting from Korea must be under 45 years of age and married at least 3 years (no single applicants are allowed). Although the specific eligibility requirements vary from country to country, on the whole, IA parents are very well educated, financially secure, and highly motivated to parent (e.g., McGuiness, 1998). They are also quick to seek evaluations and advocate for services for their children if problems are identified. IA parents are predominantly monolingual English speakers, and therefore the vast majority of children have little or no continued exposure to the language of their birth country.

Preadoption care

Johnson and Dole (1999) estimated that 88 percent of IA children have spent at least some time in an orphanage prior to adoption. In many countries, such as Russia and Haiti, children typically remain in state-run orphanages until adoption. Other countries, such as Korea, have well-established foster care programs. China, which has traditionally relied on orphanages for care, appears to be increasing the use of foster care or other programs (e.g., hugging grannies) that provide more one-on-one attention and care (Johnson, 2004).

Reports of the quality of care provided in orphanages range from accusations of extreme neglect or abuse to descriptions of dedicated caregivers "doing the best they can with limited resources." Many are overcrowded and inadequately staffed, with high child-to-caregiver ratios. Access to medical care is limited, and many studies have documented that orphanage care often results in growth failure and developmental delays (e.g., Johnson and Dole, 1999; Miller and Hendrie, 2000). Even under the best conditions, where physical and medical needs are met, orphanages do not provide an environment conducive to language learning. For example, when observing her daughter's orphanage in Russia, Glennen (2002a) noted that children were grouped by age, caregivers changed from day to day, and caregivers rarely talked to the children except to express simple commands such as "sit down," and "don't do that."

Health and developmental status (at time of adoption)

IA children often arrive with a host of medical concerns (e.g., Hepatitis B, parasites, latent tuberculosis, anemia, elevated lead levels) and developmental issues (e.g., fine and gross motor delays, attachment, speech and language delays) (e.g., Edelsward, 2005; Mason and Narad, 2005). In addition, in many cases no information is available concerning birth or family history and the actual health of children on arrival does not always match the preadoption medical reports (Edelsward, 2005). Children adopted at older ages tend to have more issues, presumably related to longer periods of institutionalization (e.g., Miller and Hendrie, 2000).

Outcomes for IA children

Given the varying quality of preadoption care across institutions and countries, and changing conditions over time, there are likely to be significant cohort effects, making it difficult to generalize outcomes for IA children. For example, reports of children adopted from Romania in the early 1990s have found that as many as 65 percent had long-term difficulties with attachment, behavior, social skills, or cognitive development (e.g., Fisher, Ames, Chisholm, and Savoie, 1997). In a follow-up study of children adopted from Romania in the early 1990s, Groze and Ileana (1996) described the children as falling into three categories: the "resilient rascals," who had little or no continuing negative effects; the "wounded warriors," who were making good progress but still lagged behind their peers; and the "challenged children," who continued to have multiple problems related to early deprivation. In their study, 60 percent of the children fell into the middle category and 20 percent in each of the other two categories. However, studies of children adopted from China and Russia, and even children adopted more recently from Romania, have found more positive outcomes and suggest that despite severe delays at the time of adoption, many catch up quickly and match expectations for nonadopted peers within a year or two postadoption (e.g., Hendrie, 1995; Rutter et al., 1998). These findings have left many to marvel at the remarkable resilience of many IA children and the ameliorative effects of an enriched family environment (e.g., McGuinness, 1998). But it is important to remember that even though the majority of IA children seem to be doing well in all aspects of development, some IA children do have more significant problems and will require short- or long-term intervention.

In the area of language development, several recent studies have found that by one or two years postadoption, children adopted as infants or toddlers have "caught up" to their monolingual English-speaking peers on measures of expressive vocabulary and utterance length (e.g., Glennen and Masters, 2002; Krakow and Roberts, 2003). Roberts et al. (2005) found a low rate (5.5 percent) of persistent language problems in a group of preschoolers who had been adopted from China two or more years earlier. Children adopted at older ages have also been shown to learn English quickly (e.g., Geren et al., 2005; Krakow, Tao, and Roberts, 2005), but they have farther to go to catch up to peers exposed to English from birth.

Although there is a growing body of literature on language (e.g., vocabulary, morphosyntax) development, there have been only a handful of studies focusing on speech acquisition in Second First Language learners. These studies are reviewed below.

Speech acquisition

Example 1: Mike, adopted from Korea

The first published report of speech development in an IA child was a longitudinal account of Mike, a young boy with a severely disordered phonological system (Pollock, 1983). Mike was adopted from Korea at 2;2, after having spent 8 months in an orphanage and foster home. No information was available on his history prior to 18 months of age. At the time of his adoption, he was reported to be in good health but was delayed in many aspects of development, including speech and language. Orphanage reports indicated that he could understand and follow simple commands in Korean, respond to his name, babble, and produce simple words, but unclearly. During the first year postadoption, Mike quickly learned to understand his parents' expressions and to follow directions in English. However, he expressed himself primarily through pointing, gestures, and a high-pitched squeal or grunt. By age 3, he had a vocabulary of approximately 20 English words, recognizable to his parents in context, and was beginning to use some word combinations. By age 4, Mike performed at or above age level on receptive language tests, but his expressive language was presumed delayed but difficult to assess due to a severely restricted phonological system. Spontaneous speech was less than 10 percent intelligible to unfamiliar adults and only 50 percent intelligible to his mother. At 4;8, analyses indicated that Mike had CV and reduplicated CV word shapes, two initial consonants, [d] and [n], and one final consonant, [n]. [m] was acquired in both initial and final position at 5;6. Attempts to produce other initial consonants were largely unsuccessful, although Mike could produce a variety of consonants (e.g., [p, t, ʔ, f, s]) in isolation and in syllable final position. Pollock and Schwartz (1988) summarized Mike's progress from 3;5 to 7;3, and noted that most consonants were acquired

first in syllable final position, but later generalized to other positions, and his restrictions on syllable harmony were gradually reduced. However, by 7;3 Mike still had no word-initial consonant clusters, few word-final clusters, no affricates or interdental fricatives in any position, and no initial liquids. A contrastive analysis of Korean and English phonology indicated that Mike's errors were not the result of cross-linguistic interference (i.e., there were no structural or segmental characteristics of Korean that could account for his error patterns). More likely, his delays were rooted in unknown early trauma (e.g., neurological damage) or deprivation prior to his adoption.

Example 2: MX and GY, adopted from China

Pollock, Price, and Fulmer (2003) reported phonetic inventory data in a longitudinal investigation of two children adopted from China, MX (adopted at 13½ months) and GY (adopted at 20 months). Both girls were healthy at the time of adoption, but not yet speaking in Chinese. Differences were observed in their prelinguistic vocalizations at the time of adoption, with MX exhibiting a high proportion of canonical babbling involving a range of different consonant types ([b, d, g, m, j]) and GY producing primarily precanonical utterances (e.g., grunting, whining). Over the next year, as the girls began to acquire English words, MX showed a larger and more diverse phonetic inventory. For example, at nine months postadoption, MX (CA = 22½ months) had 11 initial consonants and 9 final consonants in her inventory, compared to GY's (CA = 29 months) 7 initial and 4 final consonants. The initial consonant inventories for both girls included nasals, glides, and voiced. MX's initial inventory also included voiceless plosives and fricatives. In final position, MX used nasals, voiced and voiceless plosives, and voiced and voiceless fricatives, but GY produced only nasals and voiceless plosives. Not surprisingly, the size of their phonetic inventories appeared to be more closely related to their vocabulary size than to chronological age or length of time postadoption. For example, at nine months postadoption, MX had over 200 words and GY had approximately 50 words. Despite the early differences in their development, by 27 months postadoption (CA = 3;5 for MX, 3;11 for GY), both girls tested within normal limits on the *GFTA-2: Goldman-Fristoe Test of Articulation–2nd Edition* (Goldman and Fristoe, 2000) and other standardized language tests. Thus, by about two years postadoption, GY had essentially "caught up" to nonadopted monolingual English-speaking peers.

Both exhibited common developmental speech errors, including difficulties with liquids and interdental fricatives. GY also exhibited some sibilant distortions (dentalization of [s] and [z]). GY's early delays may have been attributable to her older age at time of adoption and the longer amount of time spent in an institution. In addition, the results of this study suggested that quality of vocalizations at the time of adoption might be a predictor of early phonological growth, but not longer-term outcomes.

Example 3: Six girls adopted from China

In order to further explore this relationship between early vocalizations and phonological development, Price (2003) followed six girls adopted from China at 9–17 months of age with speech samples collected every 3 months, and compared their vocalizations at six months postadoption to their phonological skills at 3 years of age. At 6 months postadoption, canonical babbling ratios ranged from .22 to .83, indicating that all children had reached the canonical babbling stage, with only one child's ratio below .50. Syllable structure development appeared within the range of expectations for 1- to 2-year-old English-speaking children, with the proportion of monosyllables ranging from .42 to .94, and the proportion of closed syllables ranging from 0 to .16. Phonetic inventories included 3 to 7 different initial consonants and 0 to 2 final consonants. The most common consonants were stops, nasals, and glides. Two children also produced [s] in both initial and final position. In general, vocalizations at six months postadoption were not predictive of later phonological behaviors. Only one child fell below normal limits on standardized (*GFTA-2* SS = 57) and nonstandardized measures (PCC = 68) of phonological development at age 3. Her phonetic inventory was limited (9 initial consonants, 4 final consonants, no velars or postalveolars, only one fricative), she showed frequent use of cluster reduction (40 percent) and stopping (47 percent), and she also exhibited unusual errors such as the addition of consonants. This child's poor performance at age 3 was not predicted by any of her speech behaviors at six months postadoption; for example, she had an average Canonical Babbling Ratio of .53 and her phonetic inventory, although limited, was not unlike that of other children in the sample. However, she had the slowest rate of vocabulary development over the course of the study and was delayed in other areas of receptive and expressive language development at age 3, including vocabulary and morphosyntax.

Example 4: Children adopted from China

In a larger (nonlongitudinal) study of 55 preschoolers (3 to 6 years old) adopted from China as infants/toddlers, Roberts et al. (2005) found a low percentage of children with persistent language delays, as measured by a variety of standardized tests. Included in their test battery was the *GFTA-2*. Only four children (7 percent) scored below average (i.e., more than 1.25 SD below the mean) on the *GFTA-2*, suggesting that by two or more years postadoption, children adopted from China as infants/toddlers did not experience a high rate of articulation/phonological disorders. *GFTA-2* scores were not correlated with age at adoption or length of exposure to English, although other language scores were.

Using a subset of 25 children from the Roberts et al. (2005) sample, Pollock, Chow, and Tamura (2004) completed detailed analyses of spontaneous speech samples using the *PROPH: Profile of Phonology* component of *Computerized Profiling* (Long, Fey, and Channell, 2003). Measures included Percent Consonants Correct – Revised (PCC-R), Percent Vowels Correct – Revised (PVC-R), Phonological Mean Length of Utterance (PMLU), and phonological process usage. Three children had low scores on one or more measures, but all had different profiles of strengths and weaknesses. One child, 3;2 at testing, had been home only 26 months and had shown many developmental delays at the time of adoption. She also had had multiple ear infections and pressure equalization tubes placed. She had difficulty with fricatives, affricates, liquids, and clusters and used processes such as Cluster Reduction, Palatal Fronting, and Stopping. She never received speech-language therapy, but was retested 23 months later (at 5;1) and scored within normal limits on all language and phonological measures. A second child, who was 5;3 at testing, exhibited primarily distortion errors on fricatives and liquids, both singly and in clusters. She was enrolled in speech therapy for 3 to 4 months, and remediated all of her errors prior to beginning kindergarten. The third child exhibited a severe phonological and language disorder but had nonverbal cognitive scores within normal limits. All of her scores (PCC-R, PVC-R, PMLU) were below expectations, and she used numerous phonological processes including Final Consonant Deletion, Cluster Reduction, Stopping, and Gliding. A reassessment at 6;4 (20 months later) revealed little change in her system, despite having received speech-language services for over 2 years. The same 25 children's speech samples were also reviewed for the appropriateness of prosody, using the *PVSP: Prosody-Voice Screening Profile* (Shriberg, Kwiatkowski, & Rasmussen, 1990). Only one child failed the *PVSP*, in the area of phrasing. She exhibited numerous word, syllable, and sound repetitions. This child had no other language or phonological delays. Pollock et al. (2004) concluded that preschool children adopted from China as infants or toddlers were having little difficulty with

English phonological development, and those who did exhibited developmental errors commonly seen in non-adopted peers. They saw no evidence of cross-linguistic interference, but suggested that greater interference might be expected in children adopted at older ages. Unfortunately, there are no published data on speech acquisition in children adopted from other countries or children adopted at older ages.

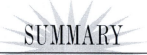

SUMMARY

- Internationally adopted (IA) children experience a unique language-learning situation sometimes referred to as Second First Language (SFL) learning.
- IA children are at risk for speech-language delays due to a history of institutionalization and associated medical and developmental concerns.
- Although there are a growing number of reports of language acquisition in IA children, very few studies have specifically addressed speech acquisition.
- Small group and case studies indicate that there is a low incidence of persistent articulation/phonological delays or disorders in IA children.
- Two or more years postadoption, preschool-aged IA children exhibit common developmental speech error

- patterns similar to their nonadopted peers, with little evidence of interference from the birth language.
- Factors such as age at adoption, length of exposure to English, or quality of vocalizations at six months post-adoption do not appear to predict speech outcomes for IA children.
- Early assessment (during the first few months post-adoption) should focus on universal aspects of speech development, such as quality of vocalizations or size and diversity of phonetic repertoire.
- Two or more years postadoption, IA children's speech may be assessed with tests normed on monolingual English-speaking children, but should still be interpreted cautiously, taking into account the child's age at adoption and other risk factors.

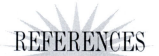

REFERENCES

Adoption Council of Canada. (2005). China leads adoption statistics for 2004. Retrieved August 28, 2005, from http://www.adoption.ca/news/050527stats04.htm.

Australian Institute of Health and Welfare. (2005). Adoptions Australia 2004–2005. *Child Welfare Series, Number 37.* Retrieved January 10, 2006, from http://www.aihw.gov.au/publications/cws/aa04-05/aa04-05.pdf. Child Welfare League of America. (2003). International adoption: Trends and issues. Retrieved January 10, 2005, from http://ndas.cwla.org.

Edelsward, L. M. (2005). *Challenges experienced by intercountry adopted children: A survey of the issues.* Report from Intercountry Adoption Services, Social Development Canada. Retrieved January 10, 2006, from http://www.adoption.ca/pdfs/ias/IASchall05_e.pdf.

Fisher, L., Ames, E., Chisholm, K., and Savoie, L. (1997). Problems reported by parents of Romanian orphans adopted to British

Columbia. *International Journal of Behavioral Development, 20,* 67–82.

Geren, J., Snedeker, J., and Ax, L. (2005). Starting over: A preliminary study of early lexical and syntactic development in internationally adopted preschoolers. *Seminars in Speech and Language, 26*(1), 44–53.

Glennen, S. (2002a). Orphanage care and language. Retrieved September 1, 2005, from http://pages.towson.edu/sglennen/OrphanageCareandLanguage.htm.

Glennen, S. (2002b). Language development and delay in internationally adopted infants and toddlers: A review. *American Journal of Speech-Language Pathology, 11,* 333–339.

Glennen, S. (2005). New Arrivals: Speech and language assessment for internationally adopted infants and toddlers within the first months home. *Seminars in Speech and Language, 26*(1), 10–21.

Glennen, S., and Masters, G. (2002). Typical and atypical development in infants and toddlers adopted from Eastern Europe. *American Journal of Speech-Language Pathology, 11*, 417–433.

Goldman, R., and Fristoe, M. (2000). *Goldman-Fristoe Test of Articulation – 2nd ed.* Circle Pines, MN: American Guidance Service.

Groze, V., and Ileana, D. (1996). A follow-up study of adopted children from Romania. *Child and Adolescent Social Work Journal, 13*, 541–565.

Hendrie, N. (1995). Follow up medical study of 263 Chinese babies and children adopted by American families. Appeared in *China Connection*, May 1995 issue. Retrieved July 7, 2005, from http://www.fccne.org.

Johnson, D., and Dole, K. (1999). International adoptions: Implications for early intervention. *Infants and Young Children, 11*(4), 34–45.

Johnson, K. (2004). *Wanting a daughter, needing a son: Abandonment, adoption, and orphange care in China.* St. Paul, MN: Yeong & Yeong.

Krakow, R., and Roberts, J. (2003). Acquisition of English vocabulary by young Chinese adoptees. *Journal of Multilingual Communication Disorders, 1*(3), 169–176.

Krakow, R., Tao, S., and Roberts, J. (2005). Adoption age effects on English language acquisition: Infants and toddlers from China. *Seminars in Speech and Language, 26*(1), 33–43.

Long, S., Fey, M., and Channell, R. (2003). Computerized Profiling (CP). Version 9.5.0. Retrieved May 20, 2004, from www.computerizedprofiling.org.

Mason, P., and Narad, C. (2005). International adoption: A health and developmental prospective. *Seminars in Speech and Language, 26*(1), 1–9.

McGuiness, T. (1998). Risk and protective factors in children adopted from the former Soviet Union. Retrieved January 10, 2006, from http://www.adoption-research.org/parent.html.

Miller, L. C., and Hendrie, N. W. (2000). Health of children adopted from China. *Pediatrics, 105*(6), 1–6.

Nicoladis, E., and Grabois, H. (2002). Learning English and losing Chinese: A case study of a child adopted from China. *International Journal of Bilingualism, 6*, 441–454.

Pollock, K. E. (1983). Individual preferences: Case study of a phonologically delayed child. *Topics in Language Disorders, 3*, 1–23.

Pollock, K. E. (2005). Early language growth in children adopted from China: Issues and preliminary normative data. *Seminars in Speech and Language, 26*(1), 22–32.

Pollock, K. E., Chow, E., and Tamura, M. (2004, May). *Phonological outcomes for preschoolers adopted from China as infants/toddlers.* Paper presented at the Child Phonology Conference, Tempe, AZ.

Pollock, K. E., Price, J. R., and Fulmer, K. C. (2003). Speech-language acquisition in children adopted from China: A longitudinal investigation of two children. *Journal of Multilingual Communication Disorder, 1*, 184–193.

Pollock, K. E., and Schwartz, R. G. (1988). Structural aspects of phonological development: Case study of a disordered child. *Language, Speech, and Hearing Services in Schools, 19*, 5–16.

Price, J. R. (2003). *Speech and language development in infants adopted from China.* Unpublished doctoral dissertation, University of Memphis, Memphis, TN.

Roberts, J., Pollock, K., Krakow, R., Price, J., Fulmer, K., and Wang, P. (2005). Language development in preschool-aged children adopted from China. *Journal of Speech, Language, and Hearing Research, 48*, 93–107.

Rutter, M., and the English and Romanian Adoptees (ERA) Study Team (1998). Developmental catch-up, and deficit, following adoption after severe global early deprivation. *Journal of Child Psychology and Psychiatry and Allied Disciplines, 39*(4), 465–476.

Shriberg, L., Kwiatkowski, J., and Rasmussen (1990). *The Prosody-Voice Screening Profile.* Tucson, AZ: Communication Skill Builders.

U.S. Department of State (2005). Immigrant visas issued to orphans traveling to the U.S. Retrieved August 28, 2005, from http://travel.state.gov/family/adoption/stats/stats_451.html.

Chapter 20

Accent Modification

Nicole Müller and Jacqueline A. Guendouzi

INTRODUCTION

Assisting persons without speech impairments in the clinically defined sense to modify their speech patterns may be on the fringe of the scope of practice for speech-language pathologists (SLPs). However, it is also an activity in which many SLPs engage very profitably. In this chapter, we will argue that SLPs planning to facilitate accent modification should acquire considerable skills in areas that are typically not at the core of the SLP curriculum, namely sociolinguistics, practical phonetics/phonology beyond their own language, and second language learning and teaching. In fact, some of the core skills of SLPs, namely the diagnosis and treatment of speech and language impairments, should be backgrounded in accent modification, because this is not a clinical intervention. In fact, accent modification in many cases will overlap with the role of a teacher of English as a second language (ESL), and we hope that some of the practical considerations discussed in the rest of this chapter will also be of interest to ESL teachers.

Terminologies

Throughout this chapter, we shall refer to *accent modification*, rather than *accent reduction*, a term also found in the scholarly and marketing literature. The term *modification* is a more accurate reflection of the goal of the intervention, that is, an alteration of the client's speech patterns. In the term *speech patterns* we include all patterned characteristics of an individual's speech, segmental and suprasegmental. An *accent*, as used here, refers to speech patterns that characterize a group of people. We distinguish accent from *dialect*, a dialect being defined as the patterns of both speech and language (for example, features of syntax, morphology, or the lexicon, as well as of phonology/phonetics) that are characteristic of a group of people. Both accents and dialects manifest in different spheres of human life; for example, there are regional accents or dialects (and even national, or countrywide, ones), as well as socially delimited ones. We refer to accent modification as a *facilitation* or an *intervention*, but we stress that this intervention is strictly a nonclinical one, since it does not address a clinically defined and diagnosed impairment of speech or language.

Accent modification and scope of practice

One may argue that the typical program of studies that leads to the certification of clinical competence does not necessarily equip the SLP with all the skills necessary to become a successful facilitator of accent modification. However, in several English-speaking countries, accent modification is considered part of the scope of practice of SLPs. For example, the Web site of the American Speech-Language-Hearing Association (ASHA) lists accent modification as one of the activities carried out by qualified SLPs (ASHA, n.d.), as do the Canadian Association of Speech-Language Pathologists (2002), and the Speech Pathology Association of Australia (2002). ASHA stresses that "accents are not a speech or language disorder" (ASHA, n.d., p.1), but the same document goes on to say that "some people may encounter difficulties communicating because of their accents" (p. 1), and that "with lots of hard work, practice, and the help of a qualified speech-language pathologist, you can learn how to change your speech pronunciation" (p. 2). The ASHA scope of practice statement published in 1996 includes in the practice of speech language pathology, "Enhancing speech and language proficiency and communication effectiveness, including but not limited to accent reduction, [and] collaboration with teachers of English as a second language ..." (ASHA, 1996, p. 18). In other countries, accent modification services are considered not to be strictly part of the jurisdiction of SLPs as SLPs. For example, in the United Kingdom, accent modification is not considered a clinical service, but some certified SLPs undertake it in private practice, independent of their clinical practice (A. Patterson, personal communication).

Powell (2000), who gives a historical overview of accent modification by SLPs in the United States and its position with regard to scope of practice, identifies a "logical inconsistency between the philosophical position that dialectal variation and foreign accent represent communicative differences (not disorders), and the fact that many SLPs provide such treatment" (p. 148). There is, as Powell states (p. 148), an obvious demand for accent modification and related services. The question is, who should provide these services? Or, to rephrase the question, what competencies should a service provider have, and what exactly should the nature of the service be? In various publications one finds the taken-for-granted expectation that SLPs are the logical choice of service provider. Sikorski (2005b, p. 118) states that "most of us ... did not actively seek out this work: those with accents [i.e. regional accents] sought us out," because, according to Sikorski, those clients were unhappy with any of the available alternatives. While Sikorski (2005a, b) stresses that SLPs need to acquire additional skills and knowledge in order to be successful as providers of accent modification, she argues that SLPs can be "viable and effective accent trainers" (2005a, p. 127). In the newsletter of the Arkansas Speech-Language-Hearing Association (Wallace, 2004), we read that "speech pathologists are uniquely qualified to assist this population" [i.e., second-language English speakers], and that "when working in the area of accent modification, a speech pathologist uses many of the same skills as in articulation therapy." This is problematic, in essence because it constructs the facilitation of accent reduction with a therapeutic intervention, and because it takes for granted that clinical skills are sufficient for the job. Sikorski (2005b) clearly states that the "therapeutic intervention model (especially its usual/customary vocabulary and its typical dynamics), while integral to rehabilitation efforts, is not appropriate for working with language/dialect-different adults" (p. 119).

Possible motivations of clients to seek out accent modification services, and of SLPs to provide them

According to ASHA's fact sheet on accent modification (ASHA, n.d.), clients who receive accent modification services include: "Non-native English speakers, speakers who want to reduce a regional accent, business and medical professionals who want to improve their communication skills because of a foreign and regional accent, [and] actors who need to learn a new accent for a role or performance" (p. 2). With the exception of the last group, what is implied here is that for these client groups, their existing accents represent a problem. Further, there is an explicit link between accent and "communication skills," and what appears to be implied is intelligibility and comprehensibility.

It is necessary to stress that accent modification should always be a truly *elective* service: In other words, whether or not a client seeks out the services of an SLP (or any other professional) to modify her or his speech patterns must truly be the choice of that individual. In reality, this is not always the case: "Corporate speech pathology" (e.g., Fitch, 2000) operates quite regularly at the level of the employer. For example, a company may engage accent modification services as part of a package of conditions of service that employees are expected to follow. Similarly, university departments may require both students and employees to attend accent modification services as part of their conditions of acceptance into a program or employment. In such situations, SLPs should ask themselves whether the elective nature of the services provided is truly guaranteed. Of course, intelligible speech is necessary for, as an example, health professionals such as nurses or nursing assistants whose first language is not English, or company employees who interact with a wide variety of clients beyond their own region. However, this presupposes a direct link between accent and intelligibility; as will be discussed below, this link is in fact rather tenuous. One might further advance the argument that having speech that is pleasing to the ear will be a great advantage for people who rely on speech as a substantial tool of their trade (anyone from teachers, university professors, and marketing personnel, to health professionals and politicians, to name only a few). This, however, begs the question of what makes anyone's speech pleasing to the ear?

A view informed by sociolinguistics would state that SLPs (or indeed anyone else) should not engage in activities that reinforce social stereotyping or discrimination, whether overt or covert, on the basis of a person's speech (see Müller, Ball, and Guendouzi, 2000; also Ball, 2005). A view informed by the marketplace of "corporate speech pathology" would counter this argument by stating that (a) a market for accent modification services clearly exists, (b) someone will fill that market niche, and (c) why should SLPs not be the ones to fulfill this role and carve out what can be a very profitable business in the process? (see e.g., Fitch, 2000; Sikorski, 2005a, b; Winkworth, 2000). A confrontation of these two opposing views leads to further questions that SLPs providing accent modification services should consider: If the business of an SLP is "enhancing speech and language proficiency and communication effectiveness" (see ASHA scope of practice document, quoted above), what is the link between accent and speech proficiency, or communication effectiveness? Further, one needs to consider how elective the service

is. Who is the actual client? Or, to formulate the question differently: How much pressure is there on a client to conform to someone else's ideal of speech that is pleasing to the ear, and are the client's existing speech patterns construed (whether inadvertently or deliberately) as defective? Moreover, one needs to ask what the chances of success are and, indeed, what the intervention goals should be. Last, but most important, the SLP needs to ask: Do I have the knowledge and skills necessary to do a good job in this undertaking? These questions will be briefly discussed in the remainder of this chapter.

Accents and intelligibility

It is not uncommon to hear people complain about, for example, teaching assistants at universities or nurses at hospitals whose first language is other than English, saying something like, "her accent is so strong, I can't understand what she's saying." A link between accent and intelligibility is more often presupposed than questioned in publications on accent modification. Thus Sikorski (2005a, p. 128), quotes Morley (1994) stating, "Intelligible pronunciation is an essential component of communicative competence," and advocates the use of the term "communicative pronunciation" as the ultimate goal of intervention. However, she also uses the metaphor of a "darkly tinted glass" for accented speech that the listener finds it impossible to "read through" (p. 127), and thus fails to keep separate two dimensions of speech that should be distinguished from one another, namely accentedness and intelligibility.

Intuitively, there appears to be a commonsensical link between accent and intelligibility. However, on closer examination, this link becomes quite a lot less straightforward. First, what makes for a "strong" accent? Above, we defined an accent as the patterned characteristics of speech that characterize a group of people. These patterns include both segmental and suprasegmental characteristics, and therefore an accent is a very complex combination of features. How, then, do we measure the strength of an accent? While there are studies that have asked participants to rate accents by using multi-item Likert scales (e.g., Munro and Derwing, 1999), there is, to our knowledge, to date no reliable and straightforward way of measuring or quantifying the strength or degree of an accent. It may well be that such an undertaking is not possible, due to the complex nature of the patterns involved in an accent. Neither is it particularly desirable or useful, since individuals' perceptions of accent features (and indeed their tolerance of those features) will vary quite considerably.

More importantly, one needs to ask whether a perceived "strong" accent (however this verdict is obtained) necessarily equates with low intelligibility. It turns out that this is not the case. For example, Munro and Derwing (1999) investigated the English produced by native speakers of Chinese with respect to intelligibility (defined as the listeners' ability to correctly write down what a speaker had said), accentedness (judged on a nine-point Likert scale), and comprehensibility (defined as the ease or difficulty of understanding the speaker's speech; also judged on a nine-point Likert scale). While there were positive correlations between accentedness and comprehensibility, there was a very wide range of significant correlations "indicating that the strength of the relationship between perceived comprehensibility and accent varied a great deal from listener to listener" (p. 298). Further, some speech samples that participants scored as heavily accented nevertheless achieved perfect comprehensibility scores, and there were fewer significant correlations between accentedness and intelligibility, than between intelligibility and perceived comprehensibility. Munro and Derwing conclude that there is no evidence that accent modification "necessarily enhances intelligibility" (p. 287), and that there is "little empirical evidence [that] indicates which particular aspects of foreign-accented speech are most detrimental to comprehensibility and intelligibility" (p. 305). In a study involving native and nonnative speakers of English from 9 countries, and listeners from 11 countries, Smith and Rafiqzad (1979) found that native speakers were regularly found to be among the less intelligible ones, showing that nonnative accentedness of participants' speech was not a reliable pointer toward low intelligibility.

Such findings have important implications for anyone offering accent modification services. If the goal of the intervention is enhanced intelligibility, or enhanced communicative effectiveness, then both the SLP and client need to realize that work on isolated splinter skills will not necessarily achieve this goal. It may be tempting for SLPs to first target the obvious segmental markers of either a foreign or a regional accent, for example, accurate realization of English fricatives or approximants, simply because they are the most obvious markers. One needs to keep in mind, however, that modifying these splinter skills does not necessarily enhance overall intelligibility. In order to assist, for example, a speaker of English as a second language to become a more efficient communicator in her role as a teacher or nurse, it is likely that all aspects of speech and communication need to be addressed: not only the client's speech patterns, but her overall communicative style.

Attempting to modify the retroflex realizations of target English /t/, /d/, /n/ of a Tamil speaker, for example, may not make her speech any more intelligible if, for example, her intonation, speech rate, and intensity also warrant (potential) modification, and her English language skills are less than proficient.

Efficacy and ethics

It would be unethical for any SLP to offer services without at least reasonable expectations that such services will be successful. However, to our knowledge, reliable data on the success of accent modification services, or systematic investigations of different methods, are not readily available. Powell (2000) reports on several studies that have investigated different aspects of efficacy and intervention methods, citing for example Schmidt and Meyers's (1995) study of traditional and minimal-pair intervention approaches for teaching English fricatives to native speakers of Korean; Gibbon, Hardcastle, and Suzuki's (1991) work on the use of electropalatography to facilitate Japanese speakers in the learning of English liquids; and Ferrier, Reid, and Chenausky's (1999) report on the use of computer-assisted accent modification. As Powell points out, there appear to be the beginnings of a scientific basis for accent modification services, but "there remain many questions regarding the efficacy of accent modification programmes in speech-language pathology" (2000, p. 147).

The lack, to date, of a solid basis for the efficacy of accent modification is not really surprising, given the complexity of what makes an accent, but also the wide area of what falls under the heading of accent modification. The latter includes everything from the modification of certain traits of, typically, nonstandard accents of native speakers, to intervention in the acquisition of the sound system of a second language by nonnative speakers of English.

Modifying native accents of English

Fitch (2000, p. 137) points out that he has "been fairly impressed with the facility with which people switch from one style to another" in the context of teaching employees at a company that teleconferences phone calls to use a non-Southern accent when dealing with customers. It is also our experience that it is, indeed, possible to modify one's speech style and accent, and moreover, that the help of an SLP or a speech coach is not necessarily required. This appears, at first sight, to contradict our contention, above, that comparatively little is known about the efficacy of accent modification programs. In fact, what we wish to stress is the existence of great individual variation in the ability to accommodate and adapt one's speech patterns to the requirements of individual contexts. Furthermore, making adjustments to one's speech patterns is likely to be considerably easier when the adaptation is required only for certain fixed or semi-formulaic interactions that are highly repetitive. Fitch (2000) advocates accent modification as a part of employee training in order to maximize the profits of the companies engaging such services. In such a context, the question of the true electivity of the service arises again.

Modifying foreign accents of English

Learning the pronunciation patterns of a second language is part of the overall language learning process, and SLPs working with speakers of English as a second language (ESL)[1] must acknowledge this fact. A client's overall language proficiency will obviously have a large impact on the practicalities of language intervention, as will the SLP's knowledge of the client's first language (more on this below). Many studies support the view that typically, adult learners of a second language are unlikely to acquire nativelike pronunciation skills, especially in suprasegmental aspects of speech, and even though their performance in other areas of the target language (e.g., grammar or overall fluency) may be very proficient, their accent will show the influence of their first language (see Baetens Beardsmore, 1986; Gass and Selinker, 2001, for detailed discussions). While it may be possible, with intensive training, to coach adult speakers of ESL to "pass" for native speakers in isolated tasks (see Neufeld, 1979, as cited in Gass and Selinker, 2001), it is highly unlikely that the skills thus acquired will carry over into natural, spontaneous, day-to-day language use.

The facts that the acquisition of pronunciation skills is an integral part of second language learning (especially for less proficient speakers of ESL), and that adult learners of ESL are unlikely to be able to shed all vestiges of their native language, has important implications for SLPs working with this potential client group. Furthermore, the motivations underlying a client's seeking (or being gently pushed toward) accent modification services have to be considered.

For a speaker of ESL who still has considerable gaps in, for example, grammar and lexicon, concentrating on splinter skills of pronunciation while other aspects of second language acquisition are neglected or relegated to the background is likely to be a waste of time in terms of that speaker's acquisition of comprehensible and functional communication skills. Unless, however, an SLP is qualified to teach ESL, she or he should not engage in providing services for ESL speakers with only a basic proficiency in English. The teaching of pronunciation skills has to be integrated with the teaching of overall language skills, and this is rightly the job of a second language teacher, who should also have in-depth knowledge about the student's first language, in order to be aware of potential areas of cross-language influence.

For most adult (or post-puberty) learners of ESL, the speech patterns of their first language will always have an influence on their second language. This fact calls into question the possible efficacy of accent modification in the narrow sense for these speakers. If it is an unrealistic goal for the great majority of speakers of German, Chinese, Punjabi, French, or any other language to "sound like" Americans, Australians, or whichever the English target accent may be, then intervention toward this goal is equally unrealistic. In addition, there is the question why a speaker of ESL should have to sound like a native speaker of English (see Baxter, 1991).

Furthermore, which variety of English should be the target accent? There are numerous well-established varieties of English spoken, in the majority, by second-language speakers of English (such as in India, Singapore, or Malaysia, for example). Rajadurai (2002, p. 366) argues that "the practice of adhering to native-speaker norms in ESL settings is both inappropriate and counterproductive," both in terms of communicative effectiveness (intelligibility), since it is unclear which aspects of pronunciation are the most crucial in terms of intelligibility, and in terms of cultural adequacy and respect for a speaker's national and cultural identity, which expresses itself through, among other things, speech patterns.

As we saw above, the relationship between intelligibility, comprehensibility, and accentedness is far from straightforward. If a speaker of ESL is intelligible and comprehensible, addressing splinter skills of pronunciation (for example, the correct production of target consonants, or intonation contours) may not be very efficacious. As

---

1 For the sake of simplicity, we do not distinguish between English as a second language and English as an additional language. Nor do we discuss the theoretical and practical implications of learning a language as a second or a foreign language (see Gass and Selinker, 2001), as this would go beyond the limited space available for this chapter. In practical terms, it can be assumed that many SLPs will encounter ESL speakers who have experienced English as both a foreign language and a second language.

pointed out above, while it may be possible to teach accurate performance on certain limited tasks, it is doubtful whether total generalization will be achieved (see again Neufeld, 1979; Gass and Selinker, 2001). If speakers of foreign-accented English face overt or covert discrimination, for example, in education or in the workplace (see Munro and Derwing, 1999; Sato, 1991), then the job becomes one for educators and policymakers, and incidentally phoneticians, sociolinguists, and other advocates (among them SLPs) to help erode language-based prejudice.

Conclusion: What makes for ethical, efficacious accent modification?

We conclude with a few recommendations regarding the skills anyone who offers accent modification should possess. In essence, the recommendations boil down to one general maxim: Be knowledgeable, be very knowledgeable. The professionals thus engaged should also be (in no particular order):

Sociolinguists

One needs to be aware of issues of culture and identity that are expressed in language and speech; how language and speech define the societies for which they are a primary means of communication. This is not an area of concern we have discussed in this chapter; readers are referred to Ball (2005), and Müller et al. (2000), for further discussions, and to Scollon and Scollon (2001) for an account of intercultural communication from a discourse perspective.

Phoneticians and phonologists

Those engaged in facilitating the modification of speech patterns need to have superior skills in the perception and analysis of speech patterns *other than their own* (see Schmidt and Meyers, 1995, for a discussion of evaluator error and its impact on the quality of assessment and, ultimately, intervention). Knowledge of the target alone is far from sufficient; a thorough knowledge of the source is required, too. Especially when working with speakers of ESL, it is essential that the facilitator can identify possible sources of cross-language influence and view the phonological target system in relation to the source system.

Comparative linguists

It is imperative that SLPs have the linguistic wherewithal to analyze their clients' language, not only their speech

patterns. In the case of speakers of ESL, this will have to include a knowledge of the structural properties of the client's first language, and the ability to compare and contrast this with the structure of the target language (typically a form of standard English). This ability is necessary in order to evaluate whether characteristics of a client's speech are due to phonological interference or to grammatical interference and incomplete acquisition of the target grammatical system. The question of grammatical versus phonological interference arises, for example, in the context of a Chinese speaker who does not produce past tense or third person singular inflections in English. Is this the case because she has difficulties with producing word-final plosives, fricatives, and consonant clusters (which do not occur in Chinese), or because she has not mastered the inflectional system of English for past tense and third person singular in the present tense (which does not have a counterpart in Chinese, either)? Drilling word final consonants and clusters is likely to be unsuccessful if the grammatical underpinning of these endings has not been mastered.

Those knowledgeable in ESL, second language acquisition, and bilingualism

Whether one works with clients who wish to acquire an accent of English other than their native accent, or with speakers of ESL, the study of second language acquisition and bilingualism will provide many fruitful insights into what is and is not likely to be successful. Issues of age of acquisition and the likelihood that most adult learners of ESL will never acquire nativelike accents has already been discussed. Other useful insights relate, for example, to the notions of additive or subtractive bilingualism, and thereby relate back to the ethics of accent modification: Additive bilingualism refers to a process whereby a speaker acquires a second communication system (be it a new language, or a new accent) without detriment to the first language (or accent). On the other hand, subtractive bilingualism refers to the process whereby a second language (the principle is equally applicable to a new accent) gradually replaces the speaker's first language. This can have far-reaching negative effects for the individual, ranging from identity crises to rejection by her or his original speech community. SLPs engaged in accent modification should always embrace the principle of additive bilingualism. Also see Sikorski's (2005b) discussion of facilitating a client's ability to code switch between accents and communicative styles.

The discussion above has, we hope, shown that modifying accents is a complex and demanding undertaking, for both client and provider. There is no doubt that there is a market for accent modification services, just as there is a market for teaching English as a second language.

Either service should be undertaken only by professionals who are adequately prepared and knowledgeable, and have the skills required.

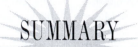

SUMMARY

- In some countries (but not everywhere) accent modification is considered part of the professional scope of practice of SLPs.
- Accent modification is a nonclinical facilitation and must not be approached from a perspective of disorder and 'therapy', and in order to be ethically sound, has to be truly elective on the part of the client.
- SLPs will typically need to acquire considerable additional skills and knowledge including sociolinguistics, a thorough knowledge of the phonetics and phonology of the clients' source and target languages, ESL, second language acquisition, and bilingualism.
- Accentedness of a client's speech does not necessarily correlate with intelligibility.
- Modification of splinter skills (such as certain speech sounds) is likely to be less effective in achieving communicative intelligibility than targeting overall

communicative strategies (including segmental and suprasegmental aspects of speech, and nonspeech strategies).
- To date, there are no reliable data available on the efficacy of accent modification intervention.
- Especially adult speakers may find it difficult or impossible to permanently and reliably modify certain aspects of their speech, which raises questions about the efficacy of accent modification intervention.
- In ESL contexts where students have limited proficiency in English, the teaching of speech skills has to be integrated with the teaching of overall language skills, which requires that the service provider (SLP or ESL teacher) has the required proficiencies.
- SLPs working outside their native country will have to carefully consider which accent of English is the appropriate target for their clients.

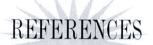

REFERENCES

American Speech-Language-Hearing Association. (1996, Spring). Scope of practice in speech-language pathology. *Asha, 39* (Suppl. 16), 16–20.

American Speech-Language-Hearing Association. (n.d.). Accent modification. Retrieved August 30, 2005, from http://www.asha.org/public/speech/development/accent_mod.htm

Baetens Beardsmore, H. (1986). *Bilingualism: Basic principles* (2nd ed.). Clevedon, UK: Multilingual Matters.

Ball, M. J. (Ed.) (2005). *Clinical sociolinguistics.* Oxford: Blackwell.

Baxter, J. (1991). How should I speak English? American-ly, Japanese-ly, or internationally? In A. Brown (Ed.), *Teaching English pronunciation: A book of readings* (pp. 53–71). London: Routledge.

Canadian Association of Speech-Language Pathologists. (2002). Careers in SLP / Aud. Retrieved September 1st, 2005, from http://www.caslpa.ca/english/careers/careers.asp

Ferrier, L. J., Reid, L. N., and Chenausky, K. (1999). Computer-assisted accent modification: A report on practice effects. *Topics in Language Disorders, 19*(4), 35–48.

Fitch, J. (2000). Accent reduction: A corporate enterprise. *Advances in Speech-Language Pathology, 2,* 135–137.

Gass, S. M., and Selinker, L. (2001). *Second language acquisition* (2nd ed.). Mahwah, NJ: Lawrence Erlbaum.

Gibbon, F., Hardcastle, W., and Suzuki, H. (1991). An electropalatographic study of the /r/, /l/ distinction for Japanese learners of English. *Computer Assisted Language Learning, 4,* 153–171.

Morley, J. (Ed.). (1994). *Pronunciation pedagogy and theory: New views, new directions.* Alexandria, VA: Teachers of English to Speakers of Other Languages.

Müller, N., Ball, M. J., and Guendouzi, J. A. (2000). Accent reduction programmes: Not a role for speech-language pathologists? *Advances in Speech-Language Pathology, 2,* 119–129.

Munro, M. J., and Derwing, T. M. (1999). Foreign accent, comprehensibility, and intelligibility in the speech of second language learners. *Language Learning, 49* (Suppl. 1), 285–310.

Neufeld, G. (1979). Towards a theory of language learning ability. *Language Learning, 29,* 227–241.

Powell, T. W. (2000). The turn of the Scrooge: One Yank's perspective on accent reduction. *Advances in Speech-Language Pathology, 2,* 145–149.

Rajadurai, J. (2002). L2 pronunciation: Sociolinguistic and pedagogical concerns. *The English Teacher, 5,* 366–387.

Sato, C. J. (1991). Sociolinguistic variation and language attitudes in Hawaii. In J. Cheshire (Ed.), *English around the world: Sociolinguistic perspectives* (pp. 647–663). Cambridge, UK: Cambridge University Press.

Schmidt, A. M., and Meyers, K. A. (1995). Traditional and phonological treatment for teaching English fricatives and affricates to Koreans. *Journal of Speech and Hearing Research, 38,* 828–838.

Scollon, R., and Scollon, S. B. (2001) *Intercultural communication: A discourse perspective* (2nd ed.). Oxford: Blackwell.

Sikorski, L. D. (2005a). Foreign accents: Suggested competencies for improving communicative pronunciation. *Seminars in Speech and Language, 26*(2), 126–130.

Sikorski, L. D. (2005b). Regional accents: A rationale for intervening and competencies required. *Seminars in Speech and Language, 26*(2), 118–125.

Smith, L., and Rafiqzad, K. (1979). English for cross-cultural communication: The quest of intelligibility. *TESOL Quarterly, 13*(3), 371–380.

Speech Pathology Association of Australia. (2002). *Scope of practice in speech pathology.* Melbourne: Author.

Wallace, S. M. (2004). Considering offering accent modification training? There's a need in Arkansas! *Sound Expressions, 4*(3), 7.

Winkworth, A. (2000). Promoting intelligibility not terminology: The role of speech-language pathologists in accent reduction programmes. *Advances in Speech-Language Pathology, 2,* 139–143.

Chapter 21

Working with Interpreters

Kim M. Isaac

INTRODUCTION

Cross-cultural communication involves an intertwining of experiences, attitudes, beliefs, and perceptions that can be complex, unpredictable, and unique to every interaction. Working with children and families from diverse cultural and language backgrounds presents many challenges to speech-language pathologists (SLPs), from choosing the most appropriate toys to use, to differentiating between language impairment and language difference, and on to providing intervention that carefully considers the child's cultural and language experiences and the family's cultural reality (including their perceptions and expectations about the child's communication impairment and how it should be managed). Gathering accurate and reliable information about the child's communication and the family's perceptions and expectations is one of the most important parts of any clinical contact. Communication is inextricably linked to culture, making it vulnerable to breakdown between people who are able to speak the same language but do not share a similar-enough cultural reality (Isaac, 2002). When shared language is removed, communication becomes more difficult and we need to make choices about how we will manage the interaction.

Interpreting in SLP

Gathering accurate and reliable information from children and their families in SLP practice requires complex communication. There are four communication options available to SLPs:

- Using simple English with additional nonverbal cues (e.g., gestures)
- Using an English-speaking family member or friend
- Using a bilingual staff member
- Using a professional health care interpreter

Relying on limited shared language and additional gestures has the advantage that it is immediately available in any health care context. However, given that such a limited shared language will not meet the requirements of a complex health care interaction, and given that nonverbal communication is culture bound (so that one gesture may have very different meanings across cultural and language groups), how well you are understood by the family and how well you are able to understand them is highly questionable. In addition, such a method has the potential to disempower the family by not giving them the opportunity to express their concerns and needs clearly and fully. Overall, relying on limited shared language is not an ethical practice.

Using a bilingual family member or friend as interpreter also has the advantage that it can be immediately available. It may also be the family's preference to have someone familiar to them (and who, therefore, already has an understanding and relationship of trust with the child and family) acting as the language mediator. Finally, a family member or family friend is likely to have an exact, or very close, language and cultural match with the child and family. However, the family member's or friend's proficiency in English (and even the home language) will not be clear, especially where a more complex and technical form of language is required, as in health care communication. This method may also disrupt family dynamics and place undue strain on relationships. Ad hoc interpreters, such as these, will not be working to any ethical standards addressing accuracy, impartiality, or confidentiality. Finally, family members and friends will not usually have any professional training in working as an interpreter or with interpreting medical and health care terminology.

Bilingual workers in health care settings are sometimes called upon to perform language mediation between patients and health care staff. This management option may be an immediate solution, and, unlike using family members or friends, the chosen mediator is more likely to have knowledge of and experience in the health care context and, perhaps, the health care provider's field. However, such a solution creates disruption for the staff members constantly called upon to act as interpreter, and they may perceive the role as being outside their normal range of professional responsibilities. The staff's proficiency in English and the language of the patient cannot be qualified, and there may not be an exact language or cultural match between the child's family and the staff member acting as interpreter. As with other untrained interpreters, such as family members and friends, bilingual staff will not be working to any ethical standards of accuracy, impartiality, or confidentiality.

Another option, when available, is for the health care provider to choose a professionally trained health care interpreter. The resources of health care interpreter services are usually stretched, meaning that professionally trained health care interpreters are not always available immediately or as soon as they are needed. Professional interpreters receive training in interpreting and, sometimes, health care interpreting, and may receive recognition and accreditation of skills. SLPs can be more confident in the interpreters' proficiency in all languages they are accredited for, including English. SLPs can also be confident that they have a depth of cultural knowledge related to the languages they are accredited for. Professional interpreters may also be bound by an ethical code addressing the issues of accuracy, impartiality, and confidentiality. Many studies and reports in the literature address the impact of using no interpreter or ad hoc and untrained interpreters, and describe the benefits of using professionally trained interpreters in health care (Baker, Parker, Williams, Coates, and Pitkin, 1996; Cambridge, 1999; Garcia, Roy, Okada, Perkins, and Wiebe, 2004; Gerrish, 2004; Giacomelli, 1997; Hornberger, Itakura, and Wilson, 1997; Isaac, 2002; Laws, Heckscher, Mayo, Li, and Wilson, 2004; Monroe and Shirazian, 2004; Pochhacker and Kadric, 1999; Tang, 1999; Woloshin, Bickell, Schwartz, Gany, and Welch, 1995).

Organization of interpreting services

Ozolins (1998, 2000) describes the organization of interpreting services along a progressive continuum, from ad hoc services through comprehensive services. Nowadays, only a few countries lack interpreting services.

Ad hoc interpreting services

Many countries offer informal and unmonitored interpreting services, which are usually established by individual organizations in response to community demand. Ozolins describes this as an ad hoc approach to interpreting services. In these services, bilingual individuals called upon to act as language mediators for a particular institution (such as a hospital or police station) often have no training in interpreting and have not had their skills in interpreting assessed or accredited. Ozolins (2000) suggested that the countries of Belgium, Austria, and Germany and many health care institutions in the United States offer this type of ad hoc interpreting service.

Generic interpreting services

Generic language services (Ozolins, 1998, 2000) develop when government and/or private sector bodies begin establishing broad-based interpreting services that reach beyond a single organization to address a wider public need. Telephone Interpreting Services (TIS), which exist in several countries, are one example of such a push for a broad-covering language service. Countries such as the United Kingdom, Holland, France, Norway, Finland, and Canada fall into this description (Ozolins, 2000).

Comprehensive interpreting services

Few countries have achieved a comprehensive interpreting service, where broad-based generic services are enhanced by training, accreditation, and registration of interpreters, and where government policy addressing the rights of people from culturally and linguistically diverse backgrounds is acknowledged and responded to by all sectors of the community. Training for professionals using interpreter services, and ongoing monitoring and evaluation of interpreter services, may also feature in comprehensive language services, although they are not necessarily defining characteristics. Ozolins (2000) suggested that only Sweden and Australia had achieved this level of service, although she argued that the services offered in the United Kingdom and Holland were approaching this degree of comprehensiveness.

Role of the interpreter in speech-language pathology

Even when interpreters are professionally trained, accredited, and bound by a comprehensive code of ethics, many find the field of speech-language pathology challenging. Interpreters often find that their role boundaries are blurred in speech-language pathology.

Most interpreters would suggest that their primary role is to facilitate communication. However, this can become very difficult in speech-language pathology, especially when one of the parties has a communication impairment. In addition, as SLPs are concerned about a child's communication development, their expectations of and needs from the interpretation and the interpreter move beyond the level of words. SLPs want to find out information that will help them make more reliable and valid decisions about a child's communication and the most appropriate way to manage any difficulties. Interpreters may be more used to conveying what a child is saying in terms of meaning or intent, whereas in a speech assessment context what is more important to the SLP is how the words are produced. It becomes far more important for the SLP to understand specific features or characteristics of the child's speech, how that compares with peers or siblings, and how cultural and language (and other background) experiences may impact on performance and behavior. Not uncommonly, SLPs ask questions of the interpreter to gather this type of information (Were the sounds all there? Did it sound clear? Were any sounds left out or substituted with other sounds?). So, while interpreters may describe their role as facilitating communication between the SLP and child (and/or child's family), SLPs may actually be asking interpreters to facilitate communication, facilitate the SLP's understanding of the child's background and cultural influences on the session, and facilitate their diagnosis by providing description of and commentary on the child's speech and language characteristics. To make this even more challenging for the interpreter, this often happens in the context of a disabled communication dyad (one party has a communication impairment) and probably with very little information from the speech-language pathologist before the session.

SLP-interpreter interaction has received a growing level of interest in recent years as cultural and linguistic diversity becomes an issue of increasing importance in clinical practice. However, there is still much to be investigated, and clinicians remain relatively uninformed about the ways in which clinicians and interpreters can work together most effectively to ensure the best outcomes for patients. Many studies and reports in past literature have focused on the act of interpreting itself, describing and discussing the quality of the interpreted session from the viewpoint of interpreting error and communication breakdown. Such breakdowns have been attributed to the use of confusing professional jargon by clinicians, dialectal and/ or cultural mismatch between the patient and interpreter, or the use of untrained or inexperienced interpreters (see Isaac, 2002, for a detailed overview in this area). Several studies are now addressing the deeper issues in interpreter-mediated communication, by looking behind the scenes and analyzing the behavior of and interaction between the health care provider and interpreter (Isaac, 2002, 2005; Wadensjo, 1998).

Information sharing

Perceptions and expectations about interpreter-mediated communication greatly influence how each professional (SLP and interpreter) will view their own and each other's role in a clinical session. When role perceptions and expectations clash, there is greater risk of the interaction failing. Approaching interpreter-mediated interactions with the view to actively seek and share information with the interpreter in preparation for the session increases the likelihood that a collaborative partnership will be established with the interpreter, enhancing the success of the session for all involved. Presession information sharing between the health care provider and interpreter has been identified as a crucial component of any interpreter-mediated encounter (Isaac, 2002; Langdon and Cheng, 2002; Langdon and Quintanar-Sarellana, 2003). It has been suggested that

presession briefing between the SLP and interpreter provides the opportunity to discuss the client's background (including culture, language, and communication impairment), the purpose of the session, session plans (including procedures and assessment or therapy materials, and the influence of the client's culture and language), and to negotiate interpreting style (Isaac, 2002; Langdon and Cheng, 2002). However, an additional crucial component of a presession briefing may be to discuss and negotiate role, not just in terms of interpreting style but in terms of negotiating how the interpreter can facilitate the SLP's understanding of the client's communication characteristics by making metalinguistic comments about the client's speech or language presentation, independently or in response to specific questions asked by the SLP (Ferguson, Candlin, Armstrong, Isaac, and Roger, 2005). This recurring process of assessment/therapy activity and metalinguistics comment helps the SLP guide the session based on his or her emerging understanding of the client's difficulties and needs. However, in order for this process to be effective, the interpreter needs to understand what to expect from the client, what speech and language characteristics the SLP is looking for in each assessment or therapy activity, and how to describe those characteristics. This information can be shared as part of the presession briefing.

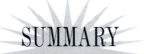

SUMMARY

- The key to working effectively with interpreters in SLP practice is to develop with them a strong collaborative partnership built on respect for each other's experiences, knowledge, and skills.
- Information sharing is an essential two-way process between the SLP and interpreter.
- Presession briefing should aim to encompass background, plans, and roles in detail.
- Be aware of what you need from the interpretation and consider how that can be achieved.

- Negotiate a system for discussing the child's speech online in the session.
- Be explicit with what types of speech errors the child may present with and how you would like the interpreter to describe the child's speech.
- The importance of sharing information becomes even greater when working with untrained interpreters, such as bilingual staff or family members. Be mindful of the limitations of the interpreter, exercise caution in diagnostic judgment, and attempt to gather as much information as possible to ensure accuracy.

REFERENCES

Baker, D. W., Parker, R. M., Williams, M. V., Coates, W. C., and Pitkin, K. (1996). Use and effectiveness of interpreters in an emergency department. *Journal of the American Medical Association, 275*(10), 783–788.

Cambridge, J. (1999). Information loss in bilingual medical interviews through an untrained interpreter. *The Translator, 5*(2), 201–219.

Ferguson, A., Candlin, C. N., Armstrong, E., Isaac, K., and Roger, P. (2005, July). *Speech pathologists and interpreters: Partners in action.* Paper presented at the 14th World Congress of Applied Linguistics, Madison, Wisconsin.

Garcia, E. A., Roy, L. C., Okada, P. J., Perkins, S. D., and Wiebe, R. A. (2004). A comparison of the influence of hospital-trained, ad-hoc, and telephone interpreters on perceived satisfaction of limited English-proficient parents presenting to a pediatric emergency department. *Pediatric Emergency Care, 20*(6), 373–378.

Gerrish, K. (2004). Bridging the language barrier: The use of interpreters in primary care nursing. *Health and Social Care in the Community, 12*(5), 407–413.

Giacomelli, J. (1997). A review of health interpreter services in a rural community: A total quality management approach. *Australian Journal of Rural Health, 5*, 158–164.

Hornberger, J., Itakura, H., and Wilson, S. R. (1997). Bridging language and cultural barriers between physicians and patients. *Public Health Reports, 112*(5), 410–417.

Isaac, K. M. (2002). *Speech pathology in cultural and linguistic diversity.* London: Whurr.

Isaac, K. M. (2005). Managing linguistic diversity in the clinic: Interpreters in speech-language pathology. In M. J. Ball (Ed.), *Clinical sociolinguistics* (pp. 265–280). Malden, MA: Blackwell.

Langdon, H. W., and Cheng, L. L. (2002). *Collaborating with interpreters and translators.* Eau Claire, WI: Thinking Publications.

Langdon, H. W., and Quintanar-Sarellana, R. (2003). Roles and responsibilities of the interpreter in interactions with speech-language pathologists, parents, and students. *Seminars in Speech and Language, 24*(3), 235–244.

Laws, M. B., Heckscher, R., Mayo, S. J., Li, W., and Wilson, I. B. (2004). A new method for evaluating the quality of medical interpretation. *Medical Care, 42*(1), 71–80.

Monroe, A. D., and Shirazian, T. (2004). Challenging linguistic barriers to health care: Students as medical interpreters. *Academic Medicine, 79*(2), 118–122.

Ozolins, U. (1998). *Interpreting and translating in Australia: Current issues and international comparisons.* Melbourne, Australia: Language Australia.

Ozolins, U. (2000). Communication needs and interpreting in multilingual settings: The international spectrum of response. In R. P. Roberts, S. E. Carr, D. Abraham, and A. Dufour (Eds.), *The critical link 2: Interpreters in the community* (pp. 21–33). Amsterdam: John Benjamins.

Pochhacker, F., and Kadric, M. (1999). The hospital cleaner as healthcare interpreter. *The Translator, 5*(2), 161–178.

Tang, S. (1999). Interpreter services in healthcare: Policy recommendations for healthcare agencies. *JONA: The Journal of Nursing Administration, 29*(6), 23–29.

Wadensjo, C. (1998). *Interpreting as interaction.* London: Longman.

Woloshin, S., Bickell, N. A., Schwartz, L. M., Gany, F., and Welch, G. (1995). Language barriers in medicine in the United States. *Journal of the American Medical Association, 273*(9), 724–727.

Part 2

Speech Acquisition Around the World

Chapter 22

General American English Speech Acquisition

Ann Bosma Smit

INTRODUCTION

Across the United States of America (USA), the dialect of English that most people understand is General American English (GAE), and it is likely that a majority also speak GAE. However, the USA is a large country settled primarily by immigrants from many different countries; consequently, it is not surprising that there are both regional and ethnic/cultural variations across the country. Several of these dialects are covered in subsequent chapters of this book, including African American English (AAE), Appalachian English, and Spanish-influenced English. There are other variants as well, including Eastern American English, Pennsylvania Dutch English, and Southern American English. Nevertheless, the variant used by most media announcers, TV personalities, and others in public telecommunications is typically GAE or close to it, regardless of the geographic origin or the ethnicity of the speaker. As a result, GAE is used routinely by most of the population of the western and midwestern regions as well as by many, if not most speakers in the northern half of the eastern USA. GAE is also spoken at least some of the time by many speakers whose native dialect is not GAE.

At the same time, ongoing immigration from many regions around the world continues to influence the English spoken in the USA In the 2000 census, about 11 percent of the population over 5 years of age was foreign born (U.S. Census Bureau, 2002a). As is typical, recent immigrants usually speak a version of English that is heavily influenced by their first language. Usually, the children of these immigrants speak whatever the regional English dialect happens to be, but in some cases, such as in certain Latino communities, the whole community speaks Spanish-influenced English (see Chapter 33).

Linguistic diversity characterizes the USA as a whole, although it is fair to say that the coasts and the southwest part of the country are far more diverse than the inland areas. About 18 percent speak a language other than English in the home (U.S. Census Bureau, 2002b). Spanish is the most common language, after English, and about 11 percent of persons over the age of 5 speak Spanish. All other languages covered by the Census are used by less than 1 percent of the population, but this includes at least 60 languages or language groups. See the Resources section in the chapter for resources pertaining to GAE.

Where General American English is spoken

GAE is spoken and understood in the continental USA, Alaska, and Hawaii (see accompanying map and Appendix D).

Components of General American English

Consonants

GAE has 24 consonant phonemes and two prominent additional consonant articulations (the flap and the glottal stop). In addition, GAE has at least two versions of /ɹ/, namely [ɹ] in syllable-initial position and the [ɹ] in r-colored vowels. GAE has its origin in British English, but it has developed separately for hundreds of years. At present, GAE is probably most closely related to Canadian English (see Chapter 26). See Table 22-1 for a list of the consonants in GAE.

Vowels and diphthongs

GAE has 18 or 19 vowels, depending on whether /ɔ/ is used (see Table 22-2). The tense vowels /i, e, u, o,

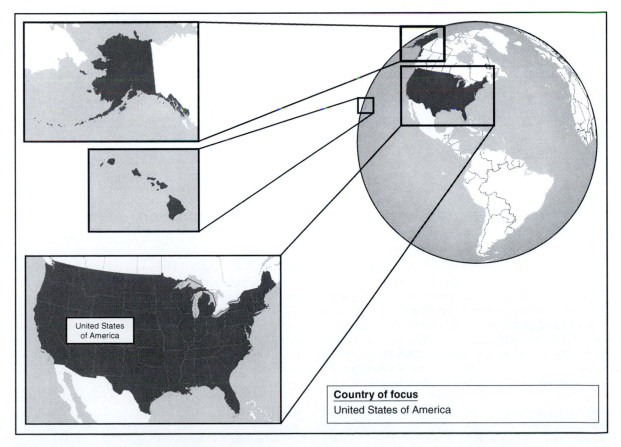

Country of focus
United States of America

United States
of America

TABLE 22-1 Consonants produced in General American English

	Bilabial	Labiodental	Dental	Alveolar
Plosive	p b			t d
Nasal	m			n
Trill				
Tap or flap				
Fricative		f v	θ ð	s z
Lateral fricative	■			
Affricate				
Approximant	w (labiovelar)			
Lateral approximant	■			l

Black = articulations judged impossible

Based on the International Phonetic Alphabet. Courtesy of the International Phonetic Association (c/o Department of Linguistics, University of Victoria, Victoria, British Columbia, Canada).

ɔ, ɑ/ are typically either lengthened or diphthongized in stressed syllables. The language also has 3 or 4 phonemic diphthongs, depending on whether /ju/ is considered a diphthong. GAE is also notable for a large number of r-colored vowels. Finally, vowel reduction is a prominent characteristic of GAE.

At present, some of the vowel articulations of GAE are changing in a process called chain shifting (Labov, 1991). The most notable effect on GAE is a tendency for /ɔ/ to be pronounced as /ɑ/, so that, for example, *caught* and *cot* are both pronounced as /kɑt/. The other vowels are expected to shift somewhat in quality so as to maintain perceptual distinctiveness.

Phonotactic restrictions

Syllables

Like other English dialects, GAE has a large inventory of syllable structures. Permissible syllables range from a single vowel, as in the word *I*, to very complex syllables such as CCCVCCC (e.g., *sprints*). Words range from 1 syllable in length to 9 or 10 syllables. Unlike languages that are based primarily on CV syllables, GAE is particularly rich in monosyllables, due to the possibility of using singleton consonants and clusters at both the beginning and the end of the word. For example, if we choose the first two sounds in the syllable as /bi/, then there are at least 23 real monosyllabic words beginning with those two sounds, including *be* (*bee*), *beep, beam, beat* (*beet*), *bead, bean, beak, beef, beach, beer, beast,* and *beard*, as well as the plural forms of many of these words.

Consonants and consonant clusters

The consonants of GAE are similar to those of other English dialects. A prominent allophone of intervocalic /t, d/ is the flap [ɾ], and a common allophone of post-vocalic /t/ and sometimes post-vocalic /k/ is the glottal stop [ʔ].

As is the case for all English dialects, GAE permits many consonant clusters, but not word-initial /tl/ or /dl/, and not /pw/ or /bw/. Also, in final position, clustered obstruents must agree in voicing.

Tones

GAE does not use tones to differentiate meaning.

Stress and intonation

Like all versions of English, GAE is stress-timed. That is, the basic unit of rhythm is a foot that consists of one stressed syllable and 0–2 unstressed syllables. In effect this means that most multisyllabic words and most multiword utterances in GAE show alternating stress. For example, the word *computer* is pronounced as *comPUTer*, and the sentence *Sarah left already* could be pronounced *SArah LEFT alREADy*. These alternating stress patterns are often implicated in moderate to severe speech disorders and in poor intelligibility of English spoken by nonnative speakers.

The alternating stress pattern of GAE can greatly affect vowel quality. Specifically, vowels in unstressed syllables tend to be reduced, that is, to change in the direction of the middle of the vowel quadrilateral. For example,

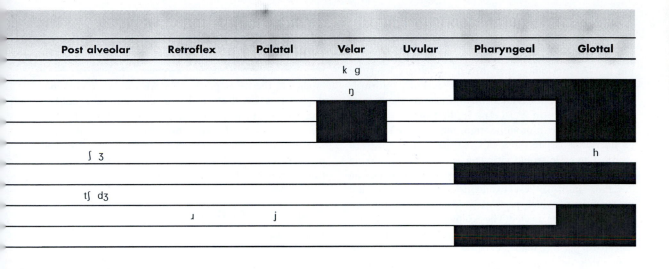

	Post alveolar	Retroflex	Palatal	Velar	Uvular	Pharyngeal	Glottal
				k g			
				ŋ			
	ʃ ʒ						h
	tʃ dʒ						
		ɻ	j				

the word *university* has an /ɪ/ vowel in the second syllable when produced as a citation form: /junɪvɝsɪtɪ/. However, in connected speech, the /ɪ/ in this unstressed syllable most often becomes /ə/. The /ə/, of course, is in the center of the vowel quadrilateral, while the /ɪ/ is near the periphery.

Writing system

The writing system of GAE is based primarily on the Latin alphabet. Although English orthography often relates inconsistently to the way the words are pronounced, English spelling has the positive feature that words that are related in meaning usually have common elements in the spelling, even if they are pronounced differently. For example, readers know that the words *wise* and *wisdom* are related because the first three letters are the same, even though the vowels in the spoken forms differ. In addition, the spelling often suggests the language of origin of a word, which gives cues to which morphological additions are appropriate. An example is the noun form of the Latinate verb *remediate,* which is *remediation,* whereas the noun form of the Old English verb *shoot* is not **shootation* but *shoot* or *shooting.*

TABLE 22-2 Vowels produced in General American English (GAE)

GAE Location	GAE Vowels	GAE Examples	GAE Location	GAE Vowels	GAE Examples
High-front	i	b*ea*t	Central (unstressed)	ə	*u*pon
	ɪ	b*i*t			sod*a*
	e	r*ai*d	[r]-colored	ɝ	f*ur*
Mid-low front	ɛ	b*e*d		ɚ	nev*er*
	æ	b*a*d			col*or*
High-back, rounded	u	bl*ue*		ɪɹ	*ear*
	ω or ʊ	b*oo*k		ɛɹ	*air*
Mid-back, rounded	o	b*oa*t		ʊɹ	t*our*
	ɔ	c*aw*			s*ure*
Low back	ɑ	dr*o*p		ɔɹ	f*or*ty
Central (stressed)	ʌ	c*u*t		ɑɹ	c*ar*
			Diphthongs	aɪ	m*y*
					b*i*ke
				aʊ	*ou*t
					m*ou*se
				ɔɪ	b*oy*

Varieties of General American English

Calvert (1980) distinguishes three levels or styles of speaking in GAE, including the "formal" or literary level, the "cultivated colloquial" level, and the "everyday informal" level. These three levels are defined largely on the basis of situation rather than social class. In the "formal" style, the speaker uses care in pronunciation, and this care results in productions that are often close to the citation forms of words. This style would characterize the public speaking of educated persons such as preachers and attorneys. The "everyday informal" level would include regional slang and productions in which parts of words and also unstressed syllables might be deleted. The "cultivated colloquial" level is in between these two levels, and it would typify the speech of persons who are native speakers in situations where they do not think they can speak casually. Wolfram and Schilling-Estes (2006) make similar distinctions, but they have named the variants the Formal Standard level, the Informal Standard level, and the Vernacular level.

The phonological changes from level to level affect both consonants and vowels. Here are two examples:

Utterance	*Did you eat yet?*	*I think so.*
Formal	[dɪdjuitjɛt]	[aɪθɪŋksoʊ]
Cultivated colloquial	[dɪdʒʊiʔjɛʔ]	[aθɪŋsoʊ]
Everyday informal	[dʒiʔdʒɛʔ]	[ahĩʔsoʊ]

Eastern American English

Several dialects of American English are treated separately in this volume, including African American, Appalachian, and Cajun English. One that is not is the Eastern American variant, which is spoken in New England and adjacent states (Small, 1999; Wolfram and Schilling-Estes, 2006). The primary phonological differences from GAE affect vowels, especially the /ɹ/-colored vowels. One of the most prominent changes is the production of the /æ/ as [a] or [ɑ] when it precedes /ɹ, f, v, s, θ, ð/. In addition, speakers of this dialect often delete post-vocalic /ɹ/, so that *barn* may be produced as [baːn] and *doctor* as [dɑktə]. On the other hand, some speakers of the Eastern dialect may *add* [ɹ] to vowels that are not r-colored in GAE. Thus *soda* may become [sodɚ]. This addition of [ɹ] is particularly likely to occur when a word ending in schwa is followed by a word beginning with a vowel, e.g., *Canada or Maine* said as [kænədɚɔːmen].

Typical acquisition of General American English

Studies of the development of GAE can be divided into those that deal with the early part of acquisition (ages 1 to 3 years), most of which are descriptive and some of which are longitudinal, and studies that are cross-sectional (ages 3 to 8 or 9 years). The Summary of Studies Table at the end of this chapter contains studies of the acquisition of GAE that provide benchmark information.

Acquired sounds

Consonants

The documentation of the early stages of speech development with respect to consonants depends on a variety of studies that include cross-sectional and longitudinal data, as well as both phonetic and phonemic use of consonant articulations. Studies of children younger than age 3 tend to report on phonetic inventories (to be described next), while the studies of older children tend to be cross-sectional examinations of the phonemic inventory.

Starting at the age of 3 years, there are several sources of cross-sectional data on consonant development, including Wellman, Case, Mengert, and Bradbury (1931) and Poole (1934) and others. Table 22-3 summarizes these data, based on studies conducted since 1950. The ages shown are the ages of acquisition, which in some cases are based on 75 percent correct performance and in some cases on 90 percent correct performance.

Consonant clusters

Consonant clusters are very common in GAE, as they are in all forms of English. In fact, English appears to have an affinity for clusters, because so many of its morphological endings produce clusters. Nevertheless, clusters seem to pose special problems for children learning them, which may account for the relatively late acquisition of correct production and for the considerable variability in cluster production from child to child in the early years. Many children learning GAE use at least one initial-position cluster by the age of 2;6 (Dyson, 1988; Stoel-Gammon, 1987; Watson and Scukanec, 1997a). These early initial clusters tend to be of the form [f]- or stop-consonant-plus-[w]. By about age 3, more variety of clusters is evident, at least among the children who produce them, and some children even use clusters with [s] (Dyson, 1988).

A few word-final clusters are used by many children by the age of about 2;6 (Stoel-Gammon, 1987; Dyson, 1988; Watson and Scukanec, 1997a). Many of these productions include a stop and a fricative (Dyson). By age 3;3, the final clusters tend to include some combination of a nasal and a stop or a nasal and a fricative or affricate (Dyson).

Templin (1957) and Smit, Hand, Freilinger, Bernthal, and Bird (1990) reported cross-sectional data on word-initial

TABLE 22-3   Age of acquisition for General American English consonants

Consonant	Templin (1957)	Prather, Hedrick, and Kern (1975)	Arlt and Goodban (1976)	Smit, Hand, Freilinger, Bernthal, and Bird (1990)
Criteria	3 word positions, 75% criterion, ages 3;0 – 8;0	2 word positions, 75% criterion (based on total attempts, not total possibilities), ages 2;0 – 4;0	3 word positions, 75% criterion, ages 3;0 – 6;0	2 word positions, 90% criterion, ages 3;0 – 9;0
m	3;0	2;0	3;0	3;0
n	3;0	2;0	3;0	3;6 (F) 3;0 (M)
ŋ	3;0	2;0	3;0	7;0 – 9;0
h	3;0	2;0	3;0	3;0
w	3;0	2;8	3;0	3;0
j	3;6	2;4	Not tested	4;0 (F) 5;0 (M)
p	3;0	2;0	3;0	3;0
b	4;0	2;8	3;0	3;0
t	6;0	2;8	3;0	4;0 (F) 3;6 (M)
d	4;0	2;4	3;0	3;0
k	4;0	2;4	3;0	3;6
g	4;0	3;0	3;0	3;6 (F) 4;0 (M)
f	3;0	2;4	3;0	/f-/ 3;6 /-f/ 5;6
v	6;0	4 +	3;6 (F) 3;0 (M)	5;6
θ	6;0	4 +	5;0	6;0 (F) 8;0 (M)
ð	7;0	4;0	5;0	/ð-/ 4;6 (F) 7;0 (M)
s	4;6	3;0	3;0 (F) 4;0 (M)	7;0 – 9;0[1]
z	7;0	4 +	4;0	7;0 – 9;01[1]
ʃ	4;6	3;8	4;0 (F) 3;6 (M)	6;0 (F) 7;0 (M)
ʒ	7;0	4;0	4;0	Not tested
tʃ	4;6	3;8	4;0 (F) 3;6 (M)	6;0 (F) 7;0 (M)
dʒ	7;0	4 +	4;0 (F) 3;6 (M)	6;0 (F) 7;0 (M)
l	6;0	3;4	4;0 (F) 4;6 (M)	/l-/ 5;0 (F) 6;0 (M), /-l/ 6;0 (F) 7;0 (M)
ɹ	4;0	3;4	5;0	/ɹ-/ 8;0, /-Vɹ/ 8;0

Note: The M and F symbols refer to males and females, respectively.

These late ages of acquisition apply only when the child is using dentalized /s, z/. Other types of errors should be corrected by age 3;6.

cluster use by children age 3;0 and older. Templin also reported on word-final clusters. Olmsted (1971) studied clusters in all word positions in children ages 1;0–4;0, but those data are not reported in a format that makes them readily comparable to the other studies. Table 22-4 shows age of acquisition data for consonant clusters.

Vowels and diphthongs

Data on vowel acquisition in GAE can be pulled together from multiple sources. Lieberman (1980) followed the vowel productions of five children between the ages of about 4 months and 14 months. He reported that some of the back vowels and [i] were quite rare throughout this period, even at the oldest ages. Of course, these data reflect phonetic tendencies rather than phonemic events. Otomo and Stoel-Gammon (1992) followed six children between the ages of 22 and 30 months with respect to the accuracy of the unrounded vowels. As part of a cross-sectional study, Paschall (1983), Hare (1983), and Larkins (1983) reported on phonemic vowel production of 20 children at 18 months, 2 years, and 3 years of age, respectively. The 18-month-old children attempted all English vowels and diphthongs, but the error rate for the nonrhotic vowels was between 20 and 50 percent. By the age of 2 years, most of the nonrhotic vowels were produced correctly, with error rates in the range of 1–14 percent. All of these studies suggest that the vowels most likely to be produced in error during the early years are /ɪ/ and /ɛ/.

It is apparent from these data that production of vowels in mono- and disyllabic words is essentially accurate by the age of 3, except for the r-colored vowels. Templin (1957) included vowels in her extensive normative study of phoneme development, but she did not document much improvement between the ages of 3 and 8. The percentage of 3-year-olds who produced correct vowels was already in the 90–95 percent range for most of the vowels and diphthongs, and 100 percent accuracy was reached by age 6 or 7 years of age. The vowels that were most frequently in error were /ɔ/ and /ə/ (70 percent and 66 percent, respectively, at age 3), as well as the diphthong /ju/ at 77 percent at age 3. The rhotic vowels were produced correctly by 75 percent of children at age 3;6 and by 90 percent of children at age 6;0.

Percent correct

Consonants

Developmental information about Percentage of Consonants Correct (PCC) (Shriberg and Kwiatkowski, 1982) in children speaking GAE comes from varied sources using different methodology and response definitions. In an unpublished thesis, Hoffman (1982) reported cross-sectional data for PCC data taken from conversational speech of children ages 3;3 to 5;9. In addition, Watson and Scukanec (1997b) reported on the PCC in conversational speech for children in the age range of 2;0 to 3;0 in a longitudinal design, and Stoel-Gammon (1987) provided a PCC measure for 2-year-olds. Finally, Pollock (2002) has reported the PCC scores of a control group of children who participated in the Memphis Vowel Project, basing these PCC scores on single-word productions. The PCC data are shown in the first four columns of Table 22-5. It is not clear why the Hoffman PCC data are generally lower than the data from the other two studies for comparable age groups; however, the methods for selecting participants and the criteria for correct vs. error consonants are likely to play a role.

Consonant clusters

There are no data on the Percentage of Clusters Correct for GAE-speaking children. The PCC for consonants noted above undoubtedly includes cluster productions.

Vowels

Benchmark information about the Percentage of Vowels Correct (PVC) has been reported by Pollock and Berni (2003), who included typically developing controls in a cross-sectional control-group study of children between the ages of 18 months and 83 months, with and without disordered phonologies. The percentages were based on production of vowels in single words. The fifth column in Table 22-5 shows the PVC data.

Phonological processes

There have been a number of studies of phonological process use by children acquiring GAE (Haelsig and Madison, 1986; Preisser, Hodson, and Paden, 1988; Roberts, Burchinal, and Footo, 1990; Watson and Scukanec, 1997a). In addition, there are several commercial tests of phonological processes that are standardized on the population of the USA, and these also provide information about the developmental course with respect to phonological processes (see the later section on speech assessment for additional information). Unfortunately, these sources have not always used consistent terminology and criteria for process use. However, some generalizations can safely be made:

- Processes involving omission of singleton final consonants are rare after the age of 3 (e.g., [bi] for *bead*).
- Stopping of fricatives is rare after the age of 3 (e.g., [pit] for *feet*).

TABLE 22-4 Age of acquisition for General American English consonant clusters

Word-initial cluster	Templin (1957), 75% criterion	Smit et al. (1990), 90% criterion	Word-final cluster	Templin (1957), 75% criterion
tw-	4;0	4;0 (F) 5:6 (M)	-sp	7;0
kw-	4;0	4;0 (F) 5:6 (M)	-st	6;0
sp-	4;0	7;0 – 9;0*	-sk	5;0
st-	4;0	7;0 – 9;0*	-ks	3;5
sk-	4;0	7;0 – 9;0*	-lp	4;0
sm-	4;0	7;0 – 9;0*	-lb	5;0
sn-	4;0	7;0 – 9;0*	-lt	3;5
sw-	7;0	7;0 – 9;0*	-lk	6;0
sl-	7;0	7;0 – 9;0*	-lf	4;5
pl-	4;0	5;6 (F) 6;0 (M)	-lθ	7;0
bl-	4;0	5;6 (F) 6;0 (M)	-lz	7;0
kl-	4;0	5;6 (F) 6;0 (M)	-ɹp	4;5
gl-	4;0	5;6 (F) 6;0 (M)	-ɹb	6;0
fl-	5;0	5;6 (F) 6;0 (M)	-ɹt	4;5
pɹ-	4;0	8;0 (F) 8:0 (M)	-ɹd	5;0
tɹ-	4;0	8;0 (F) 8:0 (M)	-ɹk	3;5
dɹ-	4;0	8;0 (F) 8:0 (M)	-ɹg	6;0
kɹ-	4;0	8;0 (F) 8:0 (M)	-ɹf	5;0
gɹ-	4;6	8;0 (F) 8:0 (M)	-ɹθ	6;0
fɹ-	4;6	8;0 (F) 8:0 (M)	-ɹtʃ	6;0
θɹ-	7;0	9;0 (F) 9:0 (M)	-ɹdʒ	6;0
skw-	6;0	7;0 – 9;0*	-ɹm	3;5
spl-	7;0	7;0 – 9;0*	-ɹn	4;0
sp-	7;0	7;0 – 9;0*	-mp	3;5
st-	5;0	7;0 – 9;0*	-nt	3;5
sk-	7;0	7;0 – 9;0*	-nd	6;0
			-ŋk	3;0
			-pt	3;5
			-kt	7;0
			-ft	4;0
			3-element final clusters	Typically age 5;0 or older

Note: Smit et al. (1990) provided separate data for females (F) and males (M) when necessary. The asterisk near all /s/-containing elements indicates that only certain types of errors are developmental up to age 9;0, e.g., dentalized productions. Information about word-final clusters was taken from Appendix IV, Table 2 in the Templin (1957) monograph. Smit et al. (1990) did not provide data on word-final clusters.

TABLE 22-5 Percent correct for General American English consonants (PCC) and vowels (PVC)

Age	Percentage Consonants Correct (PCC)	PCC	PCC	PCC	Percentage Vowels Correct (PVC)
	Pollock (2002)	Watson and Scukanec (1997a)	Hoffman (1982)	Stoel-Gammon, (1987)	Pollock and Berni, (2003)
	single words	conversational speech	conversational speech	conversational speech	single words
1;6–1;11	53%				82% (SD: 8.3)
2;0–2;5	70%	2;0 = 69% 2;3 = 70%		2;0 = 70%	92% (SD: 5.5)
2;6–2;11	81%	2;6 = 75% 2;9 = 92%			94% (SD: 6.4)
3;0–3;5	92%	3;0 = 86%	3;3 = 77% (M) 76% (F)		97% (SD: 3.0)
3;6–3;11	93%		3;9 = 72% (M) 77% (F)		97% (SD: 2.2)
4;0–5;5	93%		4;3 = 77% (M) 76% (F)		98% (SD: 2.2)
4;6–4;11	94%		4;9 = 78% (M) 81% (F)		99% (SD: 1.8)
5;0–5;5	93%		5;3 = 78% (M) 74% (F)		99% (SD: 0.8)
5;6–5;11	96%		5;9 = 83% (M) 78% (F)		99% (SD: 0.8)
6;0–6;5	97%				98% (SD: 1.3)
6;6–6;11	93%				99% (SD: 1.3)

Note: PCC data are taken from Table 3-1 in Pollock (2002) and PVC data from Table 3-3 in Pollock and Berni (2003), with ages in months converted to ages in years and months and with means rounded to whole percentage points. Data on PCC within restricted age ranges from Watson and Scukanec (1997a), Hoffman (1982), and Stoel-Gammon (1987) are also shown. Means for Hoffman (1982) are estimated from graphs.

- Fronting may be seen up to the age of 4;0 (e.g., [tæp] for *cap*).
- Depalatalization is used up to the age of 4;6 (e.g., [sip] for *sheep*).
- Weak syllable deletion and cluster reduction are relatively common up to the age of 5 (e.g., [ɛfənt] for *elephant*; [gɹin] for *green*).
- Liquid deviations (gliding and vocalization or vowelization) may persist in a few children up to age 7 (e.g., [wʌn] for *run*; [kændə] for *candle*).

In addition, some processes are very rare, and if they are seen in typically developing children, are seen only in children no older than 2;0 or 2;6, including:

- Glottal replacement (e.g., [ʔɪʔmɪʔ] for *Christmas*.
- Deletion of initial singleton consonants (e.g., [in] for *bean*).
- Assimilation (e.g., [ŋiŋ] for *king*).
- Metathesis (e.g., [æks] for *ask*).
- Epenthesis (e.g., [səmaɪl] for *smile*).

TABLE 22-6	Estimates of percentage of words that are understood by strangers
Age	**Intelligibility Level**
19–24 months	25–50%
2–3 years	50–75%
4–5 years	75%–90%
5+ years	90–100% (a few articulation errors may persist)

Source: Peña-Brooks and Hegde, 2000

Intelligibility

Systematic studies of the intelligibility expected at particular ages for children speaking GAE have not been done, except possibly as part of the standardization process for a test that has long been out of print (Weiss, 1982). However, Peña-Brooks and Hegde (2000) have put together data derived in relatively standardized ways from several studies of young children to provide guidelines for intelligibility to strangers (p. 159) found in Table 22-6.

Using entirely different methodology, Coplan and Gleason (1988) asked parents of preschoolers to fill out a questionnaire about how much of their child's speech to strangers was intelligible. The parents had the following choices: less than half, about half, three quarters, and all or almost all. The authors developed curves for "ages of emergence" for 50, 75 and 100 percent intelligibility. The resulting cutoffs (based on 90 percent of reports) for these three levels of intelligibility were as follows (p. 449):

- 50 percent intelligible by 22 months
- 75 percent intelligible by 37 months
- 100 percent intelligible by 48 months

These ages correspond reasonably well to the upper ends of the ranges seen in Table 22-6.

Phonetic inventory

The phonetic inventory of consonants at about 1 year typically includes nasals, voiced stops, and possibly a glide (Robb and Bleile, 1994). Information on consonant inventories at ages 2 and 3 years can be found in Dyson (1988), Robb and Bleile (1994), Stoel-Gammon (1985), and Watson and Scukanec (1997b). In addition, studies by Hare and by Larkins (both in Irwin and Wong, 1983) showed consonants that were correct in about 50 percent or more of tokens produced. Consonant inventories tend to look like those reported in Table 22-7, with the term *place* representing *place of articulation*. It should be noted that the correspondence among these sources is better at age 2 than at age 3, where there appears to be more variability in the accumulated data.

TABLE 22-7	Consonants in the phonetic inventories of children at the ages of 2 and 3 years	
	2 years	**3 years**
Initial consonants	Two glides	Three glides
	Nasals at two places	Nasals at two places
	Stops at three places (voiced)	Stops at three places
	One fricative	Fricatives at two places
	Zero affricates	Zero affricates
	Zero or one liquid	One liquid
Final consonants	Nasals at one or two places	Nasals at three places
	Voiceless stops at three places	Five stops
	Fricatives at two places	Five fricatives at three places
	Zero or one affricate	Zero or one affricate
	Zero or one liquid	One liquid

See sources in text.

Common mismatches

The most extensive data on common consonant mismatches are reported by Smit (1993a; 1993b) for children aged 2;0 to 9;0 years. The following summarizes these data:

1. Glides—Glides may be deleted in the youngest age groups; [w] and [d] sometimes substitute for /j/.

2. Nasals—For /m/ and /n/, the most common error in all age groups is denasalization; in all age groups the /ŋ/ may be substituted by [n] (even in nonverb forms), and it may also undergo epenthesis, (e.g., [ŋg] or [ŋk]).

3. Obstruents—Common mismatches are noted below.
   - All obstruents in final position may be deleted by children in the youngest age groups.
   - Stops are rarely in error, even in the early age groups. When they are present, but in error, the initial voiceless stops are usually voiced, and final stops are usually devoiced.
   - Among the fricatives, we find these mismatches:
     - /f-/ ⇨ [p] or [b] in youngest age groups
     - /-f/ ⇨ [s] or dentalized [s] in the youngest groups; [v] in older groups
     - /v/ ⇨ [b] in all age groups; [f] in younger age groups
     - /θ/ ⇨ [f] and variants of [s] in all age groups; [t] or [d] in younger groups
     - /ð-/ ⇨ [d]
     - /s/ ⇨ variants of [s], with dentalized versions most common; in the youngest groups, occasional substitution by stops made at the same place of articulation, i.e., [t] and [d].
     - /z-/ ⇨ [d] in younger age groups and dentalized versions of [s] in all age groups
     - /-z/ ⇨ [s] or [ts] or dentalized versions of [z] and [s] in all age groups
     - /ʃ/ ⇨ stops [t] and [d] in younger age groups; variants of [s] and [ʃ] in all age groups
     - /tʃ/ ⇨ stops [t] and [d] in younger age groups; variants of [ʃ] and [s] in all age groups
     - /dʒ/ ⇨ [d] in initial position in younger age groups; variants of [dz], [z], [tʃ], and [s] in all age groups

4. Liquids—Both /l/ and /ɹ/ in initial and intervocalic positions are commonly substituted by [w] in all age groups; in post-vocalic positions, the most common substitute is a rounded vowel or [ə].

5. Consonant clusters—Consonant cluster development has been studied extensively in a variety of English-speaking populations; however, that development can be summarized rather succinctly:
   - Clusters consisting of an obstruent plus /w/, /l/, or /ɹ/ are frequently reduced to the less marked member of the cluster up to about age 5; thereafter, the more marked member tends to be simplified, usually to [w].
   - Clusters consisting of /s/ plus a stop or nasal are frequently reduced to the stop or nasal up to about age 5; thereafter, it is relatively common for the /s/ to undergo dentalization or some other distortion.
   - Three-element clusters are usually reduced to one or two elements, none of them /s/, while /ɹ/ and /l/ tend to be substituted by [w]—up to the age of about 6;0. Thereafter three elements are likely to be present, but the /s/ may be distorted and the liquids may undergo substitution.

Syllable structure

For children acquiring GAE, the earliest syllable/word structures that occur in either babble or meaningful speech tend to be CV syllables. Early words tend to be CV in form, followed by CVCV and CVC word shapes (Stoel-Gammon and Dunn, 1985). The first systematic study of syllable structure in the meaningful speech of substantial numbers of children beyond the very early acquisition period was that of Stoel-Gammon (1987), whose participants were 24 months of age. She reported that well over half of the children used at least two exemplars of the following word structures: CV, CVC, CVCV, CVCVC, and syllables with word-initial consonant clusters. Somewhat fewer children used consonant sequences elsewhere in words.

Subsequently, Dyson (1988) reported on word shapes of slightly older children learning GAE (ages 2;5 and 3;3), using different criteria for acquisition. She found that both groups of children used predominantly CV and CVC syllables, with occasional use of V and VC and two-syllable words, and with rare use of three-syllable words. Data covering the period from 2;0 to 3;0 from Watson and Scukanec (1997a) tend to support Dyson's findings. After the age of 3 years, the large majority of children use most of the possible word shapes in English, although they may substitute for some clustered phonemes and they may delete syllables in multisyllabic words.

Prosody

The development of prosody in children who are acquiring GAE is of interest because of the stress-timed nature of English. It is commonplace that preschoolers leave out syllables when they talk, and that these left-out syllables are usually weak syllables; for example, *banana* said as [nænə], *elephant* said as [ɛfənt], and *watermelon* said as [wɑːmen]. This process, which goes by the name of weak syllable deletion, reflects something more general about the child's use of prosody.

Many writers have noted that around the first year and later, children learning GAE often embed their jargon into adultlike intonation contours. Subsequently, the early words tend to be produced with falling contours, although during the first-50-word period, a single-syllable word can be said with a variety of pitch contours that seem to carry pragmatic information, such as anticipation or demand.

The relationship between prosodic tendencies and weak syllable deletion has been subject to considerable debate (Kehoe, 2001), but one prominent theory suggests that children respond to the perceptual salience of the syllables in the intended word. Obviously, syllables with strong stress are salient, but so are word- or utterance-final syllables, whether weak or strong, because of the pervasive phenomena of final-syllable lengthening and pitch declination. Actually, Snow (1994) found that between the ages of 16 and 25 months, children learn to control first the intonation contours of final syllables and then the durational aspects.

Another factor in the pattern of children's syllable deletions is that many baby words in English are disyllables with a strong-weak structure, e.g., *baby, mommy, blanket*, and *doggie*. Kehoe (1999/2000) observed the following order of acquisition of weak syllables in children acquiring GAE:

- Weak syllables in word-final position (e.g., *kitty*),
- Weak syllables in word-internal position when produced with "strong" onsets, e.g., obstruent onsets (e.g., *crocodile*),
- Weak syllables in word-initial position (e.g., *banana*), and finally,
- Weak syllables in word-internal position with less "strong" onsets, such as sonorant onsets (e.g., *telephone*).

Older preschoolers generally appear to preserve weak syllables, although they may not produce either the phonemic content or the prosodic envelope correctly, exemplified in the case of the Winnie the Pooh stories, where the elephant is called the Heffalump (Milne, 1954).

Phonological awareness

There is relatively little systematic information about the development of phonological awareness in children learning GAE. There are several standardized tests of phonological awareness for use with children starting at age 5 years (Robertson and Salter, 1997; Torgeson and Bryant, 2004; Wagner, Torgeson, and Rashotte, 1999), but there is apparently only one explicitly developmental study of this ability in children younger than age 5 (Lonigan, Burgess, Anthony, and Barker, 1998). Studies of children at specific ages and studies of children learning other variants of English suggest that children display sensitivity first to syllables and later to phonemes, although some 3-year-olds can perform phoneme segmentation tasks (see Lonigan et al., 1998, for a review of these data).

Lonigan and colleagues (1998) studied two groups of children aged 2;1 to about 5;10, one group from a middle-income sample, and one from a lower-income sample, for a total of 356 children. They administered four types of tasks relating to what they called "phonological sensitivity": rhyme oddity detection, alliteration oddity detection, blending, and elision. They found that some children at ages 2 and 3 could perform above chance levels on all tasks, but in general, the variability in those age groups was substantial. Second, although there were clear developmental trends in performance on each of these tasks for the middle-income group, socioeconomic status had a very large effect on all but one type of task, such that the lower-income children showed far slower rates of improvement. For example, at age 2, about 9 percent of the middle-income group and 0 percent of the lower-income group performed at better than chance levels on the syllable-blending task, while at age 5, the comparable percentages were 89 percent and 27 percent. The performance of the two groups was quite similar for the rhyme oddity task, which requires awareness of syllables, but there were modest to very large differences on all the other tasks.

The authors suggest that differences in literacy-related activities in the home and elsewhere may account for these differences in the two SES groups. If their hypothesis is correct, then it seems clear that phonological awareness beyond the syllable level is not primarily a developmental phenomenon; rather it may be largely a result of environmental influences.

Speech assessment for children who speak General American English

Survey information about the most popular tests and procedures in use with children speaking GAE is not available. However, the tests that are most widely used are presumably those that are currently available commercially. These include the following instruments that focus on speech sound acquisition:

- *Goldman-Fristoe Test of Articulation-2* (GFTA-2) (Goldman and Fristoe, 2000)
- *Arizona Articulation Proficiency Scale, Third Revision (Arizona-3)* (Fudala, 2000)
- *Photo Articulation Test* (PAT) (Lippke, Dickey, Selmar, and Soder, 1997)
- *Smit-Hand Articulation and Phonology Evaluation* (SHAPE) (Smit and Hand, 1997)
- *Clinical Assessment of Articulation and Phonology* (CAAP) (Secord and Donohue, 2002)

Instruments that focus on phonology and phonological processes and that are commercially available include the following:

- *Khan-Lewis Phonological Analysis, Second Edition* (KLPA-2) (Khan and Lewis, 2002) (This analysis is used with the GFTA-2, above.)
- *Hodson Assessment of Phonological Patterns* (HAPP-3) (Hodson, 2004)
- *Bankson-Bernthal Test of Phonology* (BBTOP) (Bankson and Bernthal, 1990)
- SHAPE (see above)
- CAAP (see above)
- *Natural Process Analysis* (NPA) (Shriberg and Kwiatkowski, 1980)
- *Procedures for the Phonological Analysis of Children's Language* (Ingram, 1981)

The following computerized analyses have been designed for analyzing GAE speech and are available either commercially or as a free download:

- *Programs to Examine Phonetic and Phonologic Evaluation Records* (PEPPER) (Shriberg, 1986) (This software produces analyses like those of the NPA, above.)
- *Logical International Phonetic Programs* (LIPP)(Oller and Delgado, 1999)
- *Computerized Profiling* (CP), Version 9 (Long, Fey, and Channell, 2000)
- *Computerized Articulation and Phonology Evaluation System* (CAPES) (Masterson and Bernhardt, 2002)
- *The Macintosh Interactive System for Phonological Analysis* (ISPA) (Masterson and Pagan, 1994)

Speech intervention for children who speak General American English

A number of speech intervention techniques have been developed in the USA, as well as a number that were developed in other countries. However, with one exception, there appear to be no recent surveys of practicing speech-language pathologists to provide information on the techniques actually used by clinicians. Therefore, this section is roughly based on frequency of mention in textbooks and other books about speech sound disorders. The approaches that are typically used for disorders that are considered to be articulatory (phonetic) in nature are listed in the author's estimated order of most-frequently-used to least-frequently-used:

- Traditional articulation therapy (Van Riper, 1978)
- Behavior modification therapy using motor learning principles, either as a commercial program, for example, *Monterey Articulation Program* (Baker and Ryan, 1971), or as an adjunct to traditional intervention (Bernthal and Bankson, 1998; Smit, 2004)
- Stimulus shift approach (McLean, 1970)
- Paired stimuli (Weston and Irwin, 1971)
- McDonald sensorimotor approach (McDonald, 1964)

The intervention approaches that are often used for phonological disorders include the following:

- Cycles therapy (Hodson and Paden, 1991)
- Minimal pairs therapy (Weiner, 1981; Blache, 1982)
- Multiple oppositions therapy (Williams, 2000)
- Maximal opposition contrast therapy (Gierut, 1989)
- Metaphon therapy (Howell and Dean, 1991)

The one recent survey that has been reported was undertaken by Watson and Lof (2004). The survey dealt with one particular method of intervention. These authors reported that 85 percent of speech-language pathologists in early childhood and elementary school settings use non-speech oral-motor therapy (NS-OMT) with children who have speech sound disorders, including both "functional misarticulations" and phonological disorders. The authors note, however, that NS-OMT lacks both a theoretical basis and adequate research evidence of its effectiveness.

Working in the USA

The profession of speech-language pathology is represented in virtually every school and every health care institution in the USA, as well as in private practice and other for-profit settings. The profession is regulated in three ways. First, the American Speech-Language-Hearing Association (ASHA) has a certification program for speech-language pathologists called the Certificate of Clinical Competence (CCC). SLPs are eligible for the CCC after completing an accredited master's program or clinical doctoral program, completing a clinical fellowshipyear, and passing the Praxis Test for SLPs (Educational Testing Service, 2005). To maintain certification, SLPs must complete 30 hours of continuing education every three years. This certification program is voluntary, but many health care settings and schools explicitly require the CCC. As of January 1, 2005, ASHA entered into a quadrilateral agreement with the United Kingdom, Canada, and Australia to allow mutual recognition of certification (American Speech-Language-Hearing Association, 2005).

In addition to the ASHA certification program, 46 of the 50 states have licensure for SLPs and 38 have separate procedures for certification for SLPs working in public school settings. Typically, the state licensure laws cover either all SLPs in the state or only SLPs working in settings other than public schools. State licensure is usually modeled after the ASHA CCC standards. Typically, there are requirements for continuing education in order to renew ASHA certification, state licensure, and school certification. Sources of continuing education include the annual national convention of the ASHA and annual conventions of state associations of speech-language pathologists and audiologists.

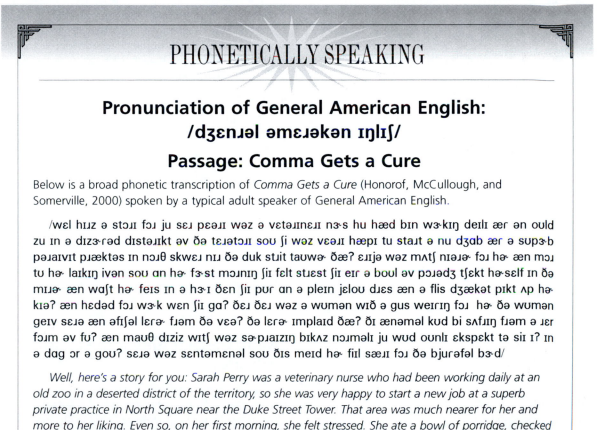

PHONETICALLY SPEAKING

Pronunciation of General American English:
/dʒɛnɹəl əmɛɹəkən ɪŋlɪʃ/
Passage: Comma Gets a Cure

Below is a broad phonetic transcription of *Comma Gets a Cure* (Honorof, McCullough, and Somerville, 2000) spoken by a typical adult speaker of General American English.

/wɛl hɪɹz ə stɔɹɪ fɔɹ ju sɛɹ pɛɹɪ wəz ə vɛtəɹɪnɛɹɪ nɝs hu hæd bɪn wɝkɪŋ deɪlɪ æt ən ould zu ɪn ə dɪzɚɹəd dɪstɹɪkt əv ðə tɛɹətɔɹɪ sou ʃi wəz vɛɹɪ hæpɪ tu staɹt ə nu dʒɑb æɹ ə supɚb pɹaɪvɪt pɹæktəs ɪn nɔɹθ skwɛɹ nɪɹ ðə duk stɹit tauwɚ ðæʔ ɛɹɪə wəz mʌtʃ nɪɹɚ fɔɹ hɚ æn mɔɹ tu hɚ laɪkɪŋ ivən sou ɑn hɚ fɝst mɔɹnɪŋ ʃi fɛlt stɹɛst ʃi eɪ ə boul əv pɔɹɪdʒ tʃɛkt hɚself ɪn ðə mɪɹɚ æn waʃt hɚ feɪs ɪn ə hɝɪ ðɛn ʃi pʊɹ ɑn ə pleɪn jɛlou dɹɛs æn ə flis dʒækət pɪkt ʌp hɚ kɪɹəʔ æn hɛdəd fɔɹ wɝk wɛn ʃi gɑʔ ðɛɹ ðɛɹ wəz ə wumən wɪð ə gus weɪɹɪŋ fɔɹ hɚ ðə wumən geɪv sɛɹə æn əfɪʃəl lɛɹɚ fɹəm ðə vɛʔ ðə lɛɹɚ ɪmplaɪd ðæʔ ðɪ ænəməl kʊd bi sʌfɹɪŋ fɹəm ə ɹɛɹ fɔɹm əv fʊʔ æn mauθ dɪziz wɪtʃ wəz sɚpɹaɪzɪŋ bɪkʌz nɔɹməlɪ ju wʊd ounlɪ ɛkspɛkt tə sii ɪʔ ɪn ə dɑg ɔɹ ə gouʔ sɛɹə wəz sɛntəmɛnəl sou ðɪs meɪd hɚ fiil sæɹɪ fɔɹ ðə bjuɹəfəl bɝd/

Well, here's a story for you: Sarah Perry was a veterinary nurse who had been working daily at an old zoo in a deserted district of the territory, so she was very happy to start a new job at a superb private practice in North Square near the Duke Street Tower. That area was much nearer for her and more to her liking. Even so, on her first morning, she felt stressed. She ate a bowl of porridge, checked herself in the mirror and washed her face in a hurry. Then she put on a plain yellow dress and a fleece jacket, picked up her kit, and headed for work. When she got there, there was a woman with a goose waiting for her. The woman gave Sarah an official letter from the vet. The letter implied that the animal could be suffering from a rare form of foot and mouth disease, which was surprising, because normally you would only expect to see it in a dog or a goat. Sarah was sentimental, so this made her feel sorry for the beautiful bird. (Honorof, McCullough, and Somerville, 2000).

RESOURCES

Books

Edwards, H. T. (1997). *Applied phonetics: The sounds of American English* (2nd ed.) San Diego: Singular.

Labov, W., Ash, S., and Boberg, C. (2005). *Atlas of North American English: Phonetics, phonology and sound change.* Berlin: Mouton de Gruyter.

Small, L. H. (2005). *Fundamentals of phonetics: A practical guide for students* (2nd ed.). Boston: Allyn and Bacon.

Van Riper, C. G., and Smith, D. E. (Reprinted 1992). *An introduction to General American phonetics* (3rd ed.) Prospect Heights, IL: Waveland Press.

Wolfram, W., and Schilling-Estes, N. (2006). *American English.* Malden, MA: Blackwell.

There are at least two dictionaries that show American English pronunciations using the International Phonetic Alphabet (International Phonetic Association, 1999), including the Cambridge Dictionary of American English (Landau, 2000) and the Dictionary of American Regional English (Cassidy and Hall, 1985).

CD-ROMs

There is a CD-ROM that accompanies the book by L. H. Small (see above).

Kortmann, B., and Schneider, E. W. (2004). A handbook of varieties of English: A multimedia reference tool. Volume 1: Phonology. Berlin: Mouton de Gruyter.

Stern, D. A. *The sound and style of American English* (audiocassettes). Los Angeles: Dialect Accent Specialists. Web site: http://www.dialectaccentspecialists.com.

Journals

The American Speech-Language-Hearing Association publishes the following refereed journals, all of them available online to ASHA members through http://www.asha.org:

- American Journal of Speech-Language Pathology: A Journal of Clinical Practice (AJSLP)
- Publishes articles that are applied in nature.
- *Journal of Speech, Language, and Hearing Research (JSLHR)*

- Publishes research articles that are either basic or applied in nature.
- Language, Speech, and Hearing Services in Schools (LSHSS)
- Publishes articles that are applied in nature, with a special focus on provision of services in school settings.

Many other general interest journals are available to SLPs. Among these, the ones most closely related to phonology and phonetics are these:

- *Journal of Phonetics* http://www.elsevier.com
  Information about this journal, which publishes primarily basic research in phonetics and speech science, may be found at the Elsevier Web site.
- *Clinical Linguistics and Phonetics* http://www.informaworld.com/smpp/title~content=+73693308
  Information about this journal, which publishes both basic and applied research, may be found at the Informa site.

Professional associations

The professional association(s) of speech-language pathologists within the USA include the national organization, called the American Speech-Language-Hearing Association, http://www.asha.org, and state associations. The state organizations are typically named (Name of State) Speech-Language-Hearing Association and are abbreviated in a way comparable to ASHA; e.g., the abbreviation for the Kansas Speech-Language-Hearing Association is KSHA.

Useful General American English Web sites

- American English, http://www.absoluteastronomy.com/encyclopedia/a/american_english.htm#. Also available from http://en.wikipedia.org/wiki/American_English/Standard_American_English.
- American Speech-Language-Hearing Association, http://www.asha.org.
- Speech-Language Pathology Web sites, http://www.herring.org/speech.html. A nationally recognized resource list for speech-language pathologists maintained by Sandy and Liz Herring.
- *Merriam-Webster online dictionary,* http://www.m-w.com/cgi-bin/dictionary.

REFERENCES

American Speech-Language-Hearing Association (n.d.). Become an international affiliate. Retrieved September 24, 2005, from http://www.asha.org/about/membership-certification/international/.

Arlt, P. B., and Goodban, M. T. (1976). A comparative study of articulation acquisition as based on a study of 240 normals aged three to six. *Language, Speech, and Hearing Services in Schools, 7*, 173–180.

Baker, R. D., and Ryan, B. P. (1971). *Programmed conditioning for articulation.* Monterey, CA: Monterey Learning Systems.

Bankson, N. W., and Bernthal, J. E. (1990). *Bankson-Bernthal Test of Phonology (BBTOP).* Austin, TX: Pro-Ed.

Cassidy, F.G., and Hall, J. H. (Eds.). (1985). *Dictionary of American Regional English.* Cambridge, MA: Belknap Press of Harvard University.

Bernthal, J.E., and Bankson, N.W. (1998). *Articulation and phonological disorders* (4th ed.). Boston: Allyn and Bacon.

Blache, S. E. (1982). Minimal word pairs and distinctive feature training. In M. Crary (Ed.), *Phonological intervention: Concepts and procedures* (pp. 61–96). San Diego, CA: College-Hill Press.

Calvert, D. R. (1980). *Descriptive phonetics.* New York: Thieme-Stratton.

Coplan, J., and Gleason, J. R. (1988). Unclear speech: Recognition and significance of unintelligible speech in preschool children. *Pediatrics, 82,* 447–452. Erratum in: *Pediatrics,* 1988, *82,* 862.

Dyson, A.T. (1988). Phonetic inventories of 2- and 3-year-old children. *Journal of Speech and Hearing Disorders, 53,* 89–93.

Educational Testing Service. (2005). The PRAXIS series. Retrieved September 30, 2005, from www.ets.org.

Fudala, J. B. (2000). *Arizona articulation proficiency scale, Third Revision (Arizona-3).* Los Angeles: Western Psychological Services.

Gierut, J. (1989). Maximal opposition approach to phonological treatment. *Journal of Speech and Hearing Disorders, 54,* 9–19.

Goldman, R., and Fristoe, M. (2000). *Goldman-Fristoe Test of Articulation-2 (GFTA-2).* Circle Pines, MN: American Guidance Service.

Haelsig, P. C., and Madison, C. L. (1986). A study of phonological processes exhibited by 3-, 4-, and 5-year-old children. *Language, Speech, and Hearing Services in Schools, 17,* 107–114.

Hare, G. (1983). Development at 2 years. In J.V. Irwin and S. P.Wong (Eds.), *Phonological development in children 18 to 72 months* (pp. 55–85). Carbondale, IL: Southern Illinois University Press.

Hodson, B. W. (2004). *Hodson Assessment of Phonological Patterns (HAPP-3).* Austin, TX: Pro-Ed, Inc.

Hodson, B. W., and Paden, E. (1991). *Targeting intelligible speech: A phonological approach to remediation* (2nd ed.). Austin, TX: Pro-Ed.

Hoffman, K. A. (1982). *Speech sound acquisition and natural process occurrence in the continuous speech of three-to-six-year-old children.* Unpublished master's thesis, University of Wisconsin-Madison.

Honorof, D. N., McCullough, J., and Somerville, B. (2000). *Comma gets a cure: A diagnostic passage for accent study.* New Haven, CT: Haskins Laboratories.

Howell, J., and Dean, E. (1991). *Treating phonological disorders in children: Metaphon-theory to practice* (2nd ed.). London: Whurr.

Ingram, D. (1981). *Procedures for the phonological analysis of children's language.* Baltimore: University Park Press.

International Phonetic Association. (1999). *Handbook of the International Phonetic Association: A guide to the use of the International Phonetic Alphabet.* Cambridge, UK: Cambridge University Press.

Irwin, M. V., and Wong, S. P. (1983). *Phonological development in children 18 to 72 months.* Carbondale, IL: Southern Illinois University Press.

Kehoe, M. (1997). Stress error patterns in English-speaking children's word productions. *Clinical Linguistics and Phonetics, 11,* 389–409.

Kehoe, M. K. (1999/2000). Truncation without shape constraints: The latter stages of prosodic acquisition. *Language Acquisition, 8,* 23–67.

Kehoe, M. K. (2001). Prosodic patterns in children's multisyllabic word productions. *Language, Speech, and Hearing Services in Schools, 32,* 284–294.

Khan, L., and Lewis, N. (2002). *Khan-Lewis Phonological Analysis, (2nd ed.) (KLPA-2).* Circle Pines, MN: American Guidance Service.

Labov, W. (1991). The three dialects of English. In P. Eckert (Ed.), *New ways of analyzing sound change.* San Diego: Academic Press.

Landau, S. I. (Ed.). (2000). *Cambridge dictionary of American English.* Cambridge, UK: Cambridge University Press.

Larkins, P. (1983). Development at 3 years. In J. V. Irwin and S. P. Wong (Eds.), *Phonological development in children 18 to 72 months* (pp. 87–105). Carbondale, IL: Southern Illinois University Press.

Lieberman, P. (1980). On the development of vowel production in young children. In G. H. Yeni-Komshian, J. F. Kavanagh, and

Ferguson, C. A. (Eds.), *Child phonology, Volume 1: Production* (pp. 113–142). New York: Academic Press.

Lippke, B., Dickey, S., Selmar, J., and Soder, A. (1997). *Photo Articulation Test (PAT)*. Austin, TX: Pro-Ed.

Long, S., Fey, M., and Channell, R. (2000). *Computerized Profiling (CP), Version 9*. Cleveland OH: Department of Communication Sciences, Case Western Reserve University.

Lonigan, C. J., Burgess, S. R., Anthony, J. L., and Barker, T. A. (1998). Development of phonological sensitivity in 2- to 5-year-old children. *Journal of Educational Psychology, 90,* 294–311.

Lowe, R. J., Knutson, P. J., and Monson, M. A. (1985). Incidence of fronting in preschool children. *Language, Speech, and Hearing Services in Schools, 16,* 119–123.

Masterson, J., and Bernhardt, B. (2002). *Computerized Articulation and Phonology Evaluation System (CAPES)*. San Antonio, TX: The Psychological Corporation.

Masterson, J., and Pagan, F. (1994). *The Macintosh Interactive System for Phonological Analysis (ISPA)*. San Antonio, TX: The Psychological Corporation.

McDonald, E. T. (1964). *Articulation testing and treatment: A sensory motor approach*. Pittsburgh, PA: Stanwix House.

McLean, J. E. (1970). *Extending stimulus control of phoneme articulation by operant techniques*. Washington, DC: ASHA Monographs, vol 14.

Milne, A. A., with Shepard, E. H. (Illustrator). (1954). *Winnie the Pooh*. New York: Puffin Books.

Oller, D. K., and Delgado, R. E. (1999). *Logical International Phonetics Programs* (Windows version). Miami: Intelligent Hearing Systems Corp.

Olmsted, D. L. (1971). *Out of the mouth of babes*. The Hague: Mouton.

Otomo, K., and Stoel-Gammon, C. (1992). The acquisition of unrounded vowels in English. *Journal of Speech and Hearing Research, 35,* 604–616.

Paschall, L. (1983). Development at 18 months. In J. V. Irwin and S. P. Wong (Eds.), *Phonological development in children 18 to 72 months* (pp. 27–54). Carbondale, IL: Southern Illinois University Press.

Peña-Brooks, A., and Hegde, M. N. (2000). *Assessment and treatment of articulation and phonological disorders in children*. Austin, TX: Pro-Ed.

Pollock, K. E. (2002). Identification of vowel errors: Methodological issues and preliminary data from the Memphis Vowel Project. In M. J. Ball and F. E. Gibbon (Eds.), *Vowel disorders* (pp. 83–113). Boston: Butterworth Heinemann.

Pollock, K. E., and Berni, M. C. (2003). Incidence of non-rhotic vowel errors in children: Data from the Memphis Vowel Project. *Clinical Linguistics and Phonetics, 17,* 393–401.

Poole, I. (1934). *The genetic development of articulation of consonant sounds in children's speech*. Unpublished doctoral dissertation, University of Michigan, Ann Arbor.

Prather, E. M., Hedrick, D. L., and Kern, C. A. (1975). Articulation development in children aged 2–4 years. *Journal of Speech and Hearing Disorders, 40,* 179–191.

Preisser, D. A., Hodson, B. W., and Paden, E. P. (1988). Developmental phonology: 18–29 months. *Journal of Speech and Hearing Disorders, 53,* 125–130.

Robb, M. P., and Bleile, K. M. (1994). Consonant inventories of young children from 8 to 25 months. *Clinical Linguistics and Phonetics, 8,* 295–320.

Robbins, J., and Klee, T. (1987). Clinical assessment of oropharyngeal motor development in young children. *Journal of Speech and Hearing Disorders, 52,* 271–277.

Roberts, J. E., Burchinal, M., and Footo, M. M. (1990). Phonological process decline from 2 1/2 to 8 years. *Journal of Communication Disorders, 23,* 205–217.

Robertson, C., and Salter, W. (1997). *The phonological awareness test*. East Moline, IL: LinguiSystems, Inc.

Sax, M. R. (1972). A longitudinal study of articulation change. *Language, Speech, and Hearing Services in Schools, 3,* 41–48.

Secord, W., and Donohue, J. (2002). *Clinical Assessment of Articulation and Phonology (CAAP)*. Greenville, SC: Super Duper Publications.

Selby, J. C., Robb, M. P., and Gilbert, H. R. (2000). Normal vowel articulations between 15 and 30 months of age. *Clinical Linguistics and Phonetics, 14,* 255–265.

Shriberg, L. (1986). *Programs to examine phonetic and phonologic evaluation records (PEPPER)*. Hillsdale, NJ: Lawrence Erlbaum.

Shriberg, L. D., and Kwiatkowski, J. (1980). *Natural process analysis (NPA): A procedure for phonological analysis of continuous speech samples*. New York: John Wiley.

Shriberg, L. D., and Kwiatkowski, J. (1982). Phonologic disorders III: A procedure for assessing severity of involvement. *Journal of Speech and Hearing Disorders, 47,* 256–270.

Small, L. H. (1999). *Fundamentals of phonetics*. Boston: Allyn & Bacon.

Smit, A. B. (1993a). Phonologic error distributions in the Iowa-Nebraska Articulation Norms Project: Consonant singletons. *Journal of Speech and Hearing Research, 36,* 533–547.

Smit, A. B. (1993b). Phonologic error distributions in the Iowa-Nebraska Articulation Norms Project: Word-initial consonant clusters. *Journal of Speech and Hearing Research, 36,* 931–947.

Smit, A. B. (2004). *Articulation and phonology resource guide for school-age children and adults.* Clifton Park, NY: Thomson Delmar Learning.

Smit, A. B., and Hand, L. (1997). *Smit-Hand Articulation and Phonology Evaluation (SHAPE).* Los Angeles: Western Psychological Services.

Smit, A. B., Hand, L., Freilinger, J. J., Bernthal, J. E., and Bird, A. (1990). The Iowa Articulation Norms Project and its Nebraska replication. *Journal of Speech and Hearing Disorders, 55,* 779–798.

Snow, D. (1994). Phrase-final syllable lengthening and intonation in early child speech. *Journal of Speech and Hearing Research, 37,* 831–840.

Snow, K. (1963). A detailed analysis of articulation responses of 'normal' first grade children. *Journal of Speech and Hearing Research, 6,* 277–290.

Stoel-Gammon, C. (1985). Phonetic inventories, 15–24 months: A longitudinal study. *Journal of Speech and Hearing Research, 28,* 505–512.

Stoel-Gammon, C. (1987). Phonological skills of 2-year-olds. *Language, Speech, and Hearing Services in Schools, 18,* 323–329.

Stoel-Gammon, C., and Dunn, C. (1985). *Normal and disordered phonology in children.* Austin, TX: Pro-Ed.

Templin, M. C. (1957). *Certain language skills in children* (Monograph Series No. 26). Minneapolis, MN: University of Minnesota, The Institute of Child Welfare.

Torgeson, J. K., and Bryant, B. R. (2004). *Test of Phonological Awareness (2nd ed): PLUS (TOPA—2+).* Austin, TX: Pro-Ed.

U.S. Census Bureau. (2002a). *QT-P14: Nativity, citizenship status, year of entry, and region of birth: 2000.* Retrieved August 23, 2005, from Census 2000 Summary file 3 (SF3)-Sample Data via http://factfinder.census.gov.

U.S. Census Bureau. (2002b). *QT-P16: Language spoken at home: 2000.* Retrieved August 22, 2005, from Census 2000 Summary file 3 (SF3)-Sample Data via http://factfinder.census.gov.

Van Riper, C. G. (1978). *Speech correction: Principles and methods* (6th ed.). Englewood Cliffs, NJ: Prentice-Hall.

Wagner, R. K., Torgeson, J. K., and Rashotte, C. (1999). *Comprehensive test of phonological processing (CTOPP).* Austin, TX: Pro-Ed.

Watson, M., and Lof, G. (2004, November). *Use of nonspeech oral motor therapy: National survey results.* Paper presented at the annual convention of the American Speech-Language Hearing Association, Philadelphia, PA.

Watson, M. M., and Scukanec, G. P. (1997a). Phonological changes in the speech of two-year-olds: A longitudinal investigation. *Infant-Toddler Intervention, 7,* 67–77.

Watson, M. M., and Scukanec, G. P. (1997b). Profiling the phonological abilities of 2-year-olds: A longitudinal investigation. *Child Language Teaching and Therapy, 13,* 3–14.

Weiner, F. (1981). Treatment of phonological disability using the method of meaningful minimal pairs: Two case studies. *Journal of Speech and Hearing Disorders, 46,* 97–103.

Weiss, C. E. (1982). *Weiss Intelligibility Test.* Tigard, OR: C. C. Publications.

Wellman, B. L., Case, I. M., Mengert I. G., and Bradbury, D. E. (1931). *Speech sounds of young children.* University of Iowa studies in Child Welfare, Volume 5, No. 2. Iowa City: University of Iowa, The Iowa Child Welfare Research Station.

Weston, A. J., and Irwin, J. V. (1971). Use of paired stimuli in modification of articulation. *Perceptual and Motor Skills, 32,* 947–957.

Williams, A. L. (2000). Multiple oppositions: Theoretical foundations for an alternative contrastive intervention approach. *American Journal of Speech-Language Pathology, 9,* 282–288.

Wolfram, W., and Schilling-Estes, N. (2006). *American English.* Malden, MA: Blackwell.

SUMMARY OF STUDIES OF TYPICAL AMERICAN ENGLISH SPEECH ACQUISITION

Authors	Year	Country	No. of children	Age of children	Information	Sample type	Data collection
Arlt and Goodban	1976	USA	240	3–6 yrs	Consonants	Words	Cross-sectional
Dyson	1988	USA	20	2–3 yrs	Phonetic inventories	Play	Combined cross-sectional and longitudinal
Haelsig and Madison	1986	USA	50	3–5 yrs	Phonological processes	Modeled sentences	Cross-sectional
Hoffman	1982	USA	72	3–6 yrs	PCC; Natural Process Analysis	Conversation	Cross-sectional
Irwin and Wong	1983	USA	100	18–72 mos	Consonants, vowels, and features	Play, conversation	Cross-sectional
Kehoe	1997	USA	18	22–34 mos	Stress error patterns	Words	Cross-sectional
Lonigan, Burgess, Anthony, and Barker	1998	USA	356	25–70 mos	Phonological sensitivity	Phonological sensitivity tasks	Cross-sectional
Lowe, Knutson, and Monson	1985	USA	1048	31–54 mos	Fronting process	Words	Cross-sectional
Olmsted	1971	USA	100	1;3–4;6	Percentage of children at several age levels who produced each phoneme; mismatch information	Connected speech	Non-standardized, closest to cross-sectional
Otomo and Stoel-Gammon	1992	USA	6	22–30 mos	Acquisition of unrounded vowels	Single words	Longitudinal
Pollock	2002	USA	162 in control group	18–83 mos	Percentage Vowels Correct (PCC)	Variety	Cross-sectional
Pollock and Berni	2003	USA	165 in control group	18–83 mos	Percentage Vowels Correct (PVC); mismatches	Single words	Cross-sectional
Poole	1934	USA	140	31–96 mos	Consonants	Single words	Cross-sectional
Prather, Hedrick, and Kern	1975	USA	147	24–48 mos	Consonants	Single words	Cross-sectional
Preisser, Hodson, and Paden	1988	USA	60	18–29 mos	Phonological processes	Single words	Cross-sectional

Authors	Year	Country	No. of children	Age of children	Information	Sample type	Data collection
Robb and Bleile	1994	USA	7	8–25 mos	Consonant inventories	Play	Longitudinal
Robbins and Klee	1987	USA			Oromotor structure and function	Oral movements	Cross-sectional
Roberts, Burchinal, and Footo	1990	USA	145	2;6–8 yrs	Phonological process decline	Single words	Longitudinal
Sax	1972	USA	417	Kindergarten to Grade 5	Consonant production	Single words; imitated sentences	Longitudinal
Selby, Robb, and Gilbert	2000	USA	4	15–36 mos	Vowel inventories	Play	Longitudinal
Smit, Hand, Freilinger, Bernthal, and Bird	1990	USA	997	3–9 yrs	Consonants and clusters	Single words	Cross-sectional
Smit	1993a	USA	1014	2–9 yrs	Consonant mismatches	Single words	Cross-sectional
Smit	1993b	USA	1014	2–9 yrs	Cluster mismatches	Single words	Cross-sectional
Snow, D.	1994	USA	9	16–25 mos	Prosody	Play	Longitudinal
Snow, K.	1963	USA	438	Grade 1	Consonants; mismatches	Single words	Cross-sectional-Grade 1
Stoel-Gammon	1985	USA	34	15–24 mos	Phonetic inventory	Play-conversation	Longitudinal
Stoel-Gammon	1987	USA	34	2 yrs	Phonetic Inventory; PCC; Word-and-syllable shape inventory	Play-conversation	Cross-sectional—age 2
Templin	1957	USA	480	3–8 yrs	Consonants, clusters, vowels	Words	Cross-sectional
Watson and Scukanec	1997a	USA	12	2 yrs	Phonological processes; PCC	Conversational sample	Longitudinal, ages 24–36 mos.
Watson and Scukanec	1997b	USA	12	2 yrs	Phonological skills; PCC	Conversational sample	Longitudinal, ages 24–36 mos.
Wellman, Case, Mengert, and Bradbury	1931	USA	204	2–6 yrs	Phonemes and clusters	Phrases and words	Cross-sectional

Note: PCC = Percentage Consonants Correct.

Chapter 23

African American English Speech Acquisition

Ida J. Stockman

INTRODUCTION

In the United States of America (USA), African Americans are the second largest minority ethnic group at 12.9 percent (U.S. Census Bureau, 2000). The overt physical markers of persons in this group include darker skin tones combined with typically coarser hair texture relative to other ethnic groups. Many of these estimated 36.4 million people of African descent speak an English dialect that differs from most English varieties. This social dialect, labeled here as African American English (AAE), also is called Black English (BE), African American Vernacular English (AAVE), and Ebonics (ebony plus phonics, or "black sounds").

All African Americans do not speak AAE. But it is readily observed among those with ancestral ties to slavery in the USA and the Caribbean island nations. It may be the most controversial minority dialect spoken in the USA. Unlike other minority English varieties (e.g., Spanish-influenced English; see Chapter 33), AAE cannot be traced to a single ancestral language in Africa or elsewhere. The Anglicist hypothesis is that AAE's origin can be traced to the English spoken by British settlers in the USA and the island nations of North America. Alternatively, the Creolist hypothesis traces AAE to an earlier pidgin-creole language. A pidgin is a restricted trade language used by adult speakers of different languages, and it has no native speakers. English vocabulary would have been imposed on a drastically reduced grammar that was influenced by African languages. This language is called a creole when it is learned as children's first or native language. The English creole was elaborated to serve more of its speakers' needs and modified (i.e., de-creolized) across time to sound more like General American English (GAE). The

Gullah dialect, spoken on the coastal islands of South Carolina and Georgia, is believed to be a modern day vestige of an earlier English creole language. However, AAE's origin is likely to be more complex than the claims of either the Anglicist or the Creolist hypothesis, given the evidence for both views (Wolfram and Schilling-Estes, 1998). For example, the pronunciation of *ask* as [æks] in AAE is traced to its earlier use by British settlers. Their shift from [æks] to [æsk] was a phonological change in which AAE speakers did not participate. But substitutions for interdental fricatives (i.e., /ð/ in *this*, *bathe*) and /θ/ (*bathroom* and *bath*) may reflect African language influences, given that these consonants do not occur in west African languages.

AAE's unique history and observable differences from GAE varieties on more than just its pronunciation have led some scholars to argue that it is a separate language and not just another English dialect. Nevertheless, AAE has been evolving across time to look more like GAE in some respects (e.g., unstressed syllable deletion; Vaughn-Cooke, 1987) but less like it in others (e.g., vowel shifts; Labov and Harris, 1989). In its contemporary forms, AAE is viewed as an English dialect (albeit a nonprestige one) whose features overlap with those of GAE and other nonprestige English varieties (e.g., Appalachian English; Rickford and Rickford, 2000).

Few AAE patterns are used exclusively by African Americans, and they are most like the Southern varieties of GAE (Fasold, 1981).

Where AAE is spoken

AAE is spoken all over the USA but it is most likely observed wherever African Americans are densely populated (see accompanying map and Appendix D). They are the most populous in the South and least populous in the West. In the Midwest and Northeast (18–19 percent each), African Americans represent 27–81 percent of the populations in five cities: Chicago, Detroit, New York City, Philadelphia, and Washington, DC (U.S. Census, 2000).

Components of AAE

Consonants

AAE's consonant inventory is the same as GAE (see Chapter 22). But AAE is distinguished from GAE by its variable rule restrictions on consonant use (Rickford and Rickford, 2000; Stockman, 1996; Wolfram, 1994; Wolfram and Schilling-Estes, 1998), as described below.

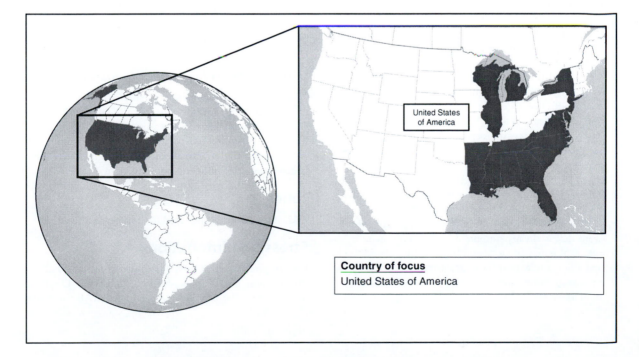

United States of America

Country of focus
United States of America

- **Interdental substitutions:** /ð/ is replaced by /d/ in word-initial position (*that* [ðæt] ⇨ [dæt]) and by /d/ or /v/ in medial and final word positions (cf. *either* [iðʌ] ⇨ [idʌ]; *bathe* [beð] ⇨ [bev]). The substituted /d/ in the initial position may be deleted altogether when it follows an alveolar nasal in the preceding word (*in that* [ɪn ðæt] ⇨ [ɪnæt]; voiceless interdental /θ/ is replaced most often by /f/ in medial and final word positions, although /t/ and /s/ substitutions also occur (cf. *bathroom* [bæfɹum], [bætɹum] or [basɹum]).
- **Other Consonant Substitutions:** Final singleton substitutions include g-dropping, that is, final /n/ replaces /ŋ/ in words ending with –ing (*swinging* [swɪŋgɪŋ] ⇨ [swɪŋgɪn], final devoicing of stops and fricatives (*bad* [bæd] ⇨ [bæt], *buzz* [bʌz] ⇨ [bʌs]); some initial clusters may be backed (/stɹ-/ in *street* [stɹit] ⇨ [skɹit]); /j/ or /l/ may be rhoticized in either word-initial position (/mj/ in *music* [mjuzɪk] ⇨ [muɚzɪk]) or final position (*milk* [mɪlk] ⇨ [mɪɚk]).
- **Initial consonant deletion** affects /ɹ/ and /j/ in some clusters. The /ɹ/ is deleted when clustered with /θ/ (*throw* [θɹo] ⇨ [θo]; *through* [θɹu] ⇨ [θu]) and when clustered with a voiceless oral stop in unstressed syllables (*professor* [pɹofɛsɚ] ⇨ [pofɛsʌ]); /j/ is deleted when clustered with an oral stop (/kj/ in *cute* [kjut] ⇨ [kut]) or a nasal stop, (/nj/ in *news* [njuz] ⇨ [nuz]).
- **Final consonant deletion:** Singleton oral and nasal stops (/b, p, d, t, g, k, m, n, ŋ/) are most deletion-prone, especially alveolar consonants (/d, t, n/). Nasal consonants may be replaced by a nasalized vowel, and voiced final stops may be replaced by lengthened vowels (Moran, 1993; Wolfram, 1989). Deletion in final consonant clusters (e.g., *risk* [ɹɪsk] ⇨ [ɹɪs]) occurs most often when the cluster (1) occurs in a word with one as opposed to two morphemes (*past* versus *passed*), (2) includes consonants with shared voicing (cf., be*st* and be*nt*), and (3) precedes words beginning with a consonant as opposed to a vowel (cf. be*st man* and be*st of*).
- **Final consonant cluster reordering** is selectively observed (e.g., ask [æsk] ⇨ [æks]).
- **Unique pronunciation patterns** can occur when a word that is already simplified by final consonant deletion is pluralized (e.g., *desk* [dɛsk] ⇨ [dɛs] ⇨ [dɛsɛs]), and when a new morphological form results from multiple assimilation and deletion processes (*fitna* derived from *fixing to*).

Vowels and diphthongs

AAE's vowel and diphthong inventory is the same as GAE (Pollock and Berni, 2001). As with consonants, vowel use in AAE is distinguished from GAE by context-sensitive rules.

- AAE speakers neutralize the contrast between /ɪ/ and /ɛ/ before nasal consonants, i.e., *pin* and *pen* sound alike; some words may be pronounced as /ɛ/ or /eɪ/ (e.g., *Sarah* [sɛɹa] or [sɛɪɹa]).
- **The vocalic allophones** of /ɹ/ and /l/ may be modified; /ɹ/ is derhoticized in stressed syllables (*bird* [bɝd] ⇨ [bɜd]), vocalized in unstressed syllables (*zipper* [zɪpɚ] ⇨ [zɪpə]), and absent in centering diphthongs (*car* [kaɚ] ⇨ [ka], *your* [joɚ] ⇨ [jo]; Pollock and Berni, 2001).
- A **diphthongal vowel** may replace /l/ in word-final position (*bell* [bɛl] ⇨ [bɛə]).

Phonotactic restrictions
Syllables

The syllable structure of AAE is the same as GAE except for the variable deletion of unstressed syllables. Unstressed syllables are most deletion-prone when they occur as a single initial vowel in words that belong to a closed grammatical class (e.g., adverbs *(a)way* and prepositions *(a)bout*), and they are preceded by a word ending in a vowel. The initial unstressed syllable in *away* is more likely to be deleted in *go away* than in *got away* (Vaughn-Cooke, 1987).

Consonants and consonant clusters

The sequential arrangement of singleton and clustered speech sounds in words is generally the same in AAE and GAE. They differ less in the initial than in medial and final word positions. The structure of words is simpler in AAE because it allows final consonants to be deleted in a larger number of phonetic contexts than does GAE.

Tones

AAE does not use tones to differentiate meaning.

Stress and intonation

Primary stress occurs on the first instead of the second syllable in some bisyllabic words (*po*lice and *ho*tel). Emphatic stress on *been* (he *been* gone) is a unique AAE form that codes remote past, that is, events that happened long before the speech act (Rickford and Rickford, 2000).

Regarding intonation, AAE speakers have a distinctive way of talking or *sounding black* that is identifiable by characteristic intonation patterns among other prosodic features (e.g., tempo and rhythm). They show wider variation in pitch and intonation (with their voices rising higher and falling lower) than do Caucasian speakers (Rickford and Rickford, 2000). This vocal signature can identify the ethnicity of African American speakers at above chance even from tape-recorded speech with standard grammar and speech articulation (Holland and Dejarnette, 2002; Tull, 1973).

Writing system

AAE is not a formally written language. But it is given written representation in the literary works of well-known African American writers (e.g., Maya Angelou and Toni Morrison). The orthography approximates the oral pronunciation of words (*before = fo; because = cuz; they = de; with = wif,* and so on; Rickford and Rickford, 2000).

Varieties of AAE

Speakers differ in the number, type, and frequency of AAE features used. The density of dialect feature use is known to vary with age, gender, social class, and regional location. However, just a few of these studies have focused on phonological patterns. Some pronunciation patterns are more common in older than in younger speakers, for example, unstressed syllable deletion (Vaughn-Cooke, 1987) and vocalic /r/ absence (Pollock and Berni, 1996). Southern AAE has a larger number and range of dialectally marked features compared to AAE spoken in the Midwest (Hinton and Pollock, 2000).

Typical acquisition of AAE

There is no published study that describes developmental changes across age for the *broad* range of speech sounds learned in AAE. A small set of studies has focused on African American children's production of a single sound or a small subset, typically just the

sounds that differ from GAE. These studies also have often sampled productions at a single age cross-section using a standard elicitation procedure such as a norm-referenced articulation test. Single-age analyses have been described even when data were collected at different ages. Consonants have been described as opposed to vowels. Therefore developmental trends must be inferred from comparisons across different data sets and data-gathering procedures.

Acquired sounds

Consonants

The available research suggests that consonants in AAE emerge in the same order and around the same ages as GAE. But /ɹ/ appears to develop earlier in AAE than in Southern GAE (Pollock and Berni, 1997; see Table 23-1). By 3;0 years, typical AAE speakers use a minimal set of 15 initial consonant singletons that include oral and nasal stops, glides, liquids, and early fricatives (Stockman, 2006a). Final consonants are present and conform already to variable deletion rules. Final nasal and oral stops are most deletion-prone for alveolar sounds /n, t, d/ that precede other consonants as opposed to vowels at word boundaries in connected speech (*put shoe* and *put on*; Stockman, 2006b; Wolfram, 1989).

Between 4;0 and 5;0 years, African American children make more errors on fricatives (3–26 percent) than on other sound classes (0–2.9 percent) when given a standardized articulation test, and they make more errors than their age-matched Caucasian peers (Seymour and Seymour, 1981).

Between 5;5 and 6;6 years, the consonant inventory expands to include later-learned fricatives and affricates plus initial /l/, /ɹ/, and /s/ clusters (Wilcox and Anderson, 1998). The /s/ sound is firmly established in this age range (Stockman, 1993), as is prevocalic /r/ (Pollock and Berni, 1997).

By third grade, most (80 percent, n = 10) African American children perceive the /θ/ and /f/ distinction in word-final position even though they do not all produce it in their speech (Seymour and Ralabate, 1985). At fourth grade, 90 percent (n = 10) produce word-final /θ/ instead of /f/ in elicited single-word productions. But in conversational speech, they continue to differ from their Caucasian, age-matched peers in producing /θ/.

Consonant clusters

Few studies have focused on consonant cluster use in AAE across age. Stockman (2006a) observed that word-initial clusters are used as early as 2;8 years of age, and the earliest ones are likely to be of the stop + sonorant type (e.g., pl-, tw-). Between 3;6 and 5;0 years, the broad range of initial consonant clusters used includes the later-learned ones such as those with two obstruents as in the case of /sk-/ and /st-/ (Wilcox and Anderson, 1998). The children's ability to reproduce initial and medial /s/ clusters in bisyllabic nonsense words increases with age such that no errors are observed by 8 years in either position (Stockman, 1993).

Vowels and diphthongs

There is no published study of vowel and diphthong acquisition in AAE. The vocalic /ɹ/ allophones (e.g., *her, horse, car*) are produced earlier by more African American children than their same-age Caucasian peers who acquire a Southern GAE variety (cf. Pollock and Berni, 1997).

Percent correct

Consonants

Pollock and Berni (1997) reported percentage of consonants correct (PCC) for Southern AAE speakers aged 3 to 6 years with mean scores ranging from 95 to 98 percent.

Consonant clusters

No PCC data appear to be available for just consonant clusters.

Vowels

No data appear to be available for the percentage of vowels correct (PVC).

Phonological processes

AAE speakers appear to use the same commonly observed developmental patterns that have been described for GAE speakers (Haynes and Moran, 1989). These include gliding of liquids, stopping of fricatives, fronting of nasals, stops, and fricatives. The number of developmental phonological processes decreases with age. But African American children make more errors on standardized articulation tests than do Caucasian children overall, and their deletion of final consonants persists beyond third grade. Final consonant deletion is likely to occur under predictable rule-governed conditions, given Wolfram's (1989) developmental study of final nasals at ages 2;0 to 4;6 years. In oral reading, AAE phonological features (e.g., consonant cluster reduction, unstressed syllable deletion, interdental fricative substitutions) account for more of the deviations from GAE pronunciation than do the grammatical features used by elementary school children (Craig, Thompson, Washington, and Potter, 2003). Fewer AAE phonological patterns are observed as age increases. They are observed more often than are morphosyntactic features in the oral reading of African American elementary school children (Thompson, Craig, and Washington, 2004).

Intelligibility

There are no known developmental studies of intelligibility for AAE speakers.

Phonetic inventory

The phonetic inventory of consonants and vowels is the same as GAE with few exceptions. The voiced interdental fricative /ð/ may be used in such restricted contexts (e.g., the biblical terms such as *thou* and *thy*) as to be virtually absent in the consonant inventory of many speakers (Stockman, 1996). The vocalic stressed and unstressed allophones of /ɹ/ as in *bird* and *better* may not be used by some AAE speakers.

Common mismatches

AAE speakers make the same kind of commonly observed developmental errors on singleton and clustered consonants that have been observed for speakers of other English varieties (Seymour and Seymour, 1981; Haynes and Moran, 1989; Stockman, 2006a). Earlier-learned sounds replace later-learned ones. For example, fronted consonant substitutions for nonfronted consonants account for the largest number of developmental errors (Stockman, 2006a). For consonant clusters, a period of deleting one consonant (typically the most marked sound such as /s/, /l/, or /ɹ/) is followed at older ages by a period of substitutions for these same marked sounds (Stockman, 1993).

Syllable structure

No developmental data appear to be available. However, the children are likely to produce words with less complex syllable codas compared to GAE, given that final single and clustered consonants are deleted in some phonetic conditions as required by AAE variable rules.

Prosody

There are no available data on prosodic development in AAE.

TABLE 23-1 Age of acquisition for AAE consonants

Consonant	Stockman (1993; 2006a, b)	Pollock and Berni (1997); Hinton and Pollock (2000)	Wilcox and Anderson (1998)	Seymour and Ralabate (1985)
m	2;8–3;0			
n	2;8–3;0			
ŋ				
b	2;8–3;0			
p	2;8–3;0			
d	2;8–3;0			
t	2;8–3;0			
g	2;8–3;0			
k	2;8–3;0			
w / hw	2;8–3;0			
j	2;8–3;0			
l	2;8–3;0			
ɹ	2;8–3;0	3;7–6;1 4;1– 5;7	5;0–6;6	
f	2;8–3;0			
v				
θ				6;0–9;0
ð				
s	2;8–3;0 5;6–6;0*		5;0–6;6	
z			5;0–6;6	
ʃ			5;0–6;6	
ʒ				
tʃ			5;0–6;6	
dʒ				
h	2;8–3;0			

Note: The table excludes studies of standardized articulation tests, oral reading, and phonological patterns.

*Production of /s/ at 5;6–6;0 years represents 80–90 percent accuracy in imitating initial and medial /s/ in nonsense bisyllables (Stockman, 1993). Word-final /p/t/k/ also are documented in Stockman (2006b).

Phonological awareness

There is little research on the development of phonological awareness by AAE speakers (Craig and Washington, 2004). Two studies of elementary school children showed that dialect influences performance on phonological awareness tasks in different ways for African American and Caucasian children (Thomas-Tate, Washington, and Edwards, 2004); and standardized tests (e.g., the *Test of Phonological Awareness*) underestimate the skills of African American children. The relationship between phonological processing skills and reading skills is less direct for AAE than GAE speakers (Sligh and Conners, 2003).

Speech assessment for children who speak AAE

No standardized test of articulation or phonology has been developed and normed on just African American children. It is generally assumed that an existing standardized test can be used with AAE speakers so long as they are included in the standardization sample in proportion to their representation in the U.S. population (i.e., 12.9 percent). However, African American children typically score lower than test norms. Although their scores do increase when adjusted for dialect bias, the adjusted scores do not always increase enough to change a speaker's diagnostic status (Washington and Craig, 1992). Earlier editions of four standardized tests have some tested validity for use with African American children:

* *Fluharty Preschool Speech and Language Screening Test* (FPSLST; Fluharty, 1978):
  Simmons (1988) reported that Southern African American children (ages 3;0 to 6;0 years, n = 166) did not fail FPSLST more often than Caucasian children (n = 94) at the same ages despite more errors.
* *Goldman-Fristoe Test of Articulation-2* (GFTA-2; Goldman and Fristoe, 2000):
  Seymour and Seymour (1981) used the earlier 1969 edition of the GFTA in their study. They concluded that a valid picture of consonant use by 4- and 5-year-old children in the northeastern USA was obtained. Although the 80 African American children made more errors than their 80 age-matched Caucasian peers, the type of developmental errors did not differ between them.
* *Photo Articulation Test* (PAT; Pendergast, Dickey, Selmar, and Sorder, 1969):
  Cole and Taylor (1990) reported that the PAT yielded no errors in predicting the normal status of 10 Southern first graders (n = 10) when scores were adjusted for dialect differences. The error rate was no more than 20 percent for two other tests (*Arizona Articulation Proficiency Scale* (AAPS; Fudala and Reynolds, 1986) and the *Templin-Darley Screening Test of Articulation* (TDST; Templin and Darley, 1969).
* *Arizona Articulation Proficiency Scale* (AAPS; Fudala and Reynolds, 1986):
  Washington and Craig (1992) observed that in spite of lower AAPS scores relative to test norms, their Midwestern sample of African American preschoolers (4;6 to 5;3) with impaired speech (n = 8) were accurately discriminated from those without impaired speech (n = 20).

Supplementary speech sampling tools for AAE speakers

Alternative assessment procedures have been created because African American children generally score lower than the norming sample on standardized articulation tests. Solutions to the problem of negative test bias have involved the modified use of existing standardized tests: when clinicians do not have adequate normative data for judging whether a clinical problem exists, they can compare child and parent performances on the same standardized test (Terrell, Arensberg, and Rosa, 1992). Alternatively, community informants such as Head Start teachers can be used to identify which children have trouble speaking and which ones do not. Clinicians can determine whether these two groups have different performance profiles on a standardized test such as the PAT (Bleile and Wallach, 1992). Local norms also could be established for performance on selected tests (Proctor, 1994; Stockman, 1996). When clinicians want to assess final consonant use in more dialect-relevant contexts than are provided on a standardized test like the GFTA, they can re-elicit test words in phonetic contexts that favor final consonant use in the dialect. For example, articulation of final consonants can be observed in a test word that precedes another word with a beginning vowel sound (*truck eyes*; *watch-eyes*, and so on; Laing, 2003).

Oral language sampling: When African American children are very young, they may not respond well to standardized tests, biased or not. Their consonant production in natural conversational speech can be screened using the *minimal competence phonetic core* (Stockman, 2006a). This screener, which identifies word-initial singleton and clustered consonant use, is now being normed on a larger sample of African American children (n = 120) in two U.S. regions (Stockman 2006c)

Speech intervention for children who speak AAE

Although no epidemiological study of the prevalence or incidence of phonological/articulatory problems has been done, the percentage of African Americans with all types of speech and language problems is estimated to be higher (16.5 percent) than that observed in other U.S. minority groups (1.2–11.6 percent; Battle, 2002, p. 23). This high percentage has been attributed to their over representation among the economically poor and medically fragile, coupled with inadequate research on their typical speech development.

No special speech intervention has been developed just for AAE speakers. Best clinical practices require all interventions to be sensitive to cultural and language differences, which can show up in many ways, for example, verbal and nonverbal interaction styles, familiarity with therapy stimuli and activities, scheduling of services, and so on. Pronunciation is not regarded as incorrect when it matches typical AAE patterns.

Clinicians should first target speech sounds that do not differ from GAE before targeting those that do (Wolfram, 1994). Shared dialect features are likely to be basic ones that could severely hamper intelligibility if incorrect. For example, intelligibility could be more diminished by word-initial than final consonant absence. In addition, the focus on noncontrastive AAE and GAE sound patterns allows clinicians to apply their own knowledge of GAE to judging disordered speech (Stockman, 1996). Proctor (1994) offers many recommendations for delivering clinical services to persons with speech impairment in minority cultural populations.

Second dialect instruction

AAE is a social dialect that is not commonly spoken by non–African Americans. Therefore, its speakers may be handicapped in employment and schooling unless they acquire proficiency in a standard dialect of wider communication. The American Speech-Language-Hearing Association views second dialect instruction as an *elective* service within the scope of practice for an SLP. This service, commonly known as *accent modification*, focuses on pronunciation patterns along with grammatical and lexical ones (see Chapter 20). Best practices for modifying accents are modeled after second language pedagogy. The goal is to expand the linguistic repertoire, not replace an existing dialect. An *additive* approach requires speakers to learn how to switch between GAE and AAE codes as a communication situation demands, much as bilingual speakers may switch languages. Therefore a speaker's linguistic repertoire includes the coexistence of two pronunciations for the same word, (e.g., *bath* [baf] and [baθ]). Intervention emphasizes contrastive analysis procedures and cultural issues that affect code switching (Taylor, 1986).

Working in the USA with AAE speakers

The professional certification of SLPs in the USA requires education about multicultural/multilingual issues inclusive of those related to accent reduction. The Multicultural Affairs office of the American Speech-Language-Hearing Association (ASHA) maintains a directory of professional experts on AAE at http://www.asha.org. Smitherman (1999) is a useful reference of terms and phrases that may be used by AAE speakers. Although AAE is an indigenous English dialect, its history of isolation from mainstream USA cultures has required speakers to create and use special terms and phrases to code specific aspects of their culture. For example, the word hotcomb refers to a tool for straightening hair.

PHONETICALLY SPEAKING

Pronunciation of African American English:
/æfɹɪkɪn əmɛɹəkɪn ɛŋlɪʃ/

Below is a broad phonetic transcription of *Comma Gets a Cure* (Honorof, McCullough, and Somerville, 2000) spoken by a typical adult speaker of African American English with high density of AAE use.

Passage: Comma Gets a Cure

/wɛə| hɪəz ə stoɹi fʌ ju|| sɛɹʌ pɛɹi wʌz ə vɛtnɹɪi nɜs hu hæd bɪn wɜkɪn deli æt ə oː zu ɪn ə dəzɜtɛ dɪskɹɪt əv də tɛɹətoɹi| so ʃi wəz vɛɹɪ hæpi tə stat ə nu dʒab æt ə səpɜb pɹəvət pɹætɪs ɪ nɔf skwæɛə nɪə də du skɹit tɑuwʌ|| dæt ɛɹə wəz mʌvʃ nɪɹə fʌ hʌ æn moə tu hʌ lakɪn|| ibɪn so| ɔn hʌ fɜs mɔnɪn| ʃi fɛl stɹɛst|| ʃi et ə boː əv pɑɹɪtʃ| tʃɛkt hʌsɛf ɪn ə mɪɹʌ æn wɑʃt hʌ fes ɪn ə hʌɹi|| dɛn ʃi put ɔn ə plaɪ jɛlə dɹɛs æn ə flis dʒækɛt| pɪkt ʌp hʌ kɪt æn hɛdəd fʌ wɜk|| ʍɪn ʃi ɡɑ dæə| dæə wʌz ə womɛn wɪd ə ɡus weɪʔn fʌ hʌ|| də womɛn ɡev sɛɹʌ ə fɪʃəl lɛtə fɹɑm də vɛt| də lɛtə ɪmplɑː dæ də ænɪmʌ kʊd bi sʌfɹɪn fɹʌm ə ɹæə fɔm ɔv fʊt æn mɑuf dəziz| ʍɪtʃ wəz səpɹaɪzɪn| bəkɔs nɔmli ju wʊd ɔnlɪ ɛspɛ tə si ɪt ɪn ə dɔɡ oə ɡoət || sɛɹʌ wʌ sɛnəmɪnəl| so dɪs med hʌ fiə sɔɹi fʌ də butəfʌ bɜd|| /

Well, here's a story for you: Sarah Perry was a veterinary nurse who had been working daily at an old zoo in a deserted district of the territory, so she was very happy to start a new job at a superb private practice in North Square near the Duke Street Tower. That area was much nearer for her and more to her liking. Even so, on her first morning, she felt stressed. She ate a bowl of porridge, checked herself in the mirror and washed her face in a hurry. Then she put on a plain yellow dress and a fleece jacket, picked up her kit and headed for work. When she got there, there was a woman with a goose waiting for her. The woman gave Sarah an official letter from the vet. The letter implied that the animal could be suffering from a rare form of foot and mouth disease, which was surprising, because normally you would only expect to see it in a dog or a goat. Sarah was sentimental, so this made her feel sorry for the beautiful bird. (Honorof, McCullough and Somerville, 2000).

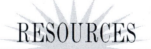

RESOURCES

Books

Labov, W. (1972). *Language in the inner city*. Philadelphia: University of Pennsylvania Press.

Luelsdorff, P. A. (1975). *A segmental phonology of Black English*. The Hague: Mouton.

Mufwene, S. S., Rickford, J. R., Bailey, G., and Baugh, J. (Eds.). (1998). *African-American English*. London: Routledge.

Rickford, J. R. (1999). *African American vernacular English*. Malden, MA: Blackwell.

Smitherman, G. (1986). *Talkin and testifying: The language of Black America*. Detroit, MI: Wayne State University Press.

Van Keulen, J. E., Weddington, G. T., and DeBose, C. E. (1998). *Speech, language, learning, and the African American child*. Boston: Allyn & Bacon.

Wolfram, W. (1969). *A sociolinguistic description of Detroit Negro speech*. Washington, DC: Center for Applied Linguistics.

CD-ROMs/Videotapes

American tongues (VHS), http://www.cnam.com/more_info/ameri3.html Directed and produced by L. Alvarez, and A. Kolker. (1987). (Available from CNAM Film Library, PO Box 1084, Harriman, NY 10926)

The story of English (VHS): Part V-Black on White (1986). Directed and produced by W. Cran. (Available from Public Media Video)

Nonbiased assessment of African American children (1995) Toya Wyatt, Infolink

Journals

• *American Speech*, http://www.dukeupress.edu/americanspeech
A publication of the American Dialect Society, printed by Duke University Press.
• *ECHO*, www.nbaslh.org
An electronic journal published by the National Black Association for Speech, Language, and Hearing.
• *Journal of Multicultural Issues*, http://www.multilingual-matters.net/jmmd/default.htm
A publication of Multilingual Matters.

• Journals of the American Speech-Language-Hearing Association (ASHA) see Chapter 22.

Professional associations

The American Speech-Language-Hearing Association: Office of Multicultural Affairs, http://www.asha.org

The National Black Association for Speech, Language and Hearing (NBASLH), http://www.nbaslh.org

The American Dialect Society, http://www.americandialect.org

The American Association for Applied Linguistics, http://www.aaal.org

The American Dialect Society, http://www.americandialect.org

The American Association for Applied Linguistics, http://www.aaal.org

Useful AAE Websites

• Phonological Features of African American Vernacular English (AAVE; Pollock, et al., 1998), http://www.rehabmed.ualberta.ca/spa/phonology/feature.htm
• The American Speech-Language-Hearing Association's Web site on Multicultural Issues, http://www.asha.org/about/Leadership-projects/multicultural
• The American Dialect Society, http://www.americandialect.org
• The American Association for Applied Linguistics, http://www.aaal.org

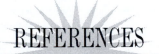

REFERENCES

Battle, D. (2002). Communication disorders in a multicultural society. In D. Battle (Ed.), *Communication disorders in multicultural populations* (pp. 3–31). Boston: Butterworth-Heinemann.

Bleile, K., and Wallach, H. (1992). A sociolinguistic investigation of the speech of African American preschoolers. *American Journal of Speech-Language Pathology, 1*, 54–62.

Cole, P., and Taylor, O. (1990). Performance of working-class African-American children on three tests of articulation. *Language, Speech, and Hearing Services in Schools, 21*(2), 171–176.

Craig, H. K., Thompson, C. A., Washington, J. A., and Potter, S. L. (2003). Phonological features of child African American English. *Journal of Speech, Language, and Hearing Research, 46*, 623–635.

Craig, H. K., and Washington, J. A. (2004). Language variation and literacy learning. In C. A. Stone, E. R. Silliman, B. J. Ehren, and K. Apel (Eds), *Handbook of literacy and literacy development and disorders* (pp. 228–247). New York: Guilford.

Fasold, R. (1981). The relationship between black and white English in the South. *American Speech, 56,* 163–189.

Fluharty, N. B. (1978). *Fluharty preschool and language screening test.* New York: Teaching Resources.

Fudala, J. B., and Reynolds, W. M. (1986). *Arizona articulation proficiency scale* (2nd ed.). Los Angeles: Western Psychological Services.

Goldman, R., and Fristoe, M. (1969; 1986; 2000). *Goldman-Fristoe test of articulation.* Circle Pines, MN: American Guidance Service.

Haynes, W., and Moran, M. (1989). A cross-sectional developmental study of final consonant production in southern black children from preschool through third grade. *Language, Speech, and Hearing Services in Schools, 20,* 400–406.

Hinton, L. N., and Pollock, K. E. (2000). Regional variations in the phonological characteristics of African American Vernacular English. *Word Englishes, 19*(1), 59–71.

Holland, R. W., and Dejarnette, G. (2002). Voice and voice disorders. In D. Battle (Ed.), *Communication disorders in multicultural populations* (3rd ed.; pp. 299–233). Boston: Butterworth-Heinemann.

Honorof, D. N., McCullough, J., and Somerville, B. (2000). *Comma gets a cure: A diagnostic passage for accent study.* New Haven, CT: Haskins Laboratories.

Labov, W., and Harris, W. A. (1989). De facto segregation of Black and White vernaculars. *American Speech, 64,* 12–39.

Laing, S. L. (2003). Assessment of phonology in preschool African American Vernacular English using an alternate response mode. *American Journal of Speech-Language Pathology, 12* (3), 273–281.

Moran, M. (1993) Final consonant deletion in African American children speaking Black English: A closer look. *Language, Speech, and Hearing Services in the Schools, 24,* 161–166.

Pendergast, K., Dickey, S., Selmar, J. W., and Sorder, A. L. (1969) *The Photo Articulation Test.* Danville, IL: Interstate.

Pollock, K. E., and Berni, M. C. (1996). *Vocalic and postvocalic /R/ in African American Memphians.* Paper presented at New Ways to Analyze Variation in English, Las Vegas, NV.

Pollock, K., and Berni, M. (1997, November). *Acquisition of /r/ by African American and European American children.* Paper presented at the annual convention of the American Speech-Language-Hearing Association, Boston, MA.

Pollock, K., and Berni, M. (2001). Transcription of vowels. *Topics in Language Disorders, 21*(4), 22–40.

Proctor, A. (1994). Phonology and cultural diversity. In R. J. Lowe (Ed.), *Phonology: Assessment and intervention: Applications in speech pathology* (pp. 207–245). Baltimore: Williams & Wilkins.

Rickford, J. R., and Rickford, R. J. (2000). *Spoken soul: The story of Black English.* New York: John Wiley.

Seymour, H. N., and Ralabate, P. K. (1985). The acquisition of a phonologic feature of Black English. *Journal of Communication Disorders, 18,* 139–148.

Seymour, H. N., and Seymour, C. (1981). Black English and Standard American English contrasts in consonantal development for four- and five-year-olds. *Journal of Speech and Hearing Disorders, 46,* 276–280.

Simmons, J. O. (1988). Fluharty preschool and language screening test: Analysis of construct validity. *Journal of Speech and Hearing Disorders, 53,* 168–174.

Sligh, A. C., and Connor, F. A. (2003). Relation of dialect to phonological processing: African American Vernacular English versus Standard American English. *Contemporary Educational Psychology, 28,* 205–228.

Smitherman, G. (1999). *Black talk: Words and phrases from the hood to the amen corner.* New York: Houghton-Mifflin.

Stockman, I. (1993). Variable word initial and medial consonant relationships in children's speech sound articulation. *Perceptual and Motor Skills, 76,* 675–689.

Stockman, I. (1996). Phonological development and disorders in African American children. In A. Kamhi, K. Pollock, and J. Harris (Eds.), *Communication development and disorders in African American children: Research, assessment and intervention* (pp. 117–153). Baltimore: Brookes.

Stockman, I. (2006a). Evidence for a minimal competence core of consonant sounds in the speech of African American children: A preliminary study [Electronic Preview Version, April 27, 2006]. *Clinical Linguistics and Phonetics, 20,* 1–27.

Stockman, I. (2006b). Alveolar segment bias in the final consonant deletion patterns of African American children. *Language, Speech, and Hearing Services in Schools, 37,* 85–95.

Stockman, I. (2006c). Cross-validation of a minimal competency phonetic core for young African American children in two regional varieties. Manuscript in preparation.

Taylor, O. (1986). Teaching English as a second dialect. In O. Taylor (Ed.), *Treatment of communication disorders in culturally and linguistically diverse populations* (pp. 153–178). San Diego, CA: College-Hill Press.

Templin, M. C., and Darley, F. L. (1969). *The Templin-Darley test of articulation* (2nd ed). Iowa City: University of Iowa, Bureau of Educational Research and Service, Division of Extension and University Services.

Terrell, S. L., Arensberg, K., and Rosa, M. (1992). Parent-child comparative analysis: A criterion-referenced method for the nondiscriminatory assessment of a child who spoke a relatively uncommon dialect of English. *Language, Speech, and Hearing Services in Schools, 23,* 34–42.

Thomas-Tate, S., Washington, J., and Edwards, J. (2004). Standardized assessment of phonological awareness skills in low-income African American first graders. *American Journal of Speech-Language Pathology, 12,* 182–190.

Thompson, C., Craig, H. K., and Washington, J. A. (2004). Variable production of African American English across oracy and literacy contexts. *Language, Speech, and Hearing Services in Schools, 35,* 269–282.

Tull, B. M. (1973). *Analysis of selected prosodic features in the speech of black and white children.* Unpublished doctoral dissertation, Ohio State University, Columbus.

U.S. Census Bureau. (2001). *The black population: 2000.* Retrieved November 14, 2006, from http://www.census.gov/prod/2001pubs/c2kbr01-5.pdf

Vaughn-Cooke, F. (1987). Are Black and White vernaculars diverging? *American Speech, 62,* 12–32.

Washington, J. A., and Craig, H. K. (1992). Articulation test performances of low-income, African-American preschoolers with communication impairments. *Language, Speech, and Hearing Services in Schools, 23,* 203–207.

Wilcox, L. D., and Anderson, R. T. (1998). Distinguishing between phonological difference and disorder in children who speak African-American vernacular English: An experimental testing instrument. *Journal of Communication Disorders, 31,* 315–335.

Wolfram, W. (1989). Structural variability in phonological development: Final nasals in vernacular Black English. In R. Fasold and D. Schiffren (Eds.), *Current issues in linguistic theory: Language change and variation* (pp. 301–332). Amsterdam: John Benjamins.

Wolfram, W. (1994). The phonology of a sociocultural variety: The case of African American Vernacular English. In J. Bernthal and N. Bankson (Eds.), *Child phonology: Characteristics, assessment, and intervention with special populations* (pp. 227–244). New York: Thieme.

Wolfram, W., and Schilling-Estes, N. (1998). *American English: Dialects and Variation.* Oxford: Blackwell.

SUMMARY OF STUDIES OF TYPICAL AFRICAN AMERICAN ENGLISH SPEECH ACQUISITION

Author	Year	States in USA	Number of children	Age of children	Information	Sample type	Data collection
Craig, Thompson, Washington, and Potter	2003	Midwestern USA	64	2nd to 5th Grades	AAE Phonological patterns	Oral reading	Cross-sectional
Haynes and Moran	1989	Southern USA	222	3;5–9;11	Phonological processes	Final consonant deletion	Cross-sectional
*Hinton and Pollock	2000	Midwestern USA	9	4;1–5;7	/ɹ/ production	Elicited words: research protocol	Single age
*Pollock and Berni	1997	Southern USA	68	3;7–6;1	/ɹ/ patterns	Elicited words: research protocol	Cross-sectional/ Single age
*Seymour and Ralabate	1985	Northeastern USA	40	1st to 4th Grades 6–9 yrs	Reception and production of /θ/	Elicited words, conversational speech	Cross-sectional

Author	Year	States in USA	Number of children	Age of children	Information	Sample type	Data collection
Seymour and Seymour	1981	Northeastern USA	160	4;0–5;0	Test score comparisons of Black and White children	Goldman-Fristoe Test of Articulation	Cross-sectional
*Stockman	1993	Northeastern USA	106	3;0–8;0	Initial and medial /s/ production	Elicited imitation nonsense bisyllables	Cross-sectional
*Stockman	2006a	Northeastern USA	7	2;8–3;0	Minimal competency core (MCC) Initial consonants	Conversational speech	Single age
*Stockman	2006b	Northeastern USA	7	2;8–3;0	Constraints on final stop deletion	Conversational speech	Single age
Stockman	2006c	Midwest and Southern USA	120	3;9–3;11	Cross validation of MCC	Conversational speech	Single age
*Wilcox and Anderson	1998	Midwestern USA	26	5;0–6;6	Initial consonant singletons and clusters varied word positions	Elicited single words	Single age
Wolfram	1989	Northeastern USA	9	1;6–4;6	Final nasal deletion	Conversational speech	Cross-sectional/ Longitudinal

* Asterisks identify studies included in Table 23-1.

Acknowledgement

The author thanks Elaina Marie Swartzlander for her help with the preparation of the map, tables, and phonetic illustrations in this chapter.

Chapter 24

Appalachian English Speech Acquisition

Peter Flipsen Jr.

INTRODUCTION

Broadly speaking, Appalachia refers to that part of the United States of America encompassing the Appalachian mountain range and nearby environs stretching from as far north as Maine to as far south as the northern parts of Alabama and Georgia. However, Appalachian English as defined here is more limited in its distribution; speakers of this dialect are found in all of West Virginia and parts of four other states—eastern Kentucky, southwestern Virginia, western North Carolina, and eastern Tennessee (Christian, Wolfram, and Dube, 1988; Richards, 2001). For current purposes, Appalachian English refers to the nonstandard (i.e., stigmatized or vernacular) dialect of American English spoken by the rural, working-class population in these areas; it is sometimes also called *mountain speech* or *Appalachian drawl* (Hazen and Fluharty, 2004; Wolfram and Christian, 1976). Speakers of this dialect are thought to be predominantly descendants of settlers who arrived in the region during the late seventeenth and early eighteenth centuries from Scotland. Many of these original settlers had previously been temporary settlers in Ireland; hence they are often referred to as Scots-Irish. Settlers also came to the area from southern Britain during this same period. The region was geographically isolated for over 200 years; socioeconomic differences also isolated the rural residents from the emerging urban centers. The isolation largely ended with the introduction of electricity, the telephone, and highway construction during the second quarter of the twentieth century.

There continues to be some debate about whether the dialect originated as a product of mostly Scots-Irish or southern British language influence; a systematic analysis of the grammatical features of the dialect (thought to be far more resistant to change than vocabulary or phonology) suggests a predominance of Scots-Irish influence (Montgomery, 1991). Regardless of its origin, the long period of relative isolation appears to have allowed for the evolution of this unique form of American English. Currently there may be as many as 2 million speakers of this dialect (Hazen, personal communication, April 9, 2002).

Similar to speakers of other nonstandard dialects such as African American English, speakers of Appalachian English are predominantly members of a stigmatized social group. As such, there has been a historical tendency to view their speech as a sign of reduced intellectual capacity (Adler, 1979). There has also been a tendency to overidentify speakers of such dialects as having speech or language disorders (Adler and Birdsong, 1983). Fortunately, misguided notions of an "impoverished" language system have been easily countered by the work of sociolinguists such as Labov as well as by our broadening understanding of the very rich oral tradition in the cultures of African American, Native American, and Appalachian populations.

As is typical of stigmatized dialects, use of Appalachian English is variable (Christian et al., 1988). Not all residents of the region speak the dialect, nor do speakers of the dialect use it all of the time. It is common for speakers of Appalachian English to code switch and use forms that are more consistent with either Southern American English (see Chapter 25) or General American English (GAE) (see Chapter 22), particularly when conversing with speakers of those other dialects. Speakers of Appalachian English as young as 5 years of age appear to be quite proficient at such code switching (Davis, 1998).

It should be noted that the notion of a single unitary entity known as Appalachian English has been the subject of some debate. There is common reference to a form of speech that is different in "every holler" (i.e., every mountain valley). After discussing a number of factors that might be considered in settling the issue, Wolfram (1984) suggests that a "cautious conclusion is that there is still an objective basis for the designation Appalachian English." (p. 224). In addition to considerations about the validity of the dialect, its continued existence has also been the subject of some question. Richards (2001), for example, demonstrated that speakers born after 1940 were much less likely to use Appalachian English vowel forms than their older relatives, even when conversing with speakers of that dialect. On the other hand, some of the differences observed by Richards and others may have reflected what Wolfram and Christian (1975) have referred to as "age-grading" or differences expected for speakers at different stages of life. See the Resources section later in the chapter for materials pertaining to Appalachian English.

Where Appalachian English is spoken

Appalachian English is spoken across the entire state of West Virginia, and portions of four other states—eastern Kentucky, southwestern Virginia, western North Carolina, and eastern Tennessee (see accompanying map and Appendix D).

Components of Appalachian English

Consonants

The consonant inventory of Appalachian English is the same as for GAE.

Appalachian English includes a number of context-specific variations for consonants and consonant clusters relative to GAE (Adler, 1979; Bailey, 1979; Davis, 1998; Wolfram and Christian, 1975, 1976). The most common of these variations include:

- Deletion of /p, d, t, k/ from word-final clusters (e.g., [dɛs] for *desk*). Such deletions are more likely when the following word begins with a consonant. Deletions in contexts where the following word begins with a vowel are more likely if the cluster also includes the lateral approximant /l/ or a nasal
- Deletion of /ɹ/ in some unstressed clusters (e.g., [pətɛkt] for *protect*)
- Deletion of /l/ in post-vocalic clusters if the following segment is a bilabial (e.g., [hɛp] for *help*)
- Deletion of word-initial /w/ in some function words (e.g., [ʌn] for *one*, [ʌz] for *was*)
- Fronting of the velar nasal /ŋ/ in unstressed –ing contexts (e.g., [ɹʌnən] for *running*)
- Deletion of word-initial /ð/ in unstressed words (e.g., [əm] for *them*). Most common when the preceding word ends in a consonant
- Substitution of /t, d/ for the dental fricatives /θ, ð/ in word-initial position
- Overgeneralization of the /əz/ allomorph to words ending in /sp, st, sk/ (e.g., [gostəs] for *ghosts*, [wɑspəz] for *wasps*)
- Intrusive /t/ at the end of a small set of words ending in fricatives (e.g. [əkɹɔst] for *across*, [klɪft] for *cliff*, [wʌnst] for *once*, [twɑst] for *twice*)
- Intrusive /ɹ/ in a small set of words (e.g., [wɑɹʃ] for *wash*, [oɹt] for *ought*)

Vowels and diphthongs

The vowel and diphthong inventory of Appalachian English is the same as for GAE.

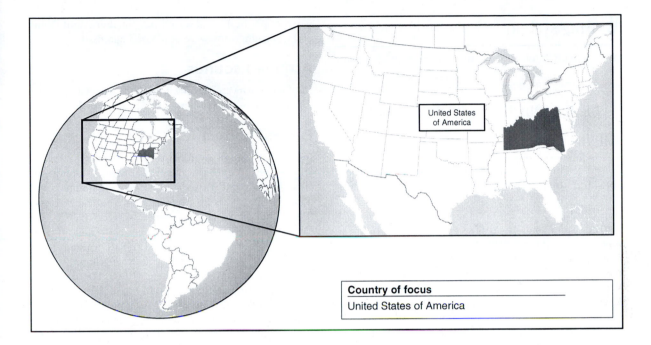

Country of focus
United States of America

As with consonants, the vowels of Appalachian English are subject to a number of context-specific variations from GAE (Adler, 1979; Davis, 1998; Richards, 2001; Wolfram and Christian, 1976). The most common of these include:

- Monophthongization of the diphthongs that include /ɪ/ (e.g., [rɑd] for *ride*, [bɔl] for *boil*)
- /ɛ/ changed to /a/ before /ɹ/ (e.g., [baɹ] for *bear*)
- Word-final ow sequences produced as /ɚ/ (e.g., [hɔlɚ] for *hollow*, [wɪndɚ] for *window*)
- Word-final unstressed schwa changed to /i/ (e.g., [sodi] for *soda*)
- /ɪ/ and /ɛ/ collapsed to /ɪ/ before nasals (e.g., *pin* and *pen* both produced as [pɪn])
- /ɪ/ changed to /i/ before /l/ or /ʃ/ (e.g., [fiʃ] for *fish*, [pil] for *pill*)
- /æ/ raised and diphthongized to /ɛə/ especially before velars and fricatives (e.g., [bɛəg] for *bag*, [gɹɛəs] for *grass*)
- Substitution of /ə/ for unstressed vocalic /ɚ/ (e.g., [faðə] for *father*)

Phonotactic restrictions

Syllables

The overall syllable structure of Appalachian English is the same as for GAE. Speakers of Appalachian English are known to regularly delete unstressed syllables such as those involving schwa (e.g., *lectrician* for *electrician*, *bout* for *about*) or some CV sequences (e.g., *fore* for *before*, *posed* for *supposed*).

Consonants and consonant clusters

The consonants and consonant clusters of Appalachian English are similar to those of GAE and other English dialects.

Tones

Appalachian English does not use tones to differentiate meaning.

Stress and intonation

Little formal research appears to have been done on the prosodic features of Appalachian English. Williams (1992) describes the rhythmic patterns of Appalachian English as "similar to those found in traditional nursery rhymes, riddles, ballads, and folk songs" (p. 17). Adler (1979), on the other hand, describes a dialect that uses monopitch, relatively level loudness, and slow, deliberate rate. There is an occasional tendency among speakers of Appalachian English to shift syllable stress in some words (e.g., *INsurance* for *inSURance*, *biCYcle* for *BIcycle*).

Writing system

Appalachian English uses the same spelling system as GAE.

Typical acquisition of Appalachian English

A very limited amount of acquisition data is available for this dialect. As far as could be determined, only two such studies exist (Davis, 1998; Flipsen and Parker, 2005), and they are summarized in the Summary of Studies Table at the end of this chapter. Davis (1998) conducted a retrospective study of recordings made during administration of the *Let's Talk Inventory for Children* (Bray and Wiig, 1987). Participants included 42 children aged 5 to 7 years from one school in Knox County, Tennessee, who were tested by adult speakers of GAE. In the other study of Appalachian English, Flipsen and Parker (2005) recorded the conversational speech of eight preschool children from Wise, Virginia. This town is situated in the heart of the Appalachian English-speaking region and (as of 2002) included approximately 3,200 residents. All of the children passed a hearing screening and achieved standard scores of at least 93 on the *Peabody Picture Vocabulary Test* (3rd ed) (Dunn and Dunn, 1997). The conversational speech samples were evoked by an adult native speaker of Appalachian English and transcribed using narrow phonetic transcription (Shriberg and Kent, 2003). Productions were compared against GAE.

Acquired sounds

Insufficient data are available to provide age of acquisition data for any of the phonemes of Appalachian English.

Percent correct

Insufficient data are available to provide reference values for percentage correct on any phoneme or phoneme class. Flipsen and Parker (2005) provide limited preliminary data. Values for percentage of consonants correct (PCC) and percentage of vowels correct (PVC) were calculated. These values were then converted to age-referenced z-scores (z-PCC and z-PVC) using reference data for children with typically developing speech provided by Austin and Shriberg (1997). Results of the analyses are shown in Table 24-1.

As indicated in Table 24-1, 7 of 8 speakers performed within two standard deviations of their reference group mean for PCC, but only 2 of 8 met this standard for PVC. This suggested (as might be expected for dialects of English that tend to vary more on vowels than consonants) that children acquiring Appalachian English show more differences relative to GAE on vowels than on consonants. This suggests the possibility that measures of consonants might therefore be less likely to overidentify children speaking this dialect as having a disorder when they present with only a dialect difference. Generalizations from such a conclusion are, however, premature given the limited sample size in this study.

TABLE 24-1 Percent correct for Appalachian English consonants (PCC) and vowels (PVC) from conversational speech

Speaker	Age in years;months	Gender	PCC	z-PCC	PVC	z-PVC
5	3;1	Female	82.0	0.21	88.6	-1.85
6	3;4	Male	80.5	0.14	84.0	-4.35
4	3;4	Male	90.0	1.34	84.2	-4.25
8	4;0	Male	74.0	-0.78	79.2	-6.80
3	4;4	Female	83.5	0.42	84.8	-3.42
7	4;10	Female	92.7	1.61	89.9	-1.78
2	5;3	Female	97.4	1.33	89.0	-2.73
1	5;11	Male	69.7	-2.17	82.9	-5.73

Source: Flipsen and Parker (2005)

Phonological processes

No specific data on the elimination of phonological processes are available for this dialect.

However, Davis (1998) examined the percentage of children using each of nine different phonological features at least once, measured from the transcripts of interactions. Results are summarized in Table 24-2. The percentage of children using the features tended to decline with age, though five of the features continued to be used by at least half of the 7-year-old participants. Davis interpreted these results to mean that as the children gained more school experience, they were becoming more proficient at code switching into GAE.

Intelligibility

No specific data on the emergence pattern for intelligible speech are available for this dialect.

Phonetic inventory

To date there is no study of the phonetic inventories produced at different ages by children who speak Appalachian English.

Common mismatches

To date there is no study of the common mismatches produced by children who speak Appalachian English.

Syllable structure

To date there is no study of the emergence of syllable structures in children who speak Appalachian English.

Prosody

To date there is no study of the development of prosody for children who speak Appalachian English.

Phonological awareness

To date there is no study of the development of phonological awareness by children who speak Appalachian English.

Speech assessment for children who speak Appalachian English

There are no available studies that have evaluated particular assessment techniques for the speech of children speaking Appalachian English. Adler (1973) noted that tests such as the *Templin-Darley Tests of Articulation* are likely biased against speakers of this and other nonstandard dialects; such tests have historically assumed that any deviation from GAE forms constitute errors. Flipsen and Parker (2005) used conversational speech samples and measured performance against GAE.

TABLE 24-2 Percentage of children speaking Appalachian English using each of nine different phonological features

Feature	5 years	6 years	7 years
Consonant cluster reduction	100	100	100
Deletion of /ɹ/	85.7	53.9	33.3
Deletion of /l/	92.9	84.6	93.3
Substitution of /ɚ/ for final "ow"	0	0	0
Deletion of initial /w/	57.1	15.4	0
Unstressed syllable deletion	85.7	69.2	66.7
Substitution of /ɪn/ for unstressed /ɪŋ/	92.9	46.2	26.7
Stopping of /θ/ and /ð/	71.4	79.6	60.0
Deletion of initial /ð/	92.9	100	93.3

Note: Data from Davis (1998).

Speech intervention for children who speak Appalachian English

No published studies of speech intervention have specifically looked at children acquiring Appalachian English.

Working in Appalachia

Working as a speech-language pathologist in regions where Appalachian English is spoken requires licensure from the appropriate state licensing body. Information on licensing requirements can be obtained from the state professional organizations (see Resources section).

PHONETICALLY SPEAKING

Pronunciation of Appalachian English: /æpəlætʃən ɪŋglɪʃ/

Appalachian English vocabulary is a veritable treasure; entire dictionaries have been created (see Garber, 1976 and Hendrickson, 1997).

Passage: Comma Gets a Cure

Below is a broad phonetic transcription of *Comma Gets a Cure* (Honorof, McCullough, and Somerville, 2000) as spoken by a 50-year-old male speaker of Appalachian English.

/wɛl hɹɪz ə stɔɹi fə juː sɛɹə pɛɹi wəz ə vɛtənɛɹi nɚs hu həd bɪn wɚkɪŋ deli æt ən oːl zu ɪn ðə dəzɚtəd dɪstɹɪk ʌ ðə tɛɹətɔɹi so ʃi wəz vɛɹi hɛpi tə stɑɹt ə nu dʒɑb ət ðə səpɚb pɹɑːvət pɹæktəs ɑn nɔɹθ skwʌɹ nɹɪ duk stɹit tɑʊ͡ɹz ðə ɚiə wəz mʌtʃ nɹɪ fə hɚ ən mɔɹ tə hɚ laːkɪŋ ivən so ɑn hɚ fɚs mɔɹnɪŋ ʃi feːlt stɹɛːst ʃi et ə bol ə pɔɹədʒ tʃɛkt hɚself ɪn ðə mɪɹə ən wɔʃt hɚ fes ɪn ə hɚi ðɛn ʃi pət ɑn ə plen jɛlə dɹɛːs ən ə flis dʒɚəkət pɪkt ʌp hɚ kɪt ən hɛdəd fə wɔɹk wɛn ʃi gat ðɛɹ ðɚ wəz ə wumən wɪθ ə gus wetɪŋ fə hɚ ði wumən gev sɛɹə ən əfɪʃəl lɛtə fɹɔm ðə vɛt ðə lɛtə ɪmplɑːɪd ðæt ðə ænəməl kəd bi sʌfɹɪŋ fɹəm ə ɹɛɹ ɹɑɹ ʌv fut æn mɑæθ dəzɪz wɪtʃ wəz səpɹɑːzən bəkɔz nɔɹmli ju wud onli ɪkspɛk tə si ət ɪn ə dɔg ɚ ə go͡ʊt sɛɹə wəz sɛnəmɛnəl so ðɪs med hɚ fil sɔɹi fɚ ðə bjutəfəl bɚd/

Well, here's a story for you: Sarah Perry was a veterinary nurse who had been working daily at an old zoo in a deserted district of the territory, so she was very happy to start a new job at a superb private practice in North Square near the Duke Street Tower. That area was much nearer for her and more to her liking. Even so, on her first morning, she felt stressed. She ate a bowl of porridge, checked herself in the mirror and washed her face in a hurry. Then she put on a plain yellow dress and a fleece jacket, picked up her kit and headed for work. When she got there, there was a woman with a goose waiting for her. The woman gave Sarah an official letter from the vet. The letter implied that the animal could be suffering from a rare form of foot and mouth disease, which was surprising, because normally you would only expect to see it in a dog or a goat. Sarah was sentimental, so this made her feel sorry for the beautiful bird. (Honorof, McCullough, and Somerville, 2000).

RESOURCES

Books

Adler, S. (1979). *Poverty children and their language: Implications for teaching and treating.* New York: Grune & Stratton.

Hendrickson, R. (1997). *Mountain range: A dictionary of expressions from Appalachia to the Ozarks.* New York: Facts on File, Inc.

Williams, C. D. (1992). *Southern mountain speech.* Berea, KY: Berea College Press.

Wolfram, W., and Christian, D. (1976). *Appalachian Speech.* Arlington, VA: Center for Applied Linguistics.

DVDs

Mountain Talk: Language and Life in Southern Appalachia (DVD). Directed by Walt Wolfram, Ph.D., North Carolina State University. Produced by Neal Hutcheson of TalkingNC Media. http://www.talkingnc.com/newpages/mountaintalk.htm

Journals

- *American Speech,* http://www.dukeupress.edu/americanspeech/. A publication of the American Dialect Society, printed by Duke University Press.
- *Journal of Sociolinguistics,* http://www.blackwellpublishing.com/journal.asp?ref=1360-6441. A publication of Blackwell Synergy.

Professional associations

The professional associations of speech-language pathologists in the areas where speakers of Appalachian English reside are:

American Speech-Language-Hearing Association, http://www.asha.org

Kentucky Speech-Language-Hearing Association, http://www.kysha.org

North Carolina Speech-Language-Hearing Association, http://www.ncshla.org

Speech-Language-Hearing Association of Virginia, http://www.shav.org

Tennessee Association of Speech-Language Pathologists and Audiologists, http://www.taaslp.org

West Virginia Speech-Language-Hearing Association, http://www.wvsha.org/

Universities that offer training for speech-language pathologists in Kentucky, North Carolina, Tennessee, Virginia, and West Virginia can be located at the following Web sites:

University Programs in Speech-Language Pathology, http://facstaff.uww.edu/bradleys/cdprograms.html

American Speech-Language-Hearing Association, http://www.asha.org/students/academic/

Useful Appalachian English Web sites

- The West Virginia Dialect Project, http://www.as.wvu.edu/dialect/
- The North Carolina Language and Life Project at North Carolina State University, http://www.ncsu.edu/linguistics/code/Research%20Sites/ncllp2.htm
- Resource page on the language of Appalachia, http://www.ferrum.edu/applit/studyg/dialect/
- An annotated bibliography on Appalachian English, developed at the University of Alabama, http://scholar.lib.vt.edu/IUSSUS/AppEngBibliography.html

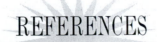

REFERENCES

Adler, S. (1973). Articulatory deviances and social class membership. *Journal of Learning Disabilities, 6,* 650–654.

Adler, S. (1979). *Poverty children and their language: Implications for teaching and treating.* New York: Grune & Stratton.

Adler, S., and Birdsong, S. (1983). Reliability and validity of standardized testing tools used with poor children. *Topics in Language Disorders, 3,* 76–87.

Austin, D., and Shriberg, L. D. (1997). Lifespan reference data for ten measures of articulation competence using the speech disorders classification system (SDCS) (Tech. Rep. No. 3). University of Wisconsin–Madison, Phonology Project, Waisman Center.

Bailey, G. H. (1979). *Folk speech on the Cumberland plateau: A phonological analysis.* Unpublished doctoral dissertation, University of Tennessee, Knoxville.

Bray, C. M., and Wiig, E. H. (1987). *Let's talk inventory for children.* New York: The Psychological Corporation.

Christian, D., Wolfram, W., and Dube, N. (1988). Variation and change in geographically isolated communities: Appalachian English and Ozark English. *Publication of the American Dialect Society, Number 74.* Tuscaloosa, AL: University of Alabama Press.

Davis, E. D. (1998). *An examination of Appalachian dialectal syntactic and phonological features used by school-age children in east Tennessee.* Unpublished master's thesis, University of Tennessee, Knoxville.

Dunn, L. M., and Dunn, L. M. (1997). *Peabody picture vocabulary test* (3rd ed.). Circle Pines, MN: American Guidance Service.

Flipsen, P., Jr, and Parker, R. G. (2005). *Speech acquisition in children learning Appalachian English.* Unpublished manuscript.

Garber, A. (1976). *Mountain-ese: Basic grammar for Appalachia.* Radford, VA: Commonwealth Press.

Hazen, K., and Fluharty, E. (2004). Defining Appalachian English. In M. Bender (Ed.), *Linguistic diversity in the south.* (pp. 50–65). Athens, GA: University of Georgia Press.

Honorof, D. N., McCullough, J., and Somerville, B. (2000). *Comma gets a cure: A diagnostic passage for accent study.* New Haven, CT: Haskins Laboratories.

Montgomery, M. (1991). The roots of Appalachian English: Scotch-Irish or British southern? *Journal of the Appalachian Studies Association, 3,* 177–191.

Richards, M. L. (2001). *An examination of change in selected vowel structures of three generations of native Appalachian speakers.* Unpublished doctoral dissertation, University of Tennessee, Knoxville.

Shriberg, L. D., and Kent, R. D. (2003). *Clinical phonetics* (3rd ed.). Boston, MA: Allyn & Bacon.

Williams, C. D. (1992). *Southern mountain speech.* Berea, KY: Berea College Press.

Wolfram, W. (1984). Is there an "Appalachian English"? *Appalachian Journal, 11,* 215–224.

Wolfram, W., and Christian, D. (1975). *Sociolinguistic variables in Appalachian dialects.* Arlington, VA: Center for Applied Linguistics.

Wolfram, W., and Christian, D. (1976). *Appalachian speech.* Arlington, VA: Center for Applied Linguistics.

SUMMARY OF STUDIES OF TYPICAL APPALACHIAN ENGLISH SPEECH ACQUISITION

Authors	Year	Country	No. of children	Age of children	Information	Sample type	Data collection
Davis	1998	USA	42	5–7 yrs	Phonological features	Conversational speech	Cross-sectional
Flipsen and Parker	2005	USA	8	3;1– 5;11	PCC, PVC	Conversational speech	Cross-sectional

Chapter 25

Cajun English Speech Acquisition

Janna B. Oetting

INTRODUCTION

The terms *Cajun English* and *Creole English* are used to describe the nonmainstream varieties of English that are spoken in the Acadian Triangle of Louisiana. Although this chapter focuses on Cajun English, information about Creole English is also presented when available. Hopefully, in the near future, additional studies will be completed on the English that is spoken by Louisiana Creoles so that a separate chapter can be devoted to this variety.

A stereotypical speaker of these dialects is an older man or woman who also speaks one of the many French varieties that are spoken in Louisiana. The historical origins of the Cajuns are typically rooted in the French-speaking Acadian migrations to the southwestern bayou and prairie areas of Louisiana in the mid-1700s, but Cajun history also includes contact and assimilation with other French immigrants, German, Irish, Italian, and Spanish immigrants, African Americans, and Native Americans. Creole history is even more varied than Cajun history, with multiple ethnic groups claiming Creole status during the French and Spanish regimes of the 1700s and during the establishment of Anglo-American governance and commerce in the area after the Louisiana Purchase of 1803 (Brasseaux, 1987; Din, 1999; Dominguez, 1986; Dormon, 1996; Hall, 1992; Henry and Bankston, 2002).

Also woven into Louisiana's history is an early tripartite system of race that consisted of whites, free people of color, and black slaves. This tripartite syste m dissolved during and after the Civil War. Current studies of Cajuns (and Cajun English) generally result in participant pools that are white. Studies of Creoles (and Creole English) often result in participant pools that are of African and French descent, but they also can include participants from other ethnic backgrounds. Whether there are substantial linguistic differences between the French and English varieties that are spoken by individuals who self-identify as either Cajun or Creole is a matter of debate and ongoing study (Dubois and Melancon, 2000; Klingler, 2002; Valdman, 1997).

In addition to the racial correlates that exist with current uses of the terms *Cajun* and *Creole* is the complex and ever-changing relation between Cajun and Creole ethnic identity and one's ability to speak French. U.S. Census data indicate that in 1970, 572,000 Louisiana residents claimed the ability to speak French whereas in 1990, only 263,000 claimed to do so (Henry and Bankston, 2001). This finding, along with those from other sociological methods of investigation, have led Henry, Bankston, and others to argue that current claims of Cajunness are now less related to speaking French than to other ethnic symbols such as ancestry, lifestyle, occupation, and activity. Indeed in 1990, 72 percent of Cajuns 50 years or older reported that they spoke French whereas only 8 percent of those under 30 reported that they did (Henry and Bankston, 2002).

Similar sociological studies of Creoleness have not been completed, but linguistic attitude and cultural identity studies of Louisiana Cajuns and Creoles are consistent with Henry and Bankston's claims. For example, Dubois and Melancon's (1997; 2000) research included 929 white and 240 African American participants who lived in the Acadian Triangle. For each group, the sample was stratified by age and gender, and participants varied in whether they could or could not speak French and whether they had or didn't have Cajun/Creole French ancestry. For all participants, having Cajun and/or Creole ancestry and having a parent or grandparent who spoke French were the two most important indicators of ethnic identity.

Few quantitative studies of Cajun English and Creole English have been completed. More prevalent are written descriptions of the stereotypic aspects of these dialects from linguists, literary scholars, folklorists, and native residents. For a comprehensive anthology on Cajun English, see Scott, 1992; for a review of scholarly works completed during the twentieth century, see Cheramie, 1998. Also widespread are uses of these dialects in books, songs, travel signs, and advertisements (for two examples, see Boudreaux, 2000; Trosclair, 1973). Within these sources, five features are often illustrated as defining characteristics of Cajun English (and perhaps Creole English as well). These are vowel pronunciation, stress change, substitutions of /t, d/ for /θ, ð/, nonaspirated /p, t, k/, and lexical differences (Melancon, 2001).

Where Cajun English and Creole English are spoken

Cajun English and Creole English are spoken in the Acadian triangle of Louisiana within the following

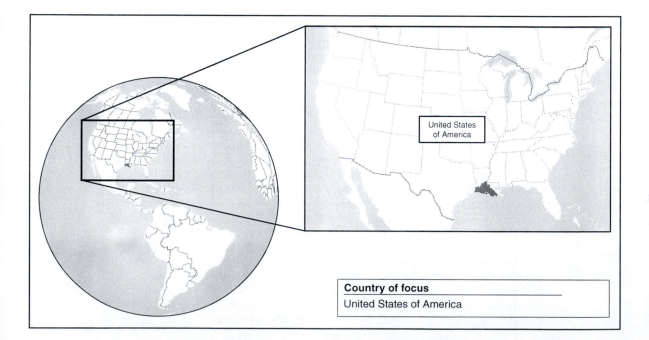

Country of focus
United States of America

22 parishes: Acadia, Ascension, Assumption, Avoyelles, Alcasieu, Cameron, Evangeline, Iberia, Iberville, Jefferson Davis, Lafayette, Lafourche, Pointe Coupee, St. Charles, St. James, St. John the Baptist, St. Landry, St. Martin, St. Mary, Terrebonne, Vermilion, and W. Baton Rouge (see accompanying map and Appendix D).

Components of Cajun English

Consonants

The consonant inventory of Cajun English is the same as for General American English (GAE; see Chapter 22).

Substitutions of /t, d/ for /θ, ð/ and nonaspiration of /p, t, k/ are considered by many to be two of the defining characteristics of Cajun English. Other features of Cajun English include word-medial and word-final consonant deletion, loss or weakening of post-vocalic /ɹ/, liaison (i.e., carrying the final sound of a word to the beginning of the next word), trilled /r/, and /h/ deletion in word-initial positions (Cheramie, 1998; Dubois and Horvath, 1998; 1999; 2003; Rubrecht, 1971; Walton, 1994). The rate at which speakers produce these patterns is variable. For example, Walton (1994) reported that in a nine-minute sample of one speaker, a 10 percent rate of /t/ for /θ/ was observed and rates of /d/ for /ð/ averaged 29 percent, but were as high as 67 percent for the word *this*; 35 cases of liaison were also documented.

Dubois and Horvath (1998; 1999) also provide information about some consonant patterns of Cajun English, but their studies examined pattern rate as a function of a speaker's age (young, middle-aged, old), gender, first language (French vs. English) and social network (open vs. closed). For nonaspirated /p, t, k/, these authors found a linear decrease from old to young regardless of a speaker's social network. In all cases, however, rates of use for men were higher than rates for women (for males, old = 60–70 percent, middle = 55–70 percent, young = 40–50 percent; for women, old = 50–55 percent, middle = 0–25 percent, young = 0–10 percent). For the middle-aged group, the speaker's first language also influenced rates of use (French L1 males = 60–70 percent and French L1 females = 20–25 percent vs. English L1 males = 55–65 percent and English L1 females = 0 percent). According to Dubois and Horvath, a linear decrease of use from the old to young speakers is consistent with a model of language interference of French for the old speakers, and with diachronic assimilation to English by the middle-aged and young speakers.

For /t, d/ substitutions of /θ, ð/, Dubois and Horvath documented very different patterns of use, and findings varied as a function of a speaker's age, gender, and social network. For closed social networks, a V-shaped pattern of use was identified, with old and young speakers producing higher rates than middle-aged speakers (old = 44–69 percent; middle = 15–39 percent; young = 35–55 percent). For open networks, a linear increase was found for men (old = 40 percent; middle = 64 percent; young = 87 percent), while a linear decrease was found for women (old = 8 percent; middle = 6 percent; young = 0 percent). Dubois and Horvath interpreted these V-shaped findings and linear increases of use as reflecting a Cajun renaissance or Francophone resurgence in Louisiana.

Vowels and diphthongs

The vowel and diphthong inventory of Cajun English is the same as for GAE.

Vowel pronunciation is considered a defining feature of Cajun English. Within this dialect, tensed vowel production, vowel lowering, and heavy glide reduction are so frequent that some describe this dialect as completely lacking a southern drawl (Melancon, 2001). Rubrecht (1971) documented a 63 percent rate of monophthongization of /aɪ/ and a 42 percent rate of vowel lowering (e.g., /i/ to /ɪ/). Dubois and Horvath (1999) documented a V-shape pattern of change for heavy nasalization of vowels in final contexts and monophthongization of /aɪ/ in both voiced contexts and final positions. In both cases, old and young males produced higher rates of use than middle-aged speakers.

In one of the few Creole English studies this author has found, Dubois and Horvath (2003) examined glide reduction of vowels. Across all vowels studied, high rates of glide reduction were documented (/oi/ = 76 percent, /au/ = 77 percent, /o/ = 74 percent, /ai/ = 72 percent, /e/ = 65 percent, /u/ = 64 percent, /i/ = 56 percent). Glide reduction rates were also found to be affected by a speaker's age and education. Rates of glide reduction were highest for speakers who were old, and in the young group, reduction was highest for those who had not attended college (old = 79 percent, middle = 69 percent, young completed high school = 74 percent, young completed college = 44 percent).

Phonotactic restrictions

Syllables

The overall syllable structure of Cajun English, like French, is stress final (e.g., when producing the word *rocking chair*, stress is placed on *chair* instead of *rock*). The tendency to stress only the final syllable is also prevalent at the phrase level. Melancon (1995) describes this as yielding an almost monotonous group of words with stress on the final one (e.g., *open the door*, with stress only on *door*).

Consonants and consonant clusters

The consonants and consonant clusters of Cajun English are similar to those of GAE and other English dialects.

Tones

Cajun English does not use tones to differentiate meaning.

Stress and intonation

Illustrations of Cajun English by native residents and folklorists often include a rhythmic pattern of prosody that is sometimes referred to as "flat speech." Walton (1994) describes this type of speech as involving shortened words that are produced with a staccato rhythm and with rising pitch at the end of utterances. Like stress-final syllable structure, Melancon (1995; 2001) ties the stress-final intonation patterns of Cajun English phrases and utterances to French.

Writing system

Cajun English uses the same spelling system as GAE.

Typical acquisition of Cajun English

Very limited data are available. The Summary of Studies Table at the end of the chapter contains a summary of studies or datasets that have examined the speech productions of children who were either classified as presenting some Cajun/Creole English features in their speech and/or classified as Cajun English speakers.

Acquired sounds

To date there is no study of the age at which children who speak Cajun English acquire consonants or vowels.

Percent correct

To date there is no study of the percentage of consonants or vowels produced correctly at different ages by children who speak Cajun English.

Phonological processes

Oetting and Garrity (in press) studied children's use of five vernacular patterns of phonology using a dataset of 93 samples (40 from African American children and 53 from Caucasian children, aged 4 to 6 years, who lived on the eastern border of the Acadian Triangle). Although all of the children were perceived to speak a variety of either Southern White English or Southern African American English, 31 of them were also perceived by listeners to present some Cajun and/or Creole English features within their dialects. Average frequency counts of the phonological patterns are presented in Table 25-1. The data show that children who were classified as sounding Cajun and/or Creole presented higher rates of vernacular phonology than the others.

Intelligibility

To date there is no study of intelligibility of children who speak Cajun English.

Phonetic inventory

To date there is no study of the phonetic inventories produced at different ages by children who speak Cajun English.

Common mismatches

Within the test development phase of the *Diagnostic Evaluation of Language Variation* (Seymour, Roeper, and de Villiers, 2003), 21 children (17 aged 5 to 8 years and 4 aged 11 years) who were classified as Cajun English speakers were administered this tool. Their consonant productions on this tool were analyzed for the purposes of this chapter by Barbara Zurer Pearson (personal communication). For the noncontrastive phoneme targets (i.e., those produced in a wide range of American English dialects, including GAE, African American English (AAE), Southern English, and Cajun and Creole English), 98 percent of the children's productions were scored as correct. Nevertheless, of the 21 speakers, two seemed to have non-dialect-related phonological problems. For example, one 6-year-old had difficulty with the /s/ phoneme and one 5-year-old simplified clusters somewhat more than expected (about 25 percent of the time, compared to an average of 4 percent for all the children).

Of the 44 contrastive phoneme targets (i.e., those that provide an opportunity for variation across American English dialects, such as /d/ for /ð/ substitutions), rates of nonmainstream productions (or those scored as different

TABLE 25-1 Average tokens of vernacular phonology in one-minute samples from children who were and were not perceived to have some Cajun/Creole English features in their speech.

Vernacular Phonology	Number of tokens	Dialect	Samples with a Cajun or Creole influence N = 31	Samples without a Cajun or Creole influence N = 62
Nonaspirated stops	41	SWE	.85 (1.21)	.10 (.38)
		AAE	1.06 (1.66)	.68 (1.13)
		All Excerpts	.97 (1.47)	.31 (.78) *
/θ, ð/ ⇨ /t, d/	91	SWE	.92 (1.15)	.60 (2.10)
		SAAE	1.44 (1.72)	1.41 (1.99)
		All Excerpts	1.23 (1.49)	.89 (2.10)
Heavy vowel nasalization	31	SWE	.08 (.28)	.25 (.77)
		SAAE	.67 (.97)	.36 (.58)
		All Excerpts	.42 (.80)	.29 (.71)
Monophthongization	50	SWE	.15 (.38)	.05 (.22)
		SAAE	.94 (1.79)	1.32 (1.36)
		All Excerpts	.61 (1.41)	.50 (1.0)
Glide weakening on vowels	110	SWE	1.31 (1.38)	.40 (1.08)
		SAAE	2.33 (2.03)	1.59 (2.67)
		All Excerpts	1.90 (1.83)	.82 (1.88) *
Vowel lowering	2	SWE	—	—
		SAAE	—	—
		All Excerpts	—	—

Note: SWE = Southern White English; SAAE = Southern African American English; * = statistical difference; Like letters = statistical difference between SWE and SAAE dialects. Vowel lowering was too infrequent to analyze.

from GAE) by the Cajun English speakers were similar to those elicited from similar-aged children who were speakers of either GAE or AAE (Cajun = 7 percent vs. GAE = 5 percent vs. AAE = 15 percent). In addition, the only two phonemes that showed a consistent dialect influence were /θ, ð/. For the former, /t/ was realized 33 percent of the time and /f/ was realized 10 percent of the time. For the latter, /d/ was realized 23 percent of the time and /v/ was realized 6 percent of the time. Realizations of /f, v/ for /θ, ð/, while not tied specifically to Cajun English, are common in other dialects (i.e., Southern English and AAE) that are spoken in Louisiana.

Syllable structure

To date there is no study of the production of syllable structures at different ages by children who speak Cajun English.

Prosody

To date there is no study of the prosody of children who speak Cajun English.

Phonological awareness

To date there is no study of the acquisition of phonological awareness skills of children who speak Cajun English.

Speech assessment for children who speak Cajun English

There are no available studies that have evaluated particular assessment techniques for children who speak Cajun English.

Speech intervention for children who speak Cajun English

There have been no published studies of speech intervention that has specifically looked at children acquiring Cajun English.

Working in the Acadian Triangle

Working as a speech-language clinician in the Acadian Triangle requires licensure from the Louisiana Board of Examiners in Speech Language Pathology and Audiology.

This licensure includes certification of Clinical Competency by the American Speech-Language-Hearing Association and the completion of 10 hours of continuing education every year.

PHONETICALLY SPEAKING

Pronunciation of Cajun English: /keɪdʒĭn ĩŋlɪʃ/

There are many words and phrases that are distinct in Cajun English and Creole English. Some of the more frequently cited words (with their source and meanings) include: *boudin* (borrowed from French, a rice and sausage mixture wrapped and fried in an intestinal sack); *lagniappe* (borrowed from French, a little something extra); *making groceries* (from French *faire les courses*, going grocery shopping); and *cher* (from French *cherie* and pronounced [ʃa], a term of endearment). See the Web sites and books that follow below.

Passage: Comma Gets a Cure

Below is a broad transcription of a 49-year-old male reading the first paragraph of Comma Gets a Cure (Honorof, McCullough, and Somerville, 2000). The speaker lives in the Acadian Triangle and self-identifies as a Cajun. The passage was transcribed by Brandi Newkirk. Although the speaker's speech output chain is a continuum where words are not physically segmented, for the sake of ease, we have chosen to segment our broad transcription into word units.

/wɛl hɪɹz ə stɔɹi fə ju: sɛɹə pɛɹi wəz eɪ vɛtnɛɹi nɹs hu hæd bɪn wəɹkɪŋ deɪli æ? ən oːl zu ɪn eɪ dɪzəɹtɪd dɪstɹɪk əv ðə tɛɹətɔɹɪ sou ʃi wəz vɛɹi hæpɪ tə stɑɹt eɪ nu: dʒɑː æt eɪ sépəɹ pɹaɪvɪt pɹæktɪs ɪn nɔɹtskwɛɹə niɹ də du stɹit tauwə dæt eɹɪə wəz mətʃ niɹə fə həɹ æn mɔɹ əf hə· tə həɹ laɪkɪn ivɪn sou ɑn həɹ mɔɹ fəɹs mouɹnɪŋ ʃi fɛlt stɹɛs ʃi eɪʔeɪ boul əv pɔɹɪʒ tʃɛkt həɹsɛf ɪn ə miɹə ɛn waʃt həɹ feɪs ɪnə həɹ dɪn ʃi: puː ɑn eɪ pleɪn jɛlə dɹɛs ɛn ɑɪ flis dʒækɪt pɪkt əp həɹ kɪt ɛn hɛdɪd fə wəɹk/

Well, here's a story for you: Sarah Perry was a veterinary nurse who had been working daily at an old zoo in a deserted district of the territory, so she was very happy to start a new job at a superb private practice in North Square near the Duke Street Tower. That area was much nearer for her and more to her liking. Even so, on her first morning, she felt stressed. She ate a bowl of porridge, checked herself in the mirror and washed her face in a hurry. Then she put on a plain yellow dress and a fleece jacket, picked up her kit and headed for work (Honorof, McCullough and Somerville, 2000).

RESOURCES

Books

Bruce, C., and Gipson, J. (2002). *Cajun French-English/ English-Cajun French: Dictionary and phrasebook.* New York: Hippocrene Books.

Daigle, J. (1992). *Cajun self-taught: Learning to speak the Cajun language.* Chelsea, MI: Book Crafters.

Wolfram, W., and Ward, B. (2006). *American voices: How dialects differ from coast to coast.* Malden, MA: Blackwell.

Useful Web sites

- Do You Speak American?
  http://pbs.org/speak/seatosea/americanvarieties/ cajun/
- Encyclopedia of Cajun Culture.
  http://cajunculture.com

Professional associations

These are the professional associations and licensure board of speech-language pathologists in the areas where speakers of Cajun English and Creole English reside:

American Speech-Language-Hearing Association, http://www.asha.org

Louisiana Board of Examiners in Speech Pathology and Audiology, http://lbespa.org

Louisiana Speech-Language-Hearing Association, http://www.lsha.org

Speech Pathologists and Audiologists in LA Schools, Inc., http://www.spals.org

Universities that offer training in speech-language pathology in Louisiana can be located at the following Web sites:

University Programs in Speech-Language Pathology and Audiology. http://facstaff.uww.edu/bradleys/cdprograms.html

American Speech-Language-Hearing Association: Academic Programs. http://www.asha.org/students/academic

REFERENCES

Boudreaux, L. (2000). *Aham gonna tell you again, dat Boudreaux ain't me, it's ma cousin.* Baton Rouge, LA: Boudreaux Cajun Store.

Brasseaux, C. A. (1987). *The founding of New Acadia.* Baton Rouge, LA: Louisiana State University Press.

Cheramie, D. (1998). *Cajun Vernacular English and the influence of vernacular on student writing in south Louisiana.* Unpublished doctoral dissertation, University of Southwestern Louisiana.

Din, G. (1999). *The Canary Islanders of Louisiana.* Baton Rouge, LA: Louisiana State University Press.

Dominguez, V. R. (1986). *White by definition: Social classification in Creole Louisiana.* New Brunswick, NJ: Rutgers University Press.

Dormon, J. (1996). *Creoles of color of the Gulf South.* Knoxville, TN: University of Tennessee Press.

Dubois, S., and Horvath, B. M. (1998). From accent to marker in Cajun English: A study of dialect formation in progress. *English World-Wide, 19,* 161–188.

Dubois, S., and Horvath, B. M. (1999). Let's tink about dat: Interdental fricatives in Cajun English. *Language Variation and Change, 10,* 245–261.

Dubois, S., and Horvath, B. M. (2003). The English vernacular of the Creoles of Louisiana. *Language Variation and Change, 15,* 255–288.

Dubois, S., and Melancon, M. (1997). Cajun is dead—Long live Cajun: Shifting from a linguistic to a cultural community. *Journal of Sociolinguistics, 1,* 63–93.

Dubois, S., and Melancon, M. (2000). Creole is, Creole ain't: Diachronic and synchronic attitudes toward Creole identity in South Louisiana. *Language in Society, 29,* 237–258.

Hall, G. M. (1992). *Africans in colonial Louisiana: The development of Afro-Creole culture in the eighteenth century*. Baton Rouge, LA: Louisiana State University Press.

Henry, J. M., and Bankston, C. L. (2001). Ethnic self-identification and symbolic stereotyping: The portrayal of Louisiana Cajuns. *Ethnic and Racial Studies, 24*, 1020–1045.

Henry, J. M., and Bankston, C. L. (2002). *Blue collar bayou: Louisiana Cajuns in the new economy of ethnicity*. Westport, CT: Praeger.

Honorof, D. N., McCullough, J., and Somerville, B. (2000). *Comma gets a cure: A diagnostic passage for accent study*. New Haven, CT: Haskins Laboratories.

Klingler, T. (2002). *Language labels and language use among Cajuns and Creoles in Louisiana*. Paper presented at NWAV 31, Stanford University.

Melancon, M. (1995). *Stress at the word level in Cajun French: Perceptual evidence using a non-linear approach*. Unpublished master's thesis. Louisiana State University.

Melancon, M. (2001). Stirring the linguistic gumbo. *Language Magazine: The Journal of Communication and Education, 5*(5), 29–32.

Oetting, J. B., and Garrity, A. W. (in press). Variation within dialects: A case of Cajun/Creole influence within child SAAE and SWE. *Journal of Speech, Language, and Hearing Research*.

Rubrecht, A. W. (1971). *Regional phonological variants in Louisiana speech*. Unpublished doctoral dissertation, University of Florida.

Scott, A. M. (Ed.; 1992). Cajun vernacular English: Informal English in French Louisiana. *Louisiana English Journal* [special issue].

Seymour, H., Roeper, T., and de Villiers, J. (2003). *Diagnostic evaluation of language variation*. San Antonio, TX: The Psychological Corporation.

Trosclair. (1973). *Cajun night before Christmas*. Gretna, LA: Pelican.

Valdman, A. (1997). *French and Creole in Louisiana*. New York: Plenum.

Walton, S. (1994). *Flat speech and Cajun ethnic identity in Terrebonne Parish*. Unpublished doctoral dissertation, Tulane University, New Orleans, LA.

SUMMARY OF STUDIES OF TYPICAL CAJUN ENGLISH SPEECH ACQUISITION

Authors	Year	Country	No. of children	Age of children	Information	Sample type	Data collection
Oetting and Garrity	in press	USA	31	4–6 yrs	Rate of vernacular pattern use	1-min. conversational excerpts	Cross-sectional
Seymour et. al.	2003	USA	21	5–11 yrs	Production within an articulation test	Single word productions	Cross-sectional

Chapter 26

Canadian English Speech Acquisition

Barbara May Handford Bernhardt and Jeff Deby

INTRODUCTION

Canada is the second largest country in the world, yet it has a relatively small population, with an estimated 32,800,000 people (U.S. Central Intelligence Agency, 2005). Approximately 58 percent of Canadians speak English as a mother tongue, 22 percent French, and 17 percent another language (with high diversity). By federal law, English and French are official languages. More than half of the provinces and territories have additional official language policies: in central and eastern Canada, Quebec, New Brunswick, Ontario, and Prince Edward Island; in northern Canada, the Northwest Territories, Nunavut, and the Yukon; and in the west, Manitoba. In Canada's newest northern territory, Nunavut, 70 percent of the people speak Inuktitut as their mother tongue; official territory languages include Inuktitut and one of its dialects, Inuinnaqtun, in addition to English and French.

The majority of Canadians live in urban centers within 300 kilometers of the 6,146-kilometer-long border with the United States of America. This proximity to the USA has had a strong influence on "English Canada's" history, culture, and language. In the early days of colonialism by Britain and France, a large influx of United Empire Loyalists (UEL) from the USA, during the American Revolution, brought the major dialect features to the then very small English-Canadian colony to the north. The majority of the Loyalist speakers had a dialect with postvocalic /ɹ/ (i.e., midland American), which became a feature of Canadian English. A war between France and Britain in the eighteenth century resulted in the ceding of the larger French colonies in Quebec and the Maritimes to Britain. The UEL group was then supplemented in subsequent years by waves of immigration from Britain, Ireland, and, to a lesser extent, elsewhere in Europe. The immigrants all added their influences to the dialect, although the UEL dialect persisted, maintaining its postvocalic /ɹ/, for example. Because Canada has remained part of the (British) Commonwealth of Nations, there are continuing British influences on Canadian English, although fewer than those from General American English (GAE). Canadian English nevertheless "can be seen as pursuing its own course, with the development of distinctive linguistics features and dialectal forms" (Brinton and Fee, 2001, p. 422). What is called "standard" Canadian English has traditionally been defined as the dialect spoken by the large middle class of educated Canadians west of Quebec (Brinton and Fee). This variant of English is generally used in government agencies and documents, and by the major media.

Other variants of Canadian English reflect regional and cultural/linguistic groupings. Regionally, the most distinctive variants are found in Newfoundland, the other eastern Maritime provinces (Prince Edward Island, New Brunswick, and Nova Scotia), and Quebec (the French-dominant province), although the variants are less distinctive than variants in other former British colonies around the world (Chambers, 1998). In terms of cultural/linguistic groupings, many Canada's First Peoples speak English dialects that reflect their cultures and heritage languages (Ball, Bernhardt and Deby, 2005). In addition, Canada's active immigration and refugee policy has led to a large influx of people from many diverse language backgrounds; over the past decade, approximately 200,000 people per year have come to Canada from other countries. Millions of Canadians consequently speak a variant of English influenced by another language. At the time of the 2001 census, 20 percent of young people between 5 and 24 in Toronto and Vancouver spoke a language other than English at home (Statistics Canada, 2001). Since 1961, the majority of immigrants have come from Asia. In 2001, 69 percent of the people of Vancouver, Canada's largest western city, spoke a Chinese language at home (Statistics Canada, 2001). Where a particular linguistic community becomes sufficiently large, so-called accents in their second language may become accepted pronunciations. In time, if the speakers of the less common variant are sufficiently numerous, those new pronunciations may affect the standard dialects of the area (Chambers, 1998). The term Global English, or English as an International Language, has been coined recently (Jenkins, 2005). Of 1.5 billion speakers of English worldwide, many speak another language as their first language and show variants of English reflecting those home languages. Canada's cultural and linguistic diversity reflects that worldwide pattern. Chambers (1998, p. 254) notes:

> *Canada … presents a linguistic situation in which the isoglosses of traditional dialectology do not have any semblance of meaning. It is a situation that is firmly rooted in the history and sociology of the land.*

Where Canadian English, French, and Aboriginal languages are spoken in Canada

Canada has both geographic and cultural/linguistic diversity. By geography, the most commonly agreed upon English variants are found in (1) Newfoundland; (2) the Maritime Provinces (New Brunswick, Nova Scotia, and Prince Edward Island); (3) Quebec; and (4) Ontario, the Western Provinces (Manitoba, Saskatchewan, Alberta, British Columbia), and the North (Yukon, the Northwest Territories, and Nunavut, see accompanying maps and Appendix D). Some additional breakdowns of areas have been noted by Boberg (2005), with Prince Edward Island splitting off from the other Maritime provinces, and Ontario (particularly the Ottawa valley) splitting off from Canada west of Quebec. Standard Canadian English is considered to be spoken in Ontario, the Western Provinces, and the North—the largest area (Brinton and Fee, 2001).

Canada also has a rich cultural/linguistic diversity, which results in diverse pronunciations of English that often cross geographical boundaries. A description of all of the diverse pronunciations of English deriving from the many heritage language groups in Canada is beyond the scope of this chapter. However, knowledge about the phonological system of the home language of a given child can inform speech-language pathology practice about a possible source of observed pronunciation differences (see Killam and Watson, 1983). Whether observed differences are considered articulation impairments may, however, reflect family and community beliefs about use of the standard and nonstandard dialects.

Components of standard Canadian English

Consonants, consonant clusters, phonotactics, stress and intonation, and tone

Because standard Canadian English is very much like General American English (GAE), the reader is directed to Smit (see Chapter 22) for discussion of consonants, consonant clusters, phonotactics, stress, tone, and intonation. The only "r"-less dialect in Canada is found in some speakers in Lunenburg, Nova Scotia, a relic of UEL New England "r"-less dialects (Chambers, 1998).

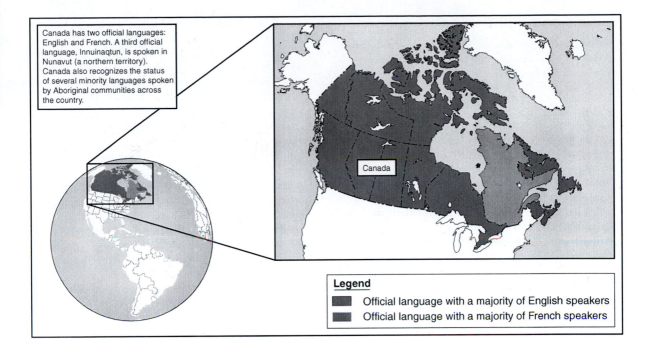

Canada has two official languages: English and French. A third official language, Innuinaqtun, is spoken in Nunavut (a northern territory). Canada also recognizes the status of several minority languages spoken by Aboriginal communities across the country.

Canada

Legend

Official language with a majority of English speakers

Official language with a majority of French speakers

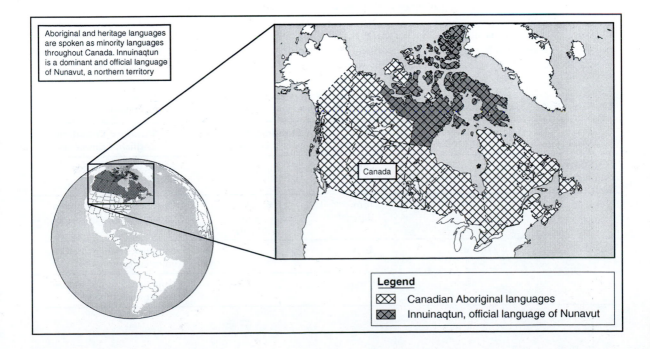

Aboriginal and heritage languages are spoken as minority languages throughout Canada. Innuinaqtun is a dominant and official language of Nunavut, a northern territory

Canada

Legend

Canadian Aboriginal languages

Innuinaqtun, official language of Nunavut

Vowels and diphthongs

Overall, vowels are also similar to those produced in GAE. However, there are a few minor differences as noted below and in Table 26-1 (Brinton and Fee, 2001).

- "Canadian" raising of the onset of the /aʊ/ and /aɪ/ diphthongs to [ʌʊ] and [ʌɪ] before voiceless consonants: This results in contrasts between *knife* (raised) and *knives* (not raised), for example. Although the raising happens elsewhere in North America, it is phonologically conditioned only in Canadian English. There has been some decline in the use of raising since the 1970s, with some fronting or lowering of the /a/ to /ɛ/ or /æ/, particularly for /aʊ/ (Chambers, 1998).

- Use of /ɔ/ only before /ɹ/: The /ɔ/ vowel is generally used only before /ɹ/ (85 percent of speakers), and elsewhere has merged with /ɑ/, as it has in many USA dialects.

- A disappearing distinction between /æ/ and /ɛ/ before /ɹ/, i.e., *merry*/*Mary*/*marry*, with some speakers still distinguishing *marry* (/æ/) and *Mary*/*merry* (/ɛ/) (Brinton and Fee, 2001).

- A possible shift relative to the front vowels /æ/, /ɛ/, and /ɪ/: Some recent studies with a small number of participants show /æ/ now to be more central rather than front, and the /ɛ/ and /ɪ/ either lowered toward the low-front space vacated by /æ/ (Clarke, Elms, and Youssef, 1995, studying 16 Ontario speakers) or retracted (Boberg, 2005, studying 35 Montreal, Quebec, speakers).

- A vowel system that is generally further back than other dialects of English, with the second formant of vowels being a little lower than the equivalent vowel in other dialects, but see below (Language Samples Project, University of Arizona, 2001)

- A tendency for the back vowel /u/ to be pronounced as a slightly diphthongized central barred [ʉ]: This is characteristic primarily of central and western Canada (Language Samples Project, University of Arizona, 2001).

- Yod dropping: Some speakers continue to use /j/ in the /juː/ sequence after the coronals /t/, /d/, and /n/, although this is becoming less common (i.e., in words like *Tuesday, news, due*).

- Variability on single lexical items: Single lexical items may show variable pronunciations, sometimes being pronounced like the GAE version, and sometimes like the British version (Chambers, 1998). Examples of more pervasive British variants are:
  - suffixes such as *-ine* or *–ile* pronounced with [aʔ], rather than a schwa as in GAE
  - full vowel use rather than schwa or lax vowels, as in, for example, *again* ([eɪ]), *been* ([i]), *lever* ([i])

There are additional different pronunciations of some lexical items (e.g., *vase* is [vɑz] in Canadian English, but [veɪs] in GAE). Words with the "a" spelling, especially Spanish, Italian, Greek, or Latin borrowings (e.g., *pasta, taco, drama*) are often pronounced with [æ] in Canadian English, compared with [a] or [ɑ] in GAE.

Writing system

The writing system has reflected British spelling historically, for example, "ou" in words such as *colour*, "re" in words such as *theatre,* and "s" in many words with the [aɪz] ending such as *analyse* (Mackey, 1998). However, American

TABLE 26-1   Vowels in standard Canadian English compared with General American English (GAE)

Vowel type	GAE Vowels Smit (2004)	Word examples	Standard Canadian English	Standard Canadian English: Comments
High, back, rounded	u	bl<u>ue</u>	ʉ	Also starting to appear in northern GAE
	ɔ	f<u>or</u>m b<u>oy</u>	Before /ɹ/ and /ɪ/ only	Open /ɔ/ context-bound in Canadian English
Diphthongs	aɪ	b<u>i</u>ke	ʌɪ	Canadian "raising" before voiceless consonants
	aʊ	<u>ou</u>t, m<u>ou</u>se	ʌʊ	Canadian "raising" before voiceless consonants

spellings are also now more commonly accepted, with some British spellings having dropped out of use (*tyre, kerb, connexion, -se* spelling of certain words, e.g., *realise*). The existence of two acceptable spellings for a word is something of a rarity in the English-speaking world.

Varieties of Canadian English

Newfoundland, the Maritime provinces, and Quebec have distinctive regional dialect variants. Newfoundland English is the most distinctive, probably because of the province's insular location and its late incorporation into Canada in 1949 (Kirwin, 2001). Overall, Newfoundlanders show less of a general tendency to retract the front vowel series. The two main English variants in Newfoundland reflect characteristics of the two main settler groups: English West Country and Irish. Examples of the English influences (Kirwin) are the following:

- No distinction between words that start with /h/ versus with a vowel, with [h] inserted before a vowel, or deleted where an "h" is in the standard target
- Voicing of some initial fricatives
- Vocalization of postvocalic /l/
- Retroflexed or constricted medial /ɹ/ in many areas, with some "r"-less dialects near the oldest settled coast at Conception Bay
- Collapse of high and mid vowel contrasts before postvocalic /ɹ/.

Examples of the Irish influences (Kirwin, 2001) are these:

- A clear /l/ (in contrast to the vocalized postvocalic /l/ mentioned above)
- Extensive substitution of the alveolar stops for the interdental fricatives
- A breathy fricative for word-final /t/
- Palatalization of /t/ and /d/ in words with /tj/ or /dj/
- A back round mid vowel where other dialects might have /ɔ/

The most notable pronunciation difference for Maritimes English (Prince Edward Island, Nova Scotia, and New Brunswick) is the use of [a] rather than [ɑ] before postvocalic /ɹ/. There is also less of a tendency to retract the front vowels than in standard Canadian English. New Brunswick has a large francophone community, which sometimes affects pronunciation of English vowels and consonants in bilinguals. Nova Scotia has a long heritage of Scottish and Irish settlement, and continues to show remnants of those pronunciations, especially in Cape Breton. (The Ottawa Valley in Ontario also shows similar Scottish and Irish influences.)

In Quebec, bilingual French-English speakers may show influences from French, for example, in lack of use of interdentals, different stress patterns (iambic rather than trochaic), or other interlanguage phenomena. In Montreal, Jewish and Italian cultural/linguistic groups may show particular English variants reflecting Hebrew or Italian. For example, a salient feature of general Montreal English is the distinction of /æ/ and /ɛ/ before /ɹ/ (*marry*/*merry*). Another is the low-front, almost low-central articulation of /æ/ before nasals (Boberg, 2004). Jewish and Italian Montreal English do not show the same pattern of lowering before nasals. Furthermore, Montreal Jewish English is characterized by a centralized and lowered /oʊ/ vowel, and Montreal Italian English by a back /u/ vowel. There are other slight vowel variants, such as a tendency for more open vowels in the Italian speech, and a fronting rather than a raising of the diphthongs that typically undergo raising (Boberg, 2004).

The influence of other heritage languages on Canadian English has not been systematically investigated in Canada, although some materials are available showing potential "accents" deriving from other heritage languages (e.g., Killam and Watson, 1983). As indicated earlier, Cantonese is a common language in Vancouver. It is now common to hear English spoken with [f] for the voiceless /θ/, with glottal stops in place of final stops and deletion of final grammatical morphemes that appear in clusters in standard English. In terms of prosody, it is common to hear a stepwise tonelike sentence intonation. Non-Cantonese residents of Vancouver are becoming attuned to such pronunciations of English. Whether there will be permanent local effects on Canadian English pronunciation remains to be seen.

For children learning English as a second language or dialect, the SLP's challenge during phonological assessment is to determine whether there is a phonological impairment, an accent, or both. If a client has both an impairment and an accent, it is relevant to know which phonological targets reflect home language phonology. Jenkins, a sociolinguist (2005), suggests that interdentals, minor vowel deviations, and minor stress and pitch variation may not contribute significantly to intelligibility in English speakers, and thus may not be of major importance in ESL teaching (or in speech therapy). Clients of course have the right to ask for help on those aspects of pronunciation if they wish to adopt the standard Canadian dialect.

Typical acquisition of Canadian English

There are no normative studies of Canadian English or its dialect variants. In a study of 1,655 children aged 5 in the Ottawa-Carleton region of Ontario (Beitchman, Nair, Clegg, and Patel, 1986), 180 were identified as having a speech and/or language delay, with 36 percent of the identified boys and 30 percent of the identified girls having *speech* delay only. These findings may be exaggerated, however, in that 5 year olds are still developing their articulatory skills, and the Ottawa region has been identified as having some of its own dialect features (Mackey, 1998).

A few studies have been published with information about children with phonological impairments living in Canada. None of these studies is norm-referenced, nor do they focus on any particular aspects of Canadian English. Bernhardt and Stemberger (2000, 2002), Major and Bernhardt (1998), and Rvachew and Andrews (2002) provide quantitative and qualitative information about the phonological systems of Canadian children with phonological impairments. These descriptions could be used as criterion reference data for other children with phonological impairments (Canadian or otherwise). Bernhardt (1992), Bernhardt and Gilbert (1992), and Rvachew and Nowak (2001) describe outcomes of intervention studies of Canadian children with phonological impairments, which again could be used to compare with data from other children with phonological impairments.

Acquired sounds

To date there is no study of the age of acquisition of consonants and vowels for children who speak Canadian English.

Percent correct

To date there is no study of the percentage of consonants and vowels produced correctly by children of different ages who speak Canadian English.

Phonological processes

To date there is no study of the production of phonological processes for children who speak Canadian English.

Intelligibility

No specific data on the emergence pattern for intelligible speech are available for this dialect.

Phonetic inventory

To date there is no study of the phonetic inventories produced at different ages by children who speak Canadian English.

Common mismatches

To date there is no study of the common mismatches produced by children who speak Canadian English.

Syllable structure

To date there is no study of the syllable structure produced by children who speak Canadian English.

Prosody

To date there is no study of the development of prosody for children who speak Canadian English.

Phonological awareness

A few studies have been published on Canadian children's phonological awareness skills. These, like studies elsewhere in the world, have observed relationships between phonological awareness and other skills, for example, perception and production, language skills, working memory, and literacy development (e.g., Bernhardt and Major, 2005; Major and Bernhardt, 1998; Rvachew, Nowak, and Cloutier, 2004). The Canadian Language and Literacy Research Network is conducting research in this area.

Speech assessment for English-speaking Canadian children

As noted, English–Canadian SLPs generally use speech assessment tools developed in the USA. The first author of this chapter, a Canadian, recently co-authored a speech sampling and analysis tool, the *Computerized Articulation and Phonology Evaluation System* (CAPES, Masterson and Bernhardt, 2001). The reference norms for the tool are USA-based, that is, the Iowa–Nebraska norms of Smit, Hand, Freilinger, Bernthal, and Bird (1990). However, in addition to common phoneme, syllable, and process analyses, the program includes nonlinear phonological analyses of children's speech as developed by Bernhardt (1990, 1992) working with Canadian children, and elaborated by Bernhardt and Stemberger (1998, 2000). Nonlinear analyses describe phonological form and patterns at multiple levels of the phonological hierarchy, from the phrase to the feature, for example:

- Word structure, including word length, word and phrasal stress patterns and word shapes in terms of CV sequences
- Segmental analyses
- Nonlinear feature analyses for vowels and consonants
- Feature sequence analyses across vowels, and between consonants and vowels

Nonlinear phonological analyses provide a comprehensive picture of a child's phonological production. However, except for the segmental level, no norms have been established for the various aspects of the phonological hierarchy, and for segments, SLPs rely on U.S. norms. Two other computerized assessment tools are under development by Canadian researchers, (1) Hodge's (2005) computer-based *TOCS.Plus* (http://www.tocs.plus.ualberta.ca), which evaluates intelligibility in addition to general phonology, and (2) *Phon,* a phonological analysis program by Rose et al. (2005, http://childes.psy.cmu.edu/phon) for the CHILDES database network.

Speech intervention for English-speaking Canadian children

Speech intervention techniques in Canada generally follow trends in the rest of the world, with individual SLPs choosing to focus more on either phonological (awareness) or motor-based approaches. Bernhardt (1990, 1994) and Bernhardt and Stemberger (2000) describe additional facilitative techniques that focus on phonological elements as defined in nonlinear phonological theory; for example,

- Syllable timing or weight units ("moras"): Attention is drawn to vowel length and final consonants using rhythm-based activities that draw attention to the number of weight units in the syllable. In English, stressed CVC monosyllables with lax vowels must have codas. The mora of the lax vowel and the mora of the coda are presented to the child with two "beats" using rhythmic support (drum, etc.). Similarly, long vowels or diphthongs are presented with two "beats."
- Syllable rimes or core syllables: Rhyme units such as VC can be alternated to target CV(C). Core syllables such as CV can be reduplicated to get CVCV.
- Feature combinations: New segments can be derived by combining features that already exist in the system: for

example, combining the [+nasal] of /n/ with the [Dorsal] of [g] to target [ŋ].

Rvachew, Nowak, and Cloutier (2004) have been developing speech perception tools that promote positive change in phonological production and awareness. Bernhardt and colleagues in the Interdisciplinary Speech Research Laboratory at Vancouver's University of British Columbia have found two-dimensional ultrasound and electropalatography to be useful adjuncts in speech habilitation of children and adults with and without hearing impairment (Adler-Bock, 2004; Bernhardt, Adler-Bock, Bacsfalvi, and Gick, 2005; Bernhardt, Gick, Bacsfalvi, and Ashdown, 2003).

Speech-language pathologists (SLPs) in Canada rely on USA-based tests for evaluating a child's age-related performance. However, there is a growing understanding of a need to develop measures and methods that are sensitive to Canada's cultural and linguistic diversity (Ball, Bernhardt, and Deby, 2005). Although there are as yet no norms or specific guidelines for practice concerning nonstandard dialects, individual SLPs have the option of exploring family and community wishes concerning dialect use. If the family and community want a child to be a speaker of the most common Canadian English dialect, standard tools and practices may continue to be useful. If a family or community wishes a child to retain use of his or her own dialect for any purpose, the SLP currently has a greater challenge in terms of assessment and intervention practice, because of the lack of tools and knowledge about the various dialects. An SLP working with someone with an uncharted dialect can learn the perspectives and dialect features of the given community and family only by spending time with community members and that family (see Chapter 18). The Resources section below contains some resources pertaining to Canadian English dialects for further study.

Working in Canada

Most current graduates find employment as soon as they finish their degree in Canada, with some positions remaining vacant for some time in isolated regions. SLPs work in schools, preschools, health centers, child development centers, hospitals, rehabilitation agencies, and private practice. The entry degree for practice in Canada is a master's degree in speech-language pathology. A recent reciprocity agreement with Britain, Australia, and the USA allows SLPs to work in the various countries with certain restrictions (see the national association guidelines for Canada, http://www.caslpa.ca).

PHONETICALLY SPEAKING

Pronunciation of Canadian English: /kʰəˈneɪdjn̩ ˈɪŋɫəʃ/

Passage: Comma Gets a Cure

Below is a broad phonetic transcription of *Comma Gets a Cure* (Honorof, McCullough, and Somerville, 2000) spoken by a typical adult speaker of standard Canadian English in Vancouver in a conversational setting. (Stress marks are indicated for primary and secondary lexical stress, for words of two or more syllables.)

/wɛɫ hɪɹz ə ˈstɔɹi fɚ jə : ˈsæɹə ˈpʰɛɹi wəz ə ˌvɛtrəˌnɛɹi nɚs hu əd bĭn ˈwɚkĭn ˈdeɪli æt?
n̩ oʊɫd zu ɪn ə dɪˈzɚ·rəd ˈdɪstɹəkt əv ðə ˈtʰɛɹəˌtɔɹi soʊ ʃi wəz ˈvɛɹi ˈhæpi tə staɹt ə nu dʒɑb
æɹ ə ˌsuˈpɚ·b ˈpɹaɪvət ˈpɹæktəs ĭn nɔɹθ skwɛɹ nɪɹ ðə dʉk stɹit ˈtʰaʊwɚ·. ðæt ˈɛɹijə wəz mʌtʃ
ˈniɚ· fɚ hɚ æn ˈmɔɹ tə hɚ ˈlʌɪkĭŋ. ˈɪvn̩ soʊ, ɑn hɚ fɚ·st ˈmɔɹnĭŋ, ʃi fɛɫt stɹɛst. ʃi eɪɹ ə boʊɫ ə
ˈpʰɔɹɪdʒ, tʃɛkt hɚ·sɛɫf ĭn ðə mɪɹ æn wɑʃt hɚ feɪs ĭn ə hɚ·i, ðɛ́n ʃi pʰʊr ɑ́n ə pleɪn̆jeloʊ dɹɛs
æn ə flis ˈdʒækət, pʰɪkt ʌp hɚ kʰɪt æn ˈhɛɹəd fɚ wɚ·k. wɛn ʃi gat ðɛɹ, ðɛɹ wəz ə ˈwʊmn̩ wɪθ
ə gus ˈweɪtʔŋ fɔɹ hɚ·. ðə ˈwʊmn̩ geɪv ˈsæɹə n̩ əˈfɪʃɫ ˈlɛɹɚ· fɹʌ́m ðə vɛt. ðə ˈlɛɹɚ· ĭmˈplaɪd ðæt
ðĭ ˈænəmɫ kʰʊd bi ˈsʌfɹ̩ĭŋ frʌ́m ə ɹæɹ fɔɹm ə fʊt n̩ mʌʊθ dəˈziz, wɪtʃ wəz səˈpɹaɪzĭŋ, bɪˈkʌz
ˈnɔɹməli jʉ wʊd ˈõʊnli ˌɛkˈspɛkt tə si ɪr ĭn ə dag ɚ· ə goʊt. sæɹə wəz ˌsɛ̃ntəˈmɛ̃ntɫ, soʊ ðɪs
meɪd hɚ· fĭɫ ˈsɔɹi fɚ ðə bɚ·d/

Well, here's a story for you: Sarah Perry was a veterinary nurse who had been working daily at an old zoo in a deserted district of the territory, so she was very happy to start a new job at a superb private practice in North Square near the Duke Street Tower. That area was much nearer for her and more to her liking. Even so, on her first morning, she felt stressed. She ate a bowl of porridge, checked herself in the mirror and washed her face in a hurry. Then she put on a plain yellow dress and a fleece jacket, picked up her kit and headed for work. When she got there, there was a woman with a goose waiting for her. The woman gave Sarah an official letter from the vet. The letter implied that the animal could be suffering from a rare form of foot and mouth disease, which was surprising, because normally you would only expect to see it in a dog or a goat. Sarah was sentimental, so this made her feel sorry for the bird. (Honorof, McCullough, and Somerville, 2000).

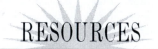

RESOURCES

Books

Algeo, J. (2001). *The Cambridge history of the English language, Volume 6, English in North America.* Cambridge, UK: Cambridge University Press.

Clarke, S. (1993). *Focus on Canada*, Amsterdam: John Benjamins.

Edwards, J. (1998). *Language in Canada.* Cambridge, UK: Cambridge University Press.

Killam, C., and Watson, B. (1983). *Thirteen language profiles.* Vancouver Community College, King Edward Campus.

Journals

- *American Speech,* http://muse.jhu.edu/journals/american_speech. This journal is dedicated to English as spoken in the western hemisphere.
- *Canadian Journal of Linguistics,* http://www.utpjournals.com/jour.ihtml?lp=cjl/cjl.html. This is the journal of the Canadian Linguistic Association, published at the University of Toronto.
- *Journal of Speech-Language Pathology and Audiology.* This is the only speech-language pathology journal published in Canada (Canadian Association of Speech-Language Pathologists and Audiologists).

- *Language Variation and Change,* http://journals.cambridge.org/action/displayJournal?jid=LVC. This journal is dedicated to dialectal variation and language change.

Professional associations

The professional association of speech-language pathologists within Canada is the Canadian Association of Speech-Language Pathologists and Audiologists (CASLPA, http://www.caslpa.ca).

Useful Web sites

- Canadian English in the Global Context, http://www.chass.utoronto.ca/canengglobal/jack.htm
- Canadian English, http://www.ic.arizona.edu/%7Elsp/CanadianEnglish.html

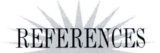

REFERENCES

Adler-Bock, M. (2004). *Visual feedback from ultrasound in remediation of persistent /r/ errors: Case studies of two adolescents.* Unpublished master's thesis, University of British Columbia, Canada.

Ball, J., Bernhardt, B., and Deby, J. (2005, May). *Implications of First Nations English dialects for supporting First Nations Children's Language Development.* Poster presented at the School Readiness Conference, Faculty of Education.

Beitchman J., Nair R., Clegg, M., and Patel, P. (1986). Prevalence of speech and language disorders in 5-year-old kindergarten children in the Ottawa-Carleton Region. *Journal of Speech and Hearing Disorders, 51,* 98–110.

Bernhardt, B. H. (1990). *The application of nonlinear phonological theory to intervention with six phonologically disordered children.* Unpublished doctoral dissertation, University of British Columbia, Canada.

Bernhardt, B. H. (1992). The application of nonlinear phonological theory to intervention with one phonologically disordered child. *Clinical Linguistics and Phonetics, 6,* 283–316.

Bernhardt, B. H. (1994). Phonological intervention techniques for syllable and word structure development. *Clinics in Communication Disorders, 4*(1), 54–65.

Bernhardt, B. H., Adler-Bock, M., Bacsfalvi, P., and Gick, B. (2005). Ultrasound in speech therapy with adolescents and adults. *Clinical Linguistics and Phonetics, 19,* 605–617.

Bernhardt, B. H., Gick, B., Bacsfalvi, P., and Ashdown, J. (2003). Speech habilitation of hard of hearing adolescents using electropalatography and ultrasound as evaluated by trained listeners. *Clinical Linguistics and Phonetics, 17*(3), 199–216.

Bernhardt, B. H., and Gilbert, J. (1992). Applying linguistic theory to speech-language pathology: The case for nonlinear phonology. *Clinical Linguistics and Phonetics, 6,* 123–145.

Bernhardt, B. H., and Major, E. (2005). Speech, language and literacy skills three years later: Long-term outcomes of nonlinear phonological intervention. *International Journal of Language and Communication Disorders, 40,* 1–27.

Bernhardt, B. H., and Stemberger, J. P. (1998). *Handbook of phonological development: From a nonlinear constraints-based perspective.* San Diego: Academic Press.

Bernhardt, B. H., and Stemberger, J. P. (2000). *Workbook in nonlinear phonology for clinical application.* Austin, TX: Pro-Ed.

Bernhardt, B. H., & Stemberger, J. (2002). Intervocalic consonants in the speech of children with phonological disorders. *Clinical Linguistics and Phonetics*, *16*(3), 199–214.

Boberg, C. (2004). Ethnic patterns in the phonetics of Montreal English. *Journal of Sociolinguistics, 8*, 538–568.

Boberg, C. (2005). The North American regional vocabulary survey: New variables and methods in the study of North American English. *American Speech*, *80*, 22–60.

Brinton, L., and Fee, M. (2001). Canadian English. In J. Algeo (Ed.), *The Cambridge history of the English Language, Volume 6, English in North America* (pp. 422–440). Cambridge, UK: Cambridge University Press.

Chambers, J. (1998). English: Canadian varieties. In J. Edwards (Ed.), *Language in Canada* (pp. 252–272). Cambridge, UK: Cambridge University Press.

Clarke, S., Elms, F., and Youssef, A. (1995). The third dialect of English: Some Canadian evidence. *Language Variation and Change, 7*, 209–228.

Hodge, M. (2005). *TOCS.plus* (2005). Retrieved August 27, 2005, from http://www.tocs.plus.ualberta.ca.

Honorof, D. N., McCullough, J., and Somerville, B. (2000). *Comma gets a cure: A diagnostic passage for accent study.* New Haven, CT: Haskins Laboratories.

Jenkins, J. (2005). *Global English.* Retrieved August 27, 2005 from www.teachingenglish.org.uk/think/pron/global_english.shtml#one.

Killam, C., and Watson, B. (1983). *Thirteen language profiles.* Vancouver, BC: Vancouver Community College, King Edward Campus.

Kirwin, W. J. (2001). Newfoundland English. In J. Algeo (Ed.), *The Cambridge history of the English Language, Volume 6, English in North America* (pp. 441–455). Cambridge, UK: Cambridge University Press.

Language Samples Project, University of Arizona. (2001). Retrieved July 15, 2005, from www.ic.arizona.edu/%7Elsp/CanadianEnglish.html.

Mackey, W. (1998). The foundations. In J. Edwards (Ed.), *Language in Canada* (pp. 13–35). Cambridge, UK: Cambridge University Press.

Major, E., and Bernhardt, B. (1998). Metaphonological skills of children with phonological disorders before and after phonological and metaphonological intervention. *International Journal of Language and Communication Disorders, 33*, 413–444.

Masterson, J., and Bernhardt, B. (2001). *Computerized Articulation and Phonology Evaluation System.* San Antonio, TX: The Psychological Corporation.

Rose, Y., MacWhinney, B., Byrne, R., Hedlund, G., Maddocks, K., O'Brien, P., and Wareham, T. (2005, November). *Introducing Phon: A software solution for the study of phonological acquisition.* 30th Annual Boston University Conference on Language Development, Boston University.

Rvachew, S., and Andrews, E. (2002). The influence of syllable position on children's production of consonants. *Clinical Linguistics and Phonetics, 16,* 183–198.

Rvachew, S., and Nowak, M. (2001). The effect of target selection strategy on sound production learning. *Journal of Speech, Language, and Hearing Research, 44,* 610–623.

Rvachew, S., Nowak, M., and Cloutier, G. (2004). Effect of phonemic perception training on the speech production and phonological awareness skills of children with expressive phonological delay. *American Journal of Speech-Language Pathology, 13*(3), 250–263.

Smit, A. B., (2004). Articulation and Phonology: Resource guide for school-age children and adullts. Clifton Park, NY: Thomas Delmar Learning.

Smit, A. B., Hand, L., Freilinger, J. J., Bernthal, J. E., and Bird, A. (1990). The Iowa Articulation Norms Project and its Nebraska replication. *Journal of Speech and Hearing Disorders, 55,* 779–798.

Statistics Canada Census. (2001). Retrieved August 27, 2005 from http://www.statcan.ca/. U.S. Central Intelligence Agency. (2005). *Canadian population.* Retrieved August 27, 2005 from www.cia.gov/cia/publications/factboook/rankorder/2119rank.html.

SUMMARY OF STUDIES OF TYPICAL CANADIAN ENGLISH SPEECH ACQUISITION

To date no studies are available.

Chapter 27

English Speech Acquisition

Sara Howard

INTRODUCTION

This chapter is concerned with the varieties of English spoken in England, one of the countries which, along with Northern Ireland, Scotland, and Wales, makes up the United Kingdom. At the risk of sounding tautologous, perhaps we should use the term "English English" to denote its specific geographical location and to reflect the fact that this is where the English language, which is now so widespread in such a rich variety of forms across the globe, originally emerged as a consequence of the Anglo-Saxon conquest of Britain in the fifth and sixth centuries AD.

Where English is spoken

The accompanying map illustrates the specific geographical area covered in this chapter and those countries of the world where English now figures as a major language (see accompanying map and Appendix D).

Components of English

Consonants

General Received Pronunciation (RP) has 24 consonants (see Table 27-1), although other regional varieties in England may have either more or fewer than this total. For example, speakers of many accents of English, including those found in London and most of the north of England, do not have the sound /h/ as part of their consonant inventory, and

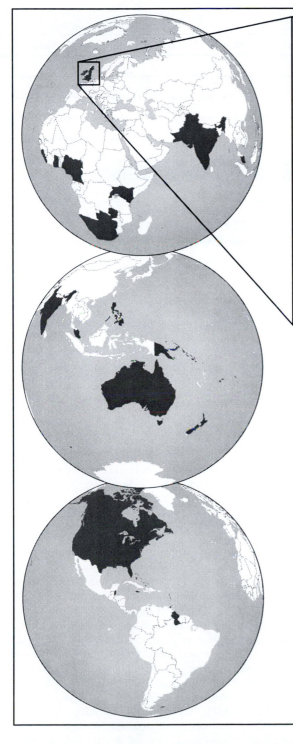

United Kingdom

Country of focus

United Kingdom

Official language of the following countries

Akrotiri, Anguilla, Antigua, Australia, Bahamas, Barbados, Bermuda, Belize, Botswana, British Virgin Islands, Cameroon, Canada, Cayman Islands, Christmas Island, Cocos (Keeling) Islands, Cook Islands, Dhekelia, Dominica, European Union, Falkaland Islands, Fiji, Gambia, Ghana, Gibraltar, Grenada, Guam, Guernsey, Guyana, Hong Kong, India, Isle of Man, Jamaica, Jersey, Kenya, Kiribati, Lesotho, Liberia, Malta, Mauritius, Marshall Islands, Federated States of Micronesia, Montserrat, Namibia, New Zealand, Nigeria, Norfolk Island, Northern Ireland, Pakistan, Palau, Papua New Guinea, Philippines, Pitcairn Islands, Republic of Ireland, Rwanda, Samoa, Seychelles, Sierra Leone, Singapore, Solomon Islands, South Africa, St Kitts and Nevis, St Lucia, St Vincent and the Grenadines, Swaziland, Tanzania, Trinidad and Tobago, Tokelau, Tonga, Turks and Caicos Islands, Tuvalu, Uganda, United Kingdom, United States of America, Virgin Islands, Zambia, Zimbabwe

TABLE 27-1 Consonants produced in English

	Bilabial	Dental	Labiodental	Alveolar
Plosive	p b			t d
Nasal	m			n
Trill				
Tap or flap				
Fricative		θ ð	f v	s z
Lateral fricative	■■■■			
Affricate				
Approximant	w (labiovelar)			ɹ
Lateral approximant	■■■■			l

Black = articulations judged impossible

Based on the International Phonetic Alphabet. Courtesy of the International Phonetic Association (c/o Department of Linguistics, University of Victoria, Victoria, British Columbia, Canada).

many speakers of the Cockney accent associated with London do not have /θ/ and /ð/ in their phonological system, producing words like *this, thin,* and *together* as [dɪs], [fɪn] and [tə'gevə]. At a phonetic level, the phoneme /r/ is usually realized by many (but not all) speakers of RP as [ɹ], the post-alveolar approximant. In some contexts and by some speakers /r/ can be realized as, among other things, a tap, a labiodental approximant, and a velar approximant. Within this chapter /ɹ/ signals a phoneme that subsumes these various phonetic realizations.

Vowels and diphthongs

General Received Pronunciation has 20 vowels, consisting of five long monophthongs, seven short monophthongs, and eight diphthongs (see Table 27-2), although currently the /ʊə/ diphthong, found in words like *poor* and *tour*, appears to be merging with the /ɔ/ vowel in words like *paw* and *north*, making, for example, *poor* and *paw* homophonous: /pɔ/. Cruttenden (2001), in *Gimson's Pronunciation of English*, and Hughes, Trudgill, and Watt (2005) provide clear accounts of the system.

Phonotactic restrictions
Syllables

The syllable structure of English is the same as for other varieties of English, including General American English (GAE; see Chapter 22). Thus a syllable has an obligatory vowel (or vocalic consonant) as its nucleus (e.g., *I* /aɪ/, *a* /eɪ/, *kettle* /kɛtl/. Syllable

onsets can contain up to three consonants (e.g., *spray* /spɹeɪ/, *straw* /stɹɔ/) and syllable codas permit up to four consonants (e.g., *twelfths* /twɛlfθs/, *strengths* /stɹɛŋkθs/, *prompts* /prɒmpts/), thus producing the following permissible structure: $C_{(0-3)}VC_{(0-4)}$. We should note that in practice, English speakers don't appear to like the long sequences of consonants found in some codas, and often reduce these in actual speech production so that *twelfths* may be realised as [twɛlθs] and *strengths* as [stɹɛŋθs]. Sequences of vowels are permissible in English only as a consequence of adjacent syllables (e.g., *trio* /'tɹiəʊ/, *dyad* /'daɪæd/).

Consonants and consonant clusters

RP can generally be said to have the same consonant system and the same consonant clusters as GAE (Ladefoged, 1999). There are, however, some significant differences of realization and distribution. For example, unlike GAE, RP is nonrhotic (Wells, 1982b), so /ɹ/ is produced only prevocalically: thus *crate* /kɹeɪt/, but *car* /kɑ/ and *cart* /kɑt/. Also note *car* /kɑ/ but *car and train* /'kɑɹ ən 'tɹeɪn/. RP produces /j/ in syllable onset clusters following an alveolar, where GAE does not: thus *intuition* RP /ɪntju'ɪʃən/ and GAE /ɪntu'ɪʃən/; *dune* RP /djun/ and GAE /dun/; *new* RP /nju/ and GAE /nu/ (Roach and Hartman, 1997). Another distributional difference in consonantal usage is that RP produces alveolar plosives intervocalically in words such as *writer* /'ɹaɪtə/ and *rider* /'ɹaɪdə/, rather than realizing them

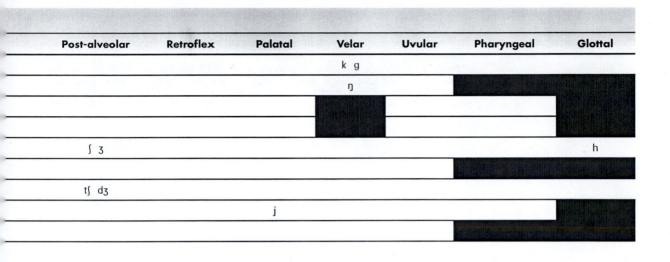

Post-alveolar	Retroflex	Palatal	Velar	Uvular	Pharyngeal	Glottal
			k g			
			ŋ			
ʃ ʒ						h
tʃ dʒ						
		j				

TABLE 27-2 Vowels of RP English compared with General American English

American English location	American English vowels (Smit, 2004)	American English examples	RP Location	RP phonetic/ phonemic symbols (Wells, 1982)	KEY WORD (Wells, 1982)	RP examples
High-front	i	*beat*	High-front	i	FLEECE	*beat*
	ɪ	*bit*	"	ɪ	KIT	*bit, hill*
	e	*raid*				
Mid-low front	ɛ	*bed*	Mid-low front	ɛ	DRESS	*bed, head*
	æ	*bad*	Low front	æ	TRAP	*bad*
High-back, rounded	u	*blue*	High-back, rounded	u	GOOSE	*blue, moon*
	ʊ	*book*	"	ʊ	FOOT	*book, sugar pull*
Mid-back, rounded	o	*boat*				
	ɔ	*form*	Mid-back, rounded	ɔ	THOUGHT, NORTH, FORCE	*form, sought, law*
			Low back, rounded	ɒ	LOT	*drop*
Low back	ɑ	*drop*	Low back,	ɑ	START, BATH, PALM	*bard, laugh, past*
[r]-colored	ɝ		Central	ɜ	NURSE	*bird, heard, fern*
	ɚ	*never, color*				

Table 27-2 continued

American English location	American English vowels (Smit, 2004)	American English examples	RP Location	RP phonetic/ phonemic symbols (Wells, 1982)	KEY WORD (Wells, 1982)	RP examples
Central	ə	*about, occur, upon,*	Front-central-mid-open	ə	COMMA, LETTER	*about, occur, upon, never, zebra*
	ʌ	*bud*	Central, mid-open	ʌ	STRUT	*bud, tough, love*
	ɪɹ					
	ɛɹ					
	ʊɹ					
	ɔɹ					
	ɑɹ					
Diphthongs	aɪ	*my, bike*	Diphthongs	aɪ	PRICE	*my, bike, sigh*
	aʊ	*out, mouse*		aʊ	MOUTH	*out, sow (pig), mouse*
	ɔɪ	*boy*		ɔɪ	CHOICE	*boy, soil*
				eɪ	FACE	*bay, bait*
				oʊ	GOAT	*boat, sow (seed)*
				ɪə	NEAR	*beer*
				ɛə	SQUARE	*bear*
				ʊə	CURE	*tour*

as flaps or voicing the /t/, as is found in GAE: thus *writer* [ˈɹaɪɾə] or [ˈɹaɪʧə] and *rider* [ˈɹaɪɾə] (Roach and Hartman; Wells, 1982c). It has also been widely noted that variants of /l/ have a different distribution in RP and GAE, with RP using a dark (or velarized) variant only preconsonantally or word-finally, whereas GAE tends to use velarized variants in more contexts. Wells (1982c, p. 490), for example, notes that "the difference ... is particularly noticeable in the environment V_V, as in *valley, jelly, rely,*" where RP would have a clear /l/ and GAE a dark /l/.

Tones

English does not use tones to differentiate meanings.

Stress and intonation

English is an intonation language, in which utterances are arranged into tone-units or intonation-groups, with one syllable within each tone-unit (called the nuclear or tonic syllable) being marked by the use of primary stress together with one of five tones (fall, rise, level, fall-rise, rise-fall) and surrounded by characteristic pitch patterns or "tunes" (Crystal, 1987; Cruttenden, 1997). Cruttenden notes that the intonation patterns of RP are quite similar to those of GAE, but that there exist significant regional differences in English, particularly in urban areas in Northern Britain (Cruttenden, 1997).

The use of the high rising tone (HRT) in sentence final position, which has been noted for many years in Australian English (Fletcher, Stirling, Mushin, and Wales, 2002; Guy, Horvath, Vonwiller, Disley, and Rogers, 1986; McGregor, 1980), appears to have become more common in England in recent years. Thus, for example, a speaker might say *I'm going to 'York tomorrow* rather than *I'm going to `York tomorrow*. Commonly referred to as "uptalk," it is described by Cruttenden (1997, p. 129) as being used "to mean 'I'm being deliberately non-assertive and checking that you are following me'." Cruttenden notes its emergence in London in the mid

1990s and observes that it is now spreading out into other areas of the UK, although Docherty and Foulkes (1999) and Stoddart, Upton, and Widdowson (1999) reported that usage was still not common. Current indications, however, are that its use is indeed becoming more widespread globally (Hughes, Trudgill, and Watt, 2005; Pratt-Johnson, 2005).

In terms of stress, differences in lexical stress patterns exist between RP and GAE for specific words. For example, RP uses the following stress patterns: *address* /əˈdɹɛs/; *ballet* /ˈbæleɪ/; *cigarette* /sɪgəˈɹɛt/; *laboratory* /ləˈbɒɹətɹi/, where GAE uses *address* /ˈædɹɛs/; *ballet* /bæˈleɪ/; *cigarette* /ˈsɪgəɹɛt/; *laboratory* /ˈlæbɹətɹi/.

Varieties of English in England

In England, accents vary along social and regional dimensions. Hughes et al. (2005, p. 9) sum the situation up succinctly:

> *In Britain, from the south-west of England to the north of Scotland, we do not have a succession of distinct accents, but an accent continuum, a gradual changing of pronunciation. Speakers of RP tend to be found at the top of the social scale, and their speech gives no clue to their regional origin. People at the bottom of the social scale speak with the most obvious, the "broadest," regional accents.*

We also need to note that even within fairly tightly defined geographical regions there will be accent differences associated with age and gender, and also between urban and rural populations (Foulkes and Docherty, 1999; Hughes et al., 2005). The situation in England, then, is complex and space will thus only permit us to look at some of the most significant accent differences in English spoken in England.

In this chapter Received Pronunciation (RP) is used at the reference accent, but it is important to note that a number of subvarieties of RP exist, related to both the social class and age of speakers. Thus Wells (1982b) adopts the categories U-RP (where U denotes "upper-crust"), Mainstream RP, and Adoptive RP, while Cruttenden (2001) outlines similar distinct varieties using the terms Refined, General, and Regional RP. Thus, for example, a speaker of U-RP might produce words like *cloth* and *off* as [klɔθ] and [ɔf], whereas in Mainstream RP these would have a short vowel: /klɒθ/ and /ɒf/. Equally, U-RP speakers would be likely to preserve a three-way distinction between *poor* [pʊə], *pore* [pɔə], and *paw* [pɔ], where the distinction is fast disappearing in Mainstream RP, with all three words

being produced as [pɔ]. Similarly, Mainstream RP speakers may produce a diphthong in words such as *tire* /taə/ and *tower* /tɒə/, where U-RP would use the more traditional triphthong: /taɪə/ and /taʊə/. Wells (1999) provides an interesting summary of changes in RP over the twentieth century.

We should also be aware that, for a reference accent, RP is actually spoken by a rather small percentage of the population. Indeed Trudgill (2002) estimates that no more than 3–5 percent of speakers in England use RP. Furthermore, as an accent traditionally associated with social prestige, wealth, education, and power, spoken as Hughes et al. (2005, p. 17) note by "those at the top of the social scale," RP is not necessarily viewed positively by speakers in England. Foulkes and Docherty (1999) bring together several sources of evidence to suggest that RP is actually regarded negatively within the UK and that some speakers brought up using RP choose later in life to modify their accent toward a more regional variety. It has been suggested that the desire of some RP speakers to "downgrade" their accents, and the desire of other speakers with more marked forms of regional accent to "upgrade" their accents, may be responsible for so-called Estuary English (EE; Coggle, 1993; Rosewarne, 1984). Estuary English is an accent variety in England that appears to contain a mixture of RP and traditional London ("Cockney") features and has gained much publicity over recent years. Cruttenden (2001, p. 81) uses the term "London regional RP" to describe EE and suggests that it "is being adopted by those wishing to avoid the stigma of RP as 'posh' and by upwardly mobile speakers of local accent." Wells (1997) discusses some of its defining features. These include the tendency for EE speakers to vocalize dark /l/ (thus *milk* RP /mɪlk/; EE [mɪʊk]); to glottalize /t/ in more contexts than would be found in RP, including some pre-vocalic positions (e.g., *that is* [ðæʔ ˈɪz]); to front, and sometimes to unround, high, back rounded vowels (e.g., *boon* RP /bun/ and EE [bʉn]; *book* RP /bʊk/ and EE [bʉk] or [bɵk]); to coalesce alveolar stops and /j/ in words such as *tune* RP /tjun/ and EE [tʃun]; *duty* RP /ˈdjuti/ and EE [ˈdʒuti], and so on. While such pronunciation changes do seem to be emerging and spreading outward from London, and being adopted by more RP speakers, Wells (1997) and Przedlacka (2001) caution that we should beware of regarding EE as an easily identifiable and coherent accent and might more usefully see it as a shorthand for accents that exist along a continuum from RP to Cockney. A further pronunciation change that is becoming more prevalent in younger speakers in England is the use of a labiodental variant for "r": thus *a red rose* [ə ˈʋed ˈʋəʊz]. Traditionally such a realization has been regarded as either immature or atypical, but it is now becoming a socially acceptable variant (Foulkes and Docherty, 2000).

There are, of course, many other important regional accent differences to be found in England. One major distinction is between northern and southern accents: Crystal (1995) and Hughes et al. (2005) suggest that a broad distinction can be made between the area including all of the north and the midlands of England on the one hand and the area comprising the southwest, the southeast, and East Anglia. Northern accents typically produce words like *cup* and *bud* with /ʊ/ rather than /ʌ/ and use /æ/ rather than /ɑ/ for words like *glass* and *path*. Southern accents, on the other hand, are similar to RP in producing *cup* [kʌp]; *bud* [bʌd]; *glass* [glɑs]; and *path* [pɑθ]. It should be noted, however, that although northern accents do not contain the vowel /ʌ/, they do contain /ɑ/, which will typically be used for words like *palm* [pɑm] and *card* [kɑd], and, to further complicate matters, that some English speakers will produce words like *cup* and *bud*, and even *put* and *sugar*, with a [ə]-type vowel: thus [kəp], [bəd], [pət], and [ˈʃəgə]. A feature common to almost all northern English accents is that they do not contain /h/, so *the ham* is produced [ðɪ ˈæm], rather than [ðə ˈhæm] and *a hog* is [ən ˈɒg] rather than [ə ˈhɒg]. However, this feature is not a clear distinguisher between northern and southern accents: the accent of Newcastle and its environs in the northeast of the country includes /h/, whereas most urban accents across the south do not.

Other significant accent features whose usage does not correspond to a neat north/south distinction in England include rhoticity, /j/-dropping, and variant realizations of /ŋ/. Although most of the regional accents of England are, like RP, nonrhotic, the southwest of England does produce post-vocalic /ɹ/, as do a small number of speakers in an area of central Lancashire in northwest England. Hughes et al. (2005) note, however, that rhoticity is gradually disappearing in England. The pattern found in GAE of dropping /j/ in prevocalic position following an alveolar consonant (e.g., *new* [nu], *tuna* [ˈtunə], *due* [ˈdu]) is also found in many Cockney speakers in London, and the dropping of prevocalic /j/ following any consonant is prevalent in the accents of East Anglia and the southeast Midlands: thus *music* [ˈmuzɪk], *huge* [hudʒ], *few* [fu], rather than [ˈmjuzɪk], [hjudʒ], [fju]. The velar nasal /ŋ/ has a number of different usage patterns in English accents. In words like *sing* or *singer* (/sɪŋ/ and /sɪŋə/ in RP), speakers in the northwest

of England (particularly Liverpool and Merseyside), as well as those in the northwest and west Midlands may produce [sɪŋg] and [sɪŋgə]. Where /ŋ/ forms part of the "-ing" suffix, (e.g., RP *falling* /ˈfɔlɪŋ/, *singing* /ˈsɪŋɪŋ/), Hughes et al. (2005) note that most regional accents use [ɪn]: thus [ˈfɔlɪn], [ˈsɪŋɪn], or [ˈsɪŋgɪn]. But there is much variation within and between regions, and Stoddart et al. (1999) and Mathisen (1999) note, respectively, that for the urban centers of Sheffield and Birmingham [ɪn], [ɪŋ], and ɪŋg] are all found.

Typical acquisition of English

Acquired sounds
Consonants

Table 27-3 contains age of acquisition data for consonants for British children from two studies (Anthony, Bogle, Ingram, and McIsaac, 1971; Dodd, Holm, Hua, and Crosbie, 2003). Dodd, Holm et al. is the only comprehensive, large group, longitudinal study of phonological acquisition of English-speaking children growing up in England. The study reports on speech samples from 684 children from across the United Kingdom, the majority of whom lived in England. The participants in the study of Anthony et al. were from Scotland. Dodd, Holm et al. use a criterion of phonetic production (regardless of phonological status) by 90 percent of children (either spontaneously or by imitation), and a comparison with the Anthony et al. data has been made using this criterion. It is worth noting, however, that the significant differences for age of acquisition for fricatives and affricates are related to the fact that Anthony et al. did not use imitation as a form of sound elicitation and also to their quite strict scoring criteria, whereby a minor realizational variant, such as [sʲ] being produced for /s/, is counted as an error.

Vance, Stackhouse, and Wells (2005), investigating speech production skills at word level in typically developing 3- to 7-year-old English children, noted a steady improvement with age in the overall accuracy of the production of words and nonwords between the ages of 3 and 6. There were no significant differences, overall, between the 6- and 7-year-old children. However, word length was a significant factor in relation to production accuracy, and although children of 5 and above showed a ceiling effect for accuracy in the production of shorter items, they still produced inaccurate realizations of test words three or more syllables in length.

TABLE 27-3 Age of phonetic acquisition for English consonants by 90 percent of children

Consonant	Anthony et al. (1971)	Dodd, Holm et al. (2003)
p	3;0–3;5	3;0–3;5
b	3;0–3;5	3;0–3;5
m	3;0–3;5	3;0–3;5
t	3;0–3;5	3;0–3;5
d	3;0–3;5	3;0–3;5
n	3;0–3;5	3;0–3;5
k	3;6–3;11	3;0–3;5
g	3;6–3;11	3;0–3;5
ŋ	3;6–3;11	3;0–3;5
f	3;6–3;11	3;0–3;5
v	3;6–3;11	3;0–3;5
θ	After 6;0	After 7;0
ð	After 6;0	After 7;0
s	5;6–5;11	3;0–3;5
z	5;6–5;11	3;0–3;5
ʃ	5;6–5;11	4;6–4;11
ʒ	5;6–5;11	4;0–4;5
tʃ	After 6;0	3;6–3;11
dʒ	After 6;0	4;0–4;5
h	3;6–4;0	3;0–3;5
w	3;0–3;5	3;0–3;5
ɹ	After 6;0	6;0–6;5
l	4;6–4;11	3;0–3;5
j	3;0–3;11	3;0–3;11

Consonant clusters

To date there are no studies of the acquisition of consonant clusters by English-speaking children living in England, although Higgs (1968) presents a study of the production of /s/ + stop clusters in a group of Scottish children aged 2;6 to 5, with data that suggest a gradual pattern of development from cluster reduction through immature segment realizations to mature productions for most children by the age of 5.

Vowels and diphthongs

Dodd, Holm et al. (2003) do not report in detail on age of acquisition for vowels, but they do note that almost all children produced almost all vowels correctly by the age of 4;0. They largely concur with Anthony et al. (1971, p. 12) who state that "by the age of 3 years, all normal children have evolved a stabilised vowel system." There has generally been relatively little attention given to vowel productions in developing speech. Howard and Heselwood (2002) discuss some of the challenges of assessing vowel development and describing vowel productions in the context of England, where there is such rich sociophonetic variation in the vowel systems of different accents.

Percent correct

Consonants

Dodd, Holm et al. (2003) report the following means for percentage of consonants correct (PCC): 82.11 percent consonants correct at age 3;0 to 3;11; 90.37 percent consonants correct at age 4;0 to 5;5; 95.86 percent consonants correct at age 5;6 to 7;0 (see Table 27-4).

Consonant clusters

There are currently no studies of the percentage of consonant clusters correct in England.

Vowels and diphthongs

Dodd, Holm et al. (2003) report the following means for percentage of vowels correct (PVC): 97.39 percent vowels correct at age 3;0 to 3;11; 98.93 percent vowels correct at age 4;0 to 5;5; 99.19 percent vowels correct at age 5;6 to 7;0 (see Table 27-4).

TABLE 27-4 Percent correct for English consonants and vowels

Age	Consonants	Vowels
3;0–3;11	82.11	97.39
4;0–5;5	90.37	98.93
5;6–7;0	95.86	99.19

Source: Dodd, Holm et al., 2003

Phonological processes

Dodd, Holm et al. (2003) report on use of phono-logical processes (which they term error patterns) by 684 typically developing English-speaking children in the UK. The simplifying processes investigated in their study include gliding, deaffrication, consonant cluster reduction, fronting, weak syllable deletion, stopping, and voicing. All of these processes, with the exception of voicing, are noted to be present in the speech produc-tion of the 3-year-olds studied. Stopping persists until 3;6, weak syllable deletion until age 4;0, fronting until 4;6, and deaffrication until 5;0. The study demonstrates that gliding is still present in typically developing English children's speech up to the age of 6;0 and notes a gradual development of the ability to produce consonant clusters, with most two-element clusters handled successfully by 4;0, but three-element clusters still being systematically partially reduced until around the age of 5;0.

Intelligibility

To date there is no study of intelligibility of English chil-dren from England.

Phonetic inventory

Dodd, Holm et al. (2003) provide data on the phonetic acquisition of consonants (regardless of the phono-logical status of the segments as produced by individual children), which are outlined in Table 27-3. To date, there are no data on the phonetic inventory of children under 3 years of age.

Common mismatches

To date there is no study of common mismatches pro-duced by English children from England.

Syllable structure

Dodd (1995) reports on the phonological development of five English-speaking children from London. In terms of syllable structure, syllables of the phonotactic form V; CV; VC; and CVC were signaled by all five children in monosyllabic and disyllabic words by 20 months. Some residual syllable simplifications persisted for some of the children up to 25 months for similar syllable forms in polysyllabic words. Two-element consonant clusters in both syllable onsets and syllable codas (e.g., CCVC and CVCC forms) were incorporated into almost all

of the children's productive systems in almost all word forms (mono-, di-, and polysyllables) by between 22 and 30 months. Three-element consonant clusters had not reliably emerged in the speech production of any of the five children by 30 months.

Prosody

Crystal (1986, 1987) provides an overview of the develop-ment of English intonation in infants and young children from birth to 18 months, setting out age-related stages through which they pass in terms of their use and under-standing of English tones and pitch patterns. Although the emergence of a contrastive system of most tones appears to take place by approximately 18 months old, a number of intonation studies carried out in England suggest that the ability to comprehend and produce intonational structures in English continues to develop throughout childhood and early adolescence (Local, 1982; Cruttenden, 1985; Wells, Peppé, and Goulandris, 2004). Wells et al. (2004), for example, studied the production and comprehension of intonation by 120 English-speaking children from the southeast of England, divided into four age groups with mean ages of 5;6, 8;7, 10;10, and 13;9. They found that although children's abilities to produce appropriate intonation patterns have largely developed by the age of 5, their ability to comprehend more complex patterns is still emerging at ages 10 and 11. Furthermore, Wells et al. identified noteworthy interspeaker variability across all age groups. This finding is echoed in the literature on atypi-cal development of intonation in English children, where considerable intersubject differences in ability profiles have been identified both in production and compre-hension tasks (Wells and Peppé, 2003; Catterall, Howard, Stojanovik, Szczerbinski, and Wells, 2006).

Phonological awareness

Burt, Holm, and Dodd (1999) investigated phonological awareness using a range of tasks in 57 typically develop-ing preschool children (aged from 46 to 58 months) from the northeast of England. Although the children in their study showed awareness of the phonological units of syllable, onset, and rime, they generally still did not display awareness of individual phonemes. The authors conclude that phonological awareness for smaller units continues to develop with age into the school years. No differences in performance were shown between girls and boys, but a significant difference did emerge for social class, with those children from higher socioeconomic backgrounds performing better than those from relatively lower backgrounds. Nathan, Stackhouse, Goulandris, and Snowling (2004) also examined phonological awareness in typical English-speaking children, who acted as controls in a longitudinal study investigating links between phonological awareness and literacy in children with specific speech difficulties. Stackhouse et al., suggest that it is phoneme awareness (or a lack of it), rather than awareness of larger phonological units such as syllable or rime, that predicts later difficulties with literacy. Stackhouse, Wells, Pascoe, and Rees (2002) provide further evidence that performance on rime awareness tasks is not a clear predictor of later literacy development. Bird and Bishop (1992) and Bird, Bishop, and Freeman (1995), comparing English children with impaired speech with those with impaired speech and language, together with a group of age-matched typical controls, also identified clear differences in phonological awareness (including awareness of onsets, rimes, and phonemes) between the typical controls and the two groups with speech and language difficulties. On all tasks the latter groups performed significantly less well than the typical controls. It is, of course, important not to overlook individual interspeaker differences in interpreting results from large group studies of phonological awareness and metaphonological abilities (Hesketh, Adams, and Nightingale, 2000; Stackhouse and Wells, 1997).

Speech assessment for British English children

The following tests are all used by British speech-language pathologists in the assessment of children with impaired speech:

- *Children's Test of Nonword Repetition* (CN – REP; Gathercole and Baddeley, 1996)
- *Diagnostic Evaluation of Articulation and Phonology* (DEAP; Dodd, Hua, Crosbie, Holm, and Ozanne, 2003)
- *Edinburgh Articulation Test* (EAT; Anthony et al., 1971)
- *Phonological Abilities Test* (PAT; Muter, Hulme, and Snowling, 1997)
- *Phonological Assessment of Child Speech* (PACS; Grunwell, 1985)
- *Phonological Awareness Procedure* (PAP; Gorrie and Parkinson, 1995)
- *Profile of Phonology* (PROPH; Crystal, 1982)
- *Profile of Prosody* (PROP; Crystal, 1982)

- *Profiling Element of Prosodic Systems—Children* (PEPS-C; Wells and Peppé, 2001)
- *Psycholinguistic Framework for Speech and Literacy* (Stackhouse and Wells, 1997)
- *South Tyneside Assessment of Phonology* (STAP; Armstrong and Ainley, 1988)

The following specialist assessments are used by British speech-language pathologists to assess speech production for specific client groups or types of speech impairment:

- *GOS.SP.ASS* (Sell, Harding and Grunwell, 1994; Revised 1998) A speech assessment for children with cleft palate and/or velopharyngeal dysfunction
- *Nuffield Centre Dyspraxia Programme* (Nuffield Centre, 1985; Revised 2004)
- *Paediatric Oral Skills Package* (POSP; Brindley, Cave, Crane, Lees, and Moffat, 1996)
- *Phonological Evaluation and Transcription of Audio-Visual Language* (PETAL; Parker, 1999) Speech assessment for speakers with hearing impairment and/or low intelligibility

Speech intervention for British English children

Speech-language pathologists in England working with children with speech impairments practice in a variety of settings including community clinics, hospitals, schools and nurseries, and private practice (Glogowska, Roulstone, Enderby, and Peters, 2000; Law et al., 2002; Lindsay et al., 2002; Hartas, 2004). There is also a wide range of service delivery models, including hands-on one-to-one therapy and group therapy, parent-skilling and home programs, and a consultative approach working with and through other professionals such as teachers, teaching assistants, and speech-language pathology assistants (Miller, 1999; Wright and Kersner, 2004; Glogowska and Campbell, 2000; McCartney et al., 2005). Law et al. (2002) discuss the recent significant shift in the UK from direct hands-on work to a consultative model whereby therapy is delivered via teachers and assistants in schools or through parents. McCartney (2000, 2004) and Sadler (2005) note the new challenges that this presents and stress the need for studies evaluating the efficacy of speech and language therapy delivered in this way.

Speech-language pathologists use a range of approaches to intervention for developmental speech impairments, including those summarized below in Table 27-5. A number of recent studies in England have suggested that no single approach is likely to be appropriate for all children with developmental speech impairments (Dodd and Bradford, 2000; Hesketh, Adams, Nightingale, and Hall, 2000) and that intervention carefully tailored to the individual child is likely to be more effective (Pascoe, Stackhouse, and Wells, 2005). Speech-language pathologists are increasingly likely, therefore, to adopt different approaches for different children or a number of different approaches presented in sequence for an individual child.

Working in the UK

The majority of speech-language pathologists working in England (known in the UK as speech and language therapists) will have trained at one of the 15 UK universities that offer qualifications in speech and language therapy, although the UK workforce also includes speech-language pathologists from all over the world. Speech and language therapy programs in the UK comprise undergraduate degrees of either three or four years' duration, or postgraduate degrees at Diploma or Masters levels of one or two years' duration respectively (see the Resources section). All practicing speech-language pathologists working in the UK are also required to be state registered with the Health Professions Council (HPC), which regulates the profession of speech and language therapy, together with other professions allied to medicine.

The Royal College of Speech and Language Therapists provides a Web page containing a very useful summary of information for therapists from overseas who wish to work in the UK (http://www.rcslt.org/international.shtml).

In general, for a speech-language pathologist from overseas to work in the UK he or she needs to have a qualification recognized as comparable to a qualification obtained in the UK. Since January 2005, there has been a mutual recognition agreement between the Royal College of Speech and Language Therapists and equivalent organizations in the USA, Canada, and Australia (ASHA, CASPLA, and Speech Pathology Australia), which allows certified members of the latter organizations to become certified members of the RCSLT without obtaining HPC registration first. A therapist whose first language is not English will need to provide proof of a specific level of competence in spoken and written English. An overseas therapist applying for work in the UK from a country outside the European Union (EU) will need a work permit; usually the prospective employer applies for this on the therapist's behalf.

TABLE 27-5   Intervention approaches commonly used by English speech-language pathologists when working with children with speech impairment

Approach	Authors
Traditional articulation therapy	Dodd and Bradford, 2000; Hesketh, Adams, Nightingale, and Hall, 2000; Van Riper and Erickson, 1996
Minimal pairs therapy	Weiner, 1981
Core vocabulary	Dodd and Bradford, 2000
Metaphon and phonological awareness	Gillon, 2004; Hesketh et al., 2000; Howell and Dean, 1994
Cycles approach	Hodson and Paden, 1991
Maximal opposition therapy	Gierut, 1989
Psycholinguistic approaches	Pascoe, Stackhouse, and Wells, in press; Stackhouse and Wells, 1997; 2001
Instrumental approaches providing visual feedback, e.g., Electropalatography; IBM Speechviewer	Hardcastle and Gibbon, 1997; Ruscello, 1995

PHONETICALLY SPEAKING

Pronunciation of English: /ˈɪŋglɪʃ/
Passage: Comma Gets a Cure

Below is a broad phonemic transcription of *Comma Gets a Cure* (Honorof, McCollough, and Somerville, 2000) spoken by a typical adult speaker of RP (Southern Standard British English).

/ ˈwel / ˈhɪəz ə ˈstɔɹi fɔ ju / ˈsɛəɹə ˈpɛɹi wəz ə ˈvɛtɹɪ ˈnɜs hʊb bin ˈwɜkɪŋ ˈdeɪli ət ən ˈəʊl ˈzu ɪn ə dɪˈzɜtɪd ˈdɪstɹɪkt əv ðə ˈtɛɹətɹi / səʊ ʃɪ wəz ˈvɛɹi hæpi tə ˈstɑːt ə ˈnjuː dʒɒb ət ə suːˈpɜːb ˈpɹaɪvəp ˈpɹæktɪs ɪn ˈnɔːθ ˈskwɛə nɪə ðə ˈdjuːk stɹɪt ˈtaə / ˈðæt ˈɛəɹɪə wəz ˈmʌtʃ ˈnɪəɹə fɹə / əm ˈmɔː tʊ ə ˈlaɪkɪŋ / ˈiːvən ˈsəʊ ɒn ə ˈfɜːs ˈmɔːnɪŋ ʃɪ fɛlt ˈstɹɛst / ʃɪ ˈɛt ə ˈbəʊl əv ˈpɒɹɪdʒ / ˈtʃɛkt əsɛlf ɪn ðə ˈmɪɹə nə ˈtʃɒ ə ˈfeɪs ɪn ə ˈhʌɪ / ðɛn ʃɪ ˈpʊt ɒn ə ˈpleɪn ˈjɛləʊ ˈdɹɛs ənd ə ˈfliːs ˈdʒækɪt / ˈpɪkt ʌp ə ˈkɪt / ən ˈhɛdɪd fə ˈwɜːk / ˈwɛn ʃɪ ˈgɒt ˈðɛə ðə wəz ə ˈwʊmən wɪð ə ˈguːs ˈweɪtɪŋ fɹə / ðə ˈwʊmən geɪv ˈsɛəɹəs ən ˈɒfɪʃəl ˈlɛtə fɹəm ðə ˈvɛt / ðə ˈlɛtəɹ ɪmˈplaɪd ðət ðɪ ˈænɪməl ˈkʊb bi ˈsʌfɹɪŋ fɹəm ə ˈɹɛə ˈfɔːm əv ˈfʊt əm ˈmaʊθ dɪˈziːz / wɪtʃ wəz səˈpɹaɪzɪŋ bɪkəz ˈnɔːməli juːd ˈəʊnli ɪksˈpɛkt tə ˈsi ɪt ɪn ə ˈdɒg ɔːɹ ə ˈgəʊt / ˈsɛəɹə wəz sɛntɪˈmɛntl̩ səʊ ˈðɪs meɪd ə fil ˈsɒɹi fə ðə ˈbjuːtɪfəl ˈbɜːd /

Well, here's a story for you: Sarah Perry was a veterinary nurse who had been working daily at an old zoo in a deserted district of the territory, so she was very happy to start a new job at a superb private practice in North Square near the Duke Street Tower. That area was much nearer for her and more to her liking. Even so, on her first morning, she felt stressed. She ate a bowl of porridge, checked herself in the mirror and washed her face in a hurry. Then she put on a plain yellow dress and a fleece jacket, picked up her kit and headed for work. When she got there, there was a woman with a goose waiting for her. The woman gave Sarah an official letter from the vet. The letter implied that the animal could be suffering from a rare form of foot and mouth disease, which was surprising, because normally you would only expect to see it in a dog or a goat. Sarah was sentimental, so this made her feel sorry for the beautiful bird. (Honorof, McCullough, and Somerville, 2000).

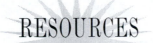

RESOURCES

Books

Foulkes, P., and Docherty, G. J. (Eds.; 1999). *Urban voices: Accent studies in the British Isles.* London: Arnold. This book provides detailed accounts of a wide range of accents associated with major cities in the UK.

Hughes, A., Trudgill, P., and Watt, D. (2005). *English accents and dialects* (4th ed.). London: Arnold. This book provides a wealth of information on social and regional varieties of English in the UK.

Roach, P., and Hartman, J. (Eds.). (1997). *English pronouncing dictionary (Daniel Jones;* 15th ed.). Cambridge,

UK: Cambridge University Press. This book provides a guide to British (RP) and U.S. word pronunciations, using the International Phonetic Alphabet.

CD-ROM

The CD accompanying Hughes et al. (2005; see above) provides a wealth of material on regional accent variation in British English.

Journals

- *The International Journal of Disorders of Communication* http://www.tandf.co.uk/journals/titles/13682822.asp An international research journal published by Taylor & Francis in conjunction with the Royal College of Speech and Language Therapists
- *Child Language Teaching and Therapy* http://www.arnoldpublishers.com/journals/pages/chi_lan/02656590.htm An international research journal published by Hodder Arnold
- *Clinical Linguistics and Phonetics* http://www.informaworld.com/smpp/title~content=t713693308 An international research journal published by Taylor & Francis in conjunction with the International Clinical Phonetics and Linguistics Association

Professional associations

The professional association of speech-language pathologists (called speech and language therapists) within the UK is the Royal College of Speech and Language Therapists, http://www.rcslt.org/ The profession of speech and language therapy is regulated by the Health Professions Council (HPC), http://www.hpc-uk.org

Universities offering courses in speech and language therapy

City University, London, http://www.city.ac.uk/

De Montfort University, Leicester, http://www.dmu.ac.uk/

Leeds Metropolitan University, http://www.lmu.ac.uk/

Manchester Metropolitan University, http://www.mmu.ac.uk/

Queen Margaret University College, Edinburgh, Scotland, http://www.qmuc.ac.uk /

University College London, http://www.ucl.ac.uk/

University of Central England in Birmingham, http://www.uce.ac.uk/

University of East Anglia, http://www.uea.ac.uk/

University of Exeter (College of St Mark and St John, Plymouth), http://www.marjon.ac.uk/

University of Manchester, http://www.manchester.ac.uk/

University of Newcastle upon Tyne, http://www.ncl.ac.uk/

University of Reading, http://www.reading.ac.uk/

University of Sheffield, http://www.sheffield.ac.uk/

University of Strathclyde (Glasgow, Scotland), http://www.strath.ac.uk/

University of Ulster (Belfast, Northern Ireland), http://www.ulster.ac.uk/

University of Wales Institute at Cardiff (Wales), http://www.uwic.ac.uk/

Useful English Web sites

The following Web sites provide a wealth of information (including audio recordings) on social and regional varieties of English:

- The Speech Accent Archive, http://accent.gmu.edu
- The Oxford English Dictionary, http://www.oed.com
- The British Sound Archive, http://www.bl.uk/collections/sound-archive/accents.html
- British Library – Collect Britain, http://www.collectbritain.co.uk/collections/dialects

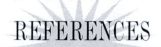

REFERENCES

Anthony, A., Bogle, D., Ingram, T. T., and McIsaac, M. W. (1971). *Edinburgh Articulation Test.* Edinburgh: Churchill Livingstone.

Armstrong, S., and Ainley, M. (1988). *South Tyneside Assessment of Phonology (STAP).* Ponteland: STASS Publications.

Bird, J., and Bishop, D. (1992). Perception and awareness of phonemes in phonologically impaired children. *European Journal of Disorders of Communication, 27*(4), 289–311.

Bird, J., Bishop, D., and Freeman, N. (1995). Phonological awareness and literacy development in children with expressive phonological impairments. *Journal of Speech and Hearing Research, 38,* 446–462.

Brindley, C., Cave, D., Crane, S., Lees, J., and Moffat, V. (1996). *The Paediatric Oral Skills Package (POSP).* London: Whurr.

Burt, L., Holm, A., and Dodd, B. (1999). Phonological awareness skills of 4-year-old British children: An assessment and development data. *International Journal of Language and Communication Disorders, 34*(3), 311–335.

Catterall, C., Howard, S., Stojanovik, V., Szczerbinski, M., and Wells, B. (2006). Investigating prosodic ability in Williams Syndrome, *Clinical Linguistics and Phonetics, 20* (7–8), 531–538.

Coggle, P. (1993). *Do you speak Estuary?* London: Bloomsbury.

Cruttenden, A. (1985). Intonation comprehension in 10-year-olds. *Journal of Child Language, 12,* 643–661.

Cruttenden, A. (1997). *Intonation* (2nd ed.). Cambridge, UK: Cambridge University Press.

Cruttenden, A. (2001). *Gimson's pronunciation of English* (6th ed.). London: Arnold.

Crystal, D. (1982). *Profiling linguistic disability.* London: Arnold.

Crystal, D. (1986). Prosodic development. In P. Fletcher and M. Garman (Eds.), *Language acquisition* (pp. 174–197), Cambridge, UK: Cambridge University Press.

Crystal, D. (1987). *Clinical linguistics* (2nd ed.). London: Edward Arnold.

Crystal, D. (1995). *The Cambridge encyclopaedia of the English language.* Cambridge, UK: Cambridge University Press.

Docherty, G. J., and Foulkes, P. (1999). Derby and Newcastle: Instrumental phonetics and variationist studies. In P. Foulkes and G. J. Docherty (Eds.), *Urban voices: Accent studies in the British Isles* (pp. 47–71). London: Arnold.

Dodd, B., and Bradford, A. (2000). A comparison of three therapy methods for children with different types of developmental phonological disorder. *International Journal of Language and Communication Disorders, 35*(2), 189–209.

Dodd, B. (1995) Children's acquisition of phonology. In B. Dodd (Ed.), *Differential diagnosis and treatment of speech disordered children* (pp. 21–48). London: Whurr.

Dodd, B., Holm, A., Hua, Z., and Crosbie, S. (2003). Phonological development: A normative study of British-speaking children. *Clinical Linguistics and Phonetics, 17*(8), 617–643.

Dodd, B., Hua, Z., Crosbie, S., Holm, A., and Ozanne, A. (2003). *Diagnostic Evaluation of Articulation and Phonology (DEAP).* London: Psychological Corporation.

Fletcher, J., Stirling, L., Mushin, I., and Wales, R. (2002). Intonational rises and dialog acts in the Australian English Map task. *Language and Speech, 45*(3), 229–253.

Foulkes, P., and Docherty, G. J. (2000). Another chapter in the story of /r/: 'Labiodental' variants in British English. *Journal of Sociolinguistics, 4*(1), 30–59.

Foulkes, P., and Docherty, G. J. (Eds.). (1999). *Urban voices: Accent studies in the British Isles.* London: Arnold.

Gathercole, S., and Baddeley, A. (1996). *Children's Test of Nonword Repetition (CN-REP).* London: Psychological Corporation.

Gierut, J. A. (1989). Differential learning of phonological oppositions. *Journal of Speech and Hearing Research, 33,* 540–549.

Gillon, G. (2004). *Phonological awareness—from research to practice.* New York: Guilford Press.

Glogowska, M., and Campbell, R. (2000). Investigating parental views of involvement in pre-school speech and language therapy. *International Journal of Language and Communication Disorders, 35*(3), 391–405.

Glogowska, M., Roulstone, S., Enderby, P., and Peters, T. (2000). Randomised controlled trial of community-based speech and language therapy in preschool children. *British Medical Journal, 321,* 923–926.

Gorrie, B., and Parkinson, E. (1995). *Phonological Awareness Procedure (PAP).* Ponteland: STASS Publications.

Grunwell, P. (1985). *PACS: Phonological assessment of child speech.* Windsor: NFER-Nelson.

Guy, G., Horvath, B., Vonwiller, J., Disley, E., and Rogers, I. (1986). An intonational change in progress in Australian English. *Language & Society, 15*(3), 23–52.

Hardcastle, W. J., and Gibbon, F. E. (1997). Electropalatography. In M. J. Ball and C. Code (Eds.). *Instrumental clinical phonetics.* London: Whurr.

Hartas, D. (2004). Teacher and speech-language therapist collaboration: Being equal and achieving a common goal. *Child Language Teaching and Therapy, 20*(1), 33–54.

Hesketh, A., Adams, C., and Nightingale, C. (2000). Metaphonological abilities of phonologically disordered children. *Educational Psychology, 20*(4), 483–498.

Hesketh, A., Adams, C., Nightingale, C., and Hall, R. (2000). Phonological awareness therapy and articulatory training approaches for children with phonological disorders: A comparative outcome study. *International Journal of Language and Communication Disorders, 35*(3), 337–354.

Higgs, J. A. W. (1968). The phonetic development of word initial /s/ plus stop clusters in a group of young children. *British Journal of Disorders of Communication, 3,* 130–138.

Hodson, B. W., and Paden, E. P. (1991). *Targeting intelligible speech: A phonological approach to remediation* (2nd ed.). Austin, TX: Pro-Ed.

Honorof, D. N., McCollough, J., and Somerville, B. (2000). *Comma gets a cure: A diagnostic passage for accent study.* New Haven, CT: Haskins Laboratories.

Howard, S. J., and Heselwood, B. C. (2002). The contribution of phonetics to the study of vowel development and disorders. In M. J. Ball and F. E. Gibbon (Eds.), *Vowel disorders* (pp. 37–82). New York: Butterworth-Heinemann.

Howell, J., and Dean, E. (1994). *Treating phonological disorders in children. Metaphon: theory to practice* (2nd ed.). London: Whurr.

Hughes, A., Trudgill, P., and Watt, D. (2005). *English accents and dialects* (4th ed.). London: Hodder Arnold.

Ladefoged, P. (1999). American English. In *The handbook of the International Phonetic Association* (pp. 41–44). Cambridge, UK: Cambridge University Press.

Law, J., Lindsay, G., Peacey, N., Gascoigne, M., Soloff, N., Radford, J., & Band, S. (2002). Consultation as a model for providing speech and language therapy in schools: A panacea or one step too far? *Child Language Teaching and Therapy, 18*(2), 145–163.

Lindsay, G., Soloff, N., Law, J., Band, S., Peacey, N., Gascoigne, M. & Radford, J. (2002). Speech and language therapy services to education in England and Wales. *International Journal of Language and Communication Disorders, 37*(3), 273–288.

Local, J. (1982). Modelling intonational variability in children's speech. In S. Romaine (Ed.), *Sociolinguistic variation in speech communities* (pp. 85–103). London: Edward Arnold.

Mathisen, A. G. (1999). Sandwell, West Midlands: Ambiguous perspectives on gender patterns and models of change. In P. Foulkes and G. J. Docherty (Eds.), *Urban voices: Accent studies in the British Isles* (pp. 107–123). London: Arnold.

McCartney, E. (2000). Include us out? Speech and language therapists' prioritization in mainstream schools. *Child Language Teaching and Therapy, 16*(2), 165–180.

McCartney, E. (2004). 'Hard health' and 'soft schools': Research designs to evaluate SLT work in schools. *Child Language Teaching and Therapy, 20*(2), 101–114.

McCartney, E., Boyle, J., Bannatyne, S., Jessiman, E., Campbell, C., Kelsey, C., Smith, J., McArthur, J. & O'Hare, A. (2005). 'Thinking for two': A case study of speech and language therapists working through assistants, *International Journal of Language and Communication Disorders, 40*(2), 221–235.

McGregor, R. L. (1980). The social distribution of an Australian English intonation contour. *Working Papers, 2*(6), 1–26. School of English and Linguistics, Macquarie University, Australia.

Miller, C. (1999). Teachers and speech and language therapists: A shared framework. *British Journal of Special Education, 26*(3), 141–146.

Muter, V., Hulme, C., and Snowling, M. (1997). *The Phonological Abilities Test (PAT)*. London: Psychological Corporation.

Nathan, L., Stackhouse, J., Goulandris, N., and Snowling, M. (2004). The development of early literacy skills among children with speech difficulties: A test of the 'Critical Age Hypothesis.' *Journal of Speech, Language, and Hearing Research, 47*(2), 377–391.

Nuffield Centre (2004). *The Nuffield centre dyspraxia programme.* London: Nuffield Centre Dyspraxia Programme Ltd (NDP).

Parker, A (1999). *Phonological Evaluation and Transcription of Audio-visual Language (PETAL)*. Bicester: Winslow Press.

Pascoe, M., Stackhouse, J., and Wells, B. (2006). *Children's speech and literacy difficulties 3: Persisting speech difficulties.* London: Wiley.

Pascoe, M., Stackhouse, J., and Wells, B. (2005). Phonological therapy within a psycholinguistic framework: Promoting changes in a child with persisting speech difficulties. *International Journal of Language and Communication Disorders, 40*(2), 189–220.

Pratt-Johnson, Y. (2005, July). *The growing use of Uptalk in the United States: Language trend or shift?* Paper presented at the Language and Global Communication Conference, Cardiff, UK.

Przedlacka, J. (2001). Estuary English and RP: Some recent findings. *Studia Anglica Posnaniensia, 36,* 35–50.

Roach, P., and Hartman, J. (1997). *Daniel Jones English pronouncing dictionary* (15th Ed.). Cambridge, UK: Cambridge University Press.

Rosewarne, D. (1984). Estuary English. *Times Educational Supplement, 19,* October 1984.

Ruscello, D. M. (1995). Visual feedback in treatment of residual phonological errors. *Journal of Communication Disorders, 28*(4), 279–302.

Sadler, J. (2005). Knowledge, attitudes, and beliefs of the mainstream teachers of children with a preschool diagnosis of speech/language impairment. *Child Language Teaching and Therapy, 21*(2), 147–163.

Sell, D., Harding, A., and Grunwell, P. (1999). Revised GOS. SP.ASS(98): Speech assessment for children with cleft palate and/or velopharyngeal dysfunction. *International Journal of Language and Communication Disorders, 34*(1), 7–33.

Stackhouse, J., and Wells, B. (1997). *Children's speech and literacy difficulties: A psycholinguistic framework.* London: Whurr

Stackhouse, J., and Wells, B. (2001). *Children's speech and literacy difficulties 2: Assessment and intervention.* London: Whurr

Stackhouse, J., Wells, B., Pascoe, M., and Rees, R. (2002). From phonological therapy to phonological awareness. *Seminars in Speech and Language, 23*(1), 27–42.

Stoddart, J., Upton, C., and Widdowson, J. D. A. (1999). Sheffield dialect in the 1990s: Revisiting the concept of NORMs. In P. Foulkes and G. J. Docherty (Eds.), *Urban voices: Accent studies in the British Isles* (pp. 72–89). London: Arnold.

Trudgill, P. (2002). *Sociolinguistic variation and change.* Edinburgh: Edinburgh University Press.

Van Riper, C., and Erickson, R. (1996). *Speech correction: An introduction to speech pathology and audiology* (9th ed.). Boston, MA: Allyn & Bacon.

Vance, M., Stackhouse, J., and Wells, B. (2005). Speech-production skills in children aged 3–7 years. *International Journal of Language and Communication Disorders, 40*(1), 29–48.

Weiner, F. (1981). Treatment of phonological disability using the method of meaningful minimal contrast: Two case studies. *Journal of Speech and Hearing Disorders, 46,* 96–103.

Wells, B., and Peppé, S. (2003). Intonation abilities of children with speech and language impairments. *Journal of Speech, Language, and Hearing Research, 46*(1), 5–20.

Wells, B., Peppé, S., and Goulandris, N., (2004). Intonation development from five to thirteen. *Journal of Child Language, 31*(4), 749–778.

Wells, J. C. (1982a). *Accents of English 1: An introduction.* Cambridge, UK: Cambridge University Press.

Wells, J. C. (1982b). *Accents of English 2: The British Isles.* Cambridge, UK: Cambridge University Press.

Wells, J. C. (1982c). *Accents of English 3: Beyond the British Isles.* Cambridge, UK: Cambridge University Press.

Wells, J. C. (1997). Whatever happened to Received Pronunciation? In C. Medina Casado and C. Soto Palomo (Eds.), *Il Jornadas de Estudio Ingleses* (pp. 19–28), Universidad de Jaén, Spain.

Wells, J. C. (1999). British English pronunciation preferences: A changing scene. *Journal of the International Phonetic Association, 29*(1), 33–50.

Wright, J., and Kersner, M. (2004). Short-term projects: The Standards Fund and collaboration between speech and language therapists and teachers. *Support for Learning, 19*(1), 19–23.

SUMMARY OF STUDIES OF TYPICAL ENGLISH SPEECH ACQUISITION

Authors	Year	Country	No. of children	Age of children	Information	Sample type	Data collection
Anthony, Bogle, Ingram, and McIsaac	1971	Scotland and England	510	3;0–6;0	Articulatory abilities for singleton consonants and consonant clusters	Single word	Cross-sectional
Burt, Holm, and Dodd	1999	NE England	57	46–58 mos	Phonological awareness	Single word	Cross-sectional
Dodd	1995	SE England	5	1;8–3;0	Age of acquisition of sounds; phonological processes	Single word and connected speech	Cross-sectional
Dodd, Holm, Hua, and Crosbie	2003	United Kingdom	684	3;0– 6;11	Age of acquisition of sounds (phonetic acquisition) and age error patterns were suppressed (phonemic acquisition)	Single word	Cross-sectional
Higgs	1968	Scotland	133	2;6–5;0	Consonant clusters (/s/ + stop)	Single word	Cross-sectional
Nathan, Stackhouse, Goulandris, and Snowling	2004	United Kingdom	47	4–7	Phonological awareness; speech perception and production; literacy skills	Single word	Longitudinal
Vance, Stackhouse, and Wells	2005	SE England	100	3;0–7;0	Speech production in real and non-words	Single word	Cross-sectional
Wells, Peppé, and Goulandris	2004	SE England	120	5;6–13;9	Intonation: comprehension and production	Connected speech	Cross-sectional

Chapter 28

Irish English Speech Acquisition

Joan Rahilly

INTRODUCTION

Like other varieties of English discussed in this collection, the term Irish English (IE) encompasses a range of dialects and accents characteristic of a specific geographical region, in this case the island of Ireland. One should note that the term Irish English itself has not been uncontroversial in the relevant literature, with alternative labels being Hiberno-English and Anglo-Irish (for a discussion of the terminological distinctions, see Rahilly, 1997). It is safe to assume equivalence among these three terms, but the choice of one or the other tends to reveal particular stances regarding the essential linguistic roots of English in Ireland, that is, whether influenced largely by the Irish language or by English. For instance, it is commonly suggested that English in Ireland demonstrates underlying influences from Irish, on various levels of structure (see Filppula, 1999; Ó Baoill, 1997), hence the appropriation of the terms *Irish-* or *Hiberno*-English. Anglo-Irish on the other hand, is the term of choice where English in Ireland is presented as a variant on British English. An Anglo-Irish orientation is common, for example, in intonation analysis, wherein authors typically apply models designed for Received Pronunciation (RP) to regional forms in Ireland (see, for instance, Cruttenden, 1995; McElholm, 1986). Recent and current accounts of the English language in Ireland use Irish English as a coverall term and that trend is followed here. In addition, this chapter also refers to Southern Irish English (SIE) and Northern Irish English (NIE) where these are a convenient means of capturing the two main varieties of IE.

Where Irish English is spoken

Irish English is spoken on the island of Ireland (see accompanying map and Appendix D). Recent censuses[1] indicate an approximate total of 5,602,470 inhabitants in Ireland, with 70 percent resident in the southern portion of the country. The map delineates the border between the northern and southern regions of Ireland. Northern Ireland consists of the province of Ulster and six counties, while Southern Ireland (also called the "Republic") consists of the three provinces of Connact, Leinster, and Munster, and a total of 26 counties.

The linguistic history of IE bears some resemblance to English as spoken in England, but it also differs in crucial respects. Most obviously, perhaps, the introduction of English to Ireland postdates that of English to Britain by approximately 100 years, arriving only in 1169 with the Anglo-Norman settlements. Also, English in Ireland shares with England, Scotland, and Wales the linguistic effects of the eighth- through eleventh-century Danish invasions, along with French influences from the eleventh- through fifteenth-century Norman rule, but it

exhibits distinctiveness because of its particular admixture of indigenous Irish and Latin alongside Scandinavian and French. (See Kallen, 1997, for a detailed history and discussion.)

Components of Irish English

Traditionally, phoneticians and speech-language pathologists (SLPs) have used RP as a convenient target variety in the analysis and transcription of IE speech. Giegerich (1992), for instance, states that SIE possesses "by and large the same vowel system as RP" (p. 82). There are indeed some basic similarities between the phonology of RP and that of IE, just as there are between RP and numerous varieties of English, but there are important differences that must be understood before embarking upon a clinical investigation. The need, moreover, to recognize the sociolinguistic factors that affect speech, for instance, is obviously relevant for SLPs working worldwide, but with specific reference to Northern Ireland, Gunn (1985, p. 22) emphasizes the necessity for "geo- and sociolinguistic attention before language attention begins." Consider the example of an

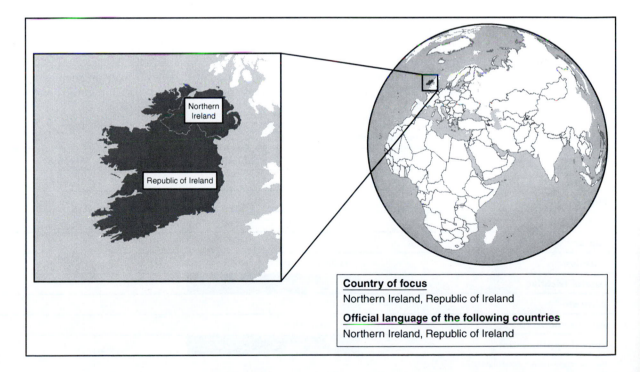

Country of focus
Northern Ireland, Republic of Ireland

Official language of the following countries
Northern Ireland, Republic of Ireland

---

1 This estimate is based on pooled figures from the separate Northern Irish and Southern Irish censuses (2001 and 2002, respectively).

SLP presented with a SIE speaker who produces [t̪] and [d̪] in place of /θ/ and /ð/, respectively. In the absence of sufficient knowledge of the ambient linguistic system in SIE, wherein dentalized alveolars are standard variants of the underlying dental fricatives, an SLP may be tempted to diagnose impairment where, in fact, none is present. Therefore, to assume that RP targets are sufficient for the IE clinical context would be a mistake. Such an assumption runs the risk of miscategorizing the output of a wide range of IE speakers. In addition to the consonantal situation, there are broad commonalities and differences between the vowels and diphthongs of IE and those of RP. Kallen (1997) refers to a "restructuring of vowel phonology" (p. 87) in IE, and Milroy (1981), referring to NIE, notes that "[I]n some respects, the phonetics of RP and other English speech is so radically different from Ulster that prior attention to RP may confuse students and make them feel that they cannot trust the evidence of their own ears" (p. 45). The rest of this chapter will offer guidance on both the phonemic and the allophonic aspects of consonants and vowels that characterize IE.

Consonants

IE has 25 consonants at its core, listed in Table 28-1, along with the voiced and voiceless labio-velar fricatives ([w] and [ʍ] in *witch* and *which* respectively). The possible realizational variation for each consonant phoneme is discussed later in this chapter. Various resources exist for listening to and gaining skill in recognizing and

transcribing these basic consonants, such as those provided by the *Sounds of the IPA* CD and the IPA's other online and interactive materials[2] (see Chapter 28). There is no audio material that sets out IE citation form consonants or vowels in the manner of the IPA CD, but readers are directed toward the IE samples that occur in the excellent CDs accompanying Hickey (2004b) and Kortmann and Schneider (2004).

Vowels and diphthongs

No single description of IE provides a detailed description of vowel variation in both NIE and SIE, although Wells's (1982) three-volume collection on a range of accents of English is a useful general starting point, as is Giegerich's (1992) account. For more comprehensive information, NI phonology is particularly well covered in a range of publications by James and Lesley Milroy, who generated groundbreaking sociolinguistic work in Ulster in the 1970s and 1980s. James Milroy's (1981) text on Belfast English, for instance, remains a core recommendation for undergraduate students in phonetics courses in NI, as does that by Harris (1985) on patterns of phonological variation and change in NIE. With reference to SIE, by far the most productive writer in the area is Raymond Hickey (see, for instance, Hickey, 1997, 2004a). One of Hickey's outstanding contributions to the field of IE is his recent (2004b) *A sound atlas of Irish English*, a collection of 1,500 DVD recordings representing all counties in Ireland. While the aim of the present

TABLE 28-1   Consonants produced in Irish English

	Bilabial	Labiodental	Dental	Alveolar
Plosive	p b			t d
Nasal	m			n
Trill				
Tap or flap				
Fricative	ʍ (labio velar)	f v	θ ð	s z
Lateral fricative	■	■		
Affricate				
Approximant	w (labio velar)			ɹ
Lateral approximant	■	■		l

Black = articulations judged impossible

Based on the International Phonetic Alphabet. Courtesy of the International Phonetic Association (c/o Department of Linguistics, University of Victoria, Victoria, British Columbia, Canada).

2 See http://www.arts.gla.ac.uk/IPA/

chapter is to highlight, for the sake of clinical convenience, stereotypical patterns in NIE and SIE, work has also been undertaken on a variety of rural and urban conurbations in Ireland (see, for instance, Kingsmore, 1995; McCafferty, 1996).

Accounts of vowel variation in Ireland tend to use RP as the reference dialect, with appropriate diacritics used, where necessary, to indicate variation. With some exceptions, the vowel system of RP more closely resembles that of SIE rather than NIE. SLPs should be aware, though, that both NIE and SIE contain examples of phonemic as well as allophonic divergence from RP, one example being mergers that characterize IE but are not present in RP. Neither NIE nor SIE shares RP's systemic distinction between /ɒ/ and /a/ or /ʀ/, for instance, so that *psalm* and *Sam* are realized as homophones [sam] in IE. This sort of phonemic neutralization can also occur optionally for target /a/ versus /ɛ/, in the environment of a following velar, as in *pack* and *peck*. Some northern varieties produce the two items as homophones, that is, either [pɛk] for both, or [pak] for both, the former being rarer but overtly more prestigious. Other phonemic distinctions in RP are often similarly dispensed with in IE: southern varieties routinely realize /ɔ/ and /ɒ/ as [ɒ], so that *cot* and *caught* are homophonous, and northern systems often collapse the /ɔ/ versus /ɒ/ distinction in *don* and *dawn*, realizing both as [ɔ]. NIE often exhibits a collapse of the RP contrast between /ɔ/ and /ɛə/ as in *burr* versus *bare*, realizing both as [bːɹ]. Furthermore, so-called Ulster Scots accents (those influenced by Scots; see Kingsmore, 1995)

often neutralize the /ɪ/ versus /ɛ/ distinction in *bit* and *bet*, realizing both as [bɛt].

The above examples illustrate where IE does not possess the same set of phonemic distinctions as RP, but the opposite situation is also the case; that is, there are vowel phonemes in IE that do not exist in RP. For instance, NIE distinguishes *days* from *daze* ([deɪz] and [deːz]/ [diːəz] respectively) while RP does not. In fact, it is axiomatic to suggest that, where the target /eɪ/ exists for RP, the NIE counterpart will be /e/ or /iə/ (*face,* for example, is [fes]/ [fiəs]). Where /iə/ occurs, the result is a set of mergers that often results in communicative problems for nonnative listeners, who have difficulty in selecting the appropriate item of the pair (reported in Millar, 1996). The pairs *meal/male, seal/sail* and *fail/feel*, for instance, are produced as homophones ([miəl, siəl, fiəl]. A comparable effect is produced, in Belfast English, when the vowel in *foot* and *feet* is fronted so that the singular and plural nouns merge to contain a slightly retracted /i/. Similarly, there are anecdotal reports of confusion among non-Belfast listeners' interpretations of *two* and *tea*, where the target phonemic distinction between /i/ and /u/ is collapsed, and the lexical items are frequently heard as homophonous (i.e. [ʉ]). A further collapse, this time in the context of the diphthongs /ai/ and /ɒʊ/, occurs in Belfast pronunciations of *high* and *how*, where both are produced as [hai], although speakers may circumvent the merger by rhoticizing *how* as [hɒːɹ] (see Harris, 1985; Millar, 1987).

With particular reference to Table 28-2 where American vowels are cited as targets, and for purposes

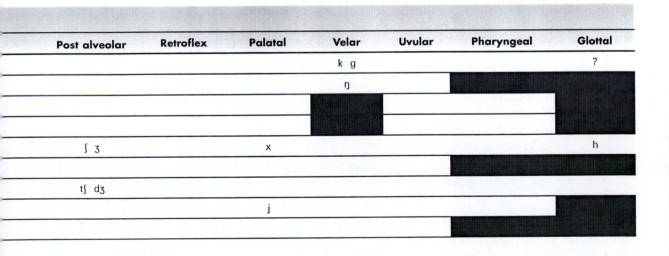

Post alveolar	Retroflex	Palatal	Velar	Uvular	Pharyngeal	Glottal
			k g			ʔ
			ŋ			
ʃ ʒ		x				h
tʃ dʒ						
		j				

TABLE 28-2 Vowels produced in Irish English compared to General American English

American English location	American English vowels (Smit, 2004)	American English examples	Northern Irish English vowels	Southern Irish English vowels	Irish English examples
High-front	i	beat	i	i	deed
	ɪ	bit	ɪ	ɪ	did
	e	raid	e/ɛ/ei/ɛi	ei/ɛi	day
Mid-low front	ɛ	bed	ɛ/eə	ɛ	bread, led
	ɒ	bad	a/ɑ	a/ɒ	and, psalm
High-back, rounded	u	blue	ʉ	u/ʊ/əu	doom, pool, fool
	ʊ	book	ʉ/ʊ/ʌ	ʊ/ʌ	pull, full
Mid-back, rounded	o	boat	o:/o ə	ɔʊ/oə/ʌʊ	goal
	ɔ	form	ɔ	ɔ/ɒ	tall
	ɑ		ɔ/ɑ	ɑ	cot, caught
Low back	ɔ/ɑ	drop	ɑ	ɑ	drop
[r]-colored			ɝ	—	hair
	ɚ	never color	ɚ	ɚ	letter
	ɪɹ		ɹ/ɜɹ/ʌɹ	ɪɹ	myrrh, spirit
	ɛɹ		ɛɹ/ɪɹ	ɛɹ/ɪɹ	hair
	ʊɹ		ʉə/ʉɹ	ʊɹ/ʉ	cure
	ɔɹ		ɔɹ/ɔɹ	ɔɹ/oɹ	hoard, support
	ɑɹ		ɒɹ	ɑɹ/ɒɹ	barn
			ʌɹ	ʌɹ	word, bird
Central	ə	about	ə	ə	about
		occur	ə	ə/o	occur
		upon	ə/ʌ	ə/	upon
			ʌ	ʌ	China
	ʌ		ʌ	ʌ	mud
Diphthongs	aɪ	my, bike	ai/ɛi	ʌi	my, bike
	aʊ	out, mouse	ɒʉ	ʌʊ	now, loud
	ɔɪ	boy	ɔi	ʌi	boy
	—		ei/e	ɛi	stay
	—		iə	iə	here, near
	—		iə/ɛi	ɛi	take, plate
	—		ɛə/ɜ:	ɛə/ɜ:	air, care
	—		ʉə	ʊə	tour, sure

Note. *V+ r-coloring is the norm for IE, but, unlike the American English r-colored vowels, IE vowels are likely to combine with [ɹ] and insert an intervening schwa, hence [ɛəɹ] for [ɛɹ], for instance.

of cross-comparison of varieties in this book, it is important to note that aspects of IPA vowel nomenclature differ from those used in American descriptions. So, the American "high" encompasses IPA "close" and "close-mid"; American "mid" also encompasses IPA open-mid. The American "mid-low" equates to "open-mid" in IPA terms, and American "mid-low" is the equivalent of IPA "open-mid." The vowels given here as targets for NIE and SIE are derived from a synthesis of published work and fieldwork, including the author's own, covering varying aspects of phonetic variation in both varieties (see, for example, Dolan, 2004; Hickey, 2003; Milroy, 1981; Wells, 1982). Apart from Wells's (1982) detailed list of the vowels that occur in standard lexical sets for "typical" Irish accents of English (p. 418), existing relevant work concentrates more narrowly on individual or small subsets of vowels.

Phonotactic restrictions

Syllables

Permissible syllable structures in IE parallel those in other varieties of English discussed in this book, that is, $C_{(0-3)}VC_{(0-4)}$. The smallest possible syllable is V (e.g., *a, oh*) and the longest legal syllable is CCCVCCCC (e.g., *strengths*). Unlike many other varieties, however, IE frequently abbreviates some structures and lengthens others, with both processes occurring in the vicinity of liquids. So, for example, the two-syllable structure of *collapse* (CV.CVCC) may be reduced to the single syllable [klaps], resulting in a complex onset and the overall structure CCVCC. The opposite case, in which syllable structures are expanded, may occur where /l/ exists as the second element in complex onsets. In the target CCVC structure for *clap* /klap/, for example, schwa may be inserted between the initial consonant and the lateral, hence [kəlap], producing an extra syllable. Of course, this syllabification of consonants is also common for word-final lateral plus nasal combinations in many varieties of English (where *film* is realized as [filɪm], for instance), but IE is additionally prone to syllabification in word-final /r/ plus nasal or /r/ plus lateral combinations. *Farm* and *farl*, therefore, may be realized as [fɒɹəm] and [fɒɹəl], respectively. Further examples of syllable addition exist for lexical items containing word-final "-*wn*," Whereas in RP the pronunciations of *shown* and *known*, for instance, are /ʃon/ and /non/, such items may be realized as [ʃowən] and [nowən] in IE. One might also note that -*ous* adjectival endings in IE are often realized as [iəs], producing two syllables rather than one, as in *mischievous* [mɪsɪtʃiviəs] and *heinous* [ɪhiniəs] for instance.

Consonants and consonant clusters

As examples so far have illustrated, both NIE and SIE typically pronounce orthographic "r" in all contexts as [ɹ], making IE a rhotic variety. Additionally, the alveolar plosives and dental fricatives are realized differently in SIE, with the so-called slit fricative being used for word-final and word-medial alveolar plosives ([θ] in *eight*; [ð] in *radiant*) and dentalized alveolars in word-initial position [t̪] in *time*. The presence of post-vocalic /ɹ/ in IE leads to a number of clusters that do not occur in nonrhotic accents (word-internal and word-final /ɹk/, /ɹt/, /ɹl/, /ɹm/, for instance) but, on the whole, the consonants and consonant clusters of IE are similar to those in RP. Nonetheless, SIE exhibits greater variability in this respect than does NIE. For example, SIE tends to alter consonant clusters involving target /θ/, with the result

that the dental fricative in *fifth, strength,* and *through* may be realized as a dental plosive, hence [fift, stɹɛnt̪, tɹʊt̪]. In NIE, it is possible for the voiced counterpart of the dental fricative, that is, /ð/, to be deleted entirely so that, for instance, [fɒː] is an acceptable realization of *father*. Also in NIE, a related deletion process occurs in target word-initial /θɹ/ contexts, although this process involves the deletion of the /ɹ/ rather than the fricative. As a result, *three* and *through* may be realized acceptably as [θi] and [θʉ]. Yet another process affecting the interdental fricative is its realization as a glottal fricative, so that, for instance, *everything* becomes [ɛvɹəhən].

IE contains word-initial consonant clusters that include the palatal approximant /j/ in, for example, *beautiful* and *music*. Exceptions are the SIE production of /hj/ in *humor* and *human*, where the initial CC may be reduced to C, that is, [jʊməɹ, jʊmən] (occasionally [hʊməɹ] and [hʊmən]). Along similar lines, SIE often deletes the palatal in word-initial /nj/ targets, with *new* and *Newry* occurring as [nʊ] and [nʊɹi]. Nonpronunciation of /j/ is also common for SIE in word-internal positions, as in adjectives ending in "-ulous," "-ular," "-urate," and "-ulate" such as *fabulous* [ˈfabələs] *spectacular* [spɛkˈtakələɹ], *accurate* [ˈakəɹət], and *immaculate* [iˈmakələt]. Conversely, /j/ insertion is common following /l/ in *column*. While the tendency of SIE toward deletion of palatal consonants follows that noted by Cruttenden (2001) for all varieties of English, NIE sometimes exhibits /j/ insertion following velar plosives where a low vowel follows ([kjan] for *can* and [gjandəɹ] for *gander*). IE also contains some examples of metathesis, that is, the reversal of segment order in "-ern" nouns and adjectives where, when the "-ern" is unstressed, the VCC order is altered to VCV, with *modern* being realized as [mɒdɹən] and *lantern* as [lantɹən]. Finally, one might encounter occasional examples of schwa deletion following /ɹ/ in vernacular varieties of northern Irish, as in [ɔɹndʒfild] for *Orangefield* and [fɔɹn] for *foreign*.

Tones

IE does not use tones to differentiate meaning.

Stress and intonation

Unusual stress patterns in IE are sometimes noticeable in both individual words and longer utterance patterns. With regard to individual words, O'Sé (1985) draws attention to some trisyllabic words in which there is a "delayed placement of stress [where] stress falls not on the initial or root position of the word, but on a subsequent suffix" (p. 98).

Examples of delayed stress placement occur in the case of verbal suffixes (*educate* [ɛdʒʊɪkeit] *advertise* [advəɹtɹaiz], *prosecute* [pɹɒsəkɪjʊt], and *justify* [dʒʌstɪfɹai]), the adverbial suffix *–arily* (*primarily* [pɹaimɹeɹɪli]), and before some medial clusters in polysyllabic nouns (*architecture* [ɒɹkəɪtɛktʃəɹ], *industry* [ɪnɹdʌstɹi], *discipline* [dɪɪsɪplɪn]). In terms of utterance-level stress patterns, many NIE utterances are altered by distinctive grammatical patterns added to the end of an utterance. They act as topic focusers (…*so I am*, …*so he was*) and take the form of unprominent syllables following the major accented syllable, as in *You'll need to be here at 8 o'CLOCK, so you will*.

Studies of intonation in IE have concentrated on NIE, focusing on the frequency and perceptual salience of rising tones followed by level stretches where RP would tend to have falling patterns (see, for instance, Cruttenden, 1997; Rahilly, 1997). There has been less published work on SIE intonation, but notable exceptions are the studies of stress and nuclear prominence among Dublin children (O'Halpin, 1994), which show that terminal falling patterns are the norm for neutral sentences. For Cork, Hickey (2004b) suggests that the intonation is particularly unusual, largely with regard to its predominance of sentence-final falling-rising contours. Most approaches to intonation in IE have presupposed the tone unit model (Crystal, 1969; Halliday, 1970) to be appropriate, but there is evidence that the phonetic criteria used to define tone units in the past may not be applicable in IE. Traditionally, for instance, the term "nucleus" refers rigidly to a single peak of prominence within a relevant stretch of speech. The fact that Belfast English, for example, often contains such stretches in which two or more syllables are equally prominent, means that it is misleading to refer to these syllables as "nuclei."

Writing system

The IE writing system is identical to that of British English, including the use of "ou" rather than "o" for *colour* and *behaviour* and "ise" rather than "ize" in *memorise*. One may occasionally encounter snippets of older Irish language text incorporated into English, in which a superscript dot appears in combination with certain consonants. This dot is known as the 'séimhiú' [ɪʃeivu] or softening mark, and its purpose was to indicate lenition of the relevant consonant, hence "c" ([k]) versus "ċ" ([x]), where the change is conditioned by grammatical criteria. The séimhiú was replaced in the 1940s by "h" following the consonant to which it relates (so, the earlier "ċ" becomes "ch").

3 Gaeltacht areas are those in which Irish is the primary language.

Varieties of Irish English

As indicated above, the main division in IE is between northern and southern varieties. Most IE speakers have learned English as a first language, although significant numbers in rural and Gaeltacht areas have learned it as a second language, with Irish as the first. Most IE speakers have no contact with Irish on a day-to-day basis and, while numbers differ depending on whether the north or south is in question, large numbers of people have little or no familiarity with Irish at all. It is difficult to be exact concerning the numbers of speakers whose first language is Irish, given that the latest available census figures for the Republic of Ireland merely probe whether respondents have a knowledge of Irish, rather than the extent of the knowledge. Nonetheless, certain inferences are possible. For example, out of a total population of 86,517 living in the Gaeltacht areas of the Republic, a total of 72.6 percent across all age groups have a knowledge of Irish. Since the ability to use the language among that group is given as 50.6 percent for 3- to 4-year-olds and 87.4 percent for 10 to 14 year olds, one can assume the latter group includes second language Irish learners and the former constitutes first language Irish, or bilingual speakers. The figures are different again for the Republic's urban and rural non-Gaeltacht contexts. In urban contexts, those who have an ability to speak Irish account for just under 40 percent of the total population, while those in rural areas who can speak Irish account for just over 45 percent (CSO, 2002). For NI, the latest census states that 89 percent of the population have no knowledge of Irish (NISRA, 2001), although continued growth in the sector of Irish medium schools in NI is likely to have some impact on this figure.

Attitudes to language variation in Ireland are traditionally colored by political and religious sensitivities, to the extent that certain linguistic variants are sometimes thought to be unambiguous indicators of religion (see, for instance, Kingsmore, 1995; Zwickl, 2002). Increasingly, though, this idea is being interrogated by many rigorous linguistic investigations and, while linguistic accounts continue to acknowledge the important relationship between language and religion in Ireland, it is no longer the overriding focus of research attention.

The border between north and south (see map, above) separates the stereotypically Nationalist and Catholic population of the south from the stereotypically Loyalist and Protestant northerners, although one should expect considerable degrees of crossover of both political and religious affiliation between northern and southern territories. Given the historically stronger influence of Catholicism and the Irish language in the south,[4] strong associations tend to exist between southern speech features and Catholicism and, in turn, between those speech features and the Irish language. One common example of this is the so-called slit-t phenomenon, otherwise known as /t/ lenition, common in SIE (see Pandeli, Eska, Ball, and Rahilly, 1997, who recommend the transcription [θ̱]). It occurs intervocalically as in *butter*, word-finally as in *but*, but not if immediately preceded or followed by another consonant, so it is impossible in *fact*. Of course, there are further divisions and, in the north of Ireland, for instance, "Mid-Ulster English" and "Ulster-Scots" (see Hickey, 2004a, for definitions) exist within the more general category of NIE. In the south, the linguistically relevant divisions are between the east coast and the west and southwest regions. As Hickey (2004b) points out, additional "dialectally indeterminate" (p. 24) regions also exist wherein the speech displays "a mixture of southern and northern features" (p. 24), particularly in the midlands, and along the connecting line from Sligo to Dundalk

Other salient characteristics of SIE, compared with NIE, are as follows:

- [t̪] for /θ/ (e.g., *heal*thy, *T*homas)
- [d̪] for /ð/ (e.g., *smooth*)
- [ʊ] for /ʌ/ (e.g., *m*uch, *c*up)
- [ɔɪ] for /aɪ/ (e.g., *del*ighted, *Fri*day)
- [a] for /ɒ/ (e.g., *honour*, *l*ots)

The salient characteristics of NIE are as follows, compared to RP targets:

- [ʉ] for /u/ (e.g., *y*ou)
- [e] or [iə] for /eɪ/ (e.g., *t*ake)
- [ɔʉ]/[ɒʉ] for /aʊ/ (e.g., *p*ound)
- [ɔ] for /ɑ/ (e.g., *p*alm)

Both NIE and SIE exhibit phonological variation along sociolinguistic lines, and readers are directed to relatively recent work in the area: McCafferty (1996) and Kingsmore (1995) for NIE and Hickey (2004a) and Kallen (1997) for SIE. In rural contexts, following more

universal sociolinguistic norms, accent differences tend to d enote regional distinctions whereas those in urban settings are usually considered to be socially relevant.

An interesting thread among studies of IE is how its speakers rate their own accents and their effects in comparison with RP, and how these assessments might influence the speakers' own habits. Milroy and McClenaghan's (1977) study of attitudes to four accents found in Ulster offers a typical interpretation of listener response patterns. On the basis of four accents, one Scottish, one Southern Irish, one RP, and one native Ulster, listeners judged RP to be "the ideal accent" (p. 5), while the Southern Irish speaker was rated as being "untrustworthy, unfriendly and ungenerous." The authors suggest that these findings are "perfectly explicable within the context of Ulster's political and cultural background." There is some evidence that perceptual standards in Ireland are changing, but it exists only for the Republic. For instance, the University of Otago's *English Accents Worldwide* project has demonstrated that, among a group of 58 third-level students in Dublin university, the lowest overall ratings were given to Southern British English females in terms of, for instance, perceived educational achievement and intelligence. Hickey (1999, p. 265) similarly states that "[f]or the southern Irish, Received Pronunciation is an extra-national norm not aspired to."

For NI, the significance of RP as a perceptually ideal form and a productive standard to which some speakers aspire derives from Milroy's (1981) investigation of Belfast English. He notes that a range of NI speakers choose to use RP in formal circumstances, or claim to use it, in spite of what Milroy says is evidence to the contrary. Whether such speakers do or do not use RP when they say they do, and irrespective of the accuracy of their production, the important factor is that RP may remain a prestigious form of English to many NI speakers. Neither is it too outlandish to suggest that NI audiences appear to adopt a wholly uncritical approach to RP, believing it to be an unimpeachable superior variety in any context. Indeed, such state of affairs seems to underlie Millar's (1987) finding that, among her informants, RP forms are "*conventionally* prestigious" (p. 59) [my italics], whether they are contextually appropriate or not.

---

4 The latest Census for Northern Ireland (NISRA, 2001) identifies just over 40 percent of the NI population as Catholic while the 2002 Census for the south (CSO, 2002) identifies just over 88 percent of the total SI population as Catholic. In relation to Irish language statistics, almost 89 percent of northerners claimed no knowledge of Irish. In the south of Ireland, the last census, out of a total of 3,917, 203, probed only whether respondents were Irish speakers or non-Irish speakers, without further investigation of particular ability in reading or writing.

Typical acquisition of Irish English

No systematic published work exists on the typical acquisition of IE, whether for northern or southern varieties. Greater research attention has been paid to the acquisition of Irish and has focused on lexical development (see, for example, Harrington, 2000). The information presented here on IE is gathered from a variety of sources that refer either to acquisition targets thought to be relevant for IE, or to more specific but isolated phonological characteristics of child language in IE (Hickey, 1997; Ní Cholmáin, 2002). The main assumption underlying relevant work is that IE follows the usual developmental patterns of other varieties of English around the world (see McLeod, 2002), with due recognition given to allophonic variants. As a result, SLPs who wish to compare the speech output of their patients with appropriate developmental norms rely on targets established for British English children, after Grunwell (1985; 1987) (also see Howard, 2006). Nonetheless, two IE-specific studies are worthy of mention here, Hickey's (1997) account of phonological development in Dublin children and Ní Cholmáin's (2002) inclusion of normative targets against which the children with Down Syndrome in her study are assessed.

Acquired sounds

Consonants

Hickey's (1997) and Ní Cholmáin's (2002) contributions to consonantal acquisition targets in IE are immensely useful, since they provide at least some information that is specific to the IE context. Nonetheless, their findings should be treated with some caution in general IE clinical settings. First, both refer to SIE, rather than NIE. Second, Hickey's account is compelling but not clinically oriented and it is based on the speech of only three children; a subject base which makes no claim to be representative of the larger population, however standard the variants seem to be. Neither is Hickey's study acquisition based in the usual sense of that term. He notes, for instance, that a distinction between /w/ and /ʌ/ emerges between the ages of 5;6 and 7;9, but not when /w/ is first acquired, or when one could expect the contrast to be well established. He is concerned with the speech in a single family of three children, aged 2;10, 5;6, and 7;9, "all of whom were emerging native speakers of Irish English" (p. 171). As particularly characteristic speech features of SIE, he considers fricativization of alveolar stops, fortition of dental fricatives, syllable final /r/, and opposition of [ʌ] versus [w]. He also notes that SIE makes a phonemic distinction between [t] and [t̪], as in *tong* versus *thong*, for

instance, but that dental stops in general are acquired late among Irish English children; only the 7;9 year old child had acquired it. With regard to dental fricative, he observes "there was not a single occurrence of /θ/ or /ð/ in the speech of any of the children" (p. 176). Apart from these features, he judges his participants speech development to follow patterns similar to British English children.

Ní Cholmáin's (2002) stated developmental levels for phoneme acquisition are "based on" (p. 138) a range of sources, but it is not clear whether her targets represent an amalgam of already published findings, or whether they have been modified to incorporate her own experience of typically developing IE children. Additionally, her useful summary table of consonant acquisition captures the stages "for *emergence*" [my italics] of consonants, rather than information on emergence versus well-established use of the phonemes in question. This focus on emergence contrasts with the developmental targets cited by Grunwell (1985; 1987), whose Developmental Assessment charts indicate the stages at which the consonant might be expected to appear, as well as the stages at which it would be expected to be stabilized. The distinction is crucial in the clinical context, especially when one notes that Ní Cholmáin's targets for emergence are often considerably earlier than those suggested by Grunwell. An extreme example is /ŋ/, which, according to Grunwell, begins to emerge during the phase from 2;0 to 2;5 years, becoming well established between 2;6 and 3;0 years. According to Ní Cholmáin, however, /ŋ/ is already present among IE children of 1;0. The compromise solution may be to interpret Ní Cholmáin's findings as an indication of children's ability in paradigmatic rather than syntagmatic production, that is, as a measure of what the children can physiologically accomplish rather than implement regularly as part of their phonological system. Details of the stated ages of acquisition in the relevant studies are given in Table 28–3.

Consonant clusters

To date, there is no study of the age of acquisition of consonant clusters in IE, although one should expect different trends that are broadly similar to those suggested by Grunwell (1985; 1987). For example, where Grunwell suggests that reductions involving initial obstruents plus approximants cease between 2;6 and 3;0 years, similar patterns exist for IE children, albeit with allophonic differences for SIE and NIE. While British English and NIE children, therefore, will begin to use the dental fricative /θ/ followed by /ɹ/, SIE acquisition of this cluster will tend to take the form of [t̪ɹ] or, simply, [tɹ].

TABLE 28-3 Consonantal acquisition targets in Irish English

Consonant	Grunwell (1985; 1987)	Ní Cholmáin (2002)	Hickey (1997)
p	1;6–2;0	1 year	–
b	1;6–2;0	1 year	–
m	1;6–2;0	1 year	–
n	1;6–2;0	1 year	–
ŋ	established between 2;6 and 3;0, although begins to emerge during 2;0–2;6	1 year	–
h	established between 2;6 and 3;0, although begins to emerge during 2;0–2;6	1 year	–
w*	1;6–2;0	1 year	/w/ versus /ʍ/ distinction emerges between 5;6 and 7;9
j	2;6–3;0	1 year	–
t		1 year	Distinction between alveolar and dental stops emerges at about 7;9 years; fricativization of /t/ and /d/ occurs "quite early" (p. 178), although not following same rules as for adults; in post-sonorant word-final position, "the voice/voiceless distinction never develops in this position" (p. 186) so, *hand* and *Raymond* are realized as [hʀnt] [ɹeːmɪnt]
d	1;6–2;0		Distinction between alveolar and dental stops emerges at about 7;9 years
k	2;6–3;0	2 years	–
g	established during 2;6–3;0, although begins to emerge between 2;0 and 2;6	2 years	–
f	2;6–3;0	2 years	–
l	established during 3;0–3;6, although begins to emerge between 2;6 and 3;0	3 years	–
ʒ	emerging in 4;6	3 years	Lip-rounded versions of /ʒ/ emerge between 5;6 and 7;9
ʃ	established during 3;6–4;6 although begins to emerge between 3;0 and 3;6	3 years	Lip-rounded versions of /ʃ/ emerge between 5;6 and 7;9
tʃ	established during 3;6–4.0, but begins to emerge during 3;0–3;6	2 years	–
dʒ	3;6–4;6	–	–
s	2;6–3;0	3 years	–
z	3;6–4;0	3 years	–

* According to Ní Cholmáin, the voiceless equivalent /ʍ/ does not exist in the target language.

Table 28-3 continued

Consonant	Grunwell (1985; 1987)	Ní Cholmáin (2002)	Hickey (1997)
ɹ	Established by 4;6, but begins to emerge during 3;6–4;0	3 years	–
v	3;6–4;6	2 years	–
ð	4;6	Notes that /θ/ occurs in restricted contexts only	No occurrences (Hickey, 1997)
θ		Notes that /ð/ occurs in restricted contexts only	No occurrences (Hickey, 1997)

- = the target consonant was not considered by the investigator

Vowels and diphthongs

In common with other varieties of English, work on IE vowel acquisition is scant. Given earlier comments in this chapter relating to IE vowel systems, SLPs should exercise caution in establishing a client's contrastive system. A child in the west of Ireland, for instance, may dispense with the /ɛ/ versus /ɪ/ contrast that distinguishes *lent* from *lint*, realizing both as [lɪnt].

Percent correct

Consonants

For her group of typically developing children, Ní Cholmáin (2002) reports PCC scores ranging from 73 to 100, with a mean of 95 and SD of 6.95.

Consonant clusters

There is no published work on IE that addresses specifically the issue of correct consonant cluster realization. While Ní Cholmáin (2002) states that cluster reduction is one of the processes that is present in her subject group, her final figures collapse cluster reduction with a range of other structural processes[5] to yield overall percentage correct figures.

Vowels

With particular reference to vowels, Hickey (1997) comments that children who are otherwise acquiring standard SIE may show "certain features of colloquial Dublin due to [their] contacts in school and with [their] peers in the neighbourhood in which they live" (p. 172). In a family of three children, the eldest, aged 7;9, showed fronting of /aʊ/ to [ɛʊ] as in *pound* and disyllabification of long vowels as in [mi:jən] for *mean*. This feature was not present in the younger children studied, aged 5;6 and 2;10.

Phonological processes

Phonological process strength, that is, the extent to which processes persist in child language, is reported by Ní Cholmáin (2002) to be relatively low for her control group of children. Hickey (1997) suggests that two main processes characterize IE children's speech, metathesis, and epenthesis, as in [mɒdɹən] *modern* and [fɪlɪm] *film*, respectively. He also notes one process that is a feature of acquisition for all children but persists into adulthood for many IE speakers, namely the lack of the voiced/voiceless distinction in post-sonorant word-final position; hence [hʀnt] and [ɹeːmɪnt] for *hand* and *Raymond*.

Intelligibility

Ní Cholmáin (2002) notes a significant relationship between intelligibility and PCC, for both children with Down Syndrome and a control group, with the Down Syndrome children showing lower scores and greater patterns of variability. She also notes a significant relationship between process strength and intelligibility, with the effect that low numbers of processes enhance intelligibility.

5 The full range of Ní Cholmáin's (2002) structural processes is unstressed/weak syllable division; reduction to monosyllables; reduplication; final-consonant deletion; initial-consonant deletion; cluster deletion; cluster reduction; epenthesis; reduction of unstressed syllable; replacement of unstressed syllable; reordering of segments.

Phonetic inventory

To date, there is no study of the phonetic inventory of consonants or vowels produced by children who speak IE. Nonetheless, some of Hickey's (1997) findings are useful in this area.

Common mismatches

To date, there is no study of mismatches produced by children speaking IE.

Syllable structure

Apart from Ní Cholmáin's consideration of syllable structure processes within the general category of structural processes, there is no published work to date on this area of IE acquisition.

Prosody

To date, the majority of work on prosodic organization has been undertaken among deaf children in Dublin, focusing on the inappropriate use of contrastive stress (O'Halpin, 1992) and pitch characteristics (see O'Halpin, 1994; 2001, respectively).

Phonological awareness

Given the caveats mentioned above in terms of the small number of participants investigated and, consequently, the degree to which one might generalize from the findings, Hickey's (1997) study nonetheless speculates usefully on children's awareness of phoneme categories in the acquisition of SIE. He notes, for instance, that the children concerned "simply learn" (p. 185) certain processes such as the metathesis and epenthesis. He also suggests that, as children acquire writing skills, "they will realize" (p. 185) that [mɒdəɹn] and [fɪlm] exist as pronunciations outside Ireland but that, until then, the children are "not necessarily aware" (p. 186) of the processes. Of course, this suggestion fits with broader ideas of language acquisition as the result of a "linguistic genotype" (Lightfoot, 1999, p. 52) combined with the effects of expanding linguistic stimuli, but it is important to note how the occasional peculiarities of the SIE system occasionally might cut across developmental norms. On the one hand, for instance, SIE-speaking children need to be aware, not just of the usual English /θ/ versus /t/ difference that distinguishes *true* from *through*. In addition, they also need to recognize and use what to many other varieties of English would be merely an allophonic distinction,

namely that between alveolar and dental stops. Hickey states that this distinction does not begin to emerge until after 7 years of age and, even then, not fully; the eldest child of his study consistently realizes both *pat* and *path* as [paːt]. That SIE children experience confusion in this area is illustrated also by the case of fricativization of alveolar stops. Hickey suggests that his 5;6-year-old child presumes /t/ to be the underlying phoneme category from which both /θ/ and /t/ derive in *worth it*. Along similar lines, de Montfort Supple (1992) relates the case of a 12-year-old boy from the west of Ireland who consistently produced [ʃ] for target /s/. While the articulation error was corrected in speech therapy, the fact that the child's ambient accent typically inserts [ʃ] for /s/ ([ʌɪʃəl] for *whistle*, for instance) meant that he continued to use the superficially nonstandard variant. Where IE children are concerned, therefore, and particularly in relation to those aspects of the phonemic system that are known to be IE-specific, SLPs should allow some flexibility in identifying awareness targets.

Speech assessment for children who speak Irish English

Little published work has emerged from clinical encounters with speech and language in Ireland, a situation partly due to heavy caseloads in pressurized clinical contexts (see NICCY, 2004/2005) and also to a traditional and natural emphasis on practice rather than research. IASLT (1993) has indicated, for instance, that "[t]he research role of the speech and language therapist is underdeveloped" (p. 14). The situation is changing, albeit slowly, with the relevant universities encouraging students and those employed in academic positions in speech-language pathology to engage in research and to publish findings.[6] Existing published work has tended to focus not on phonetic or phonological variables but on voice (see, for example, Leahy, 1989), general issues surrounding speech-language pathology (Leahy, 1989), perceptual development (Titterington, Henry, and Toner, 2001), and non-Irish specific communication tools (McCurtin and Murray, 2000).

Following international trends in speech-language pathology that recognize the effects of rapid linguistic change and broadening linguistic influences on presumed normative targets within a given language, SLPs working with IE typically assess developmental progress against the sociolinguistic background of the client. The work published to date draws on information gathered on

---

6 See http://www.rcslt.org/pdfs/ApproachingResearch-researchbooklet.pdf.

children's phonemic and phonetic inventories, phonological processes and strength of processes, consistency of speech behavior, and phonotactic constraints. The child's system is then viewed in the light of overall developmental characteristics, that is, linguistic as well as social, cognitive, and emotional, and the child's communicative needs are then established. The particular speech assessment tools used by SLPs in Ireland are similar to those in use in other countries, as follows:

- *Assessment of Phonological Patterns (HAPP-3)* (Hodson, 2004)
- *Clinical Assessment of Articulation and Phonology (CAAP)* (Secord and Donohue, 2002)
- *Diagnostic Evaluation of Articulation and Phonology (DEAP)* (Dodd, Hua, Crosbie, Holm, and Ozanne, 2003)
- *Edinburgh Articulation Test (EAT)* (Anthony et al., 1971)
- *PACS Toys* (Grunwell, 1995)
- *Phonological Assessment of Child Speech (PACS)* (Grunwell, 1985)
- *Preschool and Primary Inventory of Phonological Awareness* (Dodd, Crosbie, McIntosh, Teitzel, and Ozanne, 2000).
- *South Tyneside Assessment of Phonology (STAP)* (Armstrong and Ainley, 1988)
- *Test of Auditory Analysis Skills (TAAS)* (Rosner, 1979)
- *The Assessment of Phonological Processes (APP-R)* (Hodson, 1986)

Speech intervention for children who speak Irish English

NICCY (2004/2005) identified 333 practicing SLPs working in NI, approximately 197 of whom work within the 14 Health Care Trusts in the province. The settings in which SLPs work, both in Northern Ireland and the Republic, include mainstream school learning support centers, dedicated centers for speech-language pathology, community clinics, special schools, and Partial Hearing Units. The models for speech-language pathology consist of individual and group speech-language pathology, direct and indirect speech-language pathology, parental training, multidisciplinary assessment, home and school programs, and advisory and outreach. Pooled figures for the distribution of settings and modes of speech-language pathology are not available. The Association of Speech and Language

Therapists in Independent Practice[7] lists eight members in private practice in Northern Ireland. Specific information concerning numbers of SLPs in the Republic of Ireland is not available to the public domain.

The speech intervention techniques that are used for Irish English include traditional articulation therapy, listening therapy, electropalatography, and a variety of visual aids training.

Worthy of particular note in the Republic of Ireland is the use of the *Mayo Early Language Screening Task* (MELST), developed in 1990 as a screening procedure for children presenting in Mayo in the west of Ireland (see Dowd et al., 1992). While the test provides more comprehensive information than other protocols on children's motor skills, as well as background development and history, the linguistic aspects of the child's behavior are assessed using existing tools. McGinty (2000) has noted that MESLT enables a sensitive measure of phonological problems, although it tended to lead to overreferral.

Working in Ireland

All SLPs working in Ireland are required to be accredited members of either the Irish Association of Speech and Language Therapists (IASLT), for employment in the Republic, or the Royal College of Speech and Language Therapists (RCSLT), the latter being the UK-validated professional organization for SLPs in Northern Ireland. The norm for intending practitioners is to complete a four-year clinical degree at one of the relevant universities in Ireland (see the Resources section), or to complete a nonclinical degree, usually in a cognate discipline such as linguistics and phonetics, followed by a one- to two-year postgraduate clinical qualification. For those who wish to work within Ireland but have attained qualifications outside the Irish and UK systems, both IASLT and RCSLT offer a system for examining and validating relevant qualifications. Non-Europeans are required to be in possession of a Work Visa, or Working Holiday Visa, with the latter being valid usually for a period of up to two years. With regard to relevant journals, the School of Clinical Speech and Language Studies in Trinity College, Dublin, in collaboration with the Irish Association of Speech and Language Therapists, publishes the *Journal of Clinical Speech and Language Studies.*

---

7 See http://www.helpwithtalking.com/main.asp.

PHONETICALLY SPEAKING

Pronunciation of Irish English: /ˈaiɹɪʃ ˈɪŋlɪʃ/
Passage: The Rainbow Passage

Below are two broad transcriptions of *The Rainbow Passage* (Fairbanks, 1960), the first a representative SIE accent and the second a representative NIE version:

Southern Irish English (SIE)

Northern Irish English (NIE)

/ʍɛn t̪ə sʌnlʌiθ stɹaiks ɹeindɹɒps ɪn t̪i ɛiəɹ t̪ei akt lʌik ə pɹɪzəm ɪn foɹm ə ɹeinbo. t̪ə ɹeinbo iz ə dɪvɪʒən əv ʍʍiθ lʌiθ ɪntəu məni bjɐuθɪfəl kʌləɹz. ðiz teik ðə ʃeip əv ə lɒŋ ɹaund ɒɹtʃ wɪθ its patʃ hʌi abɒv and its to ɛnds əpaɹəntli bijɒnd t̪ə həɹaizən. t̪ɛɹ ɪz akɒɹdɪŋ t̪ə lɛdʒend ə bɒilɪŋ pɒθ əv gɒəld aθ wʊn ɛnd. pipəl lʊk bət nowən ɛvəɹ fʌindz ɪθ. ʍɛn a man lʊks fəɹ sʌmtʃɪŋ bijɒnd hɪs ɹiitʃ hiz fɹɛnds sɛi hi ɪz lʊkɪŋ fəɹ tʃə pɒθ əv gɒəld at t̪i ɛnd əv t̪ə ɹeinbo/

/wɛn ðə sʌnlait stɹaiks ɹendɹɒps ɪn ði ɛɹ ɪʒɛi akt laik ə pɹɪzəm ən fɔɹm ə ɹenbəo. ðə ɹenbəo ɪz ə dəvɪʒən əv wait lait ɪntu məni bjɐtəfəl kʌləɹz. ðiz tek ðə ʃep əv ə lɒŋ ɹaund ɒɹtʃ wɪθ ɪts paθ hai əbʌv ənd ɪts tu endz əpaɹəntli bijɒnd ðə həɹaizən. ðɛ ɹɒʒ ɪz əkɒɹdɪ t̪ə lɛdʒend ə bɒilɪŋ pɒt əvgold ət wʌn ɛnd. pipəl lʊk bət nəowʌn ɛvəɹ faindz ɪt. wɛn ə man lʊks fəɹ sʌmθɪŋ bijɒnd hɪz ɹiitʃ hɪz fɹendz sɛi hi iz lʊkɪŋ fəɹ ðə pɒt əv gold ət ði ɛnd əv ðə ɹenbəo/

When the sunlight strikes raindrops in the air, they act as a prism and form a rainbow. The rainbow is a division of white light into many beautiful colors. These take the shape of a long round arch, with its path high above, and its two ends apparently beyond the horizon. There is , according to legend, a boiling pot of gold at one end. People look, but no one ever finds it. When a man looks for something beyond his reach, his friends say he is looking for the pot of gold at the end of the rainbow.

RESOURCES

Books

Dolan, T. P. (2004). *A dictionary of Hiberno-English* (4th ed.). Dublin: Gill and Macmillan.

Hickey, R. (2002). *A source book for Irish English.* Amsterdam: John Benjamins.

Todd, J. (1990). *Words apart: A dictionary of Northern Ireland English.* Gerrards Cross: Colin Smythe.

CD-ROM

Hickey, R. (2004b). *A sound atlas of Irish English.* Berlin/ New York: Mouton de Gruyter, (book and DVD).

Journals

• *Journal of Clinical Speech and Language Studies,* http://www.iaslt.com/ie4p/pub/Journals.html. A journal published annually and jointly by the Irish Association of Speech and Language Therapists and the School of Clinical Speech and Language Studies, Trinity College, Dublin. Issues are not limited to the Irish context. According to the journal's notes for contributors, "contributions are invited from practising clinicians on all types of communication impairments and therapy ... [and] there is scope for philosophical, theoretical and practical issues to be presented."

- *Teanga* (The Irish Yearbook of Applied Linguistics), http://www.iraal.ie/pub1_en.html. Published annually by Irish Association for Applied Linguistics, *Teanga* publishes a range of papers that have an explicitly Irish and IE orientation. Its applied nature means that it contains clinical and nonclinical papers.
- *Belfast Working Papers in Language and Linguistics.* An occasional series of working papers and presentation of conference proceedings published by the University of Ulster, Belfast. Working Papers publish clinical and nonclinical work relating to any variety of English, not just IE.
- *Update* of IASLT, http://www.iaslt.com/ie4p/pub.html. A newsletter style publication that provides information on current issues affecting SLPs and services in the Republic of Ireland.

Professional associations

Irish Association of Speech and Language Therapists (IASLT), http://www.iaslt.com/.

A register of SLPs working in private practice is maintained by IASLT and is available at http://www.iasltpp.com. This site provides a valuable source of information on SLP services in the Republic of Ireland, as well as some useful links to related UK and Irish sites.

Royal College of Speech and Language Therapists (RCSLT), http://www.rcslt.org/.

Along similar lines to the Republic's register of SLPs in private practice, the UK provides information on private practitioners in Northern Ireland, under the auspices of the Association for Speech and Language Therapists in Independent Practice, http://www.asltip.co.uk/main.asp.

Like other European SLPs, those in Ireland contribute to the debate of CPLOL (Standing Liaison Committee of Speech and Language Therapists of the European Union), www.cplol.org.

Universities offering courses in speech-language pathology

National University of Ireland, Galway, http://www.nuigalway.ie (4-year BSc Hons.)

Trinity College, Dublin http://www.tcd.ie/Clinical_Speech/index.php (4-year BSc Hons.)

University College, Cork, http://www.ucc.ie/speechlang/vocational/index.php (4-year BSc Hons.)

University of Limerick, http://www/ul.ie (2-year postgraduate MSc conversion course)

University of Ulster, http://www.science.ulster.ac.uk/health/ (4-year BSc Hons.)

Useful Irish English Web sites

In addition to the Web sites listed above, SLPs working in Ireland are likely to find useful information on the following two sites:

- The Cleft Lip and Palate Association of Ireland, www.cleft.ie, offers, on a voluntary basis, guidance and help for children with cleft palate and their parents.
- Down Syndrome Ireland, http://www.downsyndrome.ie/, is a national resource center for a wide range of information, including aspects of speech relevant to Down Syndrome children.

REFERENCES

Anthony, A., Bogle, D., Ingram, T.T., and McIsaac, M. W. (1971). *Edinburgh Articulation Test*. Edinburgh: Churchill Livingstone.

Armstrong, S., and Ainley, M. (1988). *South Tyneside Assessment of Phonology (STAP)*. Ponteland: STASS Publications.

Cruttenden, A. (1995). Rises in English. In J. Windsor-Lewis (Ed.), *Studies in general and English phonetics* (pp. 155–173). London: Routledge.

Cruttenden, A. (1997). *Intonation* (2nd ed.). Cambridge, UK: Cambridge University Press.

Cruttenden, A. (2001). *Gimson's pronunciation of English* (6th ed.). London: Edward Arnold.

Crystal, D. (1969). *Prosodic systems and intonation in English.* Cambridge, UK: Cambridge University Press.

CSO (Central Statistics Office). (2002). *Census 2002: Preliminary report*. Dublin: Stationery Office.

de Montfort Supple, M. (1992). Sociolinguistics: The clinical perspective. In M. M. Leahy and J. Kallen (Eds.), *Interdisciplinary perspectives in speech and language pathology* (pp. 24–29). Dublin: Trinity College.

Dodd, B., Crosbie, S., McIntosh, B., Teitzel, T., and Ozanne, A. (2000). *Preschool and Primary Inventory of Phonological Awareness*. London: The Psychological Corporation.

Dodd, B., Hua, Z., Crosbie, S., Holm, A. and Ozanne, A. (2003). *Diagnostic Evaluation of Articulation and Phonology (DEAP)*. London: The Psychological Corporation.

Dolan, T. P. (2004). *A dictionary of Hiberno-English* (4[th.] ed.). Dublin: Gill and Macmillan.

Dowd, P., Garvey-Cecchetti, B., Heslin, C., Laundon, O., McGinty, C., O'Malley, L., and Philbin, R. (1992). Mayo screening test for early language development. In M. M. Leahy and J. Kallen (Eds.), *Interdisciplinary perspectives in speech and language pathology* (pp. 125–139). Dublin: Trinity College.

Fairbanks, G. (1960). *Voice and articulation drillbook*. New York: Harper and Row.

Filppula, M. (1999). *The grammar of Irish English*. London: Routledge.

Giegerich, H. J. (1992). *English phonology: An Introduction*. Cambridge, UK: Cambridge University Press.

Grunwell, P. (1985). *PACS: Phonological Assessment of Child Speech*. Windsor: NFER-Nelson.

Grunwell, P. (1987). *Clinical phonology* (2nd ed.). London: Croom Helm.

Grunwell, P. (1995). *PACS Toys Screening Assessment* (2nd ed.). Windsor: NFER-Nelson

Gunn, B. (1985). Geo- and socio-linguistic indicators in clinical speech analysis. *Belfast Working Papers in Language and Linguistics*, 7, 16–25.

Halliday, M. A. K. (1970). *A course in Spoken English: Intonation*. Oxford, UK: Oxford University Press.

Harris, J. (1985). *Phonological variation and change*. Cambridge, UK: Cambridge University Press.

Hickey, R. (1997). On the acquisition of Irish English phonology. In J. R. Dow and M. Wolff (Eds.), *Languages and lives: Essays in honor of Werner Enninger* (pp. 171–187). New York: Peter Lang.

Hickey, R. (1999). Dublin English: Current changes and their motivation. In P. Foulkes and G. Docherty (Eds.), *Urban voices* (pp. 265–281). London: Edward Arnold.

Hickey, R. (2004a). The phonology of Irish English. In C. Upton (Ed.), *Handbook of varieties of English: The British Isles* (pp. 47–76). Berlin: Mouton de Gruyter.

Hickey, R. (2004b). *A sound atlas of Irish English*. Berlin/New York: Mouton de Gruyter.

Hodson, B. (1986). *Assessment of Phonological Processes-Revised.* Austin, TX: Pro-Ed.

Hodson, B. (2004). *Assessment of Phonological Patterns* (3rd ed.). Austin, TX: Pro-Ed

IPA (International Phonetic Association). *The sounds of the IPA*. See http://www.arts.gla.ac.uk/IPA/ipa.html

Kallen, J. (1997). Irish English: Context and Contacts. In J. Kallen, (Ed.), *Focus on Ireland* (pp. 1–33). Amsterdam: John Benjamins.

Kingsmore, R. K. (1995). *Ulster Scots speech: A sociolinguistic study*. Tuscaloosa: University of Alabama Press.

Kortmann, B., and Schneider, E. W. (Eds.). (2004). *A handbook of varieties of English: A multimedia reference tool.* Berlin: de Gruyter.

Leahy, M. M. (1989). *Communication disorders: The science of intervention*. London: Whurr.

Lightfoot, D. (1999). *The development of language: Acquisition, change and evolution*. Cambridge, MA: Blackwell.

McCafferty, K. (1996). *Ethnicity and language change: English in (London)Derry, Northern Ireland*. Amsterdam: John Benjamins.

McCurtin, A., and Murray, G. (2000). *The manual of AAC* [Augmentative and Alternative Communication]. Oxford, UK: Windsor Press.

McElholm, D.D. (1986). Intonation in Derry English. In H. Kirkwood (Ed.), *Studies in Intonation: Occasional Papers in Linguistics and Language Learning 11* (pp. 1–58). Ulster: University of Ulster.

McGinty, C. (2000). An investigation into aspects of the Mayo Early Language Screening Test. *Child Care Health Development*, 26(2), 111–128.

McLeod (2002). The plethora of available data on children's speech development. *ACQuiring Knowledge in Speech, Language and Hearing, 4,* 141–147.

Millar, S. (1987). *Accent in the classroom: Sociolinguistic perspectives on the teaching of elocution in some Belfast secondary-level schools*. Unpublished doctoral dissertation, Queen's University, Belfast.

Millar, S. (1996). By George she's got it? Problems of modifying accent in Belfast. *Belfast Working Papers in Language and Linguistics, 13*, 287–307.

Milroy, J. (1981). *Regional accents of English: Belfast.* Belfast: Blackstaff Press.

Milroy, L., and McClenaghan, P. (1977). Stereotyped reactions to four educated accents in Ulster. *Belfast Working Papers in Language and Linguistics, 2*(4), 1–10.

Ní Cholmáin, C. (2002). *Good communicators, poor speakers.* Unpublished doctoral dissertation, Trinity College, Dublin.

NICCY (Northern Ireland Commissioner for Children and Young People). (2004/2005). *Overview of speech and language therapy provision in Northern Ireland 2004/2005.* (http://www.niccy.org/downloads/overview.pdf)

NISRA (Northern Ireland Statistics and Research Agency). (2001). *Northern Ireland census 2001.* Belfast: HMSO.

Ó Baoill, D. (1997). The emerging phonological substratum in Irish English. In J. Kallen (Ed.), *Focus on Ireland* (pp. 73–87). Amsterdam: John Benjamins.

Ó Sé, D. (1985). Word stress in Hiberno-English. In J. Harris, D. Little, and D. Singleton (Eds.), *Perspectives on the English language in Ireland* (pp. 67–81). Dublin: Centre for Language and Communication Studies, Trinity College.

O'Halpin, R. (1992). Contrastive stress in profoundly deaf children: An auditory and acoustic analysis before and after training. In M. M. Leahy and J. Kallen (Eds.), *Interdisciplinary perspectives in speech and language pathology* (pp. 266–277). Dublin: Trinity College.

O'Halpin, R. (1994). Nuclear prominence in Hiberno-English: A preliminary investigation. *Teanga, 14*, 1–14.

O'Halpin, R. (2001). Intonation issues in the speech of hearing impaired children: Analysis, transcription and remediation. *Clinical Linguistics and Phonetics, 15*(7), 529–550.

Pandeli. H., Eska, J. F., Ball, M. J., and Rahilly, J. (1997). Problems of phonetic transcription: The case of the Hiberno-English slit-t. *Journal of the International Phonetic Association, 27*, 65–75.

Rahilly, J. (1997). Aspects of prosody in Hiberno-English: The case of Belfast. In J. Kallen (Ed.), *Focus on Ireland* (pp. 109–132). Amsterdam: John Benjamins.

Renfrew, C. (2000). *The Renfrew Language Scales: The Bus Story Test.* Brackley UK: Speechmark.

Rosner, J. (1999). *Test of Auditory Analysis (TAAS).* New York: Academic Therapy.

Secord, W., and Donohue, J. (2002). *Clinical assessment of articulation and phonology.* Austin, TX: Pro-Ed.

Semel, E., Wiig, E. H., and Secord, W. (1987). *Clinical Evaluation of Language Fundamentals-Revised.* New York: Psychological Corporation.

Semel, E., Wiig, E. H., and Secord, W. (1992). *Pre-school CELF: Preschool Clinical Evaluation of Language Fundamentals.* New York: Psychological Corporation.

Smit, A. B. (2004). *Articulation and phonology: Resource guide for school-age children and adults.* Clifton Park, NY: Thomson Delmar Learning.

Titterington, J., Henry, A., and Toner, J. G. (2001). The relationship between auditory sensory memory and spoken language development in children with significant hearing impairment. *Belfast Working Papers in Language and Linguistics, 15*, 75–100.

Wells, J. C. (1982). *Accents of English: The British Isles.* Cambridge, UK: Cambridge University Press.

Zwickl, A. (2002). *Language attitudes, ethnic identity and dialect use across the Northern Ireland border: Armagh and Monaghan.* Belfast: Cló Ollscoil na Banríona.

SUMMARY OF STUDIES OF TYPICAL IRISH ENGLISH SPEECH ACQUISITION

Authors	Year	Country	No. of children	Age of children	Information	Sample type	Data collection
Hickey	1997	Republic of Ireland	3	2;10, 5;6, and 7;9	Realization of SIE-specific consonants and vowels; brief information in phonological processes.	Single words	Cross-sectional

Chapter 29

Scottish English Speech Acquisition

James M. Scobbie, Olga Gordeeva, and Ben Matthews

INTRODUCTION

Scottish English is usually characterized as "a language continuum from Broad Scots to Scottish Standard English" (Corbett, McClure, and Stuart-Smith, 2003, p. 2). A 1996 survey preparatory to the 2001 census by the General Register Office (Scotland) estimated that about 30 percent of the Scottish population use (Broad) Scots to some extent, rising to 90 percent in the northeast. The linguistic situation on the ground is complicated somewhat by population movement and dialect contact, as well as uncertainty about what constitutes Scots or Scottish Standard English (SSE) in the first place.

Scots derives from the Anglian variety of Old English spoken in the sixth century and varies regionally, whereas SSE is far more homogeneous geographically. Scots speakers still tend only to be exposed in childhood to a Scottish English continuum rooted in their own local variety of Scots and so are not influenced much by other geographically delimited broad varieties. This continuum is, of course, just one aspect of sociolinguistic variation and is itself always undergoing language change: large differences should be expected between older, more conservative speakers and the young, as well as between regional and socioeconomic levels. In the urban setting, local housing variation means that adjacent neighborhoods may have markedly different linguistic profiles. Even the two ends of the Scots-SSE continuum are largely mutually intelligible, though mastery of SSE will not prepare someone new to Scotland (or indeed naïve Scots themselves) for the difficulties they will face in understanding a broad speaker from an unfamiliar area.

In general, the closely related varieties of Scottish English can be thought of as being parallel with, but independent from, the other Englishes of the UK, with their own national focus, however vague that is. The size, proximity, and influence of England, as well as population movements, mean however that historically and synchronically, the Scottish English continuum is attracted toward its English neighbor. See the Resources section in this chapter for materials pertaining to Scottish English.

Where Scottish English is spoken

Scottish English is spoken in Scotland (see accompanying map and Appendix D). At the time of the 2001 census, 87 percent of the 5,062,011 in the Scottish population had been born in Scotland, while about 8 percent (approximately 400,000) had been born in England. In the UK as a whole, 5,229,364 million residents (9.2 percent) had been born in Scotland, so 84 percent of people born in Scotland continue to live there. In England, 408,948 (1 percent) had been born in Scotland (the majority living in London and the southeast). The Scots tongue spread to Ulster through emigration and settlement, so Scottish English and Ulster Scots share a number of features. How many people speak Scottish English is unknown, but a rough estimate would be between four and five million.

Components of Scottish English

The major authorities on the pronunciation of contemporary adult (including adolescent) Scots and Scottish English whose works are most accessible and appropriate for our readership are Stuart-Smith, Johnston, Macafee, and Macaulay. We will give specific references to these researchers' work where most relevant, but for more information on much of the adult material presented here, for useful summaries of Scottish English, for detailed exposition of their extensive empirical research, and not least for further references on Scottish English, see their works cited in the bibliography and references therein.

Consonants

Scottish English has 25 phonemes and is most closely related to English as spoken in England (see Table 29-1). Worthy of note are [ç]~[χ](/x/) and [ʍ] (here /hw/, hence not in Table 29-1, but readily analyzed as a 26th phoneme /ʍ/). These consonants are rather peripheral to the phonological system (Scobbie and Stuart-Smith, in press) and are low in frequency (Macafee, 1983; 1994;

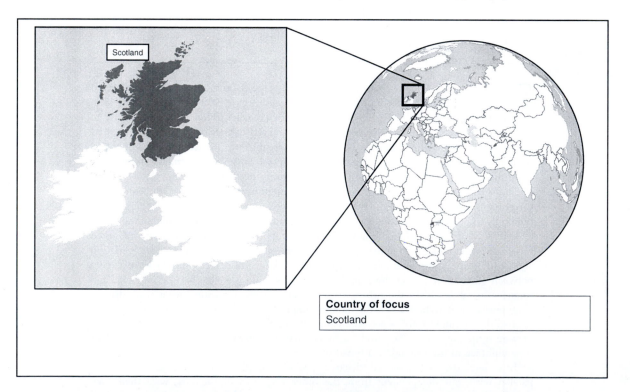

Country of focus
Scotland

Stuart-Smith, 2003) though well exemplified by minimal pairs such as *loch - lock* and *witch - which*. More controversial is [ʔ], included because it is such an extremely common phone (structurally an allophone of /t/ in medial and final positions) that it is used almost categorically for /t/ in those positions by many broad speakers, a long-standing pattern in the central belt. While a trilled or tapped realization of /r/ in adult broad Scots is typical, on the whole, /r/ in Scottish English is often an approximant [ɹ], and sometimes a tap [ɾ]; indeed, see below for discussion of further weakening of the rhotic. Any single IPA symbol for the phoneme in Table 29-1 is oversimplistic: in the text we use phonemic /r/ for convenience. Johnston (1997) says /l/ is characteristically dark ([ɫ]) in all positions, sometimes strongly pharyngealized, though Highland English and some northern and southwestern Scots varieties have a clear /l/. The "alveolar" stops /t, d, n/ are often dental under the influence of Scots. The strident fricatives display a fair amount of variation in their placement (Johnston, 1997; Stuart-Smith and Timmins, in press b). /θ, ð/ are being replaced by /f, v/ among (broad) younger speakers (Stuart-Smith and Timmins, in press a), whereas in the north /θ, ð/ remain peripheral phonemes (Johnston, 1997) and stop variants are still common in the northern isles, for example. Further south, in traditional Scots, /θ/ was replaced by /h/ and /ð/ was absent, particularly in pronouns and determiners. But as with so many other formally phonological patterns, fossilization and lexicalization (e.g. *thing* with initial /h/) is what is found in the contemporary situation rather than strictly phonological or phonotactic patterning (Macafee, 1994), though it is still common in the north (J. Smith, personal communication).

Vowels and diphthongs

Abercrombie (1979) is an excellent starting point for considering the vowel systems of Scottish English. In his scheme there are 13 vowel phonemes in SSE. Ten of them are monophthongs (see Figure 29-1), of which /ə/ (schwa) appears only in unstressed syllables. /ɪ, ɛ, ʌ/ mainly appear in closed syllables. There are three diphthongs /ai, ʌʉ, ɔe/. An unstressed word-final vowel (e.g., in *happy, baby*) tends to be [e]-like. The Scottish vowel system is small for English because it has maintained post-vocalic /r/ (but see below). However, it might be both larger and less like other varieties if we were to accept that the quasi-phonemic contrast of the Scottish Vowel Length Rule (SVLR) establishes three extra phonemes by splitting /i, ʉ, ae/ into "long" and "short" variants, of which more appear below.

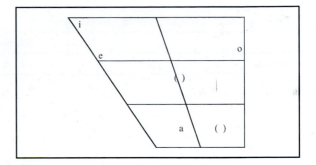

Figure 29-1 Scottish English vowel monophthongs

SSE vowels differ from Southern Standard British English (SSBE) in their phonetic realization (Figure 29-1), their system, and their lexical incidence. Table 29-2 summarizes the phonemic (and some significant allophonic) correspondences between the systems, thus addressing the first two points of difference. We have departed in some respects from traditional SSBE transcriptions to highlight similarities and dissimilarities between the systems (and see the section below on common mismatches, which stresses variation in lexical incidence as well as the phonetic similarity between pairs like SSE *coat* and SSBE *court*).

Note that widespread variation in phonetic targets even *within* SSE are found, for example in /ʉ/ (cf. also the endpoint of /aʉ/), which is variable in height, frontness and rounding, especially in the front-back dimension; in /ɪ/, which may be further lowered and backed, or raised and fronted; and in the diphthongs /ʌʉ/, /ʌi/, and /ɑːe/, which may start from a higher or lower point. A minority of SSE speakers have the phonemic contrast /a/ versus /ɑ/, but it is far more common to have just one low vowel /a/ with two allophones (see below), which may have a large phonetic distance between them. The vowels in *face* and *goat* are monophthongs ([fes], [got]). In the latter, /o/ is a close-mid back vowel with no tendency to front, and strong breaking before alveolar consonants is common in certain words (cf. *phone, don't, coat* as near disyllabic [fo.ən] [do.ənʔ] [ko.eʔ]). A minor point is that some speakers have a marginally phonemic /ë/, known as "Aitkens' vowel", in a small set of mainly "v" words such as *seven, heaven, never, devil, Shepherd* (Abercrombie, 1979, p.74). It is subtly distinct from the /ɪ/ of *divot, river, Liverpool* and is clearly different from the /e/ of *David* and the /ɛ/ of *Devon*.

The low vowel /a/ is complex. In many speakers either a tauto-syllabic post-vocalic /r/ or a word-final open syllable conditions a backish [ɑ], categorically distinct from the very different [a] in *hat*. Less systematically, speakers at

TABLE 29-1 Consonants produced in English

	Bilabial	Labiodental	Dental	Alveolar
Plosive	pʰ b̥			tʰ d̥
Nasal	m			n
Trill				r
Tap or flap				ɾ
Fricative		f v	(θ ð)	s z
Lateral fricative	███████		███████	
Affricate				
Approximant	w̜ labialvelar̯			ɹ
Lateral approximant	███████		███████	ɫ

Black = articulations judged impossible

Note. /r, ɾ, ɹ/ are variants of one phoneme, as are [ʔ, t]. [x] is peripheral. [o] is not included because it is analysed as a cluster /hw/.

Based on the International Phonetic Alphabet. Courtesy of the International Phonetic Association (c/o Department of Linguistics, University of Victoria, Victoria, British Columbia, Canada).

the SSE end of the continuum may extend the allophonic distribution of [ɑ] into contexts (at least in some common words) where /a/ precedes a voiceless fricative (*bath, grass*). Among broader speakers, a more homogeneous allophony occurs, in which /a/ in *hat* tends to be central or back-ish and, especially in the northeast of Scotland, extremely similar to the vowel in *car*. However, in Glasgow even vernacular speakers are adopting the standard variety's categorical front/back *hat/car* allophony (Stuart-Smith, 1999, p. 208). The categorical quality of this vowel allophony and its phonetic extent are likely to be important factors in development of post-vocalic /r/ derhoticization (which we discuss next, and in the consonant section below, based mainly on the findings of Stuart-Smith). Basically, a strong and categorical allophony is likely to lead to the creation of a new phoneme /ɑ/ (or /ɑː/) to replace /ar/. A merger between such pairs as *cat* [kat] and *cart* [kɑˑt] (as /kat/) appears unlikely.

Vowels in rhotic contexts are presented separately below (Table 29-3), because though post-vocalic /r/ has had only a small effect on the vowel inventory to date, this may change rapidly if the highly derhoticized variants of /r/ just introduced become established (see below). The two crucial factors needed to redefine Scottish English as a nonrhotic system with vocalized /r/ are phonetic derhoticization of coda /r/ and consequential changes in the vowel system. The main thing to be noted about the contemporary situation is the large number of vowel phonemes that are still possible before /r/. Conservative

speakers might even have a full set. If /r/ *is* derhoticized, a centering diphthong with a uvular or pharyngeal quality will generally be the result. This may ultimately lead to mergers and other effects similar to those that have previously occurred in SSBE, at which time these vowels could be phonological diphthongs rather than phonological vowel+/r/ sequences with strong transitions and weak rhoticity. As things stand, we do not seem to have reached that stage.

Even in clearly rhotic speakers, there are nevertheless some typical vowels mergers, and these are indicated in Table 29-3. An extra dimension to variation arises because broader rhotic Scottish English tends not to rigidly distinguish /er/ from /ɛr/, or less so /ɔr/ from /or/, either neutralizing the contrast or using /o/ and /ɛ/ in some of the lexemes where /ɔ/ or /e/ are used by other speakers, for example, *border* as [bordər] (homophonous with *boarder*) instead of [bɔrdər], or *air* as [ɛr] (homophonous with err) instead of [eɹ]). This distribution of /ɛr/ in particular is quite salient and may be stigmatized (cf. Macafee, 1994, pp. 225–226), but the raising of /ɔr/ to /or/ can be observed in middle class Edinburgh speakers.

Post-vocalic /l/ also impacts on vowel phonetics, because it can be very dark, and because it may lack alveolar contact and be rounded. Strong breaking occurs before /l/ after fronter/higher vowels, making *feel, fail, fool* sound disyllabic ([fiːəɫ], [feːəɫ], [fuːəɫ], or, if /l/ is not alveolar, then something like [fiːəʕ] or [fiːo]), and so on. The vowel inventory may be regarded as altered if

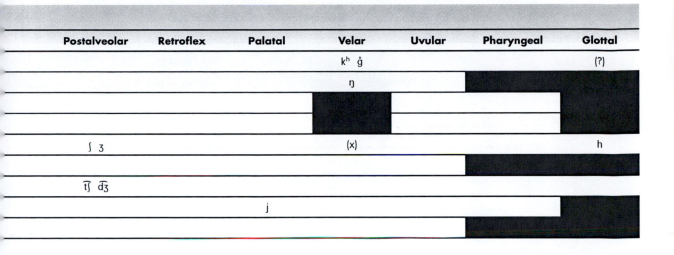

TABLE 29-2 The SSE system of vowel phonemes and major allophones, with representative phonetic labels, compared to the phonemic system of SSBE

English Examples	Scottish Standard English (SSE)	Southern Standard British English (SSBE)
greed / greet / niece	i	i ↔ i:
agreed / sea / freeze	i:	
grade / greyed / great / say	e ↔ e:	ei
bid	ɪ ↔ ɪ̈	ɪ
bed	ɛ	ɛ
Pam	a ↔ ɑ	a
palm / shah	a ↔ ɑ / ɑ	ɑ
cot	ɔ	ɒ
caught		ɔ ↔ o
coat / code / flowed / sew	o ↔ o:	əu
put	ʉ	ʊ
brood / brute / Bruce		u ↔ u:
brewed / bruise / moo	ʉ:	
queue	jʉ:	ju:
but	ʌ	ʌ
side / price	ʌi	ae
sighed / prize	ɑ:e	
bough	ʌʉ	ɑu
boy	ɔe	ɔe

Note. An arrow indicates a particularly notable range of productions; a slash separates two categorical alternatives. The SSBE symbols are not typical, and they reflect a compromise between phonetic accuracy and a desire to stress the similarities and dissimilarities with SSE phonetic targets from a Scottish English perspective, while retaining traditional transcription practice as much as possible. Recent developments in SSBE are not recorded.

TABLE 29-3 The SSE vowel system for monophthongal rhotic contexts compared to SSBE.

English Examples	Scottish Standard English (SSE)	Southern Standard British English (SSBE)
near	ir	iə ↔ ɪː
bear	er / ɛr	eə ↔ ɛː
bird	ʌr ↔ ər ↔ ɚ	3ː
word		
heard	ɛr / ʌr ↔ ər ↔ ɚ	
bard	ɑr	ɑː
cord	ɔr / or	
board	or	ɔː ↔ oː
tour	ʉr	
cure	jʉr	ʊə
fire	ɑːer	aeə
hour	ʌʉr	aʊə
Moir	ɔir	ɔic

Note. See the text for discussion of pronunciation of /ɾ/ and dipthongisation of the preceding vowel.

the vocalized /l/ is phonologically a vowel, by definition (cf. nonrhotic English), but currently some consonantal reflex of /l/ seems to be always present. Yet even if final (nonalveolar) /l/ is phonologically consonantal, the pairs *foe, foal* can be so nearly homophonous ([foː] vs. [foːˤ] or [foːʷ]) that the difference is hard to hear. Similar but lesser difficulties pertain to *law, loll* ([lɔː] vs. [lɔˤ]). If both /r/ and /l/ are very weak, then there might appear to be scope for *foal* and *four* to merge with *foe*, since all are similar to [foː], but a phonetic distance seems to be maintained at present, the precise nature of which remains to be investigated. Note that there can be an absolute absence of /l/ after historical /a/ in broad Scots (e.g., *ball, fall*, where the vowel may be either /a/ or /ɔ/ depending on the dialect), but this is a separate phenomenon.

SSE and many Scots dialects feature a highly systematic allophonic distribution of duration on word-final stressed vowels conditioned by post-vocalic consonantal voicing and manner of articulation (Aitken, 1981; Scobbie, Hewlett, and Turk, 1999; Scobbie, Turk, and Hewlett, 1999). This has been labeled the "Scottish Vowel Length Rule" (SVLR; Aitken, 1981). SVLR applies primarily to the vowels /i/, /ʉ/, /ʌi/. In closed word-final syllables the long variant is conditioned by a post-vocalic voiced fricative or /r/: all other consonants condition short vowels. Open syllables also condition long variants.

This makes possible a morphological function for duration: word-final open syllables for these three vowels are long (e.g., *brew*) and they remain so even if suffixed (e.g., *brewed*). The differences in application between the phonological and morphological conditioning factors creates a "quasi-phonemic contrast" in a limited number of words like *brood* (short) versus *brewed* (long; Scobbie and Stuart-Smith, in press). Those authors also point out that with word-internal SVLR (in words like *crisis, lycra, spider*), the distribution of long and short variants is far more complex and/or unpredictable.

As for longer-term settings, one phenomenon prevalent among young vernacular speakers is that their vowels may be heavily nasalized. Also relevant is that urban working-class speech may be characterized auditorily as sounding pharyngeal (Esling, 1978; Stuart-Smith, 1999).

As mentioned, one complex aspect of the Scots-SSE continuum is the variation in lexical incidence of vowels, which, though infrequent overall, is highly salient. For example, the choice between broad /ʉ/ and more standard /ʌʉ/ is restricted to a set of high-frequency words including *down, out, about*, etc. (Macafee, 1994; Stuart-Smith, 2003). Even more restricted mini-regularities abound, involving some different lexical splits than those implied by Table 29-2; for example *stone, floor* have /o/ in SSE, whereas in many broader varieties they have /e/. In Northern Insular Scots, *saw* has /a/ instead of /ɔ/;

and so on. /a/ rather than /ɔ/ may be found after /w/ (*wad, wander*) and in some broad varieties which kept a consonantal /l/ (*ball, wall*). In North East Scots, SSE /ʉ/ can be /wi/, for example, *school* /skwil/. Such differences (many and various) cause great problems for analysis and for materials preparation.

Phonotactic restrictions

Generally speaking, Scottish English shares a lexicon with other British English varieties but many (especially older) speakers have extensive additional Scots lexis. The structure of syllables and phonotactic restrictions on the syllable onsets and codas are largely the same.

Syllables

A more phonological pattern than the strong breaking mentioned above arises because of the way that Scottish English avoids coda /rl/, /rm/, /lm/ clusters. Instead of these clusters, Scottish English tends to have CVC sequence, making pairs such as *pearl*/*peril* into homophones ([pɛrɨɫ]). Compared to other varieties, there is an extra weak syllable in *world, farm,* or *film* ([wʌrətɫd], [farʌm], [fɪlɪm]). Such extra syllables are phonotactically obligatory in broader speech, but may be merely lexical variants in SSE.

There is some regional variability in the syllabic structure. In Shetland dialect, there is a strong tendency toward a CVCC versus CVVC rhyme pattern throughout the vocabulary such as in *fatt* 'fat' versus *faat* 'fault' ascribed to the historical 'Scandinavian' Norn influence on the syllable structure (van Leyden, 2004).

Consonants and consonant clusters

Consonant clusters are generally like those in British English. Onset /hw/ is still common in "wh" words, and /x/ is limited to codas. In more conservative, especially older broad speakers, /x/ still appears in clusters (e.g., in *daughter* [dɔxtər]; Marshall, 2004; Smith 2005). Word-initial /nj/ may be absent (so that *news* has plain /n/) while *tune* and *dune* typically have /tʃ/ and /dʒ/ rather than /tj/ and /dj/. Initial /tr/ and /dr/ are often also post-alveolar affricates, but rhoticized ones. /r/, generally an approximant, may appear as a tap medially in trochaic position (*carry*) or in initial labial clusters. In older or broader speakers a trill or tap is likely to be more common in prevocalic contexts (Marshall, 2004) but "counter to American stereotypes of what a Scottish accent is like, [a trill] is now sporadic at best" (Johnston, 1997, p. 510). Aspiration of /p, t, k/ may be generally light, and some Scots varieties may have /p/ as a voiceless unaspirated

fortis stop and /b/ as a lenis fully voiced stop. The norm for coda and ambisyllabic /t/ is often [ʔ] in the central belt of Glasgow and Edinburgh, in fact "we could even say obligatory for working class adolescents" in Glasgow (Stuart-Smith, 2003, p. 125). However, it is less common elsewhere, such as in the "heartlands" of Scots, such as rural Buchan (Marshall, 2004, p. 130), where it is appears to be an innovation, and in SSE, where it is merely optional. On the other hand, a short *voiced* stop for /t/ (not a flap) is not uncommon in ambisyllabic position. Final devoicing of obstruents is characteristic, leading in some cases (even in SSE) to /z/ being completely voiceless and /s/ being preaspirated (Gordeeva and Scobbie, 2004). Obstruent devoicing is particularly evident before silence, utterance-finally.

Reference was made above to post-vocalic /r/ being less overtly rhotic among younger vernacular speakers than either middle-class speakers or older vernacular speakers. This is quite distinct from the adoption of categorically nonrhotic productions by SSE speakers under influence from English as spoken in England. Rather, younger vernacular speakers in the central belt (at least) have an acoustically weak articulation of /r/ as a central vocoid, apparently with pharyngeal qualities (Romaine, 1978; Speitel and Johnston, 1983; Stuart-Smith, 2003). As a result, many vowel+/r/ sequences sound like diphthongs. Low vowel targets like /ar/ (*car*) may be monophthongal as [ɑ], while /ɛr/ (*herd*) and /r/ (*nurse*) may be [ɚ]. The actual articulation of the /r/ itself is highly variable and articulatorily complex: we have ourselves observed some clearly retroflex articulations in (near-)monophthongal derhoticised productions of *car, cart,* and *card* (using ultrasound tongue imaging), i.e. covert /r/ which are not detectable auditorily and have little effect on the formants (Scobbie and Stuart-Smith, 2005). This is quite unlike truly nonrhotic varieties in which any such obvious reflex of /r/ is absent. This whole Scottish situation is likely to be unstable. Post-vocalic /r/ in word-internal unstressed syllables is often completely absent, so that spelling is the only clue to its supposed existence.

Coda /l/ is dark, and may "vocalize" by losing alveolar contact in a quite radical way (Scobbie and Wrench, 2003), but a simple transcription such as [ɤ], [ɣ], or [ʕ] fails to convey the impressionistically lateral-sounding quality that is possible for this type of coda /l/. It can be very hard to distinguish from a very dark alveolar [ɫ] in which case is not like the very rounded vocalized /l/, common in SE England but less so among Scottish adults. Rounded or [o]-like vocalization of /l/ is considered below, since it seems to be more prevalent in younger speakers (Stuart-Smith, Timmins, and Tweedie, 2006). The effect on tautosyllabic vowels is considered above. In connected speech, word-final /r/ and /l/ occur as onset-like consonants before vowels, a sandhi process which can be strongly categorical.

Tones

Scottish English features no phonological tonal contrasts.

Stress and intonation

Scottish English is a stress-accent language. It uses duration, spectral characteristics, and loudness to a greater extent than pitch to encode the differences between stressed and unstressed syllables. Pitch conveys intonational meaning, and intonational events are generally aligned with stressed syllables.

The intonational system of Scottish English shows important regional variability. Most notable is that in Glasgow and western Scotland statements are pronounced as rises or rise-falls (Mayo, 1996; Ladd, 1996) in the final nuclear accent. This differs from high-rising intonation of "up-talk" statements in that the rise is preceded (and followed) by low pitch turning points. Glasgow intonation is salient for native speakers and commentators alike. The dialect of Orkney features an accent-lending rise on prenuclear accents in statements, which phonetically is shifted to a later position, in fact into the unstressed syllable (van Leyden, 2004), resulting in a fall during the stressed syllable. This dipping/rising pattern is sometimes impressionistically described as "sing-song" intonation similar to patterns also found in Welsh English (Munro, Ball, and Müller, see Chapter 56). Speakers of the Anstruther variety from the east coast of Fife produce a gradually falling slope toward the end of the intonational phrase (Aufterbeck, 2003). It differs from the nuclear slope in Southern British English, where it involves a sharp pitch change immediately after the nuclear syllable to the floor level of a speaker.

Writing system

The writing system of Scottish English is largely the same as for other British English varieties, but Scots has a range of local orthographic variants that attempt to capture phonetic and phonological aspects of the variety, especially when they diverge from SSE. An example of West Coast Scots is "Everhin, but everhin, wis ma fault. Anen it caught lik an unwantit fire. Afore lang evrubdy wis sayin it. Faimly. Mates. Schuilmaisters." (MacDonald, 2003, p. 1). MacDonald also uses "gemme" *game*, "thoosan" *thousand*,

and "hame" *home* to reflect Scottish lexical incidence of /ɛ, ʉ, e/ respectively. An example of North East Scots is "Bit o luck wis it nae, the skweel veesitin the Hame last wick, an me findin oot that Syd Paterson, their newest pensioner, wis ma verra ain Granda!" (Blackhall, 2003, p. 1). Other aspects of Doric from Blackhall are "een" /in/ *eyes*, "fit" /fɪʔ/ *what*, "eneuch" /əˈnjʉx/ *enough*. Though there is a strong and vibrant literary tradition, as evidenced by such modern writing in "dense" Scots, nevertheless for many speakers Scots is an oral variety, and any attempt to write it may elicit bafflement or hilarity.

Varieties of Scottish English

Variation in Scottish English has been highlighted throughout this chapter. Two good companion pieces on Glasgow and Edinburgh phonology are Stuart-Smith (1999) and Chirrey (1999). As well as social variation, geographical variation is particularly relevant to Broad Scots, which is usually divided into a number of geographical subvarieties (cf. for a very detailed account Johnston, 1997). Scots speakers often claim use of one of these varieties, rather than of "Scots" itself, and while rural varieties have a generally positive image, urban varieties (e.g., Glaswegian) have been excoriated by Scottish and non-Scottish observers alike and often mistaken for degenerate English. Scots are often defensive and critical in their attitude toward broad Scottish speech, and inaccurate in their intuitions and reporting of their own system under the influence of literacy, social attitudes, and partial systemization of other varieties, a situation with clear clinical implications. They may also be inconsistent in production. Stylistic variation and the process of accommodation may be particularly important in the therapeutic setting, however, and may cause difficulties in carryover of linguistic skills learned in the therapeutic context into "real life."

Typical acquisition of Scottish English

Bearing in mind the issues about variation and change which have been highlighted above, we should expect Scottish English to be comparable to other similar English varieties with respect to the acquisition of consonants (though see Scobbie, 2005). The vowel system, however, is different enough to warrant no such assumptions. Moreover, it is the vowel system that is most subject to interference between Scottish English or Scots and other varieties, most commonly the vowel system of English as spoken in England (see Chapter 27).

Scobbie, Hewlett, and Turk (1999) quantified the potential for Anglo-English parental influence. They examined the birth registrations from 1997 for children born into an "executive" or "professional" family in Scotland's two largest cities, in particular the subset of families characterized as being Scottish, English, or mixed Scottish/English (composing about 75 percent of the total). In Glasgow, 12 percent of such children have at least one English parent, but this figure rises to almost a quarter in Edinburgh (633/2728). The 2001 census shows that 13.5 percent of all Scottish households have multiple countries of birth. The actual effects of parental dialect on a Scottish child's vowel system are highly complex and have been studied only to shed light on specific theoretical questions, not to provide a broad descriptive picture (Hewlett, Matthews, and Scobbie, 1999; Scobbie, 2005). The flexibility of individuals and their context means that the specific outcomes of dialect mixture for a given individual are impossible to predict, but perhaps areas such as the SVLR, where Scottish and English systems are incompatible, are liable to most interference. Diphthongization of /e/ and /o/ as well as SSBE-style nonrhoticity is likely. Smith (2003–2005) will reveal a great deal about acquisition in North East Scots. Some initial results relevant to morphophonology are presented by Watt and Smith (2005). See the Summary of Studies Table at the end of this chapter for studies of Scottish English speech acquisition.

Acquired sounds

The *Edinburgh Articulation Test (EAT;* Anthony, Bogle, Ingram, and McIsaac, 1971) was standardized on 510 Scottish children, a process which showed that EAT scores are conditioned by the subject's age; but social class, birth rank, and sex matter hardly or not at all at the level of detail investigated.

Consonants

Normal ages of acquisition (based on 90 percent correct) are presented in Table 29-4 for various consonants, based on the work of Anthony et al. (1971).

Consonant clusters

Typical age of acquisition for a variety of consonant clusters can be worked out from Table 29-6 on page 196, depending on the criteria chosen.

TABLE 29-4 Age of phonetic acquisition of consonants by 90 percent of children

Consonant	Anthony et al. (1971)
p	3;0–3;5
b	3;0–3;5
m	3;0–3;5
t	3;0–3;5
d	3;0–3;5
n	3;0–3;5
k	3;6–3;11
g	3;6–3;11
ŋ	3;6–3;11
f	3;6–3;11
v	3;6–3;11
θ	after 6;0
ð	after 6;0
s	5;6–5;11
z	5;6–5;11
ʃ	5;6–5;11
ʒ	5;6–5;11
tʃ	after 6;0
dʒ	after 6;0
h	3;6–4;0
w	3;0–3;5
r	after 6;0
l	4;6–4;11
j	3;0–3;11

Vowels and diphthongs

In general terms, Anthony et al., (1971, p. 12) say a "stabilised vowel system" is acquired by age 3. Below that age, Matthews (2001) reports substantial phonetic variation in the realizations of vowels of seven children aged 1;9 to 2;10. Different children had different easy and difficult vowels, but of particular note, the vowels /ʉ/ and /ʌʉ/ remained non-adultlike throughout (mean 63.8 percent of adultlike realizations for /ʉ/). By the age of 3;4 to 4;9 the percentage of /ʉ/ vowels remaining non-adultlike phonetically had fallen to 17 percent (Gordeeva, 2005). The residual non-adultlike production involved lowering and backing to [ʊ̈] (11.8 percent), backing to [u] (4.3 percent), and lip unrounding (0.9 percent). The vowels that Matthews found were best acquired were far less consistent, but the following five feature most often in his lists of most accurate vowels per subject-session: /a, ʌi, i, ɔ, ʌ/ (in descending order of adultlike ranking).

On the other hand, because a vowel system is not merely its list of phonemes, it should not be surprising that particularly important nonphonemic vowel targets appear early. Matthews (2001) shows (in an instrumental study) that allophonic [a] versus [ɑ] were established structurally very early (under 2;1) in two of the three children examined (though this may be related to the fact that /ar/ and /ɔr/ were merged by two of them), as were the allophonic SVLR durational variants of /ʌi/ and /ɑːe/. The appropriate quality difference seems also to have established itself well in all three children. Interestingly, there is no statistically significant difference in duration between [i] and [iː] even by 2;6, though there is a suggestive trend in the right direction. Gordeeva (2005) shows that SVLR is acquired by the age of 3;4, based on results from an acoustic study of vowel duration of seven SSE speakers aged 3;4 to 4;9. Native Scots are less likely to acquire a strong SVLR

system if they have non-Scottish parents (Hewlett et al., 1999; Scobbie, 2005). Further information on vowels will come from Smith (2003-2005).

Percent correct

Anthony et al. (1971) in the *EAT* handbook provide very useful figures on all test items for percentage correct at different ages. The standardized *EAT* was a refinement of a preliminary test applied to 130 normally developing and 57 speech-retarded children "of high economic status and superior intelligence," which provides useful differential information on which consonants and clusters vary most by age (for those two groups studied; see Tables 29-4 to 29-6).

Consonants

In addition to the figures presented in Howard (see Chapter 27), it is useful to look in more detail at the age grading of the less readily acquired consonants from the *EAT*, particularly since these include the important consonants prevocalic /r/, /θ/ and medial /ð/ (Table 29-5).

Some of the consonants in the *EAT* (Anthony et al., 1971) are particularly good for clinical discrimination, as shown in Table 29-6 by the indicative differences

TABLE 29-5   Percentage correct for those consonants which do not reach 90 percent by age 4;6 (apart from /j/ and /l/ in *yellow* which are particularly prone to consonant harmony)

	Word	Word position	3;0	3;6	4;0	4;6	5;0	5;6
v	glove	final	54	70	89	84	83	94
r	red	initial	49	63	65	76	81	86
z	scissors	medial	40	46	65	70	73	74
ð	feather	medial	44	30	53	65	68	81
tʃ	chimney	initial	22	44	63	64	71	58
s	Christma*s*	final	24	40	53	60	66	67
dʒ	bridge	final	21	28	55	55	68	77
dʒ	garage	final	24	22	51	52	64	86
tʃ	watch	final	18	29	58	51	70	72
ʃ	sugar	initial	15	37	49	48	59	76
ʃ	toothbrush	final	15	19	55	47	66	85
ʃ	fish	final	21	26	59	46	56	71
θ	teeth	final	24	26	26	38	46	55
θ	thumb	initial	22	25	36	28	40	51

Note. Based on Anthony et al. (1971).

between matched typically developing children and children diagnosed as speech impaired in the preliminary test. These percentages are not, however, indicative of the normal population and in general are slightly higher for the typically developing children than the *EAT* scores, a notable exception being prevocalic /r/ in *red* and *garage* (see below).

Unfortunately, post-vocalic /r/ is not worth presenting, because the figures do not refer to exclusively consonantal productions of /r/: "many Scottish 2½-year-old children used a diphthong in positions where they later developed one of the many forms of [r]. *As this diphthong may also be an acceptable adult realisation, it had to be considered correct in this context.*" [Our emphasis] (Anthony et al., 1971, p. 6). Furthermore, if the /l/ in *milk, bottle,* and *pencil* was a rounded back vowel, the form was marked correct because these would still be "entirely usual local versions" (Anthony et al., 1971, p. 49), as are initial clusters of consonant plus /r/ with a transitional vowel and coda /r/ in "both [r-] and [r-]less versions." A glottal stop for /t/

TABLE 29-6 Percentage correct for selected consonants from the *EAT*, for typically developing children and children with speech impairment

	Word	Word position		2;6	3;0	3;6	4;0	4;6	5;0	5;6	6;0
r	red	initial	Typical	30	37	56	63	71	79		
			Speech impaired				11	22	29	39	
r	garage	medial	Typical	39	46	61	68	73	81		
			Speech impaired				22	28	39		58
ʃ	sugar	initial	Typical	34	42	53	69	81	81		
			Speech impaired				32	40	50		66
ʃ	fish	final	Typical	18	19	26	49	61	74		
			Speech impaired				19	15	29		29
j	yellow	initial	Typical	25	44	74	82	91	99		
			Speech impaired				30	45	53		71
l	yellow	medial	Typical	66	88	98	96	97	97		
			Speech impaired				59	62	68		68
tʃ	watch	final	Typical	30	31	48	62	69	79		
			Speech impaired				22	25	34		42
θ	teeth	final	Typical	32	41	52	51	53	50		
			Speech impaired				27	20	21		26
θ	thumb	initial	Typical	30	39	47	60	60	62		
			Speech impaired				27	28	47		50
ð	feather	medial	Typical	23	42	47	54	64	72		
			Speech impaired				19	20	42		45
g	garage	initial	Typical	91	98	97	96	99	100		
			Speech impaired				59	68	74		76
dʒ	garage	final	Typical	11	25	34	50	67	76		
			Speech impaired				19	22	32		42

Note. Based on Anthony et al. (1971).

was counted as correct in word-final and also word-medial position, and even for /p/ in *stamps*. Thus something like [b̥oʔoˠ] for the item *bottle* would be scored as correct. The exact sociolinguistic situation with post-vocalic /r/ being vocalized cannot be clarified from the published data, because the *EAT* "covered a wide range of socio-economic groups... with enormously varied phonetic influences" (Anthony et al., 1971, p. 49), and no further breakdown is given. Since pre-vocalic /r/ is — unusually — less accurate among the subjects in the preliminary test, it may be that high levels of /r/ vocalization in codas may also have been a middle-class Edinburgh feature at that time, but support for more general nonrhoticity comes from Romaine (1978) and Speitel and Johnson (1983), who found vocalized /r/ among working-class Edinburgh boys and men respectively (Table 29-7).

Stuart-Smith (2003) presents results from 14- to 15-year-old children showing that working-class girls have an overt rhotic consonant for coda /r/ in approximately 10 percent of cases, boys in about 20 percent, whereas middle-class children and all adults are rhotic. So nonrhoticity does indeed seem to be an extremely common feature, and, in children who do develop rhoticity, post-vocalic /r/ generally appears later than pre-vocalic /r/ (Matthews, 2001).

Unsurprisingly, the loss of [x] (i.e., /x/) and [ʍ] (i.e., /hw/) is more obvious among the young. In teenagers in Glasgow, these phones are in a minority (Lawson and Stuart-Smith, 1999; Stuart-Smith and Tweedie, 2000), but very high levels of coda /t/ were [ʔ], and expected /θ ð/ were largely actually /f v/. In the Doric (or North East Scots) of Huntly, Marshall (2004) found high rates of [ʔ] for /t/ among teenagers of both sexes (aged 14 to 17) and younger boys (aged 8 to 12) but not the younger girls. These child subjects were all rhotic, but trill /r/ was used less than 10 percent of the time (having been replaced by an approximant) in codas, especially by the girls, whereas it was the norm for adults. Trilled onset /r/ is now the less common option in the 8 to 17 age group, with a lot of individual variation.

Consonant clusters

Anthony et al. (1971) also contains figures for various consonant sequences, from which a selection is presented in Table 29-8. Figures from the preliminary test confirm that the clusters tested are generally very good for identifying developmental speech disorder even in items like *finger* with high scores in the *EAT* (Anthony et al., 1971).

Vowels

Matthews (2001) presents seven longitudinal case studies of Edinburgh children based on conversational speech. Overall mean performance is reported in Table 29-9.

Phonological processes

One of the very useful aspects of the *EAT* (Anthony et al., 1971) is the qualitative analysis of immature vs. atypical variations. For example, initial /tr/ has "minor" variants such as [tʃr, tər, tsr], the "immature" variants [tʃ, tw, tl, tʋ, tɥ, tð, tç, ts, tɬ, tʁ], the "very immature" variants [t, ɽr, kr, sr] and the "atypical" variants [sʋ, θ, sn, ɬ]. Such information is provided for all the consonants and clusters assessed by the test, but may be based on general principles to some extent rather than being entirely empirical. The following immature features are highlighted: consonant cluster reduction, liquid confusion, lengthening, palatalization, and fronting.

Matthews's (2001) longitudinal study of vowel acquisition in children under the age of 3 reported a number of immature secondary articulations such as nasalization, rhoticity, rounding, and more extreme processes such as consonantalization (frication and approximation) in addition to plain errors of quality. He also examined the four approximants. The processes affecting onset /j/ and /w/ were vowel-like (e.g., they gain syllabicity) though they were also susceptible to consonant harmony, especially in words with more than just one approximant. Prevocalically, /l/ was commonly stopped, deleted, or glided. /r/ was commonly glided, and possibly was a

TABLE 29-7 Percentage use of variants of coda /r/

Coda /r/	age 6		age 8		age 10	
	M	F	M	F	M	F
[r]	59	33	48	40	57	45
[ɹ]	16	50	37	54	15	54
nil	25	17	15	6	28	1

Note. Based on Romaine (1978, p. 204).

TABLE 29-8   Percentage correct for tautosyllabic and other selected clusters from the *EAT*

Consonant cluster	Word	Word position	3;0	3;6	4;0	4;6	5;0	5;6
st	*stamps*	initial	19	28	56	55	64	70
sp	*spoon*	initial	40	36	59	58	68	72
str	*string*	initial	19	36	48	53	68	70
sm	*smoke*	initial	21	15	38	45	56	57
sl	*sleep*	initial	34	33	48	57	64	79
fl	*flower*	initial	50	65	74	80	88	87
θr	*three*	initial	12	20	19	35	31	52
pl	*aeroplane*	initial	68	73	70	79	91	86
br	*bridge*	initial	50	60	66	73	82	90
tr	*train*	initial	38	47	56	67	82	81
kw	*queen*	initial	44	65	80	81	84	88
kl	*clouds*	initial	43	55	62	59	84	79
kr	*Christmas*	initial	53	66	70	75	81	85
gl	*glove*	initial	41	46	54	64	78	72
ŋg	*finger*	medial	84	88	88	91	94	98
ŋk	*monkey*	medial	74	80	87	88	90	94
nt	*tent*	final	84	91	95	99	96	95
ŋz	*wings*	final	36	31	48	50	60	81
mps	*stamps*	final	21	21	48	43	61	80
dz	*clouds*	final	16	31	45	50	56	76
sk	*desk*	final	22	33	59	58	66	72
lk	*milk*	final	78	81	87	88	89	86

Note. Based on Anthony et al. (1971).

cause of affrication in alveolar stop clusters. The glides [ɥ, w, ʋ] were particularly common, but occasionally [l] was observed, although not commonly in clusters requiring lingual contact. Post-vocalically, /l/ was vocalized as a close back vowel, often with rounding so that *milk* [mok] and *smoke* [smok] rhyme, while /r/ was commonly vocalized as schwa, or in the case of low vowels, as lengthening of the vowel.

Intelligibility

As far as we know, no formal studies of intelligibility have been made. See, however, the next section.

Phonetic inventory

Development of the significant nonphonemic vowel categories is early, with front/back /a/ and the SVLR vowels emerging contemporaneously with phonemic distinctions (Matthews, 2001).

Common mismatches

In Tables 29-2 and 29-3 we used somewhat unusual transcriptions to emphasize certain structural and phonetic facts about Scottish English and its relationship to SSBE. Additionally, our goal was to assist SSBE-accented

TABLE 29-9 Overall percentages of correct vowels, and individual variation

Age range	mean	Ben	Beth	Esther	Fionn	Fraser	Lewis	Rory
1;9–2;2	60	57	65	74	n.a.	50	36	77
2;1–2;4	68	53	65	83	n.a.	63	60	85
2;5–2;8	83	81	84	84	72	79	85	95

Note. Based on Matthews (2001).

therapists in avoiding certain common mismatches between the dialects, which particularly impact children and elderly listeners. The newer variants of SSBE in Table 29-3, for example, may lead Scots to misinterpret monophthongal *speared* or *spared* ([speːd] or [spɪːd] or similar) as *spade* or perhaps *sped*. Even more confusable is the monophthong in SSBE for *caught* and *court*, which is phonetically confusable with SSE /o/: SSBE *law* and *lore* (but not *low*) sound like Scottish *low*. On the other hand, we have avoided using fronted transcriptions for SSBE back vowels and diphthongs to emphasize the differences between the varieties. SSE's /ʉ/ is fronter and rounder than SSBE's /u/, and may be lower, but SSBE's /əʊ/ for example may itself be very fronted, though not so round (Watt and Smith, 2005; Watt and Tillotson, 2001). Indeed, frequent confusions for Scottish speakers include hearing Southern English *goat* as *gate*, *kate* as *kite*, and *kite* as having a /ɔe/ vowel (with few lexical consequences due to the rarity of that vowel). Even /u/ and /ʊ/ can be misheard as /i/. The converse case, misperception of normal Glasgow vowels by non-Scottish speakers, was investigated by Nathan, Wells, and Donlan (1998). Lexical incidence also causes problems if SSE is Scots-influenced, because *join* could be phonemically /jɒin/, *more* /mer/, *good* /gɪd/ and so on (Stuart-Smith, 2003; 2004).

Syllable structure

There have been no specifically Scottish studies on this topic.

Prosody

About intonation little is known, but informal observation clearly shows that "up-talk" can be found in primary school children whose parents do not use this feature, presumably acquired from their peer group.

Phonological awareness

Reid (2003) has developed a clinical tool intended to develop phonological awareness especially designed for the Scottish vowel system. Mayo (2000) includes a longitudinal study of phonemic awareness development in

15 monolingual and bilingual children with a starting age of between 5;2 and 6;0.

Speech assessment for Scottish English children

As mentioned earlier, the major resource, the *EAT* (Anthony et al., 1971) has also been applied widely outside Scottish English because it is a consonant assessment, and consonantal dialectal variation is minimal compared to vowel variation. Sadly, the test is now quite out of date, both in terms of some of the lexis and pictures that are used, and more problematically in the way the scoring relies on post-vocalic /r/, /θ/, and /ð/, which, as we have taken care to show, are undergoing change in Scotland.

Additional speech assessments developed in Scotland include:

- *Profiling Element of Prosodic Systems-Children* (PEPS-C; Peppé and McCann, 2003)

Speech intervention for Scottish English children

A number of studies have used Scottish children as participants or have been developed in Scotland, but there are no published packages designed specifically for Scottish English. Bates and Watson have substantial materials for the study of Scottish vowel systems (partly published as Bates, Watson, and Scobbie, 2002). Reid (2003) reports on *Vowel House*.

Electropalatography (EPG; Gibbon, 2006) is an important articulatory technique that has a tradition of research and development in Edinburgh (Hardcastle et al., 1991; Gibbon et al., 1999; Scobbie, Wood and Wrench, 2004) and now, following CE certification by Articulate Instruments Ltd. in 2005, can be used in speech therapy in a nonresearch clinical context. Treatment in cleftpalate centers is particularly highly developed (Gibbon, Smeaton-Ewins, and Crampin, 2005).

Working in Scotland

The Scottish Parliament has responsibility for health provision in Scotland, but currently there are no significant differences between Scotland and the rest of the UK. The Scottish university system offers honours undergraduate degrees over four years. The two available degree courses are validated by the Royal College of Speech and Language Therapists (RCSLT; see pg. 290) so that graduates gain a license to practice in the UK. Graduates in a relevant discipline can take a validated graduate diploma in two years. Overseas speech language therapists (SLTs) who wish to work in Scotland should consult Howard (see Chapter 27).

PHONETICALLY SPEAKING

Pronunciation of Scottish English: [ˈskoʔəʃ ˈəŋləʃ] / [ˈskɔtɪʃ ˈɪŋɡlɪʃ]

Passage: Comma Gets a Cure [ˈkʰɔmʌˌɡ̊etsəˈkˤʉˤɹ]

This is a medium-broad phonetic transcription of *Comma Gets a Cure* (Honorof, McCullough, and Somerville, 2000) which incorporates typical connected speech phenomena and intraspeaker variation for a representative "central-belt" speaker. Primary and secondary phrasal stresses are marked.

[ˈwɛɫ ˈçiˑɹz ʌ ˌstore fɔɹ jʌ ... ˈserʌ ˈpʰɛɹe wˑəzʌ ˈveɪˀtᵊnɹe ˈnʌɹs ˌʍʉd bin ˈwʌɹkɪn ˈdele ˌʔadn̩ ˌoɫ ˈdˤʉː ɪn ə dᵊˈzeɹˀtɪd ˈdːɪstɹɪkˀt ᵊf d̥ᵊ ˈtʰɛɹᵊtˑɹe ... so ʃe wɪz ˌveɹe ˈhape tʰ ˈstaˑʔt̚ ə ˌɲʉː ˈdʒɔb aɹa s̥ᵊˈpʰɛɹb̚ ˈpʰʲɹaevɪˀt̚ ˈpʰʲɹakˀtɪs n̩ ˈnɔɹθ ˈskweˑɹ n iᵊɹ ð̥ᵊ ˈdʒuk ˈstɹit̚ ˈtʰᵊuˀɹ... ˈda ˀʔeɹea wˑəz ˌmʌtʃ ˌniːᵊ foɹᵊɹ n̩ ˈmoɹ tʰᵊ ɹᵊ ˈlʌikɪn ... ˈiˑvn̩ ˈso ... ˌʔɔɹ̩ ˈfʌɹst ˈmɔɹnɪn ... ʃi ˌfɛˀ ˈstɹest ... ʃi ˌetʰ ʌ ˌbot ə ˈpʰɔɹᵊdʒ̊ ... ˈtʃɛkˀt ɹ əsˈɛɹf ᵊnə ˈmɪɹᵊ ... ⁿwɔʃt ɹ ˈfes n̩ᵊ ˈhʌɹe ... ˈden ʃi ˌpʰʉˀʔᵊnə ˈplen ˌjɛlo ˈdˤʑɛs nə ˌflis ˈdʒakɹ ... ˈpʰɪkˀ tʰʌpˀɹ ˈkʰi ... n̩ ˈhɛdɪd fɹ ˈwɪk ... ˌʍɛn ʃi ˈgoˀ ðeˑɹ ... ð̥ᵊ wˑəz e ˈwʉmɛn wɪθ ə ˈɡʉs ˌwetʰɪn fəɹ ɹ ... ð̥ᵊ ˈwʉmɛn ˈɡev ˌserʌ ʔʌn ᵊˈfɪʃɫ ˈletɹ fɹᵊm ð̥ᵊ ˈvɛt ... ðᵊ ˈlɛʔᵊɹ ɪmˈplaedˑʌˀ ðə ˈanəmɫ kʰᵊɹ bi ˈsʌfᵊʉɪɹ fɹɔm ə ˈɹeˑɹ ˌfoɹᵊm ᵊ ˈfuʔ n̩ ˈmʌʉθ d̥ᵊˈziːz̥ ... ˌʍɪtʃ wˑəz s̥ᵊˈpɹaezɪn ... b̥ᵊkʰɔz ˈnɔɹməᵊɫ ju ˌʍʉd ˀʔonle ᵊkˈspɛkˀtːhᵊ ˈsiˑ əˈtʰɪn ʌ ˌdɔɡ ... ˀʔɔɹ ˈgot ... ˈserʌ wˑəz ˌsɛnˀᵊˈmɛnˀtˌχ ... sə ˈðɪsˑmedɹ ˌfiˀt ˈsɔɹe fᵊ d̥ᵊ ˈbjuːɹʌft ˌb̥ʌˀd]

Well, here's a story for you: Sarah Perry was a veterinary nurse who had been working daily at an old zoo in a deserted district of the territory, so she was very happy to start a new job at a superb private practice in North Square near the Duke Street Tower. That area was much nearer for her and more to her liking. Even so, on her first morning, she felt stressed. She ate a bowl of porridge, checked herself in the mirror and washed her face in a hurry. Then she put on a plain yellow dress and a fleece jacket, picked up her kit and headed for work. When she got there, there was a woman with a goose waiting for her. The woman gave Sarah an official letter from the vet. The letter implied that the animal could be suffering from a rare form of foot and mouth disease, which was surprising, because normally you would only expect to see it in a dog or a goat. Sarah was sentimental, so this made her feel sorry for the beautiful bird (Honorof, McCullough, and Somerville, 2000).

RESOURCES

The identification code for Scots, defined in ISO 639, is "SCO", for English "EN", and for Scottish Gaelic "GD".

Books

An excellent starting point is Stuart-Smith (2004), which takes a broader view of Scottish English than is presented here. There are a number of books about speech and language in the UK with good sections on Scotland, such as Foulkes and Docherty (1999), Hughes, Trudgill, and Watt (2005), and Wells (1982). Specifically Scottish reference works with a strong linguistic content include Jones (1997), and especially Corbett et al., (2003). A more accessible introduction to urban Scottish English is Robinson and Crawford (2001), which provides copious exemplification as well as discussion. See also Rennie (1999) aimed at school children. To "teach yourself" Scots and as convenient references, we recommend Purves (1997) and Wilson (2002). Wilson (2002, p. 14) gives a warning, however, that "sadly, many speakers are likely to be unable at first to understand why anyone would even *want* to learn Scots, and to be suspicious of the motives of anyone who does so." Such attitudes are clearly relevant clinically, and it must not be forgotten that it is only a few decades since children even received corporal punishment at school for speaking Scots *with friends in the playground*.

Another useful clinical resource are the numerous children's books in Scots (e.g., from Itchy-coo or Merkat Press), and there are a large number of generally humorous dialect lexis books, fridge magnets, popular entertainments, and so on, which can provide information or materials for use with Scottish English speakers. More serious materials are also appearing in greater numbers, perhaps due in part to an increased interest in Scots in schools.

CD-ROMs

Robinson and Crawford (2001), Wilson (2002), Foulkes and Docherty (1999), and Hughes, Trudgill, and Watt (2005) have accompanying CDs. UK-wide acoustic resources (including Web sites as well as offline audio such as CDs) will typically include a Scottish dimension. For example, see *ABI: Accents of the British Isles corpus* (D'Arcy, Russell, Browning, and Tomlinson, 2004) and *The IvIE corpus: English Intonation in the British Isles* (Grabe, Post, and Nolan, 2001).

Journals

There are no SLT academic journals specific to Scotland. International journals published in the UK are:

- *The International Journal of Disorders of Communication*, http://www.tandf.co.uk/journals/titles/13682822.asp
- *Child Language Teaching and Therapy*, http://www.arnoldpublishers.com/journals/pages/chi_lan/02656590.htm
- *Clinical Linguistics and Phonetics*, http://www.tandf.co.uk/journals/titles/02699206.asp

Professional associations

The Royal College of Speech and Language Therapists (RCSLT) is the professional body, just as elsewhere in the UK. Two higher educational institutions train Speech and Language Therapists:

Queen Margaret University College, Edinburgh, http://www.qmuc.ac.uk/shs/default.htm

Strathclyde University, Glasgow, http://www.strath.ac.uk/eps/aboutslt.html

Useful Scottish English Web sites

- Scottish Language Dictionaries, http://www.scotsdictionaries.org.uk/
- The Scuil Wab ("school web"), http://www.scuilwab.org.uk/ Resources for children
- A Selected Classified Bibliography of the Scots Language, http://dinamico.unibg.it/anglistica/slin/scot-bib.htm
- BBC Voices, http://www.bbc.co.uk/voices/ (greatly expanded to include audio material)
- Scots Language Society, http://www.lallans.co.uk/
- The Elphinstone Kist, http://www.abdn.ac.uk/elphinstone/kist/
- Scottish Corpus of Text and Speech, http://www.scottishcorpus.ac.uk/
- Click and Listen, http://clydesdale.dcs.st-and.ac.uk/cnl3/welcome.htm
- Scots Language Resource Centre, http://www.scotsy-ett.com/
- Feasibility study for an Institute for the Languages of Scotland, http://www.arts.ed.ac.uk/celtscot/institutelanguagesscotland/
- Learning and Teaching Scotland, http://www.ltscotland.org.uk/

- 5-14 Online: Scots language, http://www.ltscotland. org.uk/5to14/specialfocus/scots/index.asp
- Scottish Cultural Resources Network, http://www. scran.ac.uk/homepage/

- The Speech Science Research Centre, http://www. qmuc.ac.uk/ssrc (This organization is putting a variety of resources online, including phonetic measurements and norms as well as reports of ongoing research on Scottish English.)

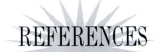

REFERENCES

Abercrombie, D. (1979). The accents of Standard English in Scotland. In A. J. Aitken and T. McArthur (Eds.), *Languages of Scotland* (pp. 65–84). Edinburgh: Chambers.

Aitken, A. J. (1981). The Scottish vowel length rule. In M. L. Benskin (Ed.), *So many people, languages, and tongues* (pp. 131–157). Edinburgh: Middle English Dialect Project.

Anthony, A., Bogle, D., Ingram, T. T. S., and McIsaac, M. W. (1971). *The Edinburgh Articulation Test.* Edinburgh: E & S Livingstone.

Aufterbeck, M. (2003). Alignment of the trailing L tone in Scottish H*+L nuclei. In M. J Solé, D. Recasens, and J. Romero (Eds.), *Proceedings of the 15ᵗʰ International Congress of Phonetic Sciences* (pp. 2937–2940). Barcelona: ICPhS.

Bates, S. A. R., Watson, J. M. M., and Scobbie, J. M. (2002). Context conditioned error patterns in disordered systems. In M. J. Ball and F. E. Gibbon (Eds.), *Vowel disorders* (pp. 145–185). London: Butterworth Heinemann.

Blackhall, S. (2003). *Loon.* Edinburgh: Itchy-Coo. [Published as S. Blackhall and H. MacDonald, *Double Heider: Twa novellas in Scots.*]

Chirrey, D. (1999). Edinburgh: descriptive material. In P. Foulkes and G. Docherty (Eds.), *Urban voices: Accent studies in the British Isles* (pp. 223–229). London: Arnold.

Corbett, J., McClure, J. D., and Stuart-Smith, J. (2003). A brief history of Scots. In J. Corbett, J. D. McClure, & J. Stuart-Smith (Eds.), *The Edinburgh companion to Scots* (pp. 1–16). Edinburgh: Edinburgh University Press.

D'Arcy, S. M., Russell, M. .J., Browning, S., and Tomlinson, M. J. (2004). The Accents of the British Isles (ABI) corpus. *Proceedings Modélisations pour l'Identification des Langues* (pp. 115–119) Paris: MIDL.

Esling, J. (1978). *Voice quality in Edinburgh: A sociolinguistic and phonetic study*, Unpublished Ph.D. thesis, University of Edinburgh.

Foulkes, P., and Docherty, G. J. (Eds.). (1999) *Urban voices: Accent studies in the British Isles.* London: Arnold.

Gibbon, F. E. (2006). *Bibliography of electropalatographic (EPG) studies in English (1957–2006).* Edinburgh: Queen Margaret University College.

Gibbon, F. E., Smeaton-Ewins, P., and Crampin, L. (2005). Tongue palate contact during selected vowels in children with cleft palate. *Folia Phoniatrica et Logopaedica, 57,* 181–192.

Gibbon, F. E., Stewart, F., Hardcastle, W. J., and Crampin, L. (1999). Widening access to electropalatography for children with persistent sound system disorders. *American Journal of Speech-Language Pathology, 8,* 319–333.

Gordeeva, O. B. (2005). *Language interaction in bilingual acquisition of sound structure: A longitudinal study of vowel quality, duration and vocal effort in pre-school children speaking Scottish English and Russian.* Unpublished Ph.D. Thesis, Queen Margaret University College, Edinburgh.

Gordeeva, O. B., and Scobbie, J. M. (2004). *Non-normative preaspiration of voiceless fricatives in Scottish English: A comparison with Swedish preaspiration.* Oral paper presented at the British Association of Academic Phoneticians (BAAP). Cambridge.

Grabe, E., Post, B., and Nolan, F. (2001). The IViE Corpus. University of Cambridge, Department of Linguistics. http://www.phon.ox.ac.uk/~esther/ivyweb

Hardcastle, W. J., Gibbon, F. E., and Jones, W. (1991). Visual display of tongue-palate contact: Electropalatography in the assessment and remediation of speech disorders. *British Journal of Disorder of Communication, 26,* 41–74.

Harris, J., Watson, J., and Bates, S. (1999). Prosody and melody in vowel disorder. *Journal of Linguistics, 35,* 489–525.

Hewlett, N., Matthews, B. M., and Scobbie, J. M. (1999). Vowel duration in Scottish English speaking children. In M. J Solé, D. Recasens, and J. Romero (Eds.), *Proceedings of the 14ᵗʰ International Congress of Phonetic Sciences* (pp. 2157–2160). San Francisco: ICPhS.

Honorof, D. N., McCullough, J., and Somerville, B. (2000). *Comma gets a cure: A diagnostic passage for accent study.* New Haven, CT: Haskins Laboratories.

Hughes, A., Trudgill, P., and Watt, D. (2005). *English accents and dialects* (4th Ed.). London: Arnold.

Johnston, P. (1997). Regional variation. In C. Jones (Ed), *The Edinburgh history of the Scots language* (pp. 433–513). Edinburgh: Edinburgh University Press.

Jones, C. (Ed.). (1997). *The Edinburgh history of the Scots language.* Edinburgh: Edinburgh University Press.

Ladd, D. R. (1996). *Intonational phonology.* Cambridge, UK: Cambridge University Press.

Lawson, E., and Stuart-Smith, J. (1999). A sociophonetic investigation of the "Scottish" consonants (/x/ and /hw/), in the speech of Glaswegian children. In J. Ohala, Y. Hasegawa, M. Ohala, D. Granville & A. Bailey (Eds.), *Proceedings of the 14th International Congress of Phonetic Sciences,* (pp. 2541–2544). San Francisco: ICPhS.

Macafee, C. (1983). *Varieties of English around the world: Glasgow.* Amsterdam: Benjamins.

Macafee, C. (1994). *Traditional dialect in the modern world: A Glasgow case study.* Frankfurt am Main: Peter Lang.

MacDonald, H. (2003). *The Girnin Gates.* Edinburgh: Itchy-Coo. [Published as S. Blackhall and H. MacDonald, *Double Heider: Twa novellas in Scots.*]

Marshall, J. (2004). *Language change and sociolinguistics: Rethinking social networks.* Basingstoke, UK: Palgrave Macmillan.

Matthews, B. M. (2001). *On variability and the acquisition of vowels in normally developing Scottish children (18–36 months).* Unpublished Ph.D. thesis, Queen Margaret University College, Edinburgh.

Mayo, C. (1996) *Transcription of Glasgow English: An evaluation study of GlaToBI.* Unpublished MSc thesis, Department of Linguistics, University of Edinburgh

Mayo, C. (2000) *The relationship between phonemic awareness and cue weighting in speech perception: Longitudinal and cross-sectional studies.* Unpublished Ph.D. thesis, Queen Margaret University College, Edinburgh.

McCann, J., Peppé, S,, Gibbon, F. E., O'Hare, A., and Rutherford, M. (2005). Prosody and its relationship to language in school-aged children with high-functioning autism. *QMUC Speech Science Research Centre Working Paper WP3.* Edinburgh: Queen Margaret University College.

Nathan, L., Wells, B., and Donlan, C. (1998). Children's comprehension of unfamiliar regional accents: A preliminary by three year olds. *Journal of Child Language, 25,* 343–365.

Peppé, S., and McCann, J. (2003). Assessing intonation and prosody in children with atypical language development: The PEPS-C test and the revised version. *Clinical Linguistics and Phonetics, 17,* 345–354.

Purves, L. C. (1997). *A Scots grammar.* Edinburgh: The Saltire Society.

Reid, J. (2003). The vowel house. *Child Language Teaching and Therapy, 19,* 152–180.

Rennie, S. (1999). *Grammar broonie.* Edinburgh: Polygon.

Robinson, C., and Crawford, C. A. (2001). *Scotspeak: A guide to the pronunciation of modern urban Scots.* Perth: Scots Language Resource Centre.

Romaine, S. (1978). Postvocalic /r/ in Scottish English: Sound change in progress. In P. Trudgill (Ed), *Sociolinguistic patterns in the British Isles* (pp. 144–157). London: Arnold.

Scobbie, J. M. (2005). Interspeaker variation among Shetland Islanders as the long term outcome of dialectally varied input: Speech production evidence for fine-grained linguistic plasticity. *QMUC Speech Science Research Centre Working Paper WP-2.* Edinburgh: SSRC.

Scobbie, J. M., Hewlett, N., and Turk, A. (1999). Standard English in Edinburgh and Glasgow: The Scottish vowel length rule revealed. In P. Foulkes and G. Docherty (Eds.), *Urban voices: Accent studies in the British Isles* (pp. 230–245). London: Arnold.

Scobbie, J. M., and Stuart-Smith, J. (2005, September). *Ongoing variation and change in Glasgow liquids: A pilot ultrasound study.* Paper presented at the Fifth Meeting of the UK Language Variation and Change Conference (UKLVC 5), University of Aberdeen.

Scobbie, J. M., and Stuart-Smith, J. (in press). Quasi-phonemic contrast and the fuzzy inventory: Examples from Scottish English. In P. Avery, E. Dresher, and K. Rice (Eds.), *Contrast: Perception and Acquisition: Selected papers from the Second International Conference on Contrast in Phonology.* Toronto: Mouton de Gruyter/University of Toronto.

Scobbie, J. M., Turk, A., and Hewlett, N. (1999). Morphemes, phonetics and lexical items: The case of the Scottish vowel length rule. In J. Ohala, Y. Hasegawa, M. Ohala, D. Granville and A. Bailey (Eds.), *Proceedings of the 14th International Congress of Phonetic Sciences* (pp. 1617–1620). San Francisco, CA: ICPhS.

Scobbie, J. M., Wood, S. E., & Wrench, A. A. (2004). Advances in EPG for treatment and research: An illustrative case study. *Clinical Linguistics and Phonetics, 18,* 373–389.

Scobbie, J. M., and Wrench, A. A. (2003). An articulatory investigation of word final /l/ and /l/-sandhi in three dialects of English. *Proceedings of the 15th International Congress of Phonetic Sciences* (pp. 1871–1874). Barcelona: ICPhS.

Scobbie, J. M., Wood, S.E., and Wrench, A.A. (2004) Advances in EPG for treatment and research; an illustrative case study, *Clinical Linguistics and Phonetics, 18, 373–389.*

Smith, J. (2003–2005). *Caregiver, community and child in the acquisition of variable dialect features.* ESRC funded project no RES-000-22-0447.

Smith, J. (2005). The sociolinguistics of contemporary Scots: Evidence from one dialect. In J. Kirk and D. P. O Baoill (Eds.), *Legislation, literature and sociolinguistics: Northern Ireland, the Republic of Ireland, and Scotland* (pp. 112–125). Belfast: Queen's University Press.

Speitel, H. H., and Johnston, P. (1983). *Socolinguistic investigation of Edinburgh speech.* Final Report to ESRC (Grant 000230023). Unpublished manuscript.

Stuart-Smith, J. (1999). Glasgow: Accent and voice quality. In P. Foulkes and G. Docherty (Eds.), *Urban voices: Accent studies in the British Isles* (pp. 203–222). London: Arnold.

Stuart-Smith, J. (2003). The phonology of modern urban Scots. In J. Corbett, J. D. McClure, and J. Stuart-Smith (Eds.), *The Edinburgh companion to Scots* (pp. 110–137). Edinburgh: Edinburgh University Press.

Stuart-Smith, J. (2004). The phonology of Scottish English. In B. Kortmann and E. W. Schneider (Eds.) A Handbook of Varieties of English, Volume 1 Phonology (pp. 47–67). Berlin Mouton de Gruyter.

Stuart-Smith, J., and Timmins, C. (in press a). "Tell her to shut her moof": The role of the lexicon in TH-fronting in Glaswegian. In G. Caie, C. Hough, and C. Kay (Eds.), *The power of words: Essays in lexicology in honour of Christian Kay.* Amsterdam: Rodopi.

Stuart-Smith, J., and Timmins, C. (in press b). Empirical evidence for gendered speech production: /s/ in Glaswegian. In J. Cole and J. Hualde (Eds.), *Change in phonology: Papers in laboratory phonology 9.* Amsterdam: Mouton de Gruyter.

Stuart-Smith, J., Timmins, C., and Tweedie, F. (2006), Conservation and innovation in a traditional dialect: L– vocalization in Glaswegian, *English World Wide, 27(1),* 71–87.

Stuart-Smith, J., and Tweedie, F. (2000). *Accent change in Glaswegian: A sociophonetic investigation.* Final Report to the Leverhulme Trust (Grant F/179/AX). Unpublished manuscript.

van Leyden, K. (2004). *Prosodic characteristics of Orkney and Shetland dialects: An experimental approach.* Utrecht, The Netherlands: LOT.

Watt, D., and Smith, J (2005). Language change. In M. J. Ball (Ed.), *Clinical sociolinguistics* (pp. 101–119). Oxford, UK: Blackwell.

Watt, D., and Tillotson, J. (2001). A spectrographic analysis of fronting in Bradford English. *English World-Wide, 2,* 269–302.

Wells, J. C. (1982). *Accents of English 2: The British Isles.* Cambridge, UK: Cambridge University Press.

Wilson, L. C. (2002). *Luath Scots language learner: An introduction to contemporary spoken Scots.* Edinburgh: Luath Press.

Windsor, F. (2002). *An acoustic investigation of gestural organisation for speech in typically developing children, phonologically disordered children and adults: A cross-sectional and longitudinal study.* Unpublished Ph.D. thesis. Queen Margaret University College, Edinburgh.

SUMMARY OF STUDIES OF TYPICAL SCOTTISH ENGLISH SPEECH ACQUISITION

Authors	Year	No.	Age	Information	Data collection	Sample type
Gibbon, Smeaton-Ewins, and Crampin	2005 onwards	30+	School age	Cleft-palate subjects from national CLEFTNET scheme	Short lists of individual words using the electropalatography (EPG) in the clinic	Clinical with intervention
Gordeeva	2001–2005	7	3;4–4;9	acoustic analysis of vowel quality, duration, vocal effort in close (-mid) vowels	Connected speech & single word, in home and laboratory	Cross-sectional & longitudinal, bilingual and monolingual
Hewlett, Matthews, and Scobbie	1999	7	6;0–9;0	Vowel duration (SVLR)	Single word, laboratory	Cross-sectional
Matthews	1999–2001	7	1;9–2;10	Transcriptional analysis of vowel system acquisition	Spontaneous speech	Longitudinal (monthly) semi-structured play

Authors	Year	No.	Age	Information	Data collection	Sample type
Peppé and McCann	2002–2006	120 controls & 70 children with Autism and Asperger's syndrome	Controls: 5–11 yearsHigh functioning Autism/Asperger's: 6–14 years	Expressive and receptive prosody, articulation errors	Speech production (single words and connected speech) and perception responses to ccomputerized PEPS-C test	Matched controls for studies on children with Autism and Asperger's syndrome
Scobbie, Gibbon, Hardcastle, and Fletcher	1993–1996	16 & 7 PD	4;0–6;0	acoustic analysis of word initial stops and clusters before /i/, /ʉ/ and /ai/	Single word in carrier phrase, laboratory and clinic, acoustic analysis.	Cross-sectional, PD longitudinal
Smith	2003–2005	24 parent-child pairs	pre-school	Buckie child speech and child-directed speech	Spontaneous carer-child speech in the home	Sociophonetic study, longitudinal
Stuart-Smith	1999–2004	44 working class and 8 middle class	10–15	consonants and vowels, spontaneous and read speech	Connected spontaneous dialogue speech and read wordlists collected in schools	Sociophonetic socially structured sample, cross-sectional
Waters	1992	12	3;8–4;10	VOT and other durations	Singlewords in carrier phases collected in the laboratory	Experimental: multiple repetitions
Windsor	2002	17 controls and 4 developmental phonological disorder	2;0–2;06 & 3;6–4;9	Phonological and acoustic measures	Connected spontaneous dialogue speech collected at home	Cross-sectional and longitudinal, structured play

Note. Studies were exclusively on normally developing (TD) children unless marked.

Future confirmed projects on Scottish children include a major MRC-funded EPG project on Down Syndrome, at QMUC.

Chapter 30

Australian English Speech Acquisition

Sharynne McLeod

INTRODUCTION

Australian English has many similarities to British English and is just over 200 years old. Australia was originally inhabited by Indigenous Australians (Aborigines) until British settlers arrived in 1788. The earliest accounts of Australian English highlight similarities with the Cockney accent from London, England (Cox, 1996). In contrast to many other countries, a similar form of Australian English is spoken throughout the entire continent of Australia.

Currently 20,000,000 people live in Australia. During the 1900s Australia changed from being a relatively homogeneous Anglo-Celtic population to "one of the world's most multicultural societies by 1996 when 16.2% had been born elsewhere" (Hugo, 2002). A further 8 percent of Australian-born people have at least one parent born in a country in which English is not the main language. Presently, Australia is experiencing an "accent shift" (Burridge and Mulder, 1998), possibly in part due to international globalization. The major language spoken in Australia is English, followed by Southern European languages (e.g., Greek, Italian) and Asian languages (e.g., Vietnamese, Cantonese). Only 20 of 200 Aboriginal languages are still spoken in Australia (Butcher, in press). See the Resources section in this chapter for materials pertaining to Australian English.

Where Australian English is spoken

Australian English is spoken by the majority of people within Australia (see the accompanying map and Appendix D).

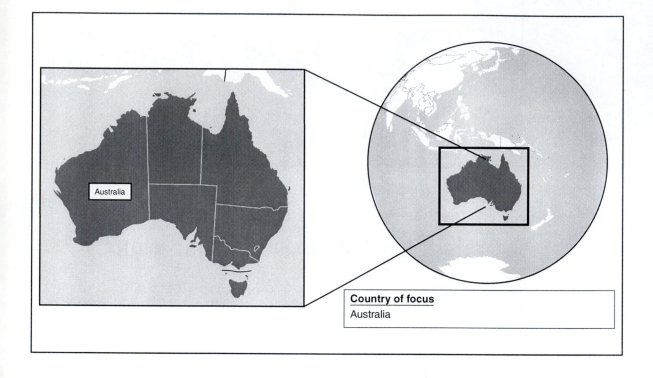

Country of focus
Australia

Components of Australian English

Consonants

Australian English has 24 consonants (see Table 30-1) and is most closely related to English as spoken in England (see Chapter 27). Saunders (2000) has produced a CD-ROM to listen to and use in transcribing Australian English using the International Phonetic Alphabet.

McLeod and Roberts (2005) documented tongue/palate contact for the production of Australian consonants (see Figure 30-1). These images provide the maximum point of contact for repeated productions of words containing lingual consonants by eight typical Australian adults using the electropalatograph (EPG). The horseshoe shape of the image is indicative of the hard palate. The circles represent electrodes that were contacted at least 50 percent of the time by the tongue during the production of each speech sound. For phonemes that are produced in word-initial and word-final position (e.g., /t/), each image represents an average of 480 productions of the sound. For phonemes that are produced in word-initial or word-final position only (e.g., /ŋ/),

each image represents an average of 240 productions of the sound.

Vowels and diphthongs

Key features of Australian English are the wide use of diphthongs and the frequent use of schwa in word-final position where speakers of General American English (GAE) would use an /r/-colored vowel. The following GAE vowels and diphthongs from Smit (2004) are not used by Australian English speakers: /o, e, ɑ, ɝ, ɚ, ɪr, ɛr, ɔr, ar/.

There are two common descriptions of Australian English vowels: one by Mitchell (1946) and the other by Harrington, Cox, and Evans (1997) (see Table 30-2). Mitchell and colleagues (1946, 1965a) documented the existence of 20 vowel sounds consisting of 12 monophthongs and 8 diphthongs in Australian speakers. The Mitchell system is still used in the *Macquarie* and *Australian Oxford* dictionaries and by many SLPs in Australia. However, Clark (1989) and later Harrington et al. argued that the Mitchell system does not accurately reflect Australian English pronunciation. Consequently, the Harrington et al. system was developed based on acoustic analysis of adults and adolescents. It has four degrees of length: high (close), high mid (half close), low mid (half open), low (open).

Phonotactic restrictions

Syllables

The syllable structure of Australian English is the same as for other varieties of English. Allowable syllable structures can be described in the following formula: $C_{(0-3)}VC_{(0-4)}$. The smallest allowable syllable is V and the largest allowable syllable is CCCVCCCC. One of the longest English words, in terms of the number of syllables is *antidisestablishmentarianism* (11 syllables). Commonly used words contain up to five syllables (e.g., *hippopotamus*).

Consonants and consonant clusters

To a large extent, the consonants and consonant clusters used within Australian English are similar to GAE. The major consonantal difference between Australian and GAE consonants is the use of the approximant /ɹ/. In Australian English "r" is not used in the word-final position in words such as *car*. This also reduces the number of allowable word-final consonant clusters (e.g., /-ɹk, -ɹt/ are not used in Australian English).

A further difference is that speakers of Australian English always use word-initial /j/ consonant clusters when followed immediately by /u/. These consonant clusters include /bj/ (e.g., *beautiful*), /mj/ (e.g., *music*), /fj/ (e.g., *few*), /dj/ (e.g., *dune*), /tj/ (e.g., *tune*), /kj/ (e.g., *cute*), /hj/ or /ç/ (e.g., *huge*).

Additionally the spirantization of final and medial /t/ in Australian English has been documented (Jones and McDougall, 2005; Horvath, 1985; Tollfree, 2001). Jones and McDougall conducted an acoustic study and found that females were likely to produce fricated /t/; and that it was more common in word-final and medial positions. They found that fricated /t/ was shorter and less intense than /s/ or /ʃ/ but had spectral qualities like /ʃ/. They indicated that the Australian frictionalized /t/ had a similarity to the Dublin Irish spirantized /t/.

Tones

Australian English does not use tones to differentiate meaning.

Stress and intonation

Speakers of Australian English often use a *high rising tone* (Fletcher, Stirling, Mushin, and Wales, 2002; Guy, Horvath, Vonwiller, Disley, and Rogers, 1986; McGregor, 1980). The high rising tone is characterized by a rising intonation on the last stressed syllable of an apparently completed statement. It does not occur consistently, but it is found more commonly in conversation, where it may seem to equate to "you know?" McGregor investigated the high rising tone and found that it occurred more often in female than in male speakers, more often in lower than in higher socioeconomic groups, and more often in younger than in older speakers.

Writing system

Australian spelling closely approximates British English spelling. Common differences between Australian English and GAE include the use of "ou" instead of "o" in words such as *colour* and *behaviour* and the use of "ise" instead of "ize" in words such as *memorise*.

Varieties of Australian English

Three accent styles of Australian English have been identified: Broad, General, and Cultivated (Mitchell and Delbridge, 1965a, b). Each is considered part of a continuum that enables a speaker to modify his or her speech into a more formal or relaxed style (Harrington et al., 1997). Mitchell and Delbridge (1965b) suggested that 11 percent of the population used Cultivated speech, which resembled the prestigious RP of British English (see Chapter 27); 34 percent used Broad speech, which possessed the stigmatized characteristics of the Australian accent; and 55 percent used General speech that was considered to be in between these two extremes. The major difference between these three varieties of Australian English relates to production of vowels and diphthongs. The differences are summarized in Table 30-3 (adapted from Burridge and Mulder, 1998, p. 63).

Additionally, there is some evidence of variants of consonant production within Australian English. Cruttenden (1994) as well as Horvarth (1985) have documented the following variations of Australian English consonants produced by some speakers, most likely with Broad speech:

- [n] for /-nd/ (e.g., *and*)
- [i] for /hi/ (e.g., *he*)
- [ɪn, ɪŋk] for /ɪŋ/ substitutions (e.g., *thing*)
- Vowelization [ʊ] of /l/ between a vowel and syllable-final consonant (e.g., *shelf*)
- Unreleased word-final plosives (e.g., *hat*)

According to McLeod and Eaton (2004) other common variants within general Australian English

TABLE 30-1   Consonants produced in Australian English

	Bilabial	Labiodental	Dental	Alveolar
Plosive	p b			t d
Nasal	m			n
Trill				
Tap or flap				(ɾ)
Fricative		f v	θ ð	s z
Lateral fricative	■	■	■	
Affricate				
Approximant	w (labiovelar)			ɹ
Lateral approximant	■	■	■	l

Black = articulations judged impossible

Based on the International Phonetic Alphabet. Courtesy of the International Phonetic Association (c/o Department of Linguistics, University of Victoria, Victoria, British Columbia, Canada).

pronunciation include [f, v] for /θ, ð/, [w] for /ɹ/ and interdentalized /s, z/ for /s, z/.

For many years it has been considered that the Australian accent has "no geographical or even cultural boundaries firmly drawn, and speakers of each of the main varieties might be found anywhere within the same city or town, and even within the same family" (Mitchell and Delbridge, 1965a, p. 13). Factors such as gender, family background, type of education, or regional differences appeared not to determine what variety of accent an

```
  /t/        /d/        /n/        /l/        /k/        /g/        /ŋ/

000000     000000     000000     000000     . . . . . .  . . . . . .  . . . . . .
00000000   00000000   00000000   00000000   . . . . . . . . . . . . . . . . . . . . . . . .
00000000   000.0000   000..000   00....00   . . . . . . . . . . . . . . . . . . . . . . . .
00....00   00....00   0......0   0......0   . . . . . . . . . . . . . . . . . . . . . . . .
0......0   0......0   0......0   .......0   0......0   0......0   0......0
0......0   0......0   0......0   . . . . . . .  0......0   0......0   0......0
0......0   0......0   0......0   . . . . . . .  00....00   00....00   00....00
0......00  0......     0......0   . . . . . . .  000.0000   00000000   000..000

  /s/        /z/        /ʃ/        /ʒ/        /r/        /j/

00..00     00..00     . . . . . .  . . . . . .  . . . . . .  . . . . . .
000..000   000..000   00......    00......    . . . . . . . . . . . . . . . .
00...000   00...000   000...00    000..000    . . . . . . . 0......0
00....00   00....00   00....00    000...00    . . . . . . . 00....00
0.....00   0.....00   00....00    00....00    0......0   00....00
0......0   0......0   00....00    00....00    0.....00   00....00
0......0   0......0   00....00    00....00    0......0   000...000
0......0   0......0   00....00    00....00    0......0   000..000
```

Figure 30-1   Tongue/palate contact for lingual consonants by Australian adults (adapted from McLeod & Roberts, 2005)

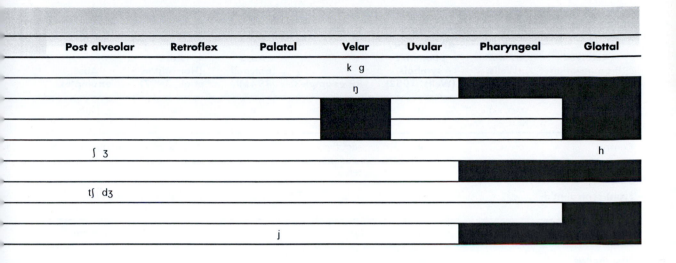

TABLE 30-2 Vowels produced in Australian English (AusE) compared to Received Pronunciation (RP)*

Received Pronunciation (RP) Location	KEY WORD (Wells, 1982)	RP phonetic/ phonemic symbols (Wells, 1982)	RP examples	AusE (Mitchell 1946)†	AusE (Harrington et al., 1997)	AusE examples
High-front	FLEECE	i	*beat*	i	iː	*b<u>ea</u>t*
	KIT	ɪ	*b<u>i</u>t*	ɪ	ɪ	*b<u>i</u>t*
Mid-low front	DRESS	ɛ	*b<u>e</u>d*	ɛ	ɘ	*b<u>e</u>d*
	TRAP	æ	*b<u>a</u>d*	æ	æ	*b<u>a</u>d*
High-back, rounded	GOOSE	u	*bl<u>ue</u>*	u	ʉː	*bl<u>ue</u>*
	FOOT	ʊ	*b<u>oo</u>k*	ʊ	ʊ	*b<u>oo</u>k*
Mid-back, rounded	THOUGHT, NORTH, FORCE	ɔ	*f<u>or</u>m*	ɔ	oː	*f<u>or</u>m*
Low back, rounded	LOT, CLOTH	ɒ	*dr<u>o</u>p*	ɒ	ɔ	*dr<u>o</u>p*

Table 30-2 continued

Received Pronunciation (RP) Location	KEY WORD (Wells, 1982)	RP phonetic/ phonemic symbols (Wells, 1982)	RP examples	AusE (Mitchell 1946)[†]	AusE (Harrington et al., 1997)	AusE examples
Low back,	START, BATH, PALM	ɑ	b<u>ar</u>d	a	ɐː	<u>car</u>, p<u>al</u>m
Central	COMMA, LETTER	ə	<u>a</u>bout, <u>o</u>ccur, <u>u</u>pon, nev<u>er</u>, zebr<u>a</u>	ə	ə	<u>a</u>bout, <u>o</u>ccur, <u>a</u>
Front-central-mid-open	NURSE	ɜ	b<u>ir</u>d	ɜ	ɜː	f<u>ur</u>, b<u>ir</u>d
	STRUT	ʌ	b<u>u</u>d	ʌ	ɐ	c<u>u</u>p, s<u>o</u>me
Diphthongs	PRICE	aɪ	m<u>y</u>, b<u>i</u>ke	aɪ	ɑe	m<u>y</u>, b<u>i</u>ke
	MOUTH	aʊ	<u>ou</u>t, m<u>ou</u>se	aʊ	æɔ	<u>ou</u>t, m<u>ou</u>se
	CHOICE	ɔɪ	b<u>oy</u>	ɔɪ	ɔɪ	b<u>oy</u>
	FACE	eɪ	b<u>ay</u>, b<u>ai</u>t	eɪ	æɪ	<u>ai</u>m, st<u>ay</u>
	GOAT	oʊ	b<u>oa</u>t, b<u>ow</u>(tie)	oʊ	əʉ	b<u>oa</u>t
	NEAR	ɪə	b<u>ee</u>r	ɪə	ɪə	h<u>e</u>re, n<u>ea</u>r
	SQUARE	ɛə	b<u>ea</u>r	ɛə	eː	<u>ai</u>r, c<u>a</u>re
	CURE	ʊə	t<u>our</u>	ʊə	ʊə	t<u>our</u>, s<u>ure</u>

Note. In Australian English the vowels corresponding to GOOSE, NURSE, COMMA, LETTER are centralized.

* Dr Felicity Cox, Macquarie University provided advice regarding the comparison between the Mitchell and Harrington et al. vowel transcription.

† Also used in the *Macquarie Dictionary*

individual used. This situation is unlike other countries such as England or the United States where diversity of regional and social accents is common (Ball, Rahilly, and Tench, 1996; Cruttenden, 1994). However, questions have arisen regarding previously drawn conclusions about the Australian English accent. More recently researchers have studied whether there are variations in accent (particularly geographical) or whether there has been a more widespread accent shift over time (Cox, 1999; Squires and McLeod, 2002, 2003). For example, Squires

TABLE 30-3 Allophonic differences between the three varieties of Australian English

	Cultivated	General	Broad	Exemplar word
/i/	[i]/[ɪi]	[əɪ]	[əɪ]	beat
/eɪ/	[ɛɪ]	[ʌɪ]	[ʌɪ]	bait
/oʊ/	[oʊ]	[ʌʊ]	[aʊ]	boat
/aɪ/	[aɪ]	[aɪ]	[ɒɪ]	bite
/aʊ/	[aʊ]	[æʊ]	[æʊ]	bout

Note. Adapted from Burridge and Mulder (1998, p. 63).

and McLeod (2003) documented that teenagers in rural Victoria produced [ɛ] for /æ/ before /l/ (e.g., [æl/əfənt] for /ɛləfənt/ *elephant)*.

Aboriginal English

More than 100 languages are spoken by Indigenous Australians; although fewer than 20 are widely used. Features of Australian languages include a small system of vowel contrasts, a large number of places of articulation for consonants, no voicing contrast, and no manner contrasts among obstruents (Butcher, in press). Approximately 80 percent of Indigenous Australians also speak a variety of Australian English: Aboriginal English (McKay, 1996). As with Australian English, there is a continuum of Aboriginal English, with variation occurring as a result of geographic location and the context of the interaction. Some of the features of Aboriginal English reflect features of Aboriginal languages (Harkins, 1994). Williams (2000, p. 70) provides a helpful summary of the features of Aboriginal English based on Kaldor and Malcolm (1991):

- Interdental fricatives may be replaced by labio-dental fricatives, or by alveolar plosives.
- The velar nasal may be replaced by an alveolar nasal (word final), or by a homorganic nasal-plosive cluster (mostly reported in the Sydney area).
- /h/ may be inserted before an initial vowel (mostly in southern metropolitan regions).
- /h/ deletion
- Alternation of voiced and voiceless plosives, particularly in nasal-plosive clusters
- Alternation of alveolar stops with a flap (e.g., *put it* – [pʊrət])
- Alternation of affricates and fricatives with palatals (e.g., *chicken* – [tjɪkən])
- Alternation of fricatives with stops
- Alternation of alveolar and palatal fricatives (e.g., *fish* – [fɪs])
- Alternation of diphthongs with short vowels (e.g., *home* – [hɒm])
- Reduction of consonant clusters, particularly in word-final position

Typical acquisition of Australian English

The Summary of Studies Table in this chapter contains studies of the Age of acquisition for Australian consonants and have been summarized in McLeod (2002).

Acquired sounds
Consonants

Table 30-4 contains age of acquisition data for males and females from studies by Chirlian and Sharpley (1982) and Kilminster and Laird (1978). Both studies used the criterion of 75 percent correct production in word-initial, -medial, and -final positions.

Consonant clusters

To date, there is no Australian cross-sectional study of the age of acquisition of consonant clusters. However, in a longitudinal study of young children, McLeod, van Doorn, and Reed (2001a) found that 2-year-old children could produce consonant clusters, but the productions often were not of the same form as the ambient language.

Vowels and diphthongs

According to James, van Doorn, and McLeod (2002), paradigmatic production of vowels (i.e., production of individual vowels) is generally mastered by 3 years. However syntagmatic production (production of vowels in contexts such as polysyllabic words) takes up to at least 6 years of age.

Percent correct
Consonants

Percentage of consonants produced correctly has been studied by two groups. Waring, Fisher, and Aitken (2001) reported that children produced a mean of 52/61 (85.2 percent) consonants correct at age 3;5–3;11. By 7;0–7;11 years of age, children produced a mean of 60/61 (98.4 percent) consonants correctly. James, van Doorn, and McLeod (2002) reported that by age 7;0–7;11, children produced 93.93 percent of consonants correctly in monosyllables and 90.99 percent of consonants correctly in polysyllables (see Table 30-5).

Consonant clusters

Percentage of consonant clusters produced correctly has been studied by Waring et al., (2001), who reported that children produced a mean of 51/59 (86.4 percent) consonant clusters correctly at age 3;5–3;11. By 7;0–7;11 years of age, children produced a mean of 58/59 (98.3 percent) consonants correctly (see Table 30-5).

Vowels

James, van Doorn, and McLeod (2002) reported that by age 7;0–7;11, children produced 95.10 percent of vowels

TABLE 30-4   Age of acquisition for Australian consonants

Consonant	Kilminster and Laird (1978)	Chirlian and Sharpley (1982)	Kilminster and Laird (1978)	Chirlian and Sharpley (1982)
	Males	Males	Females	Females
p	3;0	3;0	3;0	2;6
b	3;0	3;0	3;0	3;6
m	3;0	2;0	3;0	2;0
n	3;0	2;0	3;0	2;0
ŋ	3;0	2:6	3;0	2;6
h	3;0	3;0	3;0	2;0
w	3;0	3;0	3;0	2;6
j	3;0	3;6	3;6	3;0
t	3;0 then 4;6	3;6	3;0	2;6
d	3;0	2:6	3;0	2;6
k	3;6	3;0	3;0	2;6
g	3;0	3;0	3;6	2;0
f	3;6	3;6	3;0	3;0
l	4;6	3;6	3;6	4;0
ʒ	3;0	4;6	3;0	4;0
ʃ	4;6	3;6	4;0	3;6
tʃ	4;6	3;6	4;0	3;6
dʒ	4;6	3;6	4;0	4;0
s	4;6 then 6;6	4;0	4;6	3;6
z	4;6 then 6;6	*	4;6	9;0
ɹ	5;0	5;0	5;0	5;0
v	6;6	9;0	5;6	5;0
ð	*	7;6	7;6	7;6
θ	*	8;0	7;6	7;6

* = Sound was not produced correctly in 3 positions to criterion (75 percent)

correctly in monosyllables and 95.44 percent of vowels correctly in polysyllables (see Table 30-5).

Phonological processes

The most recent study of phonological processes in Australian children was conducted by James (2001a). She found that between 2 and 3 years of age there was a major decline of the following phonological processes: affrication, depalatization, gliding, metathesis, and prevocalic voicing. Between 3 and 4 years of age the following processes were declining: backing, cluster reduction, deaffrication, final consonant deletion, final devoicing, initial consonant deletion, labial assimilation, palatalization, stopping, unstressed syllable deletion, and fricative simplification. Between 5 and 6 years of age depaiatization, gliding, and glottal replacement were declining, and by 5 to 6 years of age deaffrication, epenthesis, metathesis, and fricative simplification of /v/ for /ð/ were declining.

TABLE 30-5 Percent correct for Australian consonants, consonant clusters, and vowels

Age	Consonants		Consonant clusters	Vowels	
	(James, van Doorn, and McLeod, 2002)		(Waring, Fisher, and Aitken, 2001)	(James, van Doorn, and McLeod, 2001)	
	Monosyllabic words	cf Monosyllabic Polysyllabic words		Monosyllabic words	cf Monosyllabic Polysyllabic words
3;0–3;11	76.77%	76.41%	86.4%	94.9%	88.28%
4;0–4;11	83.97%	82.45%	88.1%	95.2%	92.08%
5;0–5;11	89.54%	88.36%	94.9%	94.8%	94.3%
6;0–6;11	93.74%	90.76%	96.6%	95.39%	94.86%
7;0–7;11	93.93%	90.99%	98.3%	95.10%	95.44%

Intelligibility

To date there is no study of intelligibility of Australian children.

Phonetic inventory

To date there is no study of the phonetic inventory of consonants or vowels produced by Australian children. However, McLeod, van Doorn, and Reed (2001b) indicated that 2-year-olds' inventories of consonant clusters predominantly consisted of word-initial consonant clusters containing /w/ (e.g., [bw, kw]). By 3 years old, word-initial clusters predominantly contained /l/, /w/, or /s/ and common word-final clusters contained nasals (e.g., [-nd, -nt, -ŋk]).

Common mismatches

To date there is no study of common mismatches produced by Australian children.

Syllable structure

To date there is no study of syllable structure produced by Australian children, with the exception of the work of Dodd (1995), who had one Australian child among her British participants, and that child was similar to the British participants.

Prosody

To date there is no study of Australian children's prosody.

Phonological awareness

Dodd and Gillon (2001) report emerging phonological awareness skills between 3 and 4 years of age. They stated that "the majority of 4-year-old children...will not exhibit phonological awareness other than syllable segmentation and the emergence of rhyme awareness" (p.142). Typically, Australian children commence formal schooling between 5 and 6 years of age. Dodd and Gillon state that the following skills are reported to be established in Australian children between 5;0 and 6;5 years of age: syllable segmentation, rhyme awareness, alliteration awareness, and phoneme isolation. Between 6;6 and 6;11 years, phoneme segmentation is added.

Speech assessment for Australian children

Australian speech-language pathologists use many of the published tests of articulation and phonology produced in the USA and UK. However, the standardized norms are not relevant for Australian children. The target does not always correspond to Australian speech; for example, the word final /r/ in car is not produced by Australian children. Also, some test items are not readily apparent to Australian children; for example, in the Goldman-Fristoe Test of Articulation (Goldman and Fristoe, 1986), the picture of a squirrel is often misinterpreted by Australian children to be a possum.

McLeod and Baker (2004) surveyed 270 speech-language pathologists across Australia who worked with children with speech impairment and found that the most popular tests for assessing children's speech sounds were the following:

- *Articulation Survey* (Aitken and Fisher, 1996) (35.6 percent) (Australian)
- *Goldman-Fristoe Test of Articulation* (Goldman and Fristoe, 1986) (34.4 percent)

- Informal/homemade single-word tests (27.4 percent)
- Conversational speech sampling (20.7 percent)
- *Daz Roberts' Test of Articulation* (Roberts, 2000) (15.2 percent) (Australian)

Additional speech sampling tools have been developed for use with Australian children:

- *Diagnostic Evaluation of Articulation and Phonology (DEAP)* (Dodd, Hua, Crosbie, Holm, and Ozanne, 2003). Contains normative data for Australian children.
- *Assessment of Children's Articulation and Phonology* (ACAP) (James, 1995). The content of this test is documented in James (2001). It contains a representative number of polysyllabic words (including *Vegemite*).
- McLeod (1997) documented four procedures for assessing consonant clusters in Australian children. Two of these are also found in the appendix of McLeod et al. (2001b).

The following computerized analyses have been designed for Australian speech:

- *Computer Aided Speech and Language Assessment* (CASALA), http://www.medoto.unimelb.edu.au/people/blameyp/casala.html, documented in Serry, Blamey, Spain, and James (1997)
- *Computerized Profiling*, http://www.computerizedprofiling.org (Long, Fey, and Channell, 2004), includes the *Profile of Phonology* (PROPH+) component that has an Australian English option to assess pronunciation based on the Australian *Macquarie Dictionary*.

Speech intervention for Australian children

McLeod and Baker's (2004) survey indicated that the settings in which Australian speech-language pathologists worked included private practice (38.9 percent), community health centers (31.5 percent), education settings (18.2 percent), and hospitals (13.7 percent). The participants used a wide variety of service delivery models: the majority provided a mixture of individual therapy sessions (96.7 percent), parent training (71.5 percent), and home programming (73.3 percent) while some used group therapy (30.7 percent). Most worked in a clinic setting (75.2 percent) and/or in a preschool/school (61.5 percent) and were more likely to work with the child's parent (88.2 percent) than a teacher (48.9 percent) or teacher's aide (48.9 percent).

Australian speech-language pathologists are familiar with and use intervention techniques from many English-speaking countries. McLeod and Baker's (2004) survey found that the majority used traditional articulation and minimal pairs approaches during intervention. Table 30-6 summarizes the findings for the 10 most commonly used approaches.

The speech intervention techniques that have been developed in Australia include:

- *Parents and children together (PACT)* (Bowen and Cupples, 1998; 1999).
- *Cued articulation* (Passey, 1990a, b; 2003). A system of signed cues to highlight salient features of consonants and vowels. Each hand sign represents one phoneme.

TABLE 30-6 Intervention approaches commonly used by Australian speech-language pathologists when working with children with speech impairment

Approach	Authors	Use the approach
Traditional articulation therapy	Van Riper and Erickson (1996)	93.7%
Minimal pairs therapy	Weiner (1981)	91.5%
Core vocabulary	Bradford and Dodd (1997)	36.3%
Metaphon	Howell and Dean (1994)	30.0%
Combination of approaches	–	25.6%
Whole language approach	Hoffman, Norris, and Monjure (1990)	25.2%
Cycles approach	Hodson and Paden (1991)	21.1%
Maximal opposition contrast therapy	Gierut (1990)	16.3%
Psycholinguistic-based approach	Stackhouse and Wells (2001)	11.1%
Imagery approach	Klein (1996)	10.7%

• *Speech sounds on cue* (Bishop, 2000) (http://www. mmsp.com.au/ssoc.htm) A CD-ROM containing videos and photographs to facilitate production of consonants in isolation, words, and sentences.

Working in Australia

Most advertised jobs in Australia require eligibility for membership in Speech Pathology Australia (http://www.speechpathologyaustralia.org.au), the professional body for "speech pathologists." Speech pathologists who work in Australia come from around the world,

but typically their professional preparation occurs at one of the eight participating Australian universities (see the Resources section) during either a four-year undergraduate degree or a two-year postgraduate master's degree. A visa is needed from the Australian government in order for non-Australians to work in Australia. Speech Pathology Australia hosts an annual national conference attended by speech pathologists from across Australia and the world and publishes a clinical journal, *ACQuiring Knowledge in Speech, Language and Hearing,* and an international research journal, *Advances in Speech-Language Pathology* (to be renamed *International Journal of Speech-Language Pathology* in 2008) (see Resources).

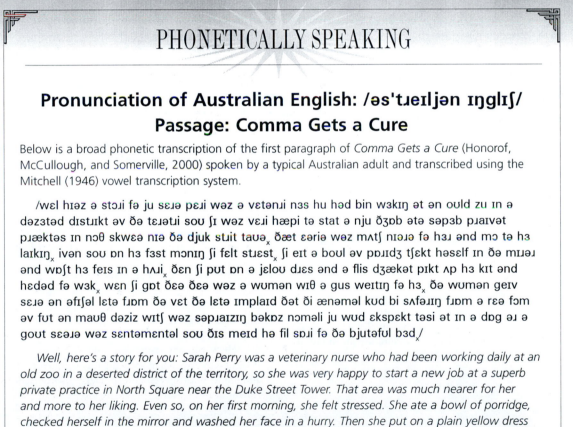

PHONETICALLY SPEAKING

Pronunciation of Australian English: /əsˈtɹeɪljən ɪŋɡlɪʃ/
Passage: Comma Gets a Cure

Below is a broad phonetic transcription of the first paragraph of *Comma Gets a Cure* (Honorof, McCullough, and Somerville, 2000) spoken by a typical Australian adult and transcribed using the Mitchell (1946) vowel transcription system.

/wɛl hɪəz ə stɔɹi fə ju sɛɹə pɛɹi wəz ə vɛtəɹɪnɹɪ nɜs hu həd bin wɜkɪŋ ət ən ould zu ɪn ə dəzɜtəd dɪstɹɪkt əv ðə tɛɹətɹi sou ʃi wəz vɛɹi hæpi tə stat ə nju dʒɒb ətə səpɜb pɹaɪvət pɹæktəs ɪn nɔθ skwɛə nɪə ðə djuk stɹit tauəx ðæt ɛəɹiə wəz mʌtʃ nɪɹ̩ə fə hɜ ənd mɔ tə hɜ laɪkɪŋx ivən sou ɒn hɜ fɜst mɔnɪŋ ʃi fɛlt stɹɛstx ʃi eɪt ə boul əv pɒɹɪdʒ tʃɛkt həsɛlf ɪn ðə mɪɹ̩ə ənd wɒʃt hɜ feɪs ɪn ə hʌɹ̩ix ðɛn ʃi pʊt ɒn ə jɛlou dɹɛs ənd ə flis dʒækət pɪkt ʌp hɜ kɪt ənd hɛdəd fə wɜkx wɛn ʃi ɡɒt ðɛə ðɛə wəz ə wʊmən wɪθ ə ɡus weɪtɪŋ fə hɜx ðə wʊmən ɡeɪv sɛɹə ən əfɪʃəl lɛtə fɹɒm ðə vɛt ðə lɛtə ɪmplaɪd ðət ði ænəməl kʊd bi sʌfɹ̩ɪŋ fɹɒm ə ɹɛə fɔm əv fʊt ən mauθ dəziz wɪtʃ wəz səpɹaɪzɪŋ bəkɒz nɔməli ju wʊd ɛkspɛkt təsi ɪt ɪn ə dɒɡ ɔɪ ə ɡout sɛɹə wəz sɛntəmɛntəl sou ðɪs meɪd hə fil sɒɹi fə ðə bjutəful bɜdx/

Well, here's a story for you: Sarah Perry was a veterinary nurse who had been working daily at an old zoo in a deserted district of the territory, so she was very happy to start a new job at a superb private practice in North Square near the Duke Street Tower. That area was much nearer for her and more to her liking. Even so, on her first morning, she felt stressed. She ate a bowl of porridge, checked herself in the mirror and washed her face in a hurry. Then she put on a plain yellow dress and a fleece jacket, picked up her kit and headed for work. When she got there, there was a woman with a goose waiting for her. The woman gave Sarah an official letter from the vet. The letter implied that the animal could be suffering from a rare form of foot and mouth disease, which was surprising, because normally you would only expect to see it in a dog or a goat. Sarah was sentimental, so this made her feel sorry for the beautiful bird (Honorof, McCullough, and Somerville, 2000).

RESOURCES

Books

Burridge, K., and Mulder, J. (1998). *English in Australia and New Zealand: An introduction to its history, structure, and use.* Melbourne: Oxford University Press.

Both *The Macquarie Dictionary* and *The Australian Concise Oxford Dictionary* contain Australian adult pronunciation of words using the International Phonetic Alphabet and the Mitchell (1946) transcription of Australian vowels.

CD-ROM

Saunders, N. (2000). [tu raɪt meɪt] 2000: Learning phonetic transcription through CD-ROM. *ACQuiring Knowledge in Speech, Language and Hearing* (October), 116–117.

Journals

- *Advances in Speech-Language Pathology,* http://www.tandf.co.uk/journals/titles/14417049.asp
  An international research journal published by Taylor and Francis in conjunction with Speech Pathology Australia (to be renamed *International Journal of Speech-Language Pathology* in 2008).
- *ACQuiring Knowledge in Speech, Language and Hearing,* http://www.speechpathologyaustralia.org.au/Content.aspx?p=46
  A clinical journal published by Speech Pathology Australia.
- *Asia-Pacific Journal of Speech Language and Hearing,* http://www.shrs.uq.edu.au/asiapacific/
  An international research journal published in conjunction with the Asia Pacific Society for the study of speech, language, and hearing.

Professional associations

The professional association of speech-language pathologists (called speech pathologists) within Australia is Speech Pathology Australia, http://www.speechpathologyaustralia.org.au

Universities

The following Australian universities offer courses to become a speech pathologist:

- Charles Sturt University
- Curtin University
- Flinders University of South Australia
- James Cook University
- LaTrobe University
- Macquarie University
- Newcastle University
- The University of Sydney
- University of Queensland

Useful Australian Web sites

- Dr Caroline Bowen, http://members.tripod.com/Caroline_Bowen/home.html
  An internationally recognized site containing resources for speech-language pathologists, teachers, parents, and children.
- Speech Hearing Language Research Centre, Department of Linguistics, Macquarie University, http://www.ling.mq.edu.au
- Extra Language Resources (eLr), http://www.elr.com.au/
  Speech pathology, language, and literacy resources, designed by Australian speech pathologists for children and adults with speech and language disorders, delayed learning, and reading support needs.

REFERENCES

Aitken, N. T., and Fisher, J. P. (1996). *Articulation survey.* Melbourne: Royal Children's Hosptial.

Ball, M. J., Rahilly, J., and Tench, P. (1996). *The phonetic transcription of disordered speech.* San Diego, CA: Singular.

Bishop, C. (2000). *Speech sounds on cue.* Miami: Queensland: Multimedia Speech Pathology.

Bowen, C., and Cupples, L. (1998). A tested phonological therapy in practice. *Child Language Teaching and Therapy,* 29–50.

Bowen, C., and Cupples, L. (1999). Parents and children together (PACT): A collaborative approach to phonological therapy. *International Journal of Language and Communication Disorders, 34,* 35–83.

Bradford, A., and Dodd, B. (1997). A treatment case study of inconsistent speech disorder. *Australian Communication Quarterly (Autumn),* 24–28.

Burridge, K., and Mulder, J. (1998). *English in Australia and New Zealand: An introduction to its history, structure, and use.* Melbourne: Oxford University Press.

Butcher, A. (in press). Australian aboriginal languages: Consonant-salient phonologies and the 'place-of-articulation imperative'. In J. M. Harrington and M. Tabain (Eds.), *Speech production: Models, phonetic processes and techniques.* New York: Psychology Press.

Chirlian, N. S., and Sharpley, C. F. (1982). Children's articulation development: Some regional differences. *Australian Journal of Human Communication Disorders, 10,* 23–30.

Clark, J. E. (1989). Some proposals for a revised phonetic transcription of Australian English. In P. Collins and D. Blair (Eds.), *Australian English: The language of a new society* (pp. 205–213). St Lucia: University of Queensland Press.

Cox, F. (1996). *An acoustic study of vowel variation in Australian English.* Unpublished doctoral thesis, Macquarie University, Sydney, Australia.

Cox, F. (1999). Vowel change in Australian English. *Phonetica, 56,* 1–27.

Cruttenden, A. (1994). *Gimson's pronunciation of English* (5th ed.). London: Arnold.

Dodd, B. (1995). Children's acquisition of phonology. In B. Dodd (Ed.), *Differential diagnosis and treatment of speech disordered children* (pp. 21–48). London: Whurr.

Dodd, B., and Gillon, G. (2001). Exploring the relationship between phonological awareness, speech impairment and literacy. *Advances in Speech-Language Pathology, 3,* 139–147.

Dodd, B., Hua, Z., Crosbie, S., Holm, A., and Ozanne, A. (2003). *Diagnostic Evaluation of Articulation and Phonology (DEAP).* London: Psychological Corporation.

Environmental Science Research Institute. (2004). Retrieved November 2, 2004 from http://www.esri.com/.

Fletcher, J., Stirling, L., Mushin, I., and Wales, R. (2002). Intonational rises and dialog acts in the Australian English Map task. *Language and Speech, 45*(3), 229–253.

Gierut, J. A. (1990). Differential learning of phonological oppositions. *Journal of Speech and Hearing Research, 33,* 540–549.

Goldman, R., and Fristoe, M. (1986). *Goldman-Fristoe Test of Articulation: Revised.* Circle Pines, MN: American Guidance Service.

Guy, G., Horvath, B., Vonwiller, J., Disley, E., and Rogers, I. (1986). An intonational change in progress in Australian English. *Language & Society, 15*(3), 23–52.

Harkins, J. (1994). *Bridging two worlds.* Brisbane: Queensland University Press.

Harrington, J., Cox, F., and Evans, Z. (1997). An acoustic phonetic study of broad, general, and cultivated Australian English vowels. *Australian Journal of Linguistics, 17,* 155–184.

Hodson, B. W., and Paden, E. P. (1991). *Targeting intelligible speech: A phonological approach to remediation* (2nd ed.). Austin, TX: Pro-Ed.

Hoffman, P. R., Norris, J. A., and Monjure, J. (1990). Comparison of process targeting and whole language treatments for phonologically delayed preschool children. *Language, Speech, and Hearing Services in Schools, 21,* 102–109.

Honorof, D. N., McCullough, J., and Somerville, B. (2000). *Comma gets a cure: A diagnostic passage for accent study.* New Haven, CT: Haskins Laboratories.

Horvath, B. M. (1985). *Variation in Australian English: The sociolects of Sydney.* Cambridge, UK: Cambridge University Press.

Howell, J., and Dean, E. (1994). *Treating phonological disorders in children. Metaphon: Theory to practice* (2nd ed.). London: Whurr.

Hugo, G. (2002). *Year book Australia: Centenary article—A century of population change in Australia.* Retrieved December, 2003, from http://www.abs.gov.au/Ausstats/abs@.nsf/Lookup/0B82C2F2654C3694CA2569DE002139D9

Ingram, J. C. L. (1989). Connected speech processes in Australian English. *Australian Journal of Linguistics, 9,* 21–49.

Ingram, J., Pittman, J., and Newman, D. (1985). Developmental and sociolinguistic variation in the speech of Brisbane school children. *Australian Journal of Linguistics, 5,* 233–246.

James, D. G. H. (1995). *Assessment of Children's Articulation and Phonology.* Adelaide: Author.

James, D. G. H. (2001a). The use of phonological processes in Australian children aged 2 to 7:11 years. *Advances in Speech-Language Pathology, 3,* 109–128.

James, D. G. H. (2001b). An item analysis of Australian English words for an articulation and phonological test for children aged 2 to 7 years. *Clinical Linguistics and Phonetics, 15,* 457–485.

James, D., McCormack, P., and Butcher, A. (1999). Children's use of phonological processes in the age range of five to seven years. In S. McLeod and L. McAllister (Eds.), *Proceedings of the 1999 Speech Pathology Australia National Conference* (pp. 48–57). Melbourne: Speech Pathology Australia.

James, D. G. H., van Doorn, J., and McLeod, S. (2001). Vowel production in mono-, di- and polysyllabic words in children aged 3;0 to 7;11 years. In L. Wilson and S. Hewat (Eds.),

Proceedings of the Speech Pathology Australia National Conference (pp. 127–136). Melbourne: Speech Pathology Australia.

James, D., van Doorn, J., and McLeod, S. (2002). Segment production in mono-, di- and polysyllabic words in children aged 3–7 years. In F. Windsor, L. Kelly, and N. Hewlett (Eds.), *Themes in clinical phonetics and linguistics* (pp. 287–298). Hillsdale, NJ: Lawrence Erlbaum.

Jones, M., and McDougall, K. (2005, September). *An acoustic study of fricated realisations of /t/ in Australian English*. Paper presented at the UK Language Variation and Change 5, University of Aberdeen.

Kaldor, S., and Malcolm, I. (1991). *Aboriginal English: An overview*. In S. Romaine (Ed.), *Language in Australia*. Cambridge, UK: Cambridge University Press.

Kilminster, M. G. E., and Laird, E. M. (1978). Articulation development in children aged three to nine years. *Australian Journal of Human Communication Disorders, 6*, 23–30.

Klein, E. S. (1996). Phonological/traditional approaches to articulation therapy: A retrospective group comparison. *Language, Speech, and Hearing Services in Schools 27*, 314–323.

Long, S., Fey, M., and Channell R. (2004). Computerized Profiling (MS-DOS version 9.6) [computer software]. Milwaukee, WI: Marquette University.

Malcolm, I., Haig, Y., Konigsberb, P., Rochecouste, J., Collard, G., Hill, A., et al. (1999). *Two way English: Towards more user-friendly education for speakers of Aboriginal English*. Perth: Education Department of Western Australia.

Masterson, J., and Bernhardt, B. H. (2001). *Computerized articulation and phonology evaluation system*. San Antonio, TX: The Psychological Corporation.

McCormack, P. F., and Knighton, T. (1996). *Gender differences in the speech patterns of two and a half year old children*. Paper presented at the Speech Science and Technology: Sixth Australian International Conference, Adelaide.

McGregor, R. L. (1980). The social distribution of an Australian English intonation contour. *Working Papers, 2*(6), 1–26. School of English and Linguistics, Macquarie University, Australia.

McKay, G. (1996). *The land still speaks*. Canberra: Australian Government Publishing Service.

McLeod, S. (1997). Sampling consonant clusters: Four procedures designed for Australian children. *Australian Communication Quarterly, Autumn*, 9–12.

McLeod, S. (2002). Part I: The plethora of available data on children's speech development. *ACQuiring Knowledge in Speech, Language and Hearing, 4*, 141–147.

McLeod, S., and Baker, E. (2004). Current clinical practice for children with speech impairment. In B. E. Murdoch, J.

Goozee, B. M. Whelan, and K. Docking (Eds.), *Proceedings of the 26th World Congress of the International Association of Logopedics and Phoniatrics*. Brisbane: University of Queensland.

McLeod, S., and Eaton, J. (2004). Speech sound production by tertiary students. *ACQuiring Knowlege in Speech, Language and Hearing, 6*, 109–112.

McLeod, S., and Roberts, A. (2005). Templates of tongue/palate contact for speech sound intervention. In C. Heine and L. Brown (Eds.), *Proceedings of the 2005 Speech Pathology Australia National Conference* (pp. 104–112). Melbourne: Speech Pathology Australia.

McLeod, S., van Doorn, J., and Reed, V. A. (2001a). Consonant cluster development in two-year-olds: General trends and individual difference. *Journal of Speech, Language, Hearing Research, 44*, 1144–1171.

McLeod, S., van Doorn, J., and Reed, V. A. (2001b). Normal acquisition of consonant clusters. *American Journal of Speech-Language Pathology, 10*, 99–110.

Mitchell, A. G. (1946). *The pronunciation of English in Australia*. Sydney: Angus & Robertson.

Mitchell, A. G., and Delbridge, A. (1965a). *The pronunciation of English in Australia*. Sydney: Angus & Robertson.

Mitchell, A. G., and Delbridge, A. (1965b). *The speech of Australian adolescents: A survey*. Sydney: Angus & Robertson.

Ozanne, A. E. (1992). Normative data for sequenced oral movements and movements in context for children aged three to five years. *Australian Journal of Human Communication Disorders, 20*, 47–63.

Passey, J. (1990a). *Cued articulation*. Melbourne: Australian Council for Educational Research.

Passey, J. (1990b). *Cued vowels*. Melbourne: Australian Council for Educational Research.

Passey, J. (2003). *Cued articulation: A handful of sounds*. Melbourne: Australian Council for Educational Research Press.

Roberts, D. (2000). *Daz Roberts' test of articulation*: Daz Roberts.

Saunders, N. (2000). [tu raɪt meɪt] 2000: Learning phonetic transcription through CD-ROM. *ACQuiring Knowledge in Speech, Language and Hearing* (October), 116–117.

Serry, T., Blamey, P., Spain, P., and James, C. (1997). CASALA: Computer Aided Speech and Language Analysis. *Australian Communication Quarterly, Spring*, 27–28.

Smit, A. B. (2004). *Articulation and phonology: Resource guide for school-age children and adults*. Clifton Park, NY: Delmar Learning.

Squires, S., and McLeod, S. (2002). The Australian accent: An historical overview of research. *ACQuiring Knowledge in Speech, Language and Hearing, 4*(3), 122–125.

Squires, S., and McLeod, S. (2003). Australian vowels produced by rural Victorian female teenagers in /hVd/ and /hVl/ contexts. In C. Williams and S. Leitao (Eds.), *Speech Pathology Australia National Conference* (pp. 65–71). Hobart: Speech Pathology Australia.

Stackhouse, J., Wells, B. (2001). *Children's speech and literacy difficulties: Identification and intervention.* London: Whurr.

Tollfree, L. (2001) Variation and change in Australian English consonants: Reduction of /t/. In D. Blair and P. Collins (Eds.), *Varieties of English around the world: English in Australia* (pp. 45–67). Amsterdam: John Benjamins.

Van Riper, C., and Erickson, R. L. (1996). *Speech correction: An introduction to speech pathology and audiology* (9th ed.). Boston, MA: Allyn & Bacon.

Waring, R., Fisher, J., and Aitkin, N. (2001). The articulation survey: Putting numbers to it. In L. Wilson. and S. Hewat. (Eds.), *Proceedings of the 2001 Speech Pathology Australia national conference: Evidence and innovation* (pp. 145–151). Melbourne: Speech Pathology Australia.

Weiner, F. (1981). Treatment of phonological disabilty using the method of meaningful minimal contrast: Two case studies. *Journal of Speech and Hearing Disorders, 46,* 97–103.

Wells, J. C. (1982). *Accents of English.* Cambridge, UK: Cambridge University Press.

Williams, C. (2000). Language in Aboriginal Australia: Aboriginal English. *ACQuiring Knowlege in Speech, Language and Hearing, 2*(2), 70–72.

SUMMARY OF STUDIES OF TYPICAL AUSTRALIAN ENGLISH SPEECH ACQUISITION

Authors	Year	Country	No. of children	Age of children	Information	Sample type	Data collection
Chirlian and Sharpley	1982	Australia	1357	2;6–9;0	Age of acquisition of consonants	Single word	Cross-sectional
Dodd	1995	UK and Australia	5	1;8–3;0	Variety	Connected speech	Longitudinal
James, McCormack, and Butcher	1999	Australia	240	5;0–7;11	Phonological processes in	Single word	Cross-sectional
Ingram	1989	Australia	26 samples	Grades 8 and 10	Phonological processes in connected speech	Connected speech	Cross-sectional
Ingram, Pittman, and Newman	1985	Australia	97	5;8–9;5	Phonological processes	Single word and connected speech	Cross-sectional
James	2001a, b	Australia	50	2;0–7;11	Phonological processes	Single word	Cross-sectional
James, van Doorn, and McLeod	2001	Australia	354	3;0–7;11	Vowels (polysyllabic words)	Single word	Cross-sectional
James, van Doorn, McLeod,	2002	Australia	354	3;0–7;11	Consonants (polysyllabic words)	Single word	Cross-sectional
Kilminster, and Laird	1978	Australia	1756	3;0–9;0	Age of acquisition of consonants	Single word	Cross-sectional
McCormack and Knighton	1996	Australia	50	2;6	Phonological processes	Single word in connected speech	Cross-sectional

Authors	Year	Country	No. of children	Age of children	Information	Sample type	Data collection
McLeod and Roberts	2005	Australia	8	adults	Tongue placement (EPG)	Single word	Cross-sectional
McLeod, van Doorn, and Reed	2001a	Australia	–	–	Consonant clusters	–	Compilation
McLeod, van Doorn, and Reed	2001b	Australia	16	2;0–3;4	Consonant clusters	Connected speech	Longitudinal
McLeod, van Doorn, and Reed	2002	Australia	16	2;0–3;4	Consonant clusters	Connected speech	Longitudinal
Ozanne	1992	Australia	180	3;0–5;5	Oromotor skills	Oromotor	Cross-sectional
Waring, Fisher, and Aitken	2001	Australia	299	3;5–7;11	Consonants and consonant clusters	Single word	Cross-sectional

Chapter 31

New Zealand English
Speech Acquisition

Margaret Maclagan and Gail Gillon

INTRODUCTION

New Zealand English is the youngest native speaker variety of English in the world, having been spoken for less than 200 years (see Gordon et al., 2004). The first English-speaking sealers and whalers came to New Zealand in the late eighteenth century, but it was not until after the Treaty of Waitangi was signed with the Maori in 1840 that English speakers arrived in any number. A recognizable variety of New Zealand English (NZE) started to appear by the 1870s (Gordon et al., 2004). NZE is similar to southern British English. A consistent variety of NZE is spoken throughout the country except for the south of the South Island, where there was a higher proportion of Scottish settlers and where post-vocalic /r/ can still be heard (Bartlett, 1992). The population of New Zealand is just over 4 million, approximately 15 percent of whom are Maori. The major language spoken in New Zealand is English, followed, especially in the North Island, by Polynesian languages (Maori, Samoan, Tongan). There has always been immigration from European countries, and in the last two decades, there has been considerable immigration from Asian countries. Although much work has been done on NZE as a variety of English, relatively little work is available on the acquisition of the variety. See the Resources section in this chapter for materials pertaining to NZE.

Where New Zealand English is spoken

New Zealand English (NZE) is spoken in New Zealand. In the Cook Islands, Cook Islands Maori and NZE are spoken (see accompanying map and Appendix D).

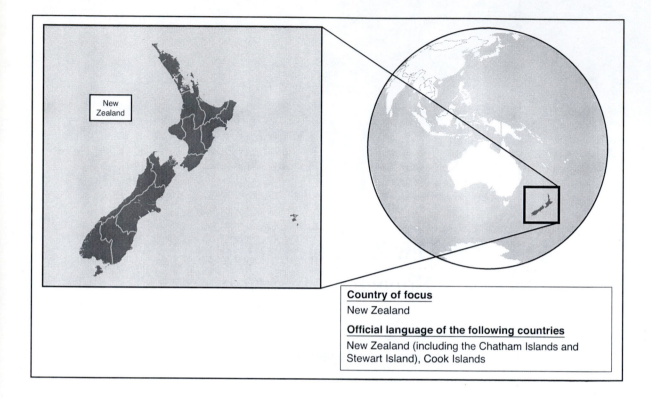

Country of focus
New Zealand

Official language of the following countries
New Zealand (including the Chatham Islands and
Stewart Island), Cook Islands

Components of New Zealand English

Consonants

NZE has 24 consonants and is most closely related to Australian English and then to British English (see Table 31-1). The rhotic consonant is usually realized as an approximant: [ɹ]. Final /p, t, k/ can have glottal reinforcement, and intervocalic /t/ is increasingly realized as a flap. Final voiced fricatives are devoiced, but the preceding vowel usually remains long.

Vowels and diphthongs

The vowels of NZE are shown in Table 31-2 together with an indication of their usual articulation. Because NZE is not rhotic and because it derives from British English, the NZE vowels have been compared with the vowels of the Received Pronunciation of Great Britain (RP) (see Chapter 27) rather than General American English (GAE) (see Chapter 22). The major differences between NZE and GAE vowels are the omission of the set of rhotic vowels from NZE and the interpretation of /ei/ FACE[1] and /oʊ/ GOAT as closing diphthongs in NZE rather than as monophthongs as in GAE. NZE has 11 monophthongs. Because of the central articulation of the KIT /ɪ/ vowel, it is questionable whether it is distinct from the neutral vowel, COMMA /ə/ realized as schwa. Nonfinal unstressed syllables are usually realized with KIT /ɪ/ (e.g., *cricket* /kɹɪkɪt/). There are five closing diphthongs, FACE /ei/, PRICE /ai/, MOUTH /aʊ/, GOAT /oʊ/, and CHOICE /ɔi/, though unrounding in the second element of MOUTH /aʊ/ means that it is realized as a centering diphthong [æə] or [ɛə] for many speakers. One of the most characteristic features of NZE is the merger of the NEAR /iə/ and SQUARE /eə/ vowels, so that

---

1 Throughout the text, words in small capitals refer to the KEY WORDS of Wells (1982). Vowels in KEY WORDS are surrounded by unique consonants, so that the consonants indicate the intended phoneme, whatever the accent in which the word is spoken. Each KEY WORD refers to its specific phoneme and also to the set of words in which the phoneme occurs. One advantage of using key words is that it shows where NZE does not make distinctions that GAE or RP do make. For example, GAE has different sounds for COMMA /ə/ and LETTER /ɚ/, or for BATH/PALM/START (all of which are /ɑ/ in NZE), whereas NZE does not.

both are now realized with a close front onset (Gordon and Maclagan, 2001). CURE /ʊə/ is relatively rare, with words that traditionally took CURE /ʊə/ being realized with GOOSE /u/ plus schwa [tʉə] or THOUGHT /ɔ/ with [tɔ] for *tour*. The long-short monophthong pairs for NZE are FLEECE /i/ ~ DRESS /ɛ/ and START /a/ ~ STRUT /ʌ/.

Phonotactic restrictions

As in other varieties of English, /ŋ/ cannot occur in the onset of a syllable and /h/, /w/, and /j/ cannot occur in the coda. NZE is a nonrhotic variety of English, so /r/ does not appear in coda position. Both linking /r/ (*car alarm*) and intrusive /r/ (*law-r-and order*) are usually present.

Syllables

The syllable structure of NZE can be described in the formula $C_{(0-3)}VC_{(0-4)}$. The smallest allowable syllable is V (e.g., *I, a*) and the largest allowable is CCCVCCCC as in *strengths* /stɹɛŋkθs/. Syllable structure in NZE is similar to Australian English.

Consonants and consonant clusters

Consonant clusters in NZE are similar to British and GAE. Three consonant clusters occur only in onsets and always start with /s/ followed by a plosive, /p, t, k/, and an approximant /ɹ, j, w/. In NZE, as in Australian English, the approximant, /ɹ/ [ɹ], does not occur in syllable final position. This reduces the number of coda clusters in that /-ɹC/ is not used (*dark* is /dak/ not [daɹk]). As in Australian English, /j/ often precedes /u/ in clusters such as /bj/ *beautiful*, /mj/ *music*, /fj/ *few*, /kj/ *cute*. /tj/ and /dj/ are usually assimilated to [tʃ] (*tune*) and [dʒ] (*duty*). TH-fronting, whereby /θ/ becomes /f/ and /ð/ becomes /v/, is increasing in NZE (Wood, 2003).

Tones

NZE does not use tones to differentiate meaning.

Stress and intonation

The most commonly noted feature of NZE intonation is the use of the high rising terminal intonation pattern (HRT) (Britain, 1992). HRT patterns are used particularly in narratives and at the beginning of conversations. They do not signal questions, but rather serve as feedback devices where speakers are checking that the listeners have understood them (see Ainsworth, 1994 for the development of HRT in children).

Writing system

The Roman alphabetic system is used for NZE.

Varieties of New Zealand English

There is only one recognized regional variety of NZE, which is spoken in Southland, in the south of the South Island (Gordon and Maclagan, 2004). This variety of NZE is partially rhotic with younger speakers using rhotic NURSE vowels only, possibly as a mark of Southland identity (see Bartlett, 1992). The most common variation within NZE is Maori English, an ethnic variety (see Holmes, 1997; King 1995, Warren and Bauer, 2004). Maori English is more common in the North Island of New Zealand, and among younger speakers, especially males. It is particularly common in the armed forces. As with other ethnic varieties of English, not all Maori speak Maori English, and non-Maori New Zealanders who live and/or work in close association with Maori may speak this variety of English. It is distinguished from General NZE by its more syllable-timed rhythm, by extremely front GOOSE /u/ vowels, by less diphthongization, especially in FACE /ei/ and GOAT /oʊ/, by devoicing of final /z/ (with shortening of the preceding vowel), and by vocabulary (*bro* for *brother, cuz* for *cousin, sis* for *sister*), and discourse features such as increased use of the high rising terminal intonation pattern and the particle *eh* at the end of utterances. None of these features is restricted to Maori English. All of them appear in General NZE, but are more common in Maori English.

Typical acquisition of New Zealand Speech

There is a paucity of research documenting the speech development of New Zealand children. In particular, little is known about early speech acquisition for Maori children who may be exposed to both English and Maori language in their home or early education environment. Speech assessments implemented as part of the Dunedin Multi-disciplinary Child Development Study in 1981 (Silva, McGee, and Williams, 1981), such as the Dunedin Articulation Check (Justin, Lawn, and Silva, 1983), provided initial insights into the speech acquisition of New Zealand 7-year-old children. This screening speech test required children to articulate 20 words and was administered

TABLE 31-1   Consonants produced in New Zealand English

	Bilabial	Labiodental	Dental	Alveolar
Plosive	p b			t d
Nasal	m			n
Trill				
Tap or flap				
Fricative		f v	θ ð	s z
Lateral fricative	███████████████████████████			
Affricate				
Approximant	w (labiovelar)			ɹ
Lateral approximant	███████████████████████████			l

Black = articulations judged impossible

Based on the International Phonetic Alphabet. Courtesy of the International Phonetic Association (c/o Department of Linguistics, University of Victoria, Victoria, British Columbia, Canada).

to 872 children from Dunedin Schools in the South Island. Girls performed significantly better than boys. Analysis indicated over 90 percent of the sample articulated the following words correctly: *fly, liked, ride, jam,* and *splashed.* Common errors occurred on words requiring the articulation of *th* (e.g., *thumb*), and the misarticulation of two multisyllabic words, *ambulance* and *hospital.* The most difficult word in the screening sample for 7-year-old children to articulate was *frothy,* with only 25 percent of the sample articulating this word correctly.

Recent research has provided further insight into the speech development of young school-aged New Zealand children in the 5- to 8-year-old age group (Gillon and Schwarz, 1999, 2001; Moyle, 2004, 2005). Gillon and Schwarz (2001) administered a spoken language-screening test including a single-word articulation subtest to 972 6-year-old children, 48 percent male and 52 percent female. The single-word articulation subtest required each child to spontaneously name the following 14 pictures: *boats, fork, glasses, game, leaf, nose, rock, soap, spoon, star, watch, car, sheep, bath.* Analysis of the children's articulation of these target words was based on the articulation of consonant sounds only, not including vowel distortion errors. The findings indicated that 20 percent of the children tested required further assessment of their articulation skills. These children presented with errors on two to eight consonant sounds in different test items or multiple error types (Gillon and Schwarz, 1999).

Moyle (2004, 2005) provided normative data for 5- to 8-year-old New Zealand children by administering the *New Zealand Articulation Test (NZAT)* to 1,013 children

aged between 5 and 8 years. The NZAT assesses all word-initial, word-medial, and word-final consonants except medial /h/, /w/, /j/, /ʒ/ and final /ʒ/, /l/, /r/, /θ/, and /w/. There were significant effects for age, gender in the 5- and 6-year-old age groups, and socioeconomic status and ethnicity in all but the 8-year-old age group. Evaluation of age-related changes in speech production showed that girls developed more complex speech sounds such as triple clusters and interdental fricatives earlier than boys. The study concluded there was no significant effect of geographical region or population density on articulation performance in New Zealand children. From analysis of the data, Moyle (2005) concluded that most New Zealand children begin school at 5 years of age with a full inventory of speech sounds. A minority of children are yet to acquire some affricate, glide, blends, and fricative sounds at 5 years.

Acquired sounds

Consonants

Age of acquisition data for children younger than 5 is not available. Moyle (2004), however, provides insight into acquisition of speech in 5- to 8-year-old children. By 5 years 6 months of age, close to 90 percent or more of both boys and girls show correct articulation of the following consonants in initial, medial, and final positions in words: /p, b, t, d, k, g, f, v, m, n, l, h, r, w, j, ŋ, s, z, ʃ, tʃ, dʒ/. The consonant that has not been mastered by this age is /θ/ (as in <u>thumb</u>). Only around 20 percent of 5-year-old children articulated this sound

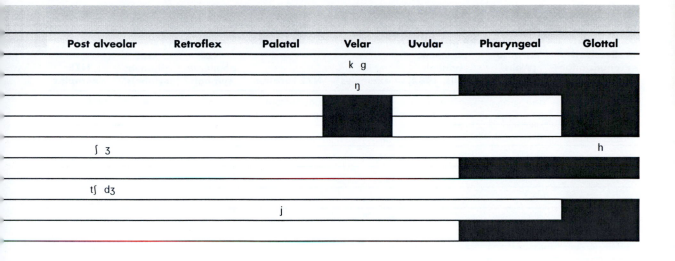

Post alveolar	Retroflex	Palatal	Velar	Uvular	Pharyngeal	Glottal
			k g			
			ŋ			
ʃ ʒ						h
tʃ dʒ						
		j				

TABLE 31-2   Vowels produced in New Zealand English (NZE) compared to Received Pronunciation (RP)

Received Pronunciation (RP) Location	KEY WORD (Wells, 1982)	RP phonetic/ phonemic symbols (Wells, 1982)	RP examples	NZE Location	NZE phonemic symbols	NZE phonetic symbols*	NZE examples
High-front	FLEECE	i	b*ea*t	high-front	i	iː ɪ̵	b*ea*t
	KIT	ɪ	b*i*t	mid-close central	ɪ	ə	b*i*t
Mid-low front	DRESS	ɛ	b*e*d	mid-close front	e	e	b*e*d
	TRAP	æ	b*a*d	mid-open front	æ	ɛ	b*a*d
High-back, rounded	GOOSE	u	bl*ue*	close central, rounded	u	ʉː	bl*ue*
	FOOT	ʊ	b*oo*k	mid-close, mid-back, rounded**	ʊ	ʊ ̝	b*oo*k
Mid-back, rounded	THOUGHT, NORTH, FORCE	ɔ	f*or*m	close, back rounded	ɔ	oə	f*or*m
Low back, rounded	LOT	ɒ	dr*o*p	mid-open, back, rounded	ɒ	ǫ	dr*o*p
Low back	START, BATH, PALM	ɑ	b*ar*d	central-front, open	a	ẹː	b*ar*d
Central	COMMA, LETTER	ə	*about*, *occur*, *upon*,	central	ə	ə	*about*, *occur*, *upon*, butt*er*
Front-central-mid-open	NURSE	ɜ	b*ir*d	front, mid-close	ɜ	ö:	b*ir*d

Table 31-2 continued

Received Pronunciation (RP) Location	KEY WORD (Wells, 1982)	RP phonetic/ phonemic symbols (Wells, 1982)	RP examples	NZE Location	NZE phonemic symbols	NZE phonetic symbols*	NZE examples
	STRUT	ʌ	*bud*	central-front, open,	ʌ	ɐ̝	*bud*
Diphthongs	PRICE	aɪ	*my, b*i*ke*	Diphthongs	ai	ɐe ɑe	*my, b*i*ke*
	MOUTH	aʊ	*out, m*ou*se*		aʊ	æə	*out, m*ou*se*
	CHOICE	ɔɪ	*b*oy		ɔɪ	oe	*b*oy
	FACE	eɪ	*bay, bait*		eɪ	ɐe	*bay, bait*
	GOAT	oʊ	*boat, bow (tie)*		oʊ	ɐʉ	*boat, bow(tie)*
	NEAR	ɪə	*beer*		iə	iə	*beer*
	SQUARE	ɛə	*bear*		iə	iə	*bear*
	CURE	ʊə	*tour*	often realized as THOUGHT /ɔ/	ʊə	ʉə oə	*tour*

Note. Data from Wells (1982).

*NZE phonetic symbols are based on Bauer and Warren (2004)

** Foot is becoming more centralized and less rounded

correctly in Moyle's study. At 8 years of age, approximately 70 percent of girls and 60 percent of boys articulate /θ/ correctly in word-initial position.

Comparison of the Moyle data with the earlier NZAT norms (based on 1957 and 1931 USA and UK data) showed that the acquisition ages for most sounds were earlier for the current New Zealand norms. This is congruent with past research showing that acquisition ages tend to become earlier over time (Smit, Hand, Freilinger, Bernthal, and Bird, 1990). The /θ/ phoneme

was the only sound that was acquired later by the New Zealand sample, with 71 percent of the 8-year-old New Zealand children producing the phoneme correctly compared with 90 percent of the earlier sample. The authors concluded that the large difference between American and New Zealand data for the acquisition of /θ/ points to a dialectal rather than a developmental difference between the two populations. The Summary of Studies Table at the end of this chapter contains studies of the acquisition of NZE.

TABLE 31-3 Percent of consonants correct for New Zealand English by children with typical speech and language development

Age (months) Mean (SD)	PCC Mean (SD)	Number of Children	Study
42 (3.6)	89 (7.2)	N = 19	Gillon (2005)
55 (2.4)	91 (7.7)	N = 20	Sutherland and Gillon (2005)
61 (3.0)	95 (5.1)	N = 20	Sutherland and Gillon (2005)
67 (3.3)	97 (2.6)	N = 20	Sutherland and Gillon (2005)
74 (4.5)	98 (2.6)	N = 30	Gillon (2000)

Consonant clusters

More than 90 percent of 5-year-old New Zealand children have mastered /l/ clusters /bl, pl, kl, gl, sl, fl/. Between 80 and 90 percent of 5-year-old girls demonstrate articulation accuracy on all common consonant clusters in word-initial position, but boys take longer to master three-element consonant clusters (i.e., /spr/, /str/, and /skr/). Between 6 and 7 years of age 80 percent or more of the male population have achieved accurate articulation of triple consonant clusters (Moyle, 2004).

Vowels and diphthongs

Data are not available for children who speak NZE.

Percent correct

Consonants

Table 31-3 provides summary information for the percentage of consonants correctly articulated (PCC score) for NZE children. In each study in Table 31-3, the PCC score was derived by combining the spontaneous production of single words in the *Goldman-Fristoe Test of Articulation* Sounds in words subtest (Goldman and Fristoe, 1986) with the 25 words from the *Phonological Variability Test* (Dodd, 1995). PCC scores were calculated using computer analysis software, *Computerized Profiling: PROPH+* (Long, Fey, and Channell, 2002).

Consonant clusters and vowels

Data are not available for children who speak NZE.

Phonological processes

Refer to discussion of typical acquisition of speech.

Intelligibility

Data are not available for children who speak NZE.

Phonetic inventory

Data are not available for children who speak NZE.

Common mismatches

Gillon and Schwarz (1999) classified errors made by the 972 6-year old children in their study into substitution, distortion, and omission errors and calculated the percentage of participants who had normal speech, one sound affected, two sounds affected, or more than two sounds affected by the respective error types. This analysis showed substitution errors (e.g., saying /baf/ for *bath* or /toʊn/ for *cone*) were more common than distortion errors (e.g., lisping) and omission errors (e.g., saying /ta/ for *star*). The authors found that 44 percent of participants exhibited substitution errors. However, most of these children (32 percent) made only one substitution error and this was typically either an /f/ for /θ/ substitution or a /w/ for /r/ substitution. A total of 9 percent of the participants exhibited distortion errors and 4 percent of participants exhibited omission errors.

Syllable structure

Data are not available for children who speak NZE.

Prosody

Data are not available for children who speak NZE.

Phonological awareness

Gillon and Schwarz (2001) investigated New Zealand children's phonological awareness development in the spoken language-screening test administered to 972 6-year-old children. The phonological awareness screening required the children to complete a phoneme blending task (e.g., blend the phonemes /l/ /ɒ/ /s/ /t/ together to make *lost*), a phoneme segmentation task (e.g., segment the word *man* into individual phonemes: /m/ /æ/ /n/), a rhyme production task (e.g., "Tell me a word that rhymes with *book*") and demonstrate the use of phonological information in the reading process through a nonword reading task of nonwords with a consonant-vowel-consonant structure (e.g., *dat*, *lek*). The results indicated that the children found the phoneme segmentation the most challenging task, but on average they still demonstrated an approximate success rate of 50 percent of the items presented. They showed the greatest success in generating rhyming words, with an average success rate of close to 75 percent. Moderate correlations between the children's performance on the phonological awareness task and the children's reading performance were obtained.

The data also showed that girls performed significantly better on the phonological awareness tasks than the boys, non-Maori children performed better than Maori children, and children who attended schools in higher socioeconomic neighborhoods performed better than children in lower socioeconomic communities. Approximately 18 percent of the total sample were identified as requiring further in-depth assessment in their phonological awareness skills due to poor performance on the screening items.

Gillon and Young (2002) investigated the phonological awareness development in 19 New Zealand children (aged between 7 and 15 years) who were blind and using only Braille as their reading medium. The *Queensland University Inventory of Literacy* (Dodd, Holm, Oerlemans, and McCormick, 1996) was administered to measure the children's phonological awareness skills at the syllable, rhyme, and phoneme level and assess their use of phonological awareness in reading and spelling nonwords. In general, the participants showed the same pattern of development as children with normal sight (i.e., they found syllable and rhyme tasks easier than phoneme segmentation tasks). They demonstrated the most difficulty in using phonological information to read and spell nonwords. A significant relationship was evident between their performance on phonological awareness tasks and on Braille reading measures.

The cross-linguistic effect of phonological awareness development demonstrated in European languages is also evident for New Zealand children who are bilingual. For example, 6-year-old New Zealand children who are bilingual in Samoan and English demonstrate comparable levels of phonological awareness in both languages after a relatively short exposure to English reading instruction (Hamilton and Gillon, 2006).

Speech assessment for children who speak New Zealand English

Speech assessment tools developed for English-speaking children in America, Australia, and Britain as well as tests that contain normative data for New Zealand children are commonly used in New Zealand. Examples of such tests are the following:

- *The New Zealand Test of Articulation* (Moyle, 2004)
- *Hodson Assessment of Phonological Patterns*, (3rd ed.) (Hodson, 2004)
- *Diagnostic Evaluation of Articulation and Phonology* (Dodd, Zhu, Crisbie, Holm, and Ozanne, 2002)
- *Goldman-Fristoe Test of Articulation-2* (Goldman and Fristoe, 2000).

Additional speech sampling tools that have been developed for use with New Zealand English children include:

- *Systematic Analysis of Language Transcripts—New Zealand version* (Gillon, Westerveld, Miller, and Nockerts, 2002)
- *New Zealand Spontaneous Language Sampling Protocol* (Westerveld and Gillon, 2002)

The following are examples of tests that have been designed for analyzing NZE speech:

- *A Speech and Language Screening Test for Academic Success* (Gillon and Schwarz, 2001).
- *New Zealand Articulation Test* (Moyle, 2004)
- *Dunedin Articulation Screening Scale* (Silva, 1980)
- *Dunedin Articulation Check* (Justin, Lawn, and Silva, 1983).

Speech intervention for children who speak New Zealand English

The speech intervention techniques that have been developed for NZE include evidence-based speech intervention techniques adopted internationally for English languages.

Phonological awareness intervention

A series of successful controlled intervention trials has demonstrated that New Zealand children with moderate or severe speech impairment respond positively to phonological awareness intervention. Interventions developed to stimulate phonological awareness at the phoneme level and integrate letter sound knowledge have proven effective for New Zealand children in these areas:

- Resolving phonological awareness deficits and improving reading and spelling development in 5- to 7-year-old children with speech impairment (Gillon, 2000, 2002; Gillon et al., 2004)
- Enhancing phonological awareness development and later literacy development in 3- to 4-year-old children with unintelligible speech (Gillon, 2005)
- Enhancing phonological and early print awareness in young preschool children with Down syndrome (Van Bysterveldt, Gillon, and Moran, 2006)
- Improving speech production, phonological awareness, and literacy development in 5- to 7-year-old children with childhood apraxia of speech (Moriarty and Gillon, 2006)

Case study data have also suggested phonological awareness treatment effectiveness for children in New Zealand who are Samoan and are bilingual in Samoan and English (Hamilton and Gillon, 2005), nonverbal children with complex communication needs using alternative communication techniques (Clendon, Gillon, and Yoder, 2005), and New Zealand children who are blind and use Braille as their reading medium (Gillon, 2004).

Working in New Zealand

Most employers of speech and language therapists in New Zealand require individuals to be members of the New Zealand Speech-Language Therapists' Association or to be eligible for membership in the Association (see the Association Web page, www.nzsta-speech.org.nz for details). The New Zealand Ministry of Education employs speech-language therapists to work with preschool and school-aged children with a range of speech and language disorders. In particular, emphasis is placed on serving the needs of school children with severe communication impairment (refer to www.minedu. org.nz, Special education, for further details). District health boards employ speech-language therapists to work across the age span from infancy to the elderly in a variety of settings. Private organizations also employ speech-language therapists to work with varying populations, for example, organizations that serve the needs of individuals with traumatic brain injury.

PHONETICALLY SPEAKING

Pronunciation of New Zealand English: [nju zɪələnd əŋgləʃ]

Passage: Comma Gets a Cure

Below is a broad phonetic transcription of *Comma Gets a Cure* (Honorof, McCullough, and Somerville, 2000) spoken by a typical adult speaker of New Zealand English.

/wɛɤ hiəz ə stoɹi fə ju. seːɹə peɹi wəz ə vetɹənɹi nɵs, hu əd bin wɵkɪŋ deeli ət ən oɤ zu ən ə dəzɤtəd dəʃtɹɪkt əv ðə teɹətʃɹi seɤ ʃi wəz veɹi hɛpi tə stät ə nju dʒǫb ət ə səpɵb pɹeəvət pɹæktəs ən nǫθ skwiə niə ðə dʒʉk ʃtrit tæə. ðɛt eɹiə wəz mʉtʃ niəɹə fo hə, ənd mǫ tə hə leekɪŋ. ivən seʉ, ən ə fɵs mǫnɪŋ, ʃi fɛɤ ʃtrest. ʃi æet ə bʉʉl əv pǫɹedʒ, tʃɛkt əsæɤf ən ðə mɹəɹ, ən wǫʃt ə fees ən ə hɐɹi. ðen ʃi put ǫn ə pleen jæləʉ dʒɹes ənd ə flɹis dʒɛkət ən hedəd fə wɵk. wen ʃi gǫt ðiə, ðə wəz ə wʉmən wəθ ə gʉs weetɪŋ fə ɹ ə. ðə wʉmən gɐev seːɹə ən əfəʃʉɤ leɹə fɹəm ðə vet. ðə leɹə ɹ əmpleəd ðə ɛnəmʉɤ kəd bi sɐfɹɪŋ fɹəm ə riə fǫm əv fut ən mæəθ dəziiz, wətʃ wəz səpɹeezɪŋ, bəkəz nǫməli jəd ɐuni əkspek tə si ət ə nə ə dǫg ǫɹ ə gɐʉt. seːɹə wəz sentəmentəɤ, seʉ ðəs mæəd ə fɪɤ sǫɹi fə ðə bjʉɤtəfʉɤ bɵd./

Well, here's a story for you: Sarah Perry was a veterinary nurse who had been working daily at an old zoo in a deserted district of the territory, so she was very happy to start a new job at a superb private practice in North Square near the Duke Street Tower. That area was much nearer for her and more to her liking. Even so, on her first morning, she felt stressed. She ate a bowl of porridge, checked herself in the mirror and washed her face in a hurry. Then she put on a plain yellow dress and a fleece jacket, picked up her kit and headed for work. When she got there, there was a woman with a goose waiting for her. The woman gave Sarah an official letter from the vet. The letter implied that the animal could be suffering from a rare form of foot and mouth disease, which was surprising, because normally you would only expect to see it in a dog or a goat. Sarah was sentimental, so this made her feel sorry for the beautiful bird. (Honorof, McCullough & Somerville, 2000).

RESOURCES

Books

Gordon, E., Campbell, L., Hay, J., Maclagan, M., Sudbury, A., and Trudgill, P. (2004). *New Zealand English: Its origins and evolution.* Cambridge, UK: Cambridge University Press.

Schneider, E., Burridge, K., Kortmann, B., Mesthrie, R., and Upton, C. (Eds.). (2004). *A handbook of varieties of English: Vol. 1. Phonology.* Berlin and New York: Mouton de Gruyter. See chapters by Bauer and Warren; Gordon and Maclagan; and Warren and Bauer referenced above.

CD-ROMs

A CD-ROM is included in Kortmann, B., and Schneider, E., with Burridge, K., and Mesthrie, R. (Eds.). (2004) *A handbook of varieties of English: A multimedia reference tool.* Berlin and New York: Mouton de Gruyter.

Journals

- *Te Reo,* http://www.vuw.ac.nz/lals/about/NZLS/NZLingSoc.html#anchor147797
- This is the official journal of the Linguistic Society of New Zealand.

- *New Zealand English Journal,* http://www.vuw.ac.nz/lals/publications/nzej.aspx
- The function of this journal is to bring research on the varieties of English spoken in New Zealand to a wider audience.
- *New Zealand Journal of Speech-Language Therapy,* http://www.nzsta-speech.org.nz/publications.htm#New%20Zealand%20Speech-Language%20Therapists%20Journal

Professional associations

The professional association of speech-language therapists within New Zealand is the New Zealand Speech-Language Therapists' Association. http://www.nzsta-speech.org.nz/

Useful New Zealand English Web site

- New Zealand English, http://www.ualberta.ca/%7Ejohnnewm/NZEnglish/home.html
- This Web site contains up-to-date information about New Zealand English, including demonstration sound files.

REFERENCES

Ainsworth, H. (1994). The emergence of the high rising terminal contour in the speech of New Zealand children. *Te Reo, 37,* 3–20.

Bartlett, C. (1992). Regional variation in New Zealand English, the case of Southland. *New Zealand English Newsletter, 6,* 5–15.

Bauer, L., and Warren, P. (2004). New Zealand English: Phonology. In E. Schneider, K. Burridge, B. Kortmann, R. Mesthrie, and C. Upton (Eds.), *A handbook of varieties of English: Vol. 1. Phonology* (pp. 580–602). Berlin and New York: Mouton de Gruyter.

Britain, D. (1992). Linguistic change in intonation, the use of high rising terminals in New Zealand English. *Language Variation and Change, 4,* 77–104.

Clendon, S., Gillon, G., and Yoder, D. (2005). Initial insights into phoneme awareness intervention for children with complex communication needs. *International Journal of Disability, Development and Education, 52*(1), 7–31.

Dodd, B. (1995). *Differential diagnosis and treatment of children with speech disorder.* London: Whurr.

Dodd, B., Holm, A., Oerlemans, M., and McCormick, M. (1996). *Queensland University Inventory of Literacy.* University of Queensland, Australia: Department of Speech Pathology and Audiology.

Dodd, B., Zhu, H., Crosbie, S., Holm, A. and Ozanne, A. (2002). *Diagnostic Evaluation of Articulation and Phonology.* London: Psychological Corporation.

Gillon, G. T. (2000). The efficacy of phonological awareness intervention for children with spoken language impairment. *Language, Speech, and Hearing Services in Schools, 31,* 126–141.

Gillon, G. T. (2002). Follow-up study investigating benefits of phonological awareness intervention for children with spoken language impairment. *International Journal of Language and Communication Disorders, 37*(4), 381–400.

Gillon, G. T. (2004). *Phonological awareness: From research to practice.* New York: Guilford Press.

Gillon, G. T. (2005). Facilitating phoneme awareness development in 3- and 4-year-old children with speech impairment. *Language, Speech, and Hearing Services in Schools, 36,* 308–324.

Gillon, G., Moran, C., Hamilton, E., Bayne, G., Smith, D., & Zens, N. (2004, August). *Phonological awareness treatment effects.* Paper presented at the International Association of Logopedics and Phoniatrics, Brisbane, Australia.

Gillon, G. T., and Schwarz, I. E. (1999). *Resourcing speech and language needs in special education: Database and best practice validation.* Wellington, New Zealand: Ministry of Education.

Gillon, G. T., and Schwarz, I. E. (2001). Screening New Zealand children's spoken language skills for academic success. In L. Wilson and S. Hewat (Eds.), *Proceedings of the 2001 Speech Pathology Australia National Conference: Evidence and Innovation* (pp. 207–214). Melbourne: Speech Pathology Australia.

Gillon, G., Westerveld, M., Miller J., and Nockerts, A. (2002). Systematic analysis of language transcripts—New Zealand Version [Computer software]. Canterbury, New Zealand: University of Canterbury, Department of Communication Disorders.

Gillon, G. T., and Young, A. A. (2002). The phonological-awareness skills of children who are blind. *Journal of Visual Impairment and Blindness, 96,* 38–49.

Goldman, R., and Fristoe, M. (1986). *Goldman-Fristoe Test of Articulation.* Circle Pines. MN: American Guidance Service.

Goldman, R., and Fristoe, M. (2000). *Goldman-Fristoe Test of Articulation.* (2nd ed). Circle Pines. MN: American Guidance Service.

Gordon, E., Campbell, L., Hay, J., Maclagan, M., Sudbury, A. & Trudgill, P. (2004). *New Zealand English: Its origins and evolution.* Cambridge, UK: Cambridge University Press.

Gordon, E., and Maclagan, M. A. (2001). Capturing a sound change: A real time study over 15 years of the NEAR/SQUARE diphthong merger in New Zealand English. *Australian Journal of Linguistics, 21*(2), 215–238.

Gordon, E., and Maclagan, M. (2004). Regional and social differences in New Zealand: Phonology. In E. Schneider, K. Burridge, B. Kortmann, R. Mesthrie, and C. Upton (Eds.), *A handbook of varieties of English: Vol. 1. Phonology* (pp. 603–613). Berlin and New York: Mouton de Gruyter.

Hamilton, E. M., and Gillon, G. T. (2005) Phoneme awareness intervention for Samoan children. *New Zealand Journal of Speech Language Therapy, 60,* 48–54.

Hamilton, E. M., and Gillon, G. T. (2006). The phonological awareness skills of school-aged children who are bilingual in Samoan and English. *Advances in Speech-Language Pathology 8*(2), 57-68.

Hodson, B. (2004). *Hodson Assessment of Phonological Patterns* (3rd ed). Austin, TX: Pro-Ed.

Holmes, J. (1997). Maori and Pakeha English: Some New Zealand social dialect data. *Language in Society, 26,* 65–101.

Honorof, D. N., McCullough, J., and Somerville, B. (2000). *Comma gets a cure: A diagnostic passage for accent study.* New Haven, CT: Haskins Laboratories.

Justin, C., Lawn, L., and Silva, P. (1983). *The Dunedin Articulation Check.* Dunedin, New Zealand: Otago Speech Therapy Association.

King, J. (1995). Maori English as a solidarity marker for te reo Maori. *New Zealand Studies in Applied Linguistics, 1,* 51–59.

Long, S. H., Fey, M. E., and Channell, R. W. (2002). *Computerized Profiling.* http://www.computerizedprofiling.org.

Moriarty, B., and Gillon, G. (2006). Phonological awareness intervention for children with childhood apraxia of speech. *International Journal for Language and Communication Disorders, 41,*713-734.

Moyle, J. (2004). *The New Zealand Articulation Test.* Lower Hutt, New Zealand: Special Education Services.

Moyle, J. (2005). The New Zealand articulation test norms project. *New Zealand Journal of Speech Language Therapy, 60,* 61–74.

Silva, P. A. (1980). *The Dunedin Articulation Screening Scale.* Dunedin, New Zealand: Otago Speech Therapy Association.

Silva, P. A., McGee, R. O., and Williams. S. M. (1981). *From birth to seven: Child development in Dunedin: A multidisciplinary study.* (Unpublished report available from the University of Otago Medical Library.)

Smit, A., Hand, L., Freilinger, J., Bernthal, J., and Bird, A. (1990). The Iowa articulation norms project and its Nebraska replication. *Journal of Speech and Hearing Disorders, 55,* 779–798.

Sutherland, D., and Gillon, G. (2005). Assessment of phonological representations in children with speech impairment. *Language, Speech, and Hearing Services in Schools, 36,* 294–307.

Van Bysterveldt, A., Gillon, G., and Moran A. (2006). Enhancing phonological awareness and letter knowledge in preschool children with Down syndrome. *International Journal of Disability, Development and Education, 53,* 301-329.

Warren, P., and Bauer, L. (2004). Maori English: Phonology. In E. Schneider, K. Burridge, B. Kortmann, R. Mesthrie, and C. Upton (Eds.), *A handbook of varieties of English: Vol. 1. Phonology* (pp. 614–624). Berlin and New York: Mouton de Gruyter.

Wells, J. C. (1982). *Accents of English.* Cambridge, UK: Cambridge University Press.

Westerveld, M., and Gillon, G. T. (2002). *A New Zealand spontaneous language sampling protocol.* University of Canterbury, Department of Communication Disorders.

Wood, E. (2003). Tн-fronting: The substitution of f/v for θ/ð in New Zealand English. *New Zealand English Journal, 17,* 50–56.

SUMMARY OF STUDIES OF TYPICAL NEW ZEALAND ENGLISH SPEECH ACQUISITION

Authors	Year	Country	No. of children	Age of children	Information	Sample type	Data collection
Gillon	2000	New Zealand	30	4;5	Percent consonants correct	Single word	Cross-sectional
Gillon	2005	New Zealand	19	3;6	Percent consonants correct	Single word	Longitudinal
Gillon and Schwarz	1999, 2001	New Zealand	972	6;5	Articulation accuracy	Single word	Cross-sectional
Justin, Lawn, and Silva	1983	New Zealand	872	7;0	Articulation accuracy	Single word	Cross-sectional
Moyle	2005	New Zealand	1013	5;0–8;0	Articulation accuracy	Single word	Cross-sectional
Sutherland and Gillon	2005	New Zealand	60	2;0 –3;6	Percent consonants correct	Single word	Longitudinal

Note. Some of these studies were not specifically designed to evaluate normal speech sound acquisition. Nevertheless, they contain relevant information.

Chapter 32

Cantonese-influenced English Speech Acquisition

Alison Holm

INTRODUCTION

Genesee (1993) considers children to be "bilingual language learners" when they are exposed to both languages within the first five years, and "second language learners" after this period. In this chapter the speech acquisition of bilingual language learners, exposed to both Cantonese and English, will be described. There is minimal information available regarding typical language exposure for children in bilingual Cantonese-English environments. In Australia, it is common for the children of bilingual Cantonese-English parents to develop stronger Cantonese skills prior to developing strong English skills through child care or school (Holm, 1998). Yavaş (1998) and Anderson (2004) suggest that this pattern of language acquisition (one language initially more dominant, but both acquired in the primary language learning period) is representative of many situations around the world. The process of second language acquisition (e.g., adult learners) of Cantonese-English is different than children's bilingual acquisition (see Fung and Roseberry-McKibbin, 1999 for an introduction to the issues surrounding Cantonese-speaking adults acquiring English).

Cantonese is one of the languages of the Chinese language family (see Chapter 36). It is mainly spoken in the southeastern part of Mainland China, Hong Kong, and Macau, by the Chinese minorities in Southeast Asia, and by many overseas Chinese of Cantonese origin worldwide (Wikipedia, 2005). Many Cantonese-speaking people have migrated throughout the world, particularly to the United States of America (USA) and Canada, Australia, the United Kingdom (UK), and Southeast Asia. Chinese immigrants were brought in as cheap laborers (e.g., to build the transcontinental railroads in North America) or were lured by gold rushes in the mid-1800s (e.g., the Australian Gold Rush and the California Gold Rush). The

White Australia Policy of the early twentieth century hindered the development of the Chinese communities in Australia. However, since changing to a multicultural government policy in the 1970s, Australia has received many immigrants from Hong Kong and southeast China. Similarly, the relaxation of immigration laws after World War II in the United States allowed for migration from both mainland China and Hong Kong. The biggest wave of Chinese immigration to the UK (mainly from Hong Kong) was in the 1950s and 1960s due to the postwar labor shortage. In Canada in the early and mid-1990s, there was a significant migration of people from Hong Kong who worried about the pending handover to the People's Republic of China (Wikipedia, 2005). See the Resources section of this chapter for materials pertaining to Cantonese English.

Countries where Cantonese-English is spoken

Australia, Canada, the Netherlands, New Zealand, Singapore, the UK, and the USA have significant numbers of bilingual Cantonese-English speakers (Gordon, 2005; see accompanying map and Appendix D). Many people in Hong Kong are also bilingual Cantonese-English speakers. The descriptions of the acquisition of Cantonese and English by bilingual Cantonese-English children presented in this chapter are based on research from an Australian context.

Components of Cantonese and English: comparisons

Both Australian English (see Chapter 30) and Cantonese (see Chapter 36) are discussed in this book. Children learning Cantonese and English in a bilingual context are able to acquire "monolingual-like" production of both languages. Bilingual children in Australia have typical Australian-English accents following adequate exposure to the language. Table 32-1 provides a comparison of the phonological structures of English and Cantonese. There are significant differences between the structure of English and Cantonese: English has many more vowel and consonant segments; English has more complex phonotactic structures and stress patterns; and Cantonese uses tones to differentiate meaning. Where phonemes occur in both languages, the sequence of Cantonese phoneme acquisition is

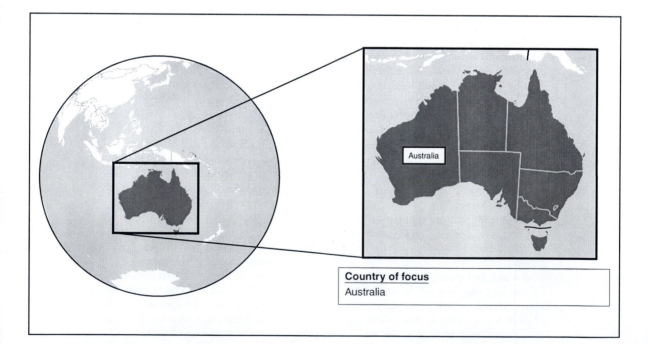

Country of focus
Australia

TABLE 32-1 Comparison of the phonological structure of English and Cantonese

	English	**Cantonese**
Vowels and diphthongs	21 monophthongs + 5 diphthongs	8 monophthongs
Consonants	24 consonants + 49 clusters	17 consonants + 2 clusters
Syllable/word structure	C_{0-3} VC_{0-4} polysyllabic	$C_{0-1}G_{0-1}VC_{0-1}/G_{0-1}$ mostly monosyllabic
Tones	None	6 tones + 3 allotones
Stress	Complex	Simple

*Note. Data from So and Dodd (1995).

similar to that of English, although the rate of acquisition is more rapid.

Despite the very different phonological structures in the two languages, monolingual developmental patterns are very similar. Table 32-2 outlines the typical and atypical phonological processes used by monolingual Cantonese- and English-speaking children. While syllable-final consonants are rarely in error in Cantonese, both

TABLE 32-2 Comparison of Cantonese and English monolingual typical and atypical processes

Process	Cantonese		English	
	Example	Status	Example	Status
Cluster reduction	/kwa/ [ka]	T	/stɛp/ [tɛp]	T
Final consonant deletion*	/suk/ [tsu]	A	/kʌp/ [kʌ]	T
Stopping	/si/ [ti]	T	/ʃu/ [du]	T
Fronting	/kam/ [tam]	T	/kʌp/ [tʌp]	T
Gliding/continuant variation*	/lɛj/ [wɛj]	A	/ɹɪŋ/ [wɪŋ]	T
Deaffrication	/tsi/ [si]	T	/tʃɪp/ [ʃɪp]	T
Affrication*	/sy/ [tsy]	T	/ʃak/ [tʃak]	A
Deaspiration*	/pʰiŋ/ [piŋ]	T	/pʰɪn/ [pɪn]	A
Aspiration*	/tɛŋ/ [tʰɛŋ]	A		
Voicing*	/pɛŋ/ [bɛŋ]	A	/tɪp/ [dɪp]	T
Weak syllable deletion*			/bənana/ [nana]	T
Assimilation	/ŋan/ [ŋaŋ]	T	/bɛd/ [bɛb]	T
Reduplication	/ji/ [jiji]	T	/bʌtʌ/ [bʌbʌ]	T
Backing	/tin/ [kin]	A	/fʊt/ [kʊt]	A
Initial consonant deletion	/mat/ [at]	A	/tɔi/ [ɔi]	A
Tone errors*	/fa̰/ [fa̱]	A		
Addition	/ap/ [tap]	A	/bæk/ [bæŋk]	A
Nasalization	/lɛj/ [nɛj]	A	/tɪp/ [mɪp]	A
Transposition	/pa si/ [sa pi]	A	bʌtən/ [tʌbən]	A

Note. Data from Grunwell (1982); So and Dodd (1995).

* indicates different status across the two languages: atypical (A) or not possible in one and typical (T) in the other.

English- and Cantonese-speaking children's errors are characterized by assimilation, cluster reduction, and simplification of the system of phoneme contrasts (e.g., fronting and stopping). Monolingual speech-impaired children's phonological processes are also similar, irrespective of language (So and Dodd, 1994).

Typical acquisition of Cantonese-influenced English

This section will give an overview of typical bilingual Cantonese-English acquisition patterns (Holm and Dodd, 1999; 2006). Normative age of acquisition data is not provided because it is not available—the age and amount of exposure to each language will impact the accuracy and proficiency of acquisition. See the Summary of Studies Table at the end of this chapter for studies of children's acquisition of Cantonese English.

Acquired sounds

The phonetic (articulatory) development of Cantonese-English bilingual children does not significantly differ from monolingual children of each language. The acquisition of speech sounds is independent of phonological development: phonemes are acquired in similar sequences and at similar times in both languages; shared phonemes (common to both languages) are stimulable in both languages. Shared phonemes are commonly evident in Cantonese slightly before English (Holm and Dodd, 2006).

Consonants

Young Cantonese-English bilingual children (e.g., <30 months) may acquire voicing contrasts differently than monolingual English-speaking children. Some Cantonese-English children will use the voiced prior to the unvoiced plosive of English plosive pairs (e.g., /b/ but not /pʰ/). In Cantonese children generally acquire unaspirated plosives before aspirated in the same way as monolingual Cantonese

speakers do. There may also be a slight delay in the age of acquisition of later-developing English phonemes (e.g., /tʃ, ɹ, ʃ, θ, ð/) (Holm and Dodd, 1999; 2006).

Consonant clusters

Cantonese-English-speaking children acquire clusters similarly to monolingual children of each language.

Vowels and diphthongs

Unlike monolingual Cantonese- or English-speaking children, vowel errors are typical in both languages for bilingual children. Tone errors are occasionally evident although still unusual in bilingual children's Cantonese. However, typically developing Cantonese-English bilingual children should be using the complete range of Cantonese and English vowels and Cantonese tones contrastively at ages similar to monolingual children of each language.

Percent correct

Differences between monolingual and bilingual speech accuracy development decrease with age (i.e., bilingual children "catch up" to their matched monolingual peers). Usually within a couple of years of exposure to the second language the bilingual children's speech accuracy in each language is comparable to monolingual development (see Table 32-3).

Phonological processes

There are differences in the phonological processes used by bilingual Cantonese-English speaking children in comparison to typical monolingual development. Table 32-4 shows a number of phonological processes evident in both English and Cantonese that are considered atypical for monolingual acquisition but are used by Cantonese-English bilingual children. For example, it is considered atypical for monolingual English-speaking and monolingual Cantonese-speaking children to make errors described by the phonological process of backing

TABLE 32-3 Percentage of phonemes correct: Comparison of bilingual and monolingual children

Age (months)	Cantonese monolingual	Cantonese bilingual	English monolingual	English bilingual
26–39	88	82	82	67
40–54	93	92	90	78
55–67	96	95	96	89

Note. Data from Holm and Dodd (2006).

TABLE 32-4 Phonological processes typically evident in Cantonese-English bilingual children's speech acquisition

Cantonese	Monolingual status	English	Monolingual status
Cluster reduction	Typical	Cluster reduction	Typical
Final consonant deletion	Typical	Final consonant deletion	Typical
Stopping	Typical	Stopping	Typical
Fronting	Typical	Fronting	Typical
Deaffrication/affrication	Typical	Deaffrication	Typical
Deaspiration	Typical	Voicing	Typical[#]
Consonant harmony	Typical	Consonant harmony	Typical
Continuant variation	Typical	Gliding	Typical
Reduplication	Typical	Weak syllable deletion	Typical
Backing	Atypical	Backing	Atypical
Voicing	Atypical	Voicing	Atypical[#]
Initial consonant deletion	Atypical	Initial consonant deletion	Atypical
Aspiration	Atypical	Addition	Atypical
Gliding	Atypical	Affrication/frication	Atypical
		Nasalisation	Atypical

Note. Data from Holm and Dodd (2006)

Note. The data refer to phonological processes used by more than 10 percent of the bilingual population.

[#] Some errors that were included within a general category of "voicing" errors are typical in English (e.g., prevocalic voicing: pig as [bɪg]) while some voicing errors are considered atypical in English (e.g., prevocalic devoicing: bed as [pɛt]).

(e.g., /tin/ as [kin]). However a large number of bilingual Cantonese-English-speaking children made backing errors in both languages. Consequently, these processes have been considered typical bilingual phonological processes for speakers of Cantonese-influenced English (Holm and Dodd, 2006). However, bilingual Cantonese-English speakers also use many of the same phonological processes as their monolingual peers. For example, cluster reduction is a typical developmental process used by monolingual English- and monolingual Cantonese-speaking children. Bilingual Cantonese-English-speaking children also reduce clusters in both languages.

Bilingual children use separate phonological systems for each language (Anderson, 2004; Holm & Dodd, 1999). Some of the evidence for separate systems from Cantonese-English bilingual children includes:

- Phonemes acquired in one language but not used in the other language
- Language-specific phonemes not used inappropriately in the other language

- The same phoneme simplified differently in each language (e.g., stopping /s/ ⇨ [d] in English but affricating /s/ ⇨ [ts] in Cantonese)
- Addition only of legal sounds (e.g., /tsi/ ⇨ [tsip] not [tsif] because final /f/ is illegal in Cantonese)
- Use of contradictory processes (e.g., backing in one language and fronting in the other)
- Use of processes specific to only one language (e.g., stopping fricatives in one language but not in the other)

The Cantonese-English children's phonological processes could be due to the bilingual children's use of underspecified rules (cf. Ellis, 1994). Atypical patterns may result from an inability to adequately process both phonological systems in enough detail to derive all the appropriate language-specific realization rules. Atypical patterns are generally transient and inconsistent in nature (Holm and Dodd, 1999). With greater exposure to English, children are able to differentiate more clearly the realization rules for each phonological system. For example, a child may hypothesize that final consonants are unreleased because that is the case in Cantonese. Limited exposure to English may not have allowed the child to identify a salient characteristic of the phonology—that final consonants are usually released—so the child simply uses the realization rules governing the release of final consonants extracted from exposure to Cantonese phonology. The bilingual children mark differences between the systems. However, occasionally the precise, specific detail of the realization rules was inaccurate or absent, resulting in unusual speech errors.

Intelligibility

To date there is no study of intelligibility of Cantonese-English bilingual children.

Phonetic inventory

To date there is no study of the phonetic inventory of Cantonese-English bilingual children.

Common mismatches

To date there is no study of common mismatches for Cantonese-English bilingual children.

Syllable structure

To date there is no study of syllable structure for Cantonese-English bilingual children.

Prosody

To date there is no study of prosody or tone acquisition of Cantonese-English bilingual children. Gong (2002) described some of the difficulties adult second language learners experience acquiring English as a second language. Some of the traces of accent evident in Cantonese-English bilingual children possibly stem from prosodic or rhythmic differences from monolingual English speakers.

Phonological awareness

The phonological awareness of Cantonese-English bilingual children may be less developed than their monolingual peers. Specifically, bilingual preschool children's English rhyme awareness may be less developed. Monolingual English-speaking school-age children may have stronger skills in terms of number of plausible spelling errors, nonword spelling, nonword reading, visual rhyme recognition, phoneme manipulation, and

spoonerisms (Bialystok, Majumder, and & Martin, 2003; Jackson, Holm, and Dodd, 1998).

Speech assessment for Cantonese-English children

To date there are no specific assessment tools for Cantonese-English bilingual children. However, standardized phonological assessments with monolingual acquisition data are available for both languages (see So, this volume for information on Cantonese and chapters by Smit, Howard, and others for information on English). Assessment of children with suspected speech impairment requires (1) investigation of whether the bilingual child has differentiated his or her phonological systems and, if so, (2) identification of the phonological error patterns for each language, and then (3) comparison of these patterns with normal bilingual developmental data for the child's specific language group. Comparison with monolingual acquisition processes is not appropriate for bilingual Cantonese-English-speaking children. The lack of clear normative quantitative data for bilingual acquisition requires that SLPs making clinical decisions must use their clinical judgment based on the child's difficulty communicating, as well as the number and, particularly, types of errors evident.

Clinical implications for assessment of speech impairment in Cantonese-English bilingual children include the following:

- Bilingual children's speech needs to be assessed in both of their languages for a clear profile of the nature of their errors.
- Articulation errors, common to both languages due to incorrect motor planning, will be evident across both languages (e.g., interdental lisp evident in both Cantonese and English).
- Bilingual children have two separate phonological systems for their two languages. This is not to suggest that the two languages are completely independent and do not interact or influence each other in any way. However, the process of acquiring two phonological systems bilingually is different from the process of acquiring each system as a monolingual.
- The deficits underlying phonological disorder are not language specific; they are the product of difficulty abstracting the phonological patterns of that language accurately. This difficulty results in different error pattern profiles across the two languages. Phonological assessment in only one language is not sufficient.

Speech intervention for Cantonese-English children

There is very limited information available regarding speech intervention for Cantonese-English bilingual children (Holm, Ozanne, and Dodd, 1997). In fact, there is very little information regarding speech intervention for bilingual children at all (Yavaş and Goldstein, 1998). The available evidence suggests that articulation errors common to both languages can be remediated in both languages by providing therapy in only one language. On the other hand, although phonological errors can be remediated in the language in which therapy is provided, this therapy probably will not affect the child's other phonological system. Phonological therapy may not generalize across languages, indicating that therapy will need to be carried out in each language separately. However, there are practical difficulties associated with offering regular intervention in a language that is not native to the SLP. The use of interpreters or other bilingual assistants is possible, but many children will be offered intervention only in English.

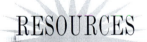

PHONETICALLY SPEAKING

Pronunciation of Cantonese-English: /kæntəniz ɪŋglɪʃ/

Unlike the other chapters in this book, it is not appropriate to include the transcription of a passage as spoken by a Cantonese-English speaker. An adult speaker exposed to Cantonese and English in a way similar to the children described in this chapter would not be noticeably different from a monolingual adult speaker from that community. Although they might take a slightly different path, monolingual and bilingual children end up speaking with a similar accent if they are bilingual from an early age.

RESOURCES

Useful Cantonese-English Web sites

- Common Pronunciation Problems for Cantonese Speakers
  http://lc.ust.hk/~sac/advice/english/pronunciation/P7.htm. Language Centre, The Hong Kong University of Science and Technology.

- Pronunciation Lessons
  http://lc.ust.hk/~material/pl/. Language Centre, The Hong Kong University of Science and Technology.

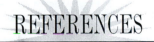

REFERENCES

Anderson, R. T. (2004). Phonological acquisition in preschoolers learning a second language via immersion: A longitudinal study. *Clinical Linguistics and Phonetics, 18,* 183–210.

Bialystok, E., Majumder, S., and Martin, M. (2003). Developing phonological awareness: Is there a bilingual advantage? *Applied Psycholinguistics, 24,* 27–44.

Ellis, R. (1994). *The study of second language acquisition.* Oxford, UK: Oxford University Press.

Fung, E., and Roseberry-McKibbin, C. (1999). Service delivery considerations in working with clients from Cantonese-speaking backgrounds. *American Journal of Speech-Language Pathology, 8,* 309–318.

Genesee, F. (1993). Bilingual language development in preschool children. In D. Bishop and K. Mogford (Eds.), *Language development in exceptional circumstances* (pp. 62–79). Hove: Lawrence Erlbaum.

Gong, J. (2002). Introducing English rhythm in Chinese EFL classrooms: A literature review. *Post-Script, 3.* Retrieved September 2005 from http://www.edfac.unimelb.edu.au/insight/pscript.shtml.

Gordon, R.G. (Ed.). (2005). *Ethnologue: Languages of the world* (15th ed.). Dallas, TX.: SIL International. Online version: http://www.ethnologue.com.

Grunwell, P. (1982). *Clinical phonology.* London: Croom Helm.

Holm, A. (1998). *Speech development and disorder in bilingual children.* Unpublished doctoral thesis, University of Newcastle upon Tyne, UK.

Holm, A., and Dodd, B. (1999). A longitudinal study of the phonological development of two Cantonese-English bilingual children. *Applied Psycholinguistics, 20,* 349–376.

Holm, A., Dodd, B. (2006); Phonological development and disorder of bilingual children acquiring Cantonese and English. In Zhu Hua & B. Dodd, (Eds.), *Phonological development and disorders in children: A multilingual perspective.* (pp. 286–325). Clevedon: Multilingual Matters.

Holm, A., Ozanne, A., and Dodd, B. (1997). Efficacy of intervention for a bilingual child making articulation and phonological errors. *International Journal of Bilingualism, 1,* 55–69.

Jackson, N., Holm, A., and Dodd, B. J. (1998). Phonological awareness and spelling abilities of Cantonese-English bilingual children. *Asia-Pacific Journal of Speech, Language and Hearing, 3,* 79–96.

So, L., and Dodd, B. (1994). Phonologically disordered Cantonese children. *Clinical Linguistics and Phonetics, 8,* 235–255.

So, L., and Dodd, B. (1995). The acquisition of phonology by Cantonese speaking children. *Journal of Child Language, 22,* 473–495.

Watson, I. (1991). Phonological processing in two languages. In E. Bialystok (Ed.), *Language processing in bilingual children* (pp. 25–48). Cambridge: Cambridge University Press.

Wikipedia (2005). *Cantonese language.* http://en.wikipedia.org/wiki/Cantonese_language. [Accessed September 2005].

Yavaş, M. (1998). *Phonology: Development and disorders.* London: Singular.

Yavaş, M. & Goldstein, B. (1998). Phonological assessment and treatment of bilingual speakers. *American Journal of Speech-Language Pathology, 7,* 49–60.

SUMMARY OF STUDIES OF TYPICAL CANTONESE-INFLUENCED ENGLISH SPEECH ACQUISITION

Authors	Year	Country	No. of children	Age of children	Information	Sample type	Data collection
Bialystok, Majumder, and Martin,	2003	Canada	16 "Chinese" children	6 yrs	Phonological awareness	Experimental and standardized tasks	Cross-sectional
Dodd, So, and Li	1996	UK	16	3–5 yrs	Speech accuracy; phonological process use	Standardized single-word speech assessments	Cross-sectional
Holm and Dodd	1999	Australia	2	2–4 yrs	Speech accuracy; phonological process use	Standardized single-word speech assessments	Longitudinal
Holm and Dodd	2006	Australia & UK	56	2–5 yrs	Speech accuracy; phonological process use	Standardized single-word speech assessments	Cross-sectional
Jackson, Holm, and Dodd	1998	UK	36	3–10 yrs	Phonological awareness	Standardized assessments	Cross-sectional

Chapter 33

Spanish-influenced English Speech Acquisition

Brian A. Goldstein

INTRODUCTION

English is the third-most common first language spoken in the world, with approximately 402 million speakers (Wikipedia, 2005). English has become the lingua franca of international business and diplomacy. Moreover, learning English as a second language is common, if not compulsory, in many countries, including those where Spanish is the first language acquired. Whenever there is contact between languages, it is likely that they will influence each other in systematic ways. Thus, the English dialect acquired by native Spanish speakers will be influenced by that ambient language (i.e., Spanish). It is also probable that the speaker's Spanish skills will be influenced by the acquisition of English, although we will not focus on that aspect of acquisition in this chapter.

Influence across languages emanates from a variety of sources: parents, peers, the dialect most common in the school system, and the influence of one phonological system on another (Wolfram, 1971). To gauge the type of influence of one linguistic system on another, Weinrich (1953) detailed types of transfer (he termed it "interference") that take place in situations of language contact. Six of seven of those patterns are recounted here along with examples from phonology.

- *Sound Substitution*. A second language learner will substitute the closest equivalent for the L1 target sound. For example, native Spanish speakers will produce [tʃ] for /ʃ/, given that /ʃ/ does not exist in most Spanish dialects.
- *Phonological Processes*. Allophonic variations are transferred from one language into the other. For example, in Spanish, voiced stops become their fricative counterparts after vowels (/laɡo/ *lake* ⇨ [laɣo]). Thus, in their production of voiced stops in English,

native Spanish speakers might misapply that process and produce a word like /lʌg/ *lugging* as [lʌɣ].

- *Underdifferentiation*. The second language makes distinctions that the first language does not. For example, English distinguishes between tense and lax vowels, although Spanish has only tense vowels. Thus, native Spanish speakers might produce lax vowels as their tense counterparts.
- *Overdifferentiation*. The first language makes distinctions that the second language does not. For example, in English /d/ and /ð/ are different phonemes, but in Spanish, they are allophones (Major, 2001). As Major points out, this distinction might not result in pronunciation differences but may indicate how speakers think about the sounds in each language.
- *Phonotactic Interference*. Syllabic patterns of the second language are modified to accommodate the syllabic patterns of the first language. Given that the majority of syllable types in Spanish are CV (Hammond, 2001), speakers may modify English syllable structure to reproduce that type (e.g., /bin/ *bean* ⇨ [bi]).
- *Prosodic Interference*. Prosodic patterns of the second language are modified to accommodate the prosodic patterns of the first language. Spanish speakers will produce utterances in a syllable-timed pattern in their English. Thus, syllables in English will tend to occur at regular intervals and neutralization (e.g., using schwa in unstressed syllables) will be uncommon.

Thus, native Spanish speakers who are acquiring English may exhibit some, or all, of these patterns. The frequency with which they exhibit these patterns depends upon on a number of factors: the amount of contact with Spanish and English speakers, the speaker's motivation, whether the speaker is learning both languages simultaneously (i.e., from birth) or sequentially (i.e., one after the other), a speaker's oral and perceptual abilities, and the prestige associated with the various dialects in which the individual comes in contact (Goldstein, 2001; Goldstein and Iglesias, 2004; Leather and James, 1996).

Where Spanish-influenced English (SIE) is spoken

Spanish-influenced English (SIE) is likely to be spoken where relatively large communities of Spanish and English speakers have contact with each other; specifically, Andorra, Belize, and the United States of America (see accompanying map and Appendix D).

Components of SIE

In the following sections, the major segmental and suprasegmental characteristics of SIE will be outlined. It should be noted that Spanish speakers learning English do not utilize all features of SIE nor do all speakers utilize all features in every context.

Consonants

SIE must be understood through the context of English, which is generally described as having 24 phonemes (Shriberg and Kent, 2003) and Spanish, which is generally described as having 18 phonemes (Hammond, 2001). The consonant phonemic inventories of General English and Spanish are listed in Table 33-1.

Characteristics of SIE Consonants

The consonant phonetic inventory of Spanish differs from that of English. Spanish contains some sounds that are not part of the English phonetic system (Table 33-2).

Given that the phonetic inventories of Spanish and English are not identical, it is possible that Spanish speakers' ambient language will influence their production of English. In terms of consonants, there are some consonants that are more likely than others to be influenced. For example, English contains sounds that do not exist in Spanish (Table 33-3).

It should be noted that some of those sounds, [ŋ], [v], [θ], [ʃ], [ʒ], and [dʒ], exist in the phonetic inventories of some Spanish dialects (Núñez-Cedeño and Morales-Front, 1999). Nonetheless, in the attempt to produce these sounds, Spanish speakers might omit them (more likely in syllable coda position) or substitute for them (Goldstein, 2001; Goldstein and Iglesias, 2004; Kayser, 1993; MacDonald, 1989; Perez, 1994; Roseberry-McKibbin, 2002). Given the differences between the English and Spanish phonological systems, speakers of SIE might modify their productions of English consonants in the ways listed in Table 33-4.

Vowels and diphthongs

Most varieties of English are described as having up to 15 monophthong vowels and five diphthong vowels (Shriberg and Kent, 2003). Monophthong vowels, depending on the specific dialect, include those in Table 33-5.

The diphthongs of General American English are /eɪ/, /oʊ/, /aɪ/, /aʊ/, and /ɔɪ/. Of all the vowels described for English, Spanish also contains /i/, /e/, /u/, and /a/, although /a/ is usually described as a low, central vowel

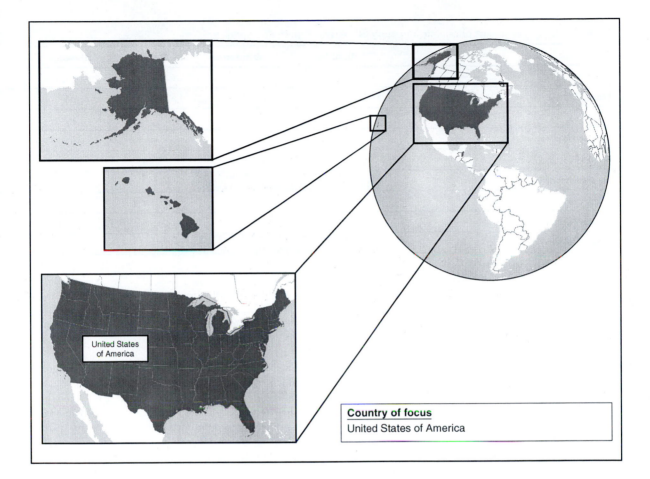

United States
of America

Country of focus
United States of America

in Spanish (Hammond, 2001). In attempting to produce these English vowels, Spanish speakers might exhibit the characteristics outlined in Table 33-6 (Goldstein, 2001; Goldstein and Iglesias, 2004; Kayser, 1993; MacDonald, 1989; Perez, 1994; Roseberry-McKibbin, 2002).

Phonotactic restrictions

The syllable structure of SIE is that of English (see Chapters 22 and 27). As noted in the section above on consonantal characteristics of SIE, however, native Spanish speakers may modify English phonotactic patterns.

Syllables

Syllable types in SIE are those inherent in English (see Chapters 22 and 27). However, native Spanish speakers

may modify that syllable structure in accordance with the patterns of SIE described previously (Table 33-4). Specifically, syllable and/or word-final consonants may be deleted and/or /s/ clusters may undergo epenthesis.

Consonants and consonant clusters

SIE is based on modifications to English, given Spanish as the speaker's ambient language. (The consonants of both Spanish and English have been described previously in Table 33-1.) Thus, speakers acquiring English as a second language may produce SIE mainly because of the absence of Spanish sounds in English (Table 33-2), the absence of English sounds in Spanish (Table 33-3), and/or the phonotactic restrictions in Spanish and English. The result of these influences may result in a number of discernable consonantal SIE patterns (Table 33-4).

TABLE 33-1 Consonant phonemic inventory of General English and Spanish

	Bilabial	Labiodental	Dental	Alveolar
Plosive	p* b*			t* d*
Nasal	m*			n*
Trill				(r)
Tap or flap				(ɾ)
Fricative		f* v	θ ð	s* z
Lateral fricative	■	■		
Affricate				
Approximant	w* (labiovelar)			ɹ*
Lateral approximant	■	■		l*

Note. *=Phonemes found in both English and Spanish are noted by an asterisk.

( ) = Phonemes specific to Spanish are indicated in parenthesis.

Phonemic and allophonic variations of English will not be covered in this chapter; see other chapters in this section for such a description.

Black = articulations judged impossible

Based on the International Phonetic Alphabet. Courtesy of the International Phonetic Association (c/o Department of Linguistics, University of Victoria, Victoria, British Columbia, Canada).

Tones

Neither English nor Spanish uses tones to differentiate meaning.

Stress and intonation

Just as there may be segmental influences across languages, there also may be suprasegmental effects. Because English and Spanish differ along stress, pitch, and intonational parameters, they may result in SIE characteristics across these dimensions.

English is considered to be a stress-timed language in which stress occurs at regular intervals, as opposed to Spanish, which is a syllable-timed language in which there is a recurrence of syllables at regular intervals (Ladefoged, 2001). There are common patterns for stress in Spanish: penultimate stress on words ending in vowels (e.g., *DEdo* 'finger') and final stress for words ending in consonants (e.g., *reLOX* 'watch') (Hochberg, 1988). In English, however, stress assignment is more complicated, depending on various factors such as syntactic category and weight of the syllable (Goodluck, 1991). Thus, in producing stress

TABLE 33-2 Spanish sounds absent in English

Description	Segment	Example
Voiced palatal nasal	[ɲ]	[niɲo] 'boy'
Voiceless bilabial fricative	[ɸ]	[emɸermo] 'sick'
Voiceless velar fricative	[x]	[relox] 'watch'
Voiced spirants	[ß] [ɣ]	[klaßo] 'nail' [laɣo] 'lake'
Alveolar trill	[r]	[pero] 'dog'
Voiced uvular trill	[ʀ]	[ʀoto] 'broken'

TABLE 33-3 English sounds absent in Spanish

Description	Segment	Example
Aspirated stops	[pʰ] [tʰ] [kʰ]	[pʰɛn] *pen* [tʰɛn] *ten* [kʰɛn] *ken*
Velar nasal	[ŋ]	[sʌŋ] *sung*
Fricatives	[v] [θ] [ʃ] [ʒ]	[vot] *vote* [mæθ] *math* [ʃu] *shoe* [mɛʒɚ] *measure*
Affricate	[dʒ]	[dʒʌmp] *jump*
Nonlateral liquid	[ɹ]	[ɹid] *read*

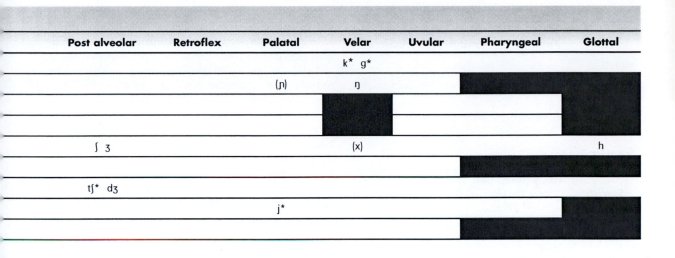

Post alveolar	Retroflex	Palatal	Velar	Uvular	Pharyngeal	Glottal
			k* g*			
		(ɲ)	ŋ			
ʃ ʒ			(x)			h
tʃ* dʒ						
		j*				

TABLE 33-4 Consonantal characteristics of SIE

English target	Likely production by a speaker of SIE	Example
Aspirated stops	Unaspirated stops	*pen* /pɛn/ ⇨ [p⁼ɛn]
Stops in intervocalic position	Fricatives	*cabin* /kæbɪn/ ⇨ [kæβɪn] *fading* /fedɪŋ/ ⇨ [feðɪŋ] *wagon* /wægən/ ⇨ [wæɣən]
Velar nasal	Alveolar nasal	*sung* /sʌŋ/ ⇨ [sʌn]
Fricatives	Stops	*vote* /vot/ ⇨ [bot] *thin* /θɪn/ ⇨ [tɪn]
Fricatives	Affricates	*shoe* /ʃu/ ⇨ [tʃu] *measure* /mɛʒɚ/ ⇨ [mɛdʒɚ]
/h/	[x]	*home* /hom/ ⇨ [xom]
Affricates	Fricatives	*chin* /tʃɪn/ ⇨ [ʃɪn] *Jack* /dʒæk/ ⇨ [ʒæk]
Prevocalic liquid "r"	Flap or trill	*read* /ɹid/ ⇨ [ɾid] or /ɹid/ ⇨ [rid]
Postvocalic liquid "r"	Flap	*fire* /fiɚ/ ⇨ [fiɛɾ]
Syllable and/or word-final consonants	Deleted	*fan* /fæn/ ⇨ [fæ]/[fæ̃] *mess* /mɛs/ ⇨ [mɛ]/[mɛʰ]
/s/ clusters	Epenthesis	*steer* /stiɚ/ ⇨ [estiɚ]
Word-final voiced consonants	Devoiced consonants	*please* /pliz/ ⇨ [pliz̥]/[plis]

TABLE 33-5 Vowel phonemic inventory of English

	Front	Central	Back
High	i, ɪ	ɨ	u, ʊ
Mid	e, ɛ	ə, ɜ	o, ʌ, ɔ
Low	æ, a		ɑ, ɒ

TABLE 33-6 Vocalic characteristics of SIE

English target	Likely production by a speaker of SIE	Example
Tense	Lax	*heat* /hit/ ⇨ [hɪt]
Lax	Tense	*bet* /bɛt/ ⇨ [bet]
Diphthongs	Monophthongs	*hose* /hoʊz/ ⇨ [hoz]
Schwa	/a/	*away* /əweɪ/ ⇨ [awe]
r-colored vowels	/e/-/ɛ/ + /r/	*tear* /tiɚ/ ⇨ [tiɛr]

patterns in English, a native Spanish speaker may exhibit SIE. For example, a native speaker of Spanish may use Spanish stress rules in English (e.g., *RIot* as *riOT*).

Pitch and intonation appear to differ in two main ways in English and Spanish (Hadlich, Holton, and Montes, 1968). First, pitch range is reported to modulate less in Spanish than in English. Second, utterances are reported to begin at a higher pitch in English than in Spanish. So, native Spanish speakers may use less robust pitch contours when speaking English, and may be perceived as relatively "monotone" compared to native English speakers.

Writing system

The writing system of SIE is that of English. There is no writing system that is unique to SIE. It is possible, however, that speakers of SIE may alter the orthography of General English in accordance with the phonology of SIE (e.g., August, Calderón, and Carlo 2002; Bebout, 1985; Fashola, Drum, Mayer, and Kang, 1996). In a study of native English- and Spanish-speaking fourth through sixth graders, Bebout organized their spelling into eight categories: (1) consonant-doubling error, (2) other consonant errors, (3) schwa errors, (4) silent "e" errors, (5) other vowel errors, (6) letter misordering, (7) unclassifiable items, and (8) correct spellings (p. 575). Her results indicated that the native

Spanish-speaking children made fewer spelling errors than the native English-speaking children. In addition, the types of errors made by the two groups differed. Native English-speaking children tended to make more errors on schwa and silent "e," and native Spanish-speaking children tended to make more consonant-doubling errors. There were no significant differences between the two groups for the other categories.

Fashola et al. (1996) tested the spelling skills of native English- and Spanish-speaking second-, third-, fifth-, and sixth-grade students. They examined the children's predicted spelling errors (i.e., those attributable to the orthographic and phonological distinctions between Spanish and English, for example, "h" ⇨ "j" in the spelling of native Spanish speakers) and nonpredicted spelling errors (i.e., those not attributable to the orthographic and phonological distinctions between Spanish and English). Results indicated that the native Spanish-speaking children made "more than four times as many predicted errors as did the English-speaking students, but the groups produced similar numbers of nonpredicted errors" (Fashola et al., 1996, p. 839). In addition, results showed that the number of nonpredicted errors decreased significantly by grade level for the native English-speaking children but not for the native Spanish-speaking children.

Zutell and Allen (1988) examined the spelling skills of Spanish-speaking second, third, and fourth graders who were enrolled in a bilingual education program. Similar to the Fashola et al. (1996) study, Zutell and Allen examined "predicted misspellings" in the English of these native Spanish-speaking children. They found that good spellers did not make significantly more "predicted misspellings" than nonpredicted misspellings. They found the opposite effect for poor spellers. Those children (i.e., poor spellers) did make significantly more "predicted misspellings" than nonpredicted misspellings.

Thus, the results of these studies indicate that native Spanish speakers who are acquiring the English orthographic system will exhibit systematic errors. Many of those errors (illustrated in Table 33-7) will be predictable given the differences between the phonology and orthography of Spanish and English (August et al., 2002; Bebout, 1985; Fashola et al., 1996; Zutell and Allen, 1988). Native Spanish-speaking children will also make errors, however, that cannot be attributed to those differences.

Varieties of SIE

As with all dialects, there will be differences in the expression of features from each language based on a

TABLE 33-7   Spanish-influenced orthography

English orthographic target	Spanish-influenced orthography	Example
Consonants		
"sh"	"ch"	shoe ⇨ choe
"j"	"ch"	badge ⇨ bache
"h"	"j"	home ⇨ jom
"c"/"cc"/"ck"/"k"	"k"/"c"/ "qu"	cat ⇨ kat blocks ⇨ blocs blocks ⇨ bloqus
"c"	"s"	decent ⇨ desent
"v"	"b"	vote ⇨ bote
"b"	"v"	boat ⇨ voat
"sk"	"sc"/ "squ"	basking ⇨ bascing, basquing
Double letters	Single letters	butter ⇨ buter
Single letters	Double letters	mining ⇨ minning
"th"	"d" or "t"	then ⇨ den
Vowels		
"ea"/"ee"	"i"	meat ⇨ mit/beet ⇨ bit
"a"	"o"	ball ⇨ boll
"a"	"ei"/"ell"/"ey"	made ⇨ meid, melld, meyd
"oo"	"o"/"u"	look ⇨ lok/luk
Silent "e"	omitted	snake ⇨ snak
Schwa	"e" or "a"	direct ⇨ derect/darect

variety of factors, including, but not limited to, age, gender, socioeconomic status, education, employment, community, and family context (Wolfram and Schilling-Estes, 1998).

Typical acquisition of SIE

There are no studies that have examined SIE from a developmental perspective.

Acquired sounds

To date there is no study of the age of acquisition of sounds for children who speak SIE.

Percent correct

To date there is no study of the percentage of correct production of consonants, consonant clusters, or vowels for children who speak SIE.

Phonological processes

To date there is no study of phonological processes produced by children who speak SIE.

Intelligibility

To date there is no study of the intelligibility of children who speak SIE.

Phonetic inventory

To date there is no study of the phonetic inventories produced at different ages by children who speak SIE.

Common mismatches

To date there is no study of the common mismatches produced by children who speak SIE.

Syllable structure

To date there is no study of the syllable structure produced by children who speak SIE.

Prosody

To date there is no study of the development of prosody for children who speak SIE.

Phonological awareness

To date there is no study of the development of phonological awareness by children who speak SIE.

Speech assessment for children who speak SIE

There are no formal assessments that examine SIE in children. To determine if a child's productions are a product of SIE, it is important to determine the set of segmental and suprasegmental characteristics of the dialect in the community in which the child lives. At a minimum, the diagnostician should examine the dialectal characteristics outlined above and those in the child's family before assessing the child. This task would involve interviewing the family (immediate and extended) about their language history, use, and proficiency and, of course, their dialect.

The diagnostician should choose the stimuli carefully. There may be certain word lists or passages that are more susceptible than others to productions of SIE. It is advisable to elicit both single-word and connected speech samples in order to differentiate SIE patterns from disordered ones. A sample of single words allows for control over phonotactic complexity and ensures that all targets will be sampled. Connected speech samples allow for the assessment of speech in context and for the assessment of suprasegmental patterns. Eliciting both types of samples will aid in conducting a least-biased assessment. It is also recommended that a family member produce the single-word stimuli that will be used to assess the child. Doing so would allow the diagnostician to determine the SIE characteristics in that particular family and decrease the likelihood that the child's dialect productions are categorized as disordered ones.

After the samples are elicited, the child's productions should be examined for instances of SIE. Subsequently, they should be scored in accordance with the patterns of SIE. That is, the examiner should mark which patterns are sensitive to dialect and which are not. Those that are attributable to dialect should *not* be scored as errors. True errors are those patterns that are not characteristic of the dialect (Goldstein and Iglesias, 2001). Other than using the patterns listed in this chapter as a guide to denoting which patterns are those of SIE, the diagnostician should review the child's productions with the family to differentiate SIE dialectal patterns from disordered ones.

Speech intervention for SIE speakers

It would not be appropriate to provide intervention for SIE speakers given that SIE is a dialect and not a disordered language variety. Individuals who speak SIE, however, may elect to modify their dialect.

PHONETICALLY SPEAKING

Pronunciation of Spanish-Influenced English:
/spænɪʃ ɪnfluənst ɪŋglɪʃ/
Passage: Comma Gets a Cure

Below is a broad phonetic transcription of *Comma Gets a Cure* (Honorof, McCullough, and Somerville, 2000) spoken by an adult speaking SIE. It should be noted that the passage was transcribed using *all* available features of SIE, even though it is *unlikely* any single speaker would produce the passage in this manner. It also should be noted that the symbol [r] is an alveolar trill.

/welirs e estori for dʒu. sara peri was e beterineri ners xu xaḏ bin workin deli at an olḏ z̩u in e dis̩erteḏ disitrikt in di teritori so tʃi waz̩ beri xapi tu estart e nu dʒab̩ at e esuperḇ praßit praktis in nort eskwer nir di duk estrit tawer. dat eria waz̩ matʃ nirer for xer anḏ mor tu xer lakin. ißen so an xer ferst mornin tʃi felt estrest. tʃi et e bol aẙ poridʒ tʃekt xerself in di miror anḏ watʃt xer fes in e xari. den tʃi put an e plen dʒelo dres anḏ e flis dʒaket pikt ap xer kit anḏ xeðiḏ for werk. wen tʃi gat der der waz̩ e wuman wit a gus wetin for xer. di wuman geẙ sara an ofsial leter fram di bet. di leter implaḏ dat di animal kuḏ bi esuferin fram e rer form aẙ fut anḏ mat disizwitʃ waz̩ surprasin bikaz̩ normali dʒu wuḏ onli espekt to si it in a dag or got. sara waz̩ esentimental so dis meḏ xer fil sari for di bijutiful berḏ/

Well, here's a story for you: Sarah Perry was a veterinary nurse who had been working daily at an old zoo in a deserted district of the territory, so she was very happy to start a new job at a superb private practice in North Square near the Duke Street Tower. That area was much nearer for her and more to her liking. Even so, on her first morning, she felt stressed. She ate a bowl of porridge, checked herself in the mirror and washed her face in a hurry. Then she put on a plain yellow dress and a fleece jacket, picked up her kit and headed for work. When she got there, there was a woman with a goose waiting for her. The woman gave Sarah an official letter from the vet. The letter implied that the animal could be suffering from a rare form of foot and mouth disease, which was surprising, because normally you would only expect to see it in a dog or a goat. Sarah was sentimental, so this made her feel sorry for the beautiful bird (Honorof, McCullough and Somerville, 2000).

RESOURCES

Books

Alvar, M. (Ed.), *Manual de dialectología Hispánica* [Manual of Hispanic dialectology]. Barcelona, Spain: Ariel.

Birdsong, D. (Ed.) (1999). *Second language acquisition and the critical period hypothesis*. Mahwah, NJ: Lawrence Erlbaum.

Bjarkman, P., and Hammond, R. (Eds.) (1989). *American Spanish pronunciation: Theoretical and applied perspective*. Washington, DC: Georgetown University Press.

Cárdenas, D. (1960). *Introducción a una comparación fonológico del español y del inglés* [Introduction to a phonological comparison of Spanish and English]. Washington, DC: Center for Applied Linguistics.

MacDonald, M. (1989). The influence of Spanish phonology on the English spoken by United States Hispanics. In P. Bjarkman and R. Hammond (Eds.), *American Spanish pronunciation: Theoretical and applied perspectives* (pp. 215-236). Washington, DC: Georgetown University Press.

Mann, D., and Hodson, B. (1994). Spanish-speaking children's phonologies: Assessment and remediation of disorders. *Seminars in Speech and Language, 15*, 137–147.

Roca, A., and Jensen, J. (Eds.) (2002). *Spanish in contact*. Somerville, MA: Cascadilla Press.

REFERENCES

August, D., Calderón, M., and Carlo, M. (2002). *Transfer of skills from Spanish to English: A study of young learners*. Washington, DC: Center for Applied Linguistics.

Bebout, L. (1985). An error analysis of misspellings made by learners of English as a first and as a second language. *Journal of Psycholinguistic Research, 14*, 569–593.

Fashola, O., Drum, P., Mayer, R., and Kang, S. (1996). A cognitive theory of orthographic transitioning: Predictable errors in how Spanish-speaking children spell English words. *American Educational Research Journal, 33*, 825–843.

Goldstein, B. (2001). Transcription of Spanish and Spanish-influenced English. *Communication Disorders Quarterly, 23*, 54–60.

Goldstein, B., and Iglesias, A. (2001). The effect of dialect on phonological analysis: Evidence from Spanish-speaking children. *American Journal of Speech-Language Pathology, 10*, 394–406.

Goldstein, B., and Iglesias, A. (2004). Language and dialectal variations. In J. Bernthal and N. Bankson (Eds.), *Articulation and phonological disorders* (5th edition, pp. 348–375). Needham Heights, MA: Allyn & Bacon.

Goodluck, H. (1991). *Language acquisition: A linguistic introduction*. Oxford, UK: Blackwell.

Hadlich, R., Holton, J., and Montes, M. (1968). *A drillbook of Spanish pronunciation*. New York: Harper & Row.

Hammond, R. (2001). *The sounds of Spanish: Analysis and application (with special reference to American English)*. Somerville, MA: Cascadilla Press.

Hochberg, J. (1988). First steps in the acquisition of Spanish stress. *Journal of Child Language, 15*, 273–292.

Honorof, D., McCullough, J., and Somerville, B. (2000). *Comma gets a cure*. New Haven, CT: Haskins Laboratories.

Kayser, H. (1993). Hispanic cultures. In D. Battle (Ed.), *Communication disorders in multicultural populations* (pp. 114–157). Boston: Andover Medical Publishers.

Ladefoged, P. (2001). *A course in phonetics* (4th ed.). Fort Worth, TX: Harcourt College.

Leather, J., and James, A. (1996). Second language speech. In W. Ritchie and T. Bhatia (Eds.), *Handbook of second language acquisition* (pp. 269–316). San Diego, CA: Academic Press.

MacDonald, M. (1989). The influence of Spanish phonology on the English spoken by United States Hispanics. In P. Bjarkman and R. Hammond (Eds.), *American Spanish pronunciation: Theoretical and applied perspectives* (pp. 215–236). Washington, D.C.: Georgetown University Press.

Major, R. (2001). *Foreign accent: The ontogeny and phylogeny of second language phonology*. Mahwah, NJ: Lawrence Erlbaum.

Núñez-Cedeño, R., and Morales-Front, A. (1999). *Fonología generativa contemporánea de la lengua española* [Contemporary generative phonology of the Spanish language]. Washington, D.C.: Georgetown University Press.

Perez, E. (1994). Phonological differences among speakers of Spanish-influenced English. In J. Bernthal and N. Bankson (Eds.), *Child phonology: Characteristics, assessment, and intervention with special populations* (pp. 245–254). New York: Thieme Medical Publishers.

Roseberry-McKibbin, C. (2002). *Multicultural students with special language needs* (2nd ed.). Oceanside, CA: Academic Communication Associates.

Shriberg, L., and Kent, R. (2003). *Clinical phonetics* (3rd ed). Allyn & Bacon.

Weinreich, U. (1953). *Languages in contact*. New York: Linguistic Circle of New York.

Wikipedia (2005). *English language*. Retrieved March 11, 2005, from http://en.wikipedia.org/wiki/English_language

Wolfram, W. (1971). *Overlapping influence and linguistic assimilation in second generation Puerto Rican English*. Paper presented at the meeting of the American Anthropological Association, New York. (ERIC Document 057665)Wolfram, W., and Schilling-Estes, N. (1998). *American English: Dialects and variation*. Oxford, UK: Blackwell.

Zutell, J., and Allen, V. (1988). The English spelling strategies of Spanish-speaking bilingual children. *TESOL Quarterly, 22,* 333–340.

SUMMARY OF STUDIES OF TYPICAL SPANISH-INFLUENCED ENGLISH SPEECH ACQUISITION

To date no studies are available.

Chapter 34

Jordanian Arabic Speech Acquisition

Alice T. Dyson and Mousa M. Amayreh

INTRODUCTION

The emphasis in this chapter is on Jordanian spoken Arabic (JSA), particularly the two major dialects, urban (*madani*) and rural (*fallahi*). Jordan is a cosmopolitan country with residents from all parts of the Arab world, but with a concentration of native Jordanians and Palestinians. See the Resources section in this chapter for materials pertaining to Jordanian Arabic.

Where Arabic is spoken

Arabic is the official language of at least 24 different countries and a minority language in many others (World Factbook, 2005; see the accompanying map and Appendix D). Over 200 million people speak some form of Arabic as a native language. In addition, it is the language of religious observances for millions of people in countries such as Pakistan, India, and Indonesia.

Components of Jordanian Arabic

Arabic is a Semitic language, which in Jordan has at least three distinct versions (see Figure 34-1). Classical Arabic (CA) is the language of Qur'an and classical literature. Modern Standard Arabic (MSA) or Educated spoken Arabic (ESA) differs from CA mainly in style and vocabulary (Amayreh, Hamdan, and Fareh, 1999) and will be called simply Standard Arabic (SA) throughout this chapter. Colloquial Arabic as spoken in Jordan will be called JSA.

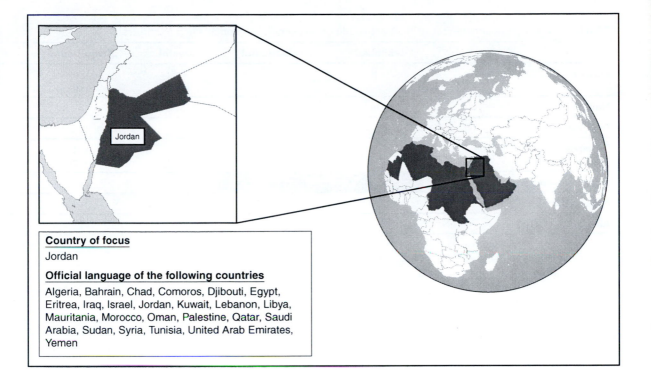

Country of focus

Jordan

Official language of the following countries

Algeria, Bahrain, Chad, Comoros, Djibouti, Egypt, Eritrea, Iraq, Israel, Jordan, Kuwait, Lebanon, Libya, Mauritania, Morocco, Oman, Palestine, Qatar, Saudi Arabia, Sudan, Syria, Tunisia, United Arab Emirates, Yemen

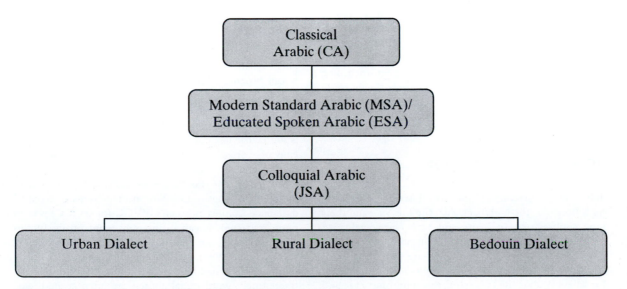

Figure 34-1 Versions of Arabic considered in this chapter.

TABLE 34-1 Consonants produced in SA with additional colloquial consonants in parentheses

	Bilabial	Labiodental	Dental	Alveo-Dental
Plosive	b			t d t̲ d̲
Nasal	m			n
Tap/Trill				r
Fricative		f (v)	θ ð ð̲	s z s̲ (z̲)
Lateral approximant	■■■■■■■■■■■■■■■■■■■■			l
Approximant	w			
Affricate				

Key. Black = articulations judged impossible.

Underlined symbols represent *emphatic* sounds with a secondary pharyngeal articulation.

Symbols in parentheses are inconsistent but acceptable replacements.

Based on the International Phonetic Alphabet. Courtesy of the International Phonetic Association (c/o Department of Linguistics, University of Victoria, Victoria, British Columbia, Canada).

Consonants

Standard Arabic has 28 consonants (see Table 34-1). In JSA, six additional consonants occur as inconsistent but acceptable replacements (in parentheses in Table 34-1) for some ESA consonants (Amayreh, 2003; Amayreh and Dyson, 1998; Dyson and Amayreh, 2000; Fareh, Hamdan, Amayreh, and Anani, 2000; Hamdan and Amayreh, in press). One unusual characteristic of Arabic is the presence of *emphatic* consonants, which have a secondary pharyngeal articulation. They are indicated symbolically in different ways by different authorities (underline, dot under, tilde through symbol, or upper case). In this chapter, the underline has been used. The /r/, /χ/, and /ʁ/ are considered emphatic in some contexts but are not underlined, as they have no non-emphatic contrasts. The /q/ is also considered emphatic because of its back articulation (Al-Ani, 1970).

Vowels and diphthongs

The vowel system of SA consists of six vowels (see Table 34-2), making up the vowel triangle with the high front /i/, the high back /u/, the low /a/, and their long counterparts /iː/, /uː/, and /aː/. The vowels vary considerably depending upon their phonetic context, especially the /a/ and /aː/, which are produced as [ɑ] and [ɑː] in the environment of emphatic consonants. In Jordanian Arabic, the two standard diphthongs /aj/ and /aw/ are produced as the prolonged monophthongs [eː]

and [oː] (Fareh et al., 2000; Huthaily, 2003; Kaye, 1987; Ladefoged and Maddieson, 1996; Mitchell, 1990).

Phonotactic restrictions

All consonants of Arabic can be used at the beginning, middle, and end of words. Some restrictions govern combinations of consonants within syllables. Syllables cannot begin with vowels.

Syllables

Standard Arabic has six types of syllables. The most frequent syllable is CV, where C can be any consonant and V can be any short vowel. The CVV (or CVː) syllable is essentially the same as the CV but includes the long vowels. CVC is also common and has no restrictions on its consonants. The very similar CVVC (or CVːC) syllable is somewhat less common and occurs most often at the ends of words. The final two syllable types include the syllable-final consonant cluster. In the CVCC syllable, the two parts of the cluster are restricted to geminates (doubled in length) and consonant pairs with maximal difference from each other. CVVCC (or CVːCC) is even more restricted. It can occur only word finally. In this kind of syllable, the CC must be geminates (Abu-Salim, 1987; Holes, 1995). In JSA the final cluster is usually simplified by epenthesis (e.g., /bint/ ⇨ [binit] 'girl'). Interestingly, word-initial clusters are often created (e.g., /ħibaːl/ ⇨ [ħbaːl] 'ropes'). In other cases, the syllable

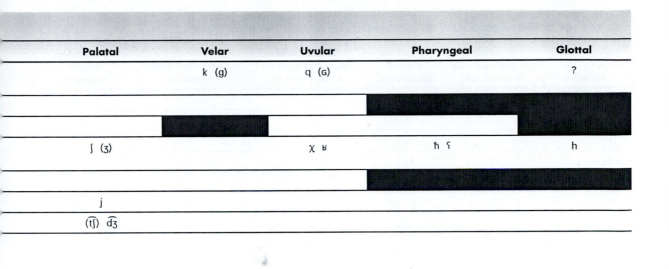

	Palatal	Velar	Uvular	Pharyngeal	Glottal
		k (g)	q (ɢ)		ʔ
	ʃ (ʒ)		χ ʁ	ħ ʕ	h
	j				
	(t͡ʃ) d͡ʒ				

structure of CVCVVC nouns is sometimes reshaped into CVCCVVC (e.g., /ħiba:l/ ⇨ [ʔiħba:l]).

Tones

Jordanian Arabic does not use tones to differentiate meaning.

Stress and intonation

Syllables in SA may be either light or heavy, generally depending upon the number of segments. There is no more than one heavy syllable in each word. When a heavy syllable occurs, it is typically stressed. If there is no heavy syllable, stress follows predictable rules. If the word has two or three syllables, the stress is on the penultimate syllable. In words with four or more syllables, the CVV syllable closest to the end of the word is stressed (Holes, 1995; Kaye, 1987). Considerable variation in stress assignment occurs from one local dialect group to another because of elision of vowels and syllables. However, within dialect groups, stress rules tend to be very regular in comparison with English. "Stress is predictable and automatic, and determined by syllable structure" (Holes, 1995, p. 65).

Because SA is primarily a written language, variations in its intonational patterns are strongly influenced by the local dialect that the speaker uses (Holes, 1995; Kaye, 1987). JSA intonation patterns are very similar to English (and many other languages of the world) with a few exceptions. These exceptions pertain primarily to question forms, where Arabic speakers rely more heavily on intonation than on structural changes (Amayreh, 1991; World Languages, 2005). For example, a falling tone in both languages indicates statements, wh-questions, commands, and exclamations, but yes-no questions are handled differently. Whereas in English they are normally signaled by syntactic changes (e.g., auxiliary verb, inversion) and a high rising tone, in JSA intonation typically signals these type of questions. The example below illustrates this principle (Amayreh, 1991, p. 106):

/ˈʔi.d͡ʒa ʔi.ˈja:d/	/ˈʔi.d͡ʒa ʔi.ˈja:d/
(mid-falling tone)	(high rising tone)
'Iyad came.'	'Did Iyad come?'

An additional example of a variation in intonation patterns occurs in wh-questions. Although both languages use a falling tone for this type of question, in Arabic the falling tone typically falls on the wh-word, whereas in English it falls near the end of the question.

Writing system

The Arabic alphabet has 28 letters, representing the consonants and long vowels. The short vowels are not written but may be specified by additional marks above or below the letters (e.g., in religious writings, children's books, and writing intended for speakers learning Arabic as a foreign language). Written

TABLE 34-2   Vowels produced in JSA compared to General American English (GAE)

American English location	American English vowels Smit (2004)	American English examples	Formal and Educated Spoken Arabic vowels	Jordanian Arabic vowels	Jordanian Arabic examples
High-front	i	b*ea*t	i:	i:	/fi:l/ 'elephant'
	ɪ	b*i*t	i	i	/bint/ 'girl'
	e	r*ai*d			
Mid-low front	ɛ	b*e*d			
	æ	b*a*d			
High-back, rounded	u	bl*ue*	u:	u:	/su:r/ 'wall'
	ʊ	b*oo*k	u	u	/kurɑ/ 'ball'
Mid-back, rounded	o	b*oa*t			
	ɔ	f*o*rm			
	–		a: ([ɑ:] with emphatic consonants)	a: ([ɑ:] with emphatic consonants)	/ba:b/ 'door' /ba:s̲/ 'bus'
	–		a ([ɑ] with emphatic consonants)	a ([ɑ] with emphatic consonants)	/jad/ 'hand' /baṭ/ 'duck'
Low-back	ɑ	dr*o*p			
Central	ə	*a*bout, *o*ccur, *u*pon			
	ʌ	c*u*p			
Diphthongs	aɪ	m*y*, b*i*ke	aj *	Becomes [e:]	/bajt/ [be:t] 'house'
	aʊ	*ou*t, m*ou*se	aw *	Becomes [o:]	/mawz/ [mo:z] 'banana'
	ɔɪ	b*oy*			

* Some disagreement exists as to whether these sounds are true diphthongs or combinations of a vowel followed by a glide. The closure for the second portion appears to be somewhat greater than that for the glides (Ladefoged and Maddieson, 1996).

text is horizontal, from right to left on the page, but numerals are written from left to right. The letters within words are joined in a cursive style with the letter before, although a few letters cannot be joined with the letter following. Letters take a distinctive shape depending upon whether they stand alone, start a word, end a word, or connect to other letters within a word. For example, the letter for the sound /b/ (/ba:ʔ/) takes the following forms: isolated form (ب); beginning of word (بـ); end of word (ـب); connected on both sides (ـبـ) (Al-Hiyari et al., 1991; Kaye, 1987).

Varieties of Jordanian Arabic

The three dialects that commonly occur in Jordan—urban, rural, and Bedouin—are mutually intelligible and widely overlapping. Because the first two are used by the majority of Jordanians (Abd-el-Jawad, 1981), the third will not be discussed further in this chapter. Phonologically the two major dialects differ in the use of only a few consonants. See Table 34-3 for a comparison of the consonants in these two dialects with SA (Amayreh, 2003; Hamdan and Amayreh, in press).

TABLE 34-3 Variants of ESA consonants that occur in JSA

SA Consonant	JSA variants (urban)	JSA variants (rural)	JSA variants (other)
/d/	[d]	[ð]	
/k/		[t͡ʃ]	
/q/	[ʔ]	[k] [g]	[ɢ]
/ʔ/	deleted when word-medial or final		
/f/	[v] in borrowed words		
/ð/	[d] [d] [z]		
/s/	[s]		
/θ/	[t]		
/ð/	[d] [z]		
/d͡ʒ/	[ʒ]	[ʒ]	
/j/	[ʔ] when word-initial in a few words		

Typical acquisition of Jordanian Arabic

The Summary of Studies Table at the end of this chapter contains the few reported studies of the acquisition of Jordanian Arabic.

Acquired sounds

Consonants

Table 34-4 contains age of acquisition data for Jordanian Arabic taken from three recent studies. The first study

TABLE 34-4 Age of acquisition for Jordanian Arabic consonants

Consonant	Amayreh and Dyson (1998)		Amayreh (2003)	Hamdan and Amayreh (in press)
b	3;0			
d	3;0			
d̪	>6;4		7;4	>6;4
t	2;6			
t̪	>6;4		8;4	≤6;4
k	2;6			
q	2;6	>6;4	7;4	>6;4
ʔ	<2;0		<6;6	≤6;4
f	2;6			
ħ	2;6			
l	3;6			
j	2;6	6;0	<6;6	≤6;4
θ	5;0	>6;4	>8;4	>6;4

Table 34-4 continued

Consonant	Amayreh and Dyson (1998)		Amayreh (2003)	Hamdan and Amayreh (in press)
ð	>6;4	>6;4	>8;4	>6;4
ð̱	6;0	>6;4	>8;4	>6;4
z	>6;4			≤6;4
s	5;0			
s̱	6;0	>6;4	>8;4	≤6;4
ʃ	5;0			
ʁ	6;0			
χ	4;6			
ʕ	>6;4		7;4	≤6;4
ħ	2;6			
h	5;0			
d̠ʒ	4;0	>6;4	>8;4	>6;4
m	<2;0			
r	5;6			
w	<2;0			

Note. The age of acquisition of any acceptable variant of the consonant is reported to the left of the column and the age of acquisition of the standard form of the consonant is reported to the right of the column. If only one age is listed, the consonant has no common variants.

(Amayreh and Dyson, 1998) reported versions of the consonants that vary in JSA. The age of acquisition of any acceptable variant of the consonant is reported to the left of the column and the age of acquisition of the standard form of the consonant is reported to the right of the column. Consonants that have no common variants have only one age listed.

Consonant clusters

To date there is no reported study of the acquisition of consonant clusters in Arabic. The study of cluster reduction is complicated by the dialectal forms used in JSA. Words that in SA would have final clusters are reduced by epenthesis as an acceptable characteristic of JSA (e.g., /χubz/ ⇨ [χubiz] 'bread'). Other words that begin with weak syllables in SA are produced with clusters in JSA (e.g., /taˈfaḏal/ ⇨ [ˈtfaḏal] 'come in'). Young children acquiring the language have been observed to delete one portion of such clusters, but no systematic study of this process is available. Dyson and Amayreh (2000) also observed that reduction of consonant sequences within words (e.g., /ˈdif.daʕ/ ⇨ [ˈdu.daʕ] 'frog') occurred about 17 percent of the time in a sample of children between 2;0

and 2;4 and was still occurring 11 percent of the time by 4;0 to 4;4. This reduction was not considered an acceptable dialectal variation. These findings included the loss of gemination of consonants within words (e.g., /ʃubˈbaːk/ ⇨ [ʃuˈbaːk]) but did not include instances in which sequences of two different consonants were combined into one geminate (e.g., /ˈʔab.jad/ ⇨ [ˈʔab.baḏ]).

Vowels and diphthongs

The process and sequence of the acquisition of vowels and diphthongs in JSA has not been reported. However, as with English, there is a general perception that they are developed earlier than consonants, and that true "errors" in vowel use are rare except in children with speech impairments such as those related to hearing or cleft palate.

Percent correct

Actual percentages of correct production of consonants, consonant clusters, and vowels typically have not been reported in acquisition studies of JSA. Only Amayreh and Dyson (1998) included data as to the percentages of overall consonants produced correctly (acceptably in the dialect) at different ages. These data are summarized in Table 34-5.

Phonological processes

The only reported study of phonological process occurrence in JSA is Dyson and Amayreh (2000) (see Table 34-6).

Intelligibility

No information is available about the intelligibility of any form of Arabic at different age levels.

Phonetic inventory

Amayreh and Dyson (2000) found certain consonants occurring in the spontaneous speech of 13 normally developing children between the ages of 14 and 24 months (see Table 34-7). All vowels expected in the dialect were observed to occur in this group.

Common mismatches

Dyson and Amayreh (2000) described the errors of normally developing children between 2;0 and 4;4 and found that one or more age groups made unacceptable consonant mismatches on more than 25 percent of their following occurrences. These are summarized in Table 34-8. In addition, clinical observations of children with speech impairments have yielded some other error substitutions that are common among young children in Jordan. These are listed at the end of Table 34-8.

Syllable structure

Errors of syllable structure have not been specifically documented for Jordanian Arabic.

TABLE 34-5 Percentage correct (acceptable production) for Jordanian Arabic consonants in elicited word naming

Age	Consonants %
2;0 – 2;4	52
2;6 – 2;10	62
3;0 – 3;4	75
3;6 – 3;10	75
4;0 – 4;4	81
4;6 – 4;10	78
5;0 – 5;4	86
5;6 – 5;10	84
6;0 – 6;10	90

Note. Data taken from Amayreh and Dyson (1998).

Prosody

Errors of prosody have not been documented for Jordanian Arabic except as they apply to the speech of hearing impaired children. Among children with hearing impairment, clinical observation indicates no errors that differentiate Arabic-speaking children from those learning English or other languages.

Phonological awareness

No studies of phonological awareness of Jordanian Arabic have been reported.

TABLE 34-6 Frequency of occurrence of selected phonological processes in elicited word naming at four age levels

Age	Syllable deletion %	Final consonant deletion %	Sequence reduction %	Stridency deletion %	Fronting %	Final devoicing %	Lateral replacement of /r/ %	De-emphasis %
2;0–2;4	6	6	17	27	7	16	35	70
2;6–2;10	8	5	18	20	5	23	16	49
3;0–3;4	4	2	12	16	3	13	13	35
3;6–3;10	4	2	11	13	1	13	8	32
4;0–4;4	3	<1	11	12	<1	18	10	30

Note. Data taken from Dyson and Amayreh (2000).

TABLE 34-7 Consonants occurring in at least three different words in the phonetic inventories of at least 5/13 participants

Manner	All positions combined
Stop	b, d, t, ʔ
Fricative	ʃ, ʕ, ħ, h
Affricate	
Nasal	m, n
Lateral	l
Tap-Trill	
Approximant	w, j
Number of consonants	13

Note. Data taken from Amayreh and Dyson (2000).

Speech assessment for Jordanian Arabic children

The only published articulation test is the *Amayreh Articulation Test* (Amayreh, 1994). It is a picture–naming test that originally included 58 pictures. Recently, some pictures have been added and others were replaced to make it more balanced (Amayreh, 2003; Hamdan and Amayreh, in press). An unpublished articulation test developed by Attiyeh (1986) is also available. Additional informal speech sampling tools that have been developed for use with Jordanian Arabic children include deep tests for frequently misarticulated sounds.

The Logical International Phonetic Programs (LIPP, Oller and Delgado, 1990) have been adapted for use in analysis of Jordanian Arabic speech (Dyson and Amayreh, 2000). Analyses for phonological processes, phonetic inventories, and percentages of consonants correct have been developed.

Speech intervention for Jordanian Arabic children

Standard procedures for speech intervention in English (traditional approach, Cycles, etc.) have been adapted

TABLE 34-8 Consonant substitutions of normally developing children in Jordan and commonly occurring error substitutions in clinical populations

Standard consonant ⇨ Unacceptable substitute
d̪ ⇨ t
t ⇨ t*
d̪ ⇨ t
d̪ ⇨ d*
s̪ ⇨ s*
s ⇨ θ
ʃ ⇨ s
ʁ ⇨ χ
ʕ ⇨ ʔ
d͡ʒ/ʒ ⇨ d

Substitution errors observed clinically
r ⇨ l, ʁ, ɹ
l ⇨ j
k, q ⇨ t
s, ʃ ⇨ t

Note. Data on consonant substitution taken from Dyson and Amayreh (2000).

*Acceptable in urban dialect, but the urban and rural dialects were not distinguished in this study.

for Jordanian Arabic. However, techniques for eliciting sounds that do not exist in English have been developed by clinicians as needed. For example, the trilled /r/ is often elicited by modifying its homorganic counterpart /l/ and the /ʁ/ sound by gurgling water.

Working in Jordan

In 1999, regulations for working in the field of speech-language pathology (SLP) in Jordan were approved. Requirements for obtaining a license and working independently in the country include the following: MA or Ph.D. in SLP, two years of experience in the field after graduation, and passing an exam given by the Ministry of Health. A person with a bachelor's degree in SLP can work as a therapist only under supervision.

PHONETICALLY SPEAKING

Pronunciation of Jordanian Arabic:
/ʔallahd͡ʒa ʔalmadanijja/ *[urban dialect]*
/ʔallhd͡ʒa ʔalfalla:hijja/ *[rural dialect]*

Relevant words for speech assessment and intervention

Word/Phrase	Formal usage	Pronunciation	Informal usage	Pronunciation
Tongue	*lisaan*	/li'sa:n/	lsaan	/ˌlsa:n/
Teeth	*asnaan*	/ʔas'na:n/	snaan	/sna:n/
Lips	*shifaah*	/ʃi'fa:h/	shafaayif	/ʃa'fa:jif/
Hard palate	*ghaar*	/ʁa:r/	saqfilfam	/'sɑqfilˌfam/
Soft palate	*tabaq*	/ʔat'tabɑq/	saqfilfamallayyin	/ˌsɑqfilˌfamil'lajjin/
Larynx	*hunjurah*	/'ħund͡ʒura/		
Lungs	*ria'taan*	/riʔa'ta:n/	ri'aten	/riʔa'te:n/
Nose	*'anf*	/ʔanf/	munkhaar	/mun'χɑ:r/
Sound	*sawt*	/sɑwt/	sowt	/so:t/
Word	*kalimah*	/'kalima/	kilmeh	/'kilmi/
Sentence	*jumlah*	/'d͡ʒumla/	jumleh	/'d͡ʒumli/
Paragraph	*fiqarah*	/'faqra/	fagra	/'fagra/

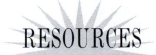

RESOURCES

Books

Al Shakhs, A. (1997). /ʔidtra:ba:t ʔannutq walkala:m/ [Speech disorders: Background, diagnosis, types, and treatment]. Riyadh, Saudi Arabia: Sharikat Al Safahat Al Thahabiya Al Mahduda.

Al Zarrad, F. (1990). /ʔalluʁa wadtra:ba:t ʔ alkala:m/ [Language and speech disorders]. Riyadh, Saudi Arabia: Dar Al Marrikh Linnashr.

Amin, S. (2000). /ʔallad͡ʒlad͡ʒa: ʔasba:buha: waʕila:d͡ʒuha:/ [Stuttering: Its causes and intervention]. Arabic Thought Series in Special Education, 2. Cairo: Dar Al Fikr Al Arabi.

Porot, D. (1996). /ʔidtraːbaːt ʔalluʁa/ [Les troubles du langue] (A. I. Hachem, Trans., 1997). Beirut, Lebanon: Editions Oueidat.

Sartawi, A., and Abu Judah, W. (2000). /ʔidtraːbaːt ʔ annutq walluʁa/ [Speech and language disorders]. Riyadh, Saudi Arabia: Saudi Academy for Autism.

CD-ROMs

The *Amayreh Articulation Test* has been adapted for CD-ROM but is not yet available commercially.

Journals

Currently, there are no journals dedicated to Arabic SLP in Jordan.

Professional associations

A professional association of speech–language pathologists within Jordan is being organized but is not yet active.

Useful Arabic Web sites

- Saudi Speech Pathology and Audiology Association, http://www.sspaa.org/en/
- Union des Phoniatrics Europeans – Egypt, http://www.uni-leipzig.de/~hno/uep/Continents/africa/egypt/
- Proceedings of the National Academy of Sciences of the USA, manuscript by Vargha-Khadem, et al., http://www.pnas.org/cgi/content/full/95/21/12695

REFERENCES

Abd-El-Jawad, H. R. (1987). Cross-dialectal variation in Arabic: Competing prestigious forms. *Language in Society, 16,* 359–367.

Abu-Salim, I. (1987). Al-bunya almaqta'iya fil lughatil 'arabiyya [Syllable structure in Arabic]. *Journal of Jordanian Academy of Arabic Language,* 45–63.

Al Khalaylah, A. R. (1980). *Tatawwur annutq 'inda atfalen Urdiniyeen bayna sin sanatyni wanisf wa sit sanawat* [Development of articulation in Jordanian children between 2½ and 6 years]. Unpublished master's thesis, University of Jordan, Amman.

Al-Ani, S. (1970). *Arabic phonology.* The Hague: Mouton.

Al-Hiyari, A., Kukhun, A., Manasrah, Y., Bakeer, U., Shahin, Y., Jardanah, B., et al. (1991). *luʁatuna l-ʕarabijja : kitaːbutʕtaːlib, d͡ʒuzʔ 1 & 2* [Our Arabic language: Student's book, Parts 1 and 2]. Amman, Jordan: Ministry of Education.

Amayreh, M. M. (1991). *A study of the basic intonational patterns in Standard and Jordanian Arabic.* Unpublished master's thesis, University of Jordan, Amman.

Amayreh, M. M. (2003). Completion of the consonant inventory of Arabic. *Journal of Speech, Language, and Hearing Research, 46,* 517–529.

Amayreh, M. M., and Dyson, A. T. (1998). The acquisition of Arabic consonants. *Journal of Speech, Language, and Hearing Research, 41,* 642–653.

Amayreh, M. M., and Dyson, A. T. (2000). Phonetic inventories of young Arabic-speaking children. *Clinical Linguistics and Phonetics, 14,* 193–215.

Amayreh, M. M., Hamdan, J., and Fareh, S. (1999). Frequency of occurrence of consonant phonemes in Arabic and English discourse. *Dirasat, Series of Human and Social Sciences, special issue,* 207–220.

Attiyeh (1986). *Articulation test.* Unpublished manuscript.

Dyson, A. T., and Amayreh, M. M. (2000). Phonological errors and sound changes in Arabic-speaking children. *Clinical Linguistics and Phonetics, 14,* 79–109.

Fareh, S., Hamdan, J. M., Amayreh, M. M., and Anani, M. (2000). *Muqaddima fil lughawiyyat al mu,asira* [Introduction to modern linguistics]. Amman, Jordan: Dar Wael.

Hamdan, J. M., and Amayreh, M. M. (in press). Consonant profile of Arabic-speaking school-age children in Jordan. *Folio Phoniatrica.*

Holes, C. (1995). *Modern Arabic: Structures, functions, and varieties.* London: Longman Linguistics Library.

Huthaily, K. (2003). *Contrastive phonological analysis of Arabic and English.* Unpublished master's thesis, University of Montana.

Kaye, A. S. (1990). Arabic. In B. Comrie (Ed.), *The world's major languages* (pp. 664–685). New York: Oxford University Press.

Ladefoged, P., and Maddieson, I. (1976). *The sounds of the world's languages.* Oxford, UK: Blackwell.

Mitchell, T. F. (1990). *Pronouncing Arabic.* Oxford, UK: Clarendon Press.

Oller, D. K., and Delgado, R. (1990). *Logical International Phonetics Programs (LIPP).* Miami, FL: Intelligent Hearing Systems.

Omar, M. K. (1973). The acquisition of Egyptian Arabic as a native language. *Janua linguarum. Series Practica, 160,* 199–205.

World Factbook (CIA). (2005). Retrieved August 15, 2005, from http://www.cia.gov/cia/publications/factbook/fields/2098.html

World Languages (2005). *A description of Arabic.* Retrieved August 15, 2005, from http://www.lerc.edu.ubc.ca/LERCcourses/489/worldlang/Abdulmanan/description.html/

SUMMARY OF STUDIES OF TYPICAL JORDANIAN ARABIC SPEECH ACQUISITION

Authors	Year	Country	No. of children	Age of children	Information	Sample type	Data collection
Al Khalaylah	1980	Eastern Jordan	120	2;6–6;0	Age of suppression of articulation errors	Single word	Cross-sectional
Amayreh and Dyson	1998	Jordan	180	2;0–6;4	Age of acquisition of consonants	Single word	Cross-sectional
Amayreh	2003	Jordan	60	6;6–8;4	Age of acquisition of consonants	Single word	Cross-sectional
Amayreh and Dyson	2000	Jordan	13	14–24 mo.	Phonetic inventories	Spontaneous speech	One observation
Dyson and Amayreh	2000	Jordan	50	2;0–4;4	Errors and sound changes	Single word	Cross-sectional
Hamdan and Amayreh	in press	Jordan	100	Mean age 6;4	Age of acquisition of consonants and effect of dialect	Single word	One observation

Chapter 35

Lebanese Arabic Speech Acquisition

Ghada Khattab

INTRODUCTION

The Lebanese Republic is just over 85 years old, but the territory of present-day Lebanon can be traced back to antiquity with the establishment of city-states along the Eastern Mediterranean coast by the Phoenicians, who spoke a Semitic language called Canaanite (Salibi, 1988), which was then replaced by Aramaic. Over the centuries, these cities, together with Mount Lebanon, Syria, Jordan, and Palestine, formed part of a wide geographical area that witnessed several ruling powers, including the Persian conquest, the Hellenistic Seleucid Kingdom, the Roman Empire, and a succession of Islamic empires (Salibi; Versteegh, 1997). Bedouin varieties of Arabic existed in the area before the early Islamic conquests in the seventh century, but the conquests introduced urban varieties that underwent fast changes and gradually acquired prestige (Versteegh). The last of the empires, the Ottoman Empire, was finally defeated by the Allies at the end of the First World War, making present-day Lebanese territory part of the French mandate. The French created the State of Greater Lebanon in 1920. This was reconstituted as the Lebanese Republic in 1926, which gained its independence from the French in 1943 (Salibi). Due to the complex historical background of Lebanon, the country came to be inhabited by people with different religions, cultures, dialects, and languages. Currently, more than 3.5 million people live in Lebanon. Lebanon is a multilingual society with three widely spoken languages, Arabic, English, and French. The three languages have experienced variation in their use over the course of the twentieth century due to historical, political, and religious events (Abou, Kasparian, and Haddad, 1996; Joseph, 2004; Shaaban and Ghaith, 2002). Currently, Standard Arabic and French are the official languages, and Arabic use is diglossic (see section on Varieties of Lebanese Arabic). Lebanon also has sizable Armenian and Kurdish communities (Gordon, 2005), and the respective languages are maintained as the first language of many of the members of these communities. See the Resources section in this chapter for materials pertaining to Lebanese Arabic.

Where Lebanese Arabic is spoken

Lebanese Arabic is mainly spoken in Lebanon (see the accompanying map and Appendix D), although there are Lebanese communities all over the world due to different waves of immigration that took place in the middle of the nineteenth century and throughout the twentieth century, especially during the Lebanese civil war (1975–1990). Sizable Lebanese communities can be found in Africa (e.g., Leichtman, 2005), Australia (e.g., Hage, 2002; Labaki, 1989; Taft and Cahill, 1989), Canada (e.g., Abu-Laban, Barclay, Walstrom, and Sweet, 1999), Europe (e.g., Hourani, 1992), and North and South America (e.g., Daher, 1988; Dweik, 1992; Samore, 1983).

Components of Lebanese Arabic

Consonants

Lebanese Arabic has 27 consonants (Nasr, 1966) and is most closely related to Central Syrian Arabic (see Table 35-1). Consonant length is phonemic in Arabic (Nasr, 1960), and all Lebanese consonants can be geminated (e.g., /sabab/ 'cause' vs. /sabːab/ 'he caused'). Emphatic consonants (/tˤ, dˤ, sˤ, zˤ, lˤ/) involve simultaneous articulatory postures, one for the primary place of articulation of the consonant and another one in the velo-pharyngeal area of the mouth (Ferguson, 1956). The primary articulatory contact of these consonants is often retracted, especially for /tˤ/ and /dˤ/ (Al-Ani, 1970; Laradi, 1983; Odisho, 1973). Varieties of Arabic differ with respect to which and how many of these emphatic consonants they possess, and there are conflicting research findings concerning whether the articulatory basis of emphasis is uvularization (Zawaydeh, 1998), velarization (Gairdner, 1925; Obrecht, 1968), or

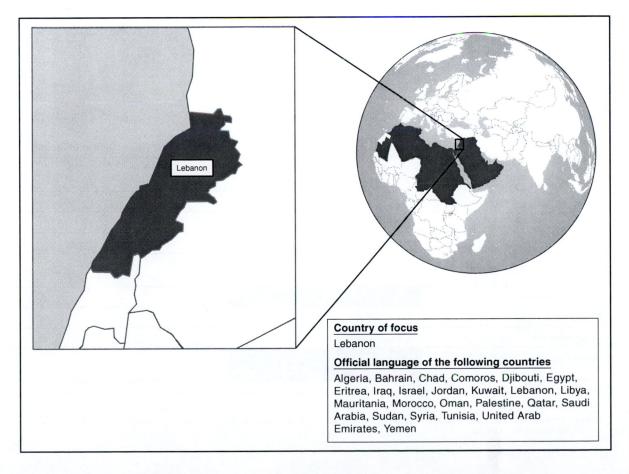

Country of focus

Lebanon

Official language of the following countries

Algeria, Bahrain, Chad, Comoros, Djibouti, Egypt, Eritrea, Iraq, Israel, Jordan, Kuwait, Lebanon, Libya, Mauritania, Morocco, Oman, Palestine, Qatar, Saudi Arabia, Sudan, Syria, Tunisia, United Arab Emirates, Yemen

pharyngealization (Al-Ani, 1970; Giannini and Pettorino, 1982; Laufer and Thomas, 1988).

Additional consonants

Table 35-1 contains a number of additional consonants (in parentheses), either to indicate that they are used in loan words or that their production is subject to dialectal and/or free variation. In Arabic, no native /p/ or /v/ exists. However, proper names and loan words, principally from French (*piscine, service*), are frequent in the Lebanese dialect and are usually produced with [p] and [v] by the majority of people, especially if they are highly educated. [b] and [f] can also be heard as realizations for /p/ and /v/, especially among the uneducated. Similarly, no native /g/ exists in Lebanese Arabic, but people usually produce it accurately in loan words (e.g., *garage, gateau*). /g/ is also familiar to the Lebanese due to its use in nearby Arabic dialects such as Palestinian and Egyptian (e.g., Al-Shareef, 2002; Ammar and Morsi, 2006). However, [k] is sometimes heard as a realization for /g/ in loan words. As for /q/, it is mainly realized as [ʔ] in Lebanese Arabic (but see the section on Varieties of Lebanese Arabic), although a handful of lexical items that are borrowed from classical Arabic have kept the original [q] pronunciation (e.g., [qʊrʔaːn] 'Koran'). /θ/ and /ð/ are restricted to

Standard Arabic usage (news reading, sermons, etc.) and are normally realized as [t] (or [s]) and [d] (e.g., [tleːte] for /θalaːta/ 'three'; [sɪʔa] for /θɪqa/ 'trust'; [danab] for /ðanab/ 'tail'). Finally, [χ] and [ʁ] are in free variation with [x] and [ɣ], while /tʃ/ and /dʒ/ are either produced in loan words (e.g., *Chernobyl*; *jeans*) or are realizations of CVC syllables with reduced vowels (e.g., [tʃamːas] for /taʃamːasa/ 'he sun-bathed').

Vowels and diphthongs

There are no instrumental studies of vowels in spoken Lebanese Arabic, and available descriptions tend to concentrate on the threefold distinction between phonologically short and long /i/, /a/, and /u/ (e.g., Abu Haidar, 1979; Haddad, 1984; Nasr, 1966). The realizations of these vowels in various dialects significantly exceed three (Mitchell, 1990). In Table 35-2, an attempt is made at presenting the rich phonetic variation that is available in the realization of Lebanese Arabic vowels compared with their familiar phonological representation in Standard Arabic.

Some of the features of Lebanese Arabic vowels are typical of many spoken dialects of Arabic. These include frequent elisions, centralizations, and/or lax realizations of short vowels in various contexts, retraction in emphatic

TABLE 35-1   Consonants produced in Lebanese Arabic

	Bilabial	Labiodental	Interdental	Dental-alveolar
Plosive	(p) b			t d tˤ dˤ
Nasal	m			n
Trill				r
Tap or flap				ɾ
Fricative		f (v)	(θ) (ð)	s z sˤ zˤ
Lateral fricative	■■■■■		■■■■■	
Affricate				
Approximant	w (labiovelar)			
Lateral approximant	■■■■■		■■■■■	l lˤ

Note. Sounds in parentheses indicate either that they are used in loan words or that their production is subject to dialectal and/or free variation

Black = articulations judged impossible

Based on the International Phonetic Alphabet. Courtesy of the International Phonetic Association (c/o Department of Linguistics, University of Victoria, Victoria, British Columbia, Canada).

contexts, and a rich variation in the realizations of /aː/ and /a/ depending on neighboring contexts. But one particular aspect of Lebanese vowels relates to the realization of /a/ as [e] in the neighborhood of an /i/ vowel (e.g., /kitaːb/ is realized as [kteːb] 'book', and /ʒaːmiʕ/ as [ʒeːmiʕ] 'mosque'). This is known as Imala (Haddad, 1984; Nasr, 1966), a historical process that has extended to other contexts in Lebanese Arabic (Table 35-2) apart from emphatic ones. As a result of that, short and long vowel systems in Lebanese Arabic (and other spoken dialects) are no longer symmetrical and have both qualitative and quantitative differences (e.g., /safar/ 'travel' vs. /seːfar/ 'he traveled'; /ʕiʃte/ 'you lived' vs. /ʕiːʃte/ 'my life'). Moreover, in most Lebanese dialects, the diphthongs /aɪ/ and /aʊ/ have developed into /eː/ and /oː/ in closed-syllable contexts, which has added to the system of long vowels (Table 35-2).

Phonotactic restrictions

Syllables

A distinction needs to be drawn between syllable structure in Standard Arabic and in Lebanese Arabic. In Standard Arabic, syllable types are divided into three quantities driven by the phonological importance of vowel and consonant length: short (CV), medium (CVV or CVC), and long (CVVC, CVCC, CVVCC). CVV, CVVC, and CVVCC contrast quantitatively with CV, CVC, and CVC due to vowel length (Mitchell, 1990). These play a role in stress placement (see the section on Stress). In Lebanese Arabic, however, elision of vowels results in a reorganization of syllables and in consonant clusters. More importantly, the short/long vowel systems are no longer complementary; for example, loss of final contrast between /ʔakala/ 'he ate' and /ʔakalaː/ 'they ate' due to elision of final short vowels in Lebanese Arabic (/ʔakal/ for 'he ate' and /ʔakalao/ for 'they ate'). Although descriptions of syllable structure in Lebanese Arabic mention five syllable types (CV, CVV, CVC, CVVC, and CVCC), phonetically, more syllable types are possible due to vowel elision (Haddad, 1984). The syllable structure of Lebanese Arabic can therefore be described phonetically in the following formula: $C_{(1-2)}V_{(1-2)}C_{(0-2)}$. The onset and the nucleus are essential constituents in Arabic whereas the coda is optional, but there is a tendency toward closed syllables at word-final positions. The nucleus of the syllable can be a short (V) or a long (VV) vowel. The smallest allowable syllable is therefore CV (e.g., /wa/ 'and'), and the largest allowable syllable is CCVVCC (e.g., /lʕaːmː/ 'the general'). Commonly used words contain up to four

	Post-alveolar	Retroflex	Palatal	Velar	Uvular	Pharyngeal	Glottal
				(k) g	(q)		ʔ
	ʃ ʒ			x ɣ (χ) (ʁ)		ħ ʕ	h
	(tʃ) (dʒ)						
			j				

TABLE 35-2 Vowels produced in Standard Arabic (SA) compared to Lebanese Arabic (LA)

SA location	SA Vowels (Mitchell, 1990)	SA examples (phonemic)	LA location	LA realization (phonetic)	LA examples
High-front	iː	tiːn 'figs'	High-front	iː	tiːn
Mid-high front	i	min 'from'	Mid-high central	ɪ	mɪn
		bajti 'my house'	Mid-high front	e	baɪte
		tˤifil 'baby'	Mid-high central	ʊ	tˤʊfl
Central low-open	aː	xaːdim 'servant'	Mid-low front	æː	xæːdim
		baːb 'door'	Mid-high front	eː	beːb
		naːr 'fire'	Central low-open	aː	naːr
		maːʔ 'water'	Diphthong	aɪ/ɔɪ	maɪ/mɔɪ
		tˤaːba 'ball'	Low-back	ɑː	tˤɑːbe
Central mid-open	a	kalb 'dog'	Central mid-open	æ	kalb
		samaka 'fish'	Mid-high front	e	samke
		jadˤrub 'he hits'	Mid-high central	ʊ	jʊdˤrub
		batˤ 'ducks'	Low back	ɑ	batˤː
High-back rounded	uː	ħuːt 'whale'	High-back, rounded	uː	ħuːt
Mid-high back rounded	u	ħur 'free'	Mid-high central	ʊ	ħʊr
		ʔakalu 'they ate'	Mid-back, rounded	o	ʔakalo
		ħuna 'here'	Mid-back rounded	oː	hoːne
		kutub 'books'	Mid-high front	ɪ	kɪtʊb
Diphthongs	aːj	naːj 'flute'	Diphthong	æːɪ	naːɪ
	aj	zaj 'outfit'	Diphthong	æɪ	zaɪ
		bajt 'house'	Monophthong	eː	beːt
	aw	ʔaw 'or'	Diphthong	aʊ	ʔaʊ
		mawt 'death'	Monophthong	oː	moːt

Note. Diphthongs in Arabic are often presented as sequences of vowels and semivowels, the latter considered as having a consonantal type of articulation (e.g., /bajt/ for 'house' and /ʔaw/ for 'or'); Source: Mitchell, 1990.

syllables (e.g., /sɪʒːeːˈdeːtna/ 'our carpets'). Note that, as can be seen in this last example, phonologically long vowels occur in both accented and unaccented syllables in Lebanese Arabic.

Consonants and consonant clusters

As mentioned in the previous section, although the onset and coda in Standard Arabic cannot consist of more than one consonant, consonant clusters are phonetically common in dialectal varieties, including Lebanese Arabic. Since these clusters are often the result of vowel reduction (e.g., Standard Arabic /kiˈtaːb/ 'book' is [kteːb] in Lebanese Arabic), the sonority principle does not always apply to the resulting syllables (e.g., [lʔaːb] 'play!'; [msaːħ] 'wipe!'; /lbaħr/ 'the sea'). Various phonological accounts have presented ways of resyllabification of these syllables so that the initial and or final consonants are considered

extrametrical (e.g., /l.baħ.r/) (e.g., Al-Ageli, 1996; Haddad, 1984; McCarthy and Prince, 1990). Exceptionally long onsets include CCC in [striːħ] for /ʔistariħ/ 'rest!' and [ʃtraɪt] for /ʔiʃtarait/ 'I bought', but these vary in their production across speakers and dialects.

Tones

Lebanese Arabic does not use tones to differentiate meaning.

Stress and intonation

Like many Eastern Arabic dialects, Lebanese Arabic has a trochaic word-stress pattern (Watson, 2002). Primary stress is placed on monosyllabic words (e.g., /ˈmɪn/ 'from'), while stress in multisyllabic words is determined by the number of syllables and their weight (Haddad, 1984;

Kenstowicz and Abdul-Karim, 1980; Nasr, 1966). A short or light syllable is one that contains a CV(C) sequence (only word-final CVC is short). A long or weighted syllable is one that contains C(C)V(V)C(C) (non-final CVC is long). In multisyllabic words, primary stress is placed on the first syllable of two or three short-syllable words (e.g., /ˈmasa/ 'evening'; /ˈʔakalit/ 'she ate'), the penultimate long syllable in a multisyllabic word (e.g., /ʔaˈkalt/ 'I ate'; /ˈmaktabe/ 'library'; /ʔawaːˈmirna/ 'our orders'), or the penultimate short syllable in a multisyllabic word (e.g., /kamaˈʃito/ 'she caught him') (Haddad, 1984; Nasr, 1966). Nasr (1966) describes two other levels of stress: secondary stress, which is placed on the other long syllables in a multisyllabic word (e.g., /sɪʒːeːˈdeːtna/ 'our carpets'), while all other short syllables take tertiary stress.

There are no studies of Lebanese Arabic intonation apart from Chahal's (2001) investigation of the intonation patterns of the Tripoli dialect using an Autosegmental-Metrical framework. Arabic is an intonational language that uses pitch postlexically to give a particular meaning to the overall utterance. Pitch accents are placed on primary stressed syllables, while phrase edges have a variety of pitch contours. For instance, declarative sentences have a falling contour, questions have a high rising edge configuration, while continuation phrases have a falling rising edge to signal that more information is on the way (Chahal, 2001).

Writing system

Like other Arab children, Lebanese children learn the writing system of Standard Arabic, the variety used in printed materials (see next section). They therefore face the challenge of learning a writing system together with being exposed to a variety of Arabic that is different from their colloquial variety spoken at home (Saiegh-Haddad, 2003). Arabic uses a Semitic system that is written from right to left and whereby short vowels (called *fatHa, damme,* and *kasra*) are represented as diacritics on consonantal letters (two above and one below), whereas long vowels have their own individual consonant letters (*alif, waw,* and *ja*). While diacritics are kept in children's scripts to aid learning, they are not normally present in adult scripts as it is assumed that skilled learners will deduce them from the overall grammatical structure of the utterance (e.g., Taouk and Coltheart, 2004). There is one-to-one grapheme-phoneme correspondence in (vowelized) Arabic, which makes it predictable and regular, but the letter used to represent a consonant differs in shape as a function of the position of that letter in the

letter sequence. There are four other reading signs to help readers process the written strings in a particular way:

- The *sukun*, which indicates that there is no short vowel to follow
- The *shaddeh*, which indicates the doubling of a consonant and is placed above it
- The *maddeh*, which indicates the doubling of the *alif*
- The *hamzeh*, which is the glottal stop

Varieties of Lebanese Arabic

Arabic use is diglossic (Ferguson, 1959), with Standard Arabic being used for educational, religious, and media purposes, and Spoken Arabic being used for everyday interaction. Standard Arabic is nobody's native language. It is learned formally at school and/or at home as part of the child's education. An Arab child's native tongue is the colloquial variety of Arabic that is particular to his or her dialect, which differs considerably from Standard Arabic in terms of its phonology, morphology, syntax, and lexicon (Watson, 2002). Lebanese Spoken Arabic belongs to the North Levantine variety of Eastern Arabic dialects and includes the following dialects: North Lebanese Arabic, South Lebanese Arabic (Shii, Metuali), North-Central Lebanese Arabic (Mount Lebanon Arabic), South-Central Lebanese Arabic (Druze Arabic), Standard Lebanese Arabic, Beqaa Arabic, Sunni Beiruti Arabic, Saida Sunni Arabic, Iqlim-Al-Kharrub Sunni Arabic, and Jdaideh Arabic (Gordon, 2005). These dialects are very much understudied, and most available descriptions are either sketchy or outdated (e.g., Abu Haidar, 1979; Cadora, 1976; El-Hajje, 1954; Elrabih, 1983; Furayhah, 1938; Lakkis, 1987). Apart from the Lebanese varieties of Arabic, Lebanon has sizable Palestinian and Syrian communities, and very little is known about how their varieties compare with those spoken in Syria and Palestine.

Apart from Arabic, French plays a great political and economic role in Lebanese identity, especially among the Christian population (Gueunier and Haddad, 1993; Joseph, 2004; Shaaban and Ghaith, 2003; Thonhauser, 2001). Arabic-French bilingualism has been maintained since independence from France in 1943 due to missionary schools and the Christian community's efforts to sustain links with the West. The Muslim population, on the other hand, has tended to defend the maintenance of Arabic in order to ascertain the Lebanese identity as an Arab one. Lebanese Muslims also tend to prefer learning English as a foreign language rather than French. Regardless of their religious affiliation, the Lebanese have always associated learning foreign languages with upward social and economic mobility (Thonhauser), and English use has recently been on the rise due to its dominance in communication and technology. Despite the use of Arabic as an official language, Lebanese governments have always stressed the importance of mastery of foreign languages. The national curriculum therefore requires that another language be taught by the seventh grade (Bahous, 1999), and many Lebanese children learn a third language from age 11. Schools are mainly divided according to whether they offer French or English first at the primary level, with the other language then being introduced at the secondary level.

Very little, however, is known about how early each of these languages is introduced to children growing up in Lebanon. There are hardly any investigations of the daily patterns of language use in the community or about the role the languages play in children's acquisition. Informal observation of child–adult interaction in several homes shows that many Lebanese children are exposed to all three languages to varying degrees from a very early age (Khattab, 2004). The input also varies between native and nonnative varieties of the three languages, depending on the type of education that the child receives (private vs. government school and/or nursery) and the nature of home care (foreign nannies and maids are employed in many households). Very little is known about how these varying types of input may influence the children's acquisition process. From a phonological perspective, the three languages are very different at both the segmental and suprasegmental level. For children acquiring these languages in combination, little is known about how the language systems interact and how the children develop communicative abilities through their growing productive and perceptive repertoires.

Typical acquisition of Lebanese Arabic

There are barely any comprehensive descriptions of the phonetics/phonology of Lebanese Arabic, let alone of typical acquisition. A lot of the information compiled for previous sections of this chapter has been gathered from unpublished theses/dissertations (e.g., Abdul-Karim, 1980; Daher, 1988; Haddad, 1984; Lakkis, 1987) or journal articles that address particular aspects of Arabic phonology (e.g., Kenstowicz and Abdul-Karim, 1980; Yeni-Komshian, Caramazza, and Preston, 1977). There are no normative studies of typical acquisition of Lebanese Arabic to date, but a handful of studies have concentrated on some aspects of phonological acquisition by Lebanese children living abroad and acquiring more than one language. For

instance, Preston, Yeni-Komshian, and Stark (1967) looked at VOT production in the prelinguistic vocalization of two infants acquiring English, one Lebanese and one American. The authors found that both infants produced their stops in the short lag region with VOT values ranging between 0 and 30 ms, and concluded that short VOT intervals may be easier for infants to accomplish as opposed to voicing lead and long lag, which require careful timing between supraglottal and glottal articulators. Khattab (2002a, b, c, 2003, 2006) investigated the phonological development of Lebanese-English bilinguals growing up in the UK and concentrated on a handful of consonantal and vocalic variables that differed in their patterning in the two languages. The bilinguals' production in each language was nativelike and exhibited developmental patterns similar to those produced by monolingual controls from each language but also patterns that were exclusive to the bilinguals and that may have been due to interaction between their languages. More interestingly, the bilinguals' production in English was shown to vary in phonetic detail depending on factors such as language base and interlocutors; this was interpreted as a sign of sociolinguistic competence by these children. Salameh, Nettelbladt, and Norlin (2003) worked with Arabic-Swedish bilinguals (including Lebanese participants) with and without phonological impairments. The authors suggested that bilinguals can develop separate phonological systems for each of their languages and that their developmental and abnormal patterns were similar to those exhibited by normal and disordered monolingual children. Various case studies have been conducted as master's dissertations by students at Lebanese universities (e.g., de Smidt, 1980; Jamous, 1981; Schmidt, 1970), but none of these has been published or has become widely available in the public domain. The Summary of Studies Table at the end of this chapter contains studies of the acquisition of Lebanese Arabic.

Acquired sounds
Consonants

To date there is no study of age of consonant acquisition by Lebanese children. Communication with speech and language therapists working in Lebanon reveals that there are no available norms that could be used to assess the speech of disordered children, and the milestones that are mentioned are purely anecdotal and based on work experience. Table 35-3 contains anecdotal rather than published data on the age of consonant acquisition for Lebanese Arabic children. The data were collected from

	TABLE 35-3 Age of acquisition for Lebanese Arabic consonants	

Consonant	Anecdotal data from speech and language therapists
b	2;0
m	2;0
n	2;0
h	2;0
ħ	5;0
w	3;0
j	4;0–5;0
t	2;0
d	2;0
tˤ	6;0 and later
dˤ	6;0 and later
k	3;0
ʔ	2;0
l	3;0
lˤ	6;0 and later
ʒ	4;0
ʃ	4;0–5;0
s	3;0
z	4;0
sˤ	6;0 and later
zˤ	6;0 and later
r	6;0 and later
ɾ	5;0
f	3;0
x	5;0
ɣ	5;0
ʕ	5;0

communications with 10 speech and language therapists working in Lebanon. No data on differences between males and females are available.

Consonant clusters

To date there is no Lebanese study of the age of acquisition of consonant clusters.

Vowels and diphthongs

To date there is no Lebanese study of the age of acquisition of vowels.

Percent correct

Consonants

To date there is no study of percentage of consonants produced correctly by Lebanese children according to age.

Consonant clusters

To date there is no study of percentage of consonant clusters produced correctly by Lebanese children according to age.

Vowels

To date there is no study of percentage of vowels produced correctly by Lebanese children according to age, whether in monosyllables or in polysyllables.

Phonological processes

To date there is no study of phonological processes in Lebanese children. Information gathered from speech and language therapists in Lebanon reveals that the following processes are the most common:

- /r/ gliding to [j] and [l]
- /k/ fronting to [t]
- /s/ fronting to [θ]
- Backing
- Stopping
- Devoicing
- De-emphasization

Intelligibility

To date there is no study of intelligibility of Lebanese children.

Phonetic inventory

To date there is no study of the phonetic inventory of consonants or vowels produced by Lebanese children.

Common mismatches

To date there is no study of common mismatches produced by Lebanese children.

Syllable structure

To date there is no study of syllable structure produced by Lebanese children.

Prosody

To date there is no study of Lebanese children's prosody.

Phonological awareness

To date there is no study of the emerging phonological awareness skills of Lebanese children.

Speech assessment for Lebanese Arabic children

The fields of speech assessment and speech therapy in Lebanon are underdeveloped in many ways. There are only two universities in Lebanon that have recently started offering Speech and Language Pathology degrees (Institut Supérieur D'orthophonie, Faculté the Médecine, Université Saint-Joseph; Département D'orthophonie, Faculté de Santé Publique, Université Libanaise). French speech-language pathologists visit both universities every year to offer intensive courses on some of the professional subjects. Around 25 students graduate from both programs every year, the first cohort having graduated in 1999. Some go on to pursue postgraduate studies abroad while others start working straight away.

As part of their work for their theses, students from these two universities normally work on descriptive aspects of language development or create speech and language assessment tools, but these tools are often tested on a small number of people and are rarely published or normalized. There are no formal, standardized Lebanese Arabic tests of articulation or phonology. All speech and language therapists who were consulted for this chapter mentioned having to rely on their experience in the field when carrying out speech assessments. Speech and language therapists use online learning resources to create their own "homemade" games and activities for speech assessment using clip art, the English Learning Centre (ELC), commercially bought toys, and professional intervention tools from the United States or Europe. Since these tools were originally created for English and/or French (and sometimes German), they are adapted to the best of the speech and language therapists' knowledge and ability and then used with Lebanese clients. The speech and language therapists are aware of the problems associated with adapted English and French tests, especially with regard to phonological tests, but they mention the need for better research facilities and resources that would enable them to conduct wide-scale normative studies on normal and disordered speech acquisition before creating appropriate tests.

The most popular tests for assessing children's speech sounds are the following:

- *EDP 4-8: épreuve de discrimination phonemiques* (French) (Autesserre, Deltour, and Lacert, 1987).
- *Logical International Phonetic Programs* (LIPP) (Dyson and Amayreh, 2000)

The following has been designed for analyzing Lebanese Arabic speech:

- *Epreuve de Discrimination Phonémique Arabe "EDiPhAr"* (Fares and Chidiac, 2000), adapted from the EDP French test and tested on 120 Lebanese children aged 5;0 to 6;0 from the Greater Beirut area.

Speech intervention for Lebanese Arabic children

Until recently speech and language therapists in Lebanon had been using their own in-house speech intervention techniques without much communication with each other and with no access to published material for Lebanese Arabic. However, a speech and language therapy association has recently been created in Lebanon (Association Libanaise des Orthophonistes, July 2, 2004) and has about 80 members. Speech and language therapists working in Lebanon are excited about this new development and have been meeting to discuss ways to improve the service. One item on the agenda is to publish existing theses that are produced by students from both universities offering speech and language therapy degrees to make them more accessible and to allow future work to build on existing resources. To date, very little is known about speech intervention techniques, if any, that have been developed for Lebanese Arabic.

Any future work on normal and disordered speech development in Lebanon will need to take into account the prevalence of multilingualism in Lebanon and the consequences for early language development. French and/or English are spoken by many families and children are exposed to more than one language from a very young age. Assessment and intervention tools should therefore be designed to cater to more than one language.

Working in Lebanon

Apart from the 80 members who have joined Association Libanaise des Orthophonistes and who have mainly graduated from the Lebanese and Saint-Joseph Universities, there are an estimated 20 to 30 speech and language therapists who have not joined yet and/or who practice without qualifications, though this may change as the association becomes more powerful. Beirut and Mount Lebanon regions have the largest number of practicing speech and language therapists (up to 25 each), while the remaining regions range between 1 and 10 registered speech and language therapists. There is a need for speech therapy services in all regions, especially in the Bekaa and the South. Most speech and language therapists work in specialized centers and institutions in the morning and in clinics in the afternoon. The average caseload is four or five cases a day. Some of the Beirut-based speech and language therapists also serve other regions, and even those permanently based in Beirut sometimes work in more than one clinic. A visa is needed for non-Lebanese speech and language therapists to work in Lebanon.

PHONETICALLY SPEAKING

Pronunciation of Lebanese: /lɛbəˈniːz/
Relevant words for speech assessment and intervention

Word/Phrase	Formal usage	Pronunciation	Informal usage	Pronunciation
Tongue	lisaan	liˈsaːn	lseen	lseːn
Teeth	asnaan	ʔasˈnaːn	sneen	sneːn
Lips	shifaf	ʃiˈfaːf	shfeef	ʃfeːf
Hard palate	alhank alsalib	ʔalħank ʔasˤːɑlɪb	halq	ħalʔ
Soft palate	alhank allajjin	ʔalħank ʔalːjːɪn	halq	ħalʔ
Larynx	alhunzhura	ʔalˈħunʒura	lhinzhra	ˈlhɪnʒra
Lungs	alriʔataan	ʔalriʔaˈtaːn	lrijjeet	lrijːeːt
Nose	anf	ʔanf	minxaar	mɪnxaːr
Sound	sawt	sˤɑʊt	sot	sˤoːt
Word	kalima	ˈkalima	kilme	ˈkilme
Sentence	zhumla	ˈʒumla	zhimle	ˈʒɪmle
Paragraph	maqtaa	ˈmaqtˤɑʕ	maqtaa	ˈmaʔtˤɑʕ

RESOURCES

Books

Abu-Haidar, F. (1979). *A study of the spoken Arabic of Baskinta*. Leiden: Brill.

Cantineau, J. (1934). *Le dialecte Arabe de palmyre*, 2 vols. Beirut: Librarie du Liban.

El-Hajje, H. (1954). *Le parler arabe de Tripoli (Liban)*. Paris: Librairie C. Klincksieck.

El-Sayed, K. (1990). *Arabic as spoken in Lebanon*. USA: El-Sayed Publications.

Feghali, M. (1928). *Syntaxe des parlers arabes actuels du Liban*. Paris: Imprimerie Nationale.

Feghali, M. N. (1999). *Spoken Lebanese*. Beirut: Parkway Publishers.

Fleisch, H. (1974). *Études d'Arabe dialectal*. Beyrouth: Dar El-Machreq.

Karam, E. (1982). *Spoken Arabic: The language of Lebanon*. Petersham, MA: St Bede's Publications.

Mattsson, E. (1910). *Études Phonologiques sur le Dialecte Arabe Vulgaire de Beyrouth*. Upsal: K.W. Appelberg.

Nasr, R. T. (1966). *Colloquial Arabic: An oral approach*. Beirut: Librarie du Liban.

Professional associations

The professional association of speech-language pathologists within Lebanon is Association Libanaise des Ortophonistes (ALO), www.orthophonistes.net/

Useful Lebanese Arabic Web sites

- The Online Lebanese Community, http://www.lebanon.com/
- Lebanese Ministry of Tourism, http://www.lebanon-tourism.gov.lb/
- Introduction to Lebanese Language, http://www.abcleb.com/
- Lebanese Language Books, http://www.berro.com/lebanese_books/lebanese_language_books.htm

REFERENCES

Abdul-Karim, K.W. (1980). *Aspects of the phonology of Lebanese Arabic*. Unpublished Ph.D. thesis, University of Illinois at Urbana-Champaign.

Abou, S., Kasparian, C., and Haddad, K. (1996). *Anatomie de la Francophony Libanaise*. Beirut: Universite Saint-Joseph.

Abu-Haidar, F. (1979). *A study of the spoken Arabic of Baskinta*. Leiden: Brill.

Abu-Laban, B., Barclay, H. B, Walstrom. N., and Sweet, L. E. (1999). *Arab Canadians*. New Haven, CT: Human Relations Area Files.

Al-Ageli, H. M. (1996). *Syllabic and metrical structure in Tripolitanian Arabic: A comparative study in standard and optimality theory (Libya)*. Unpublished Ph.D. thesis, University of Essex, UK.

Al-Ani, S. (1970). *Arabic phonology*. The Hague: Mouton.

Al-Shareef, J. (2002). *Language change and variation in Palestine*. Unpublished Ph.D. thesis, University of Leeds, UK.

Ammar, W., and Morsi, R. (2006). Phonological development and disorders: Colloquial Egyptian Arabic. In Z. Hua and B. Dodd (Eds.), *Phonological development and disorders: A cross-linguistic perspective* (pp. 204–232). Clevedon: Multilingual Matters.

Autesserre, D., Deltour, J. J., and Lacert, Ph. (1987). *Épreuve de discrimination phonemique pour enfants the 4-8 ans (EDP 4-8)*. Édition EAP.

Bahous, J. (1999, December). *What language should a Lebanese child learn first?* Paper presented at the Lebanese American University Multilingualism and Multiculturalism in Lebanon one-day international conference, Beirut, Lebanon.

Cadora, F. J. (1976). Contrastive compatibility in some Arabic dialects and their classification. *Anthropological Linguistics*, *18*(9), 393–407.

Chahal, D. (2001). *Modeling the intonation of Lebanese Arabic using the autosegmental metrical framework: A comparison with English*. Unpublished Ph.D. thesis, University of Melbourne, Australia.

Daher, Nazih Y. (1975). *Topics in the phonology of Lebanese Arabic.* Unpublished M.A. thesis, Ohio State University, Columbus.

Daher, Nazih Y. (1988). What is happening to a Lebanese dialect in Cleveland, Ohio: Language attrition in progress. *Al-Arabiyya, 21*(1-2), 3–18.

de Smidt, B.A. (1980). *First language acquisition of Arabic by a child exposed to two languages.* Unpublished M.A. thesis, American University of Beirut.

Dweik, B. S. (1992). Lebanese Christians in Buffalo: Language maintenance and language shift. In A. Rouchdy (Ed.). *The Arabic language in America* (pp. 100–118). Detroit: Wayne State University Press.

Dyson, A. T., and Amayreh, M. M. (2000). Phonological errors and sound changes in Arabic-speaking children. *Clinical Linguistics and Phonetics, 14*, 79–109.

El-Hajje, H. (1954). *Le parler arabe de Tripoli (Liban).* Paris: Librairie C. Klincksieck.

Elrabih, M. M. (1983). *The Lebanese dialect of Arabic: Southern region.* Unpublished Ph.D. thesis, Georgetown University, Washington, DC.

Fares, D., and Chidiac, W. (2000). *Epreuve de Discrimination Phonemic Arabe (E.Di.Ph.Ar.).* Unpublished B.Sc. dissertation. Département d'Orthophonie, Université Libanaise.

Ferguson, C.A. (1956). The emphatic l in Arabic. *Language, 32*(3), 446–452.

Ferguson, C.A. (1959). Diglossia. *Word, 15*, 325–337.

Furayhah, A. (1938). *Quadriliterals from the dialect of Ras al-Matn (Lebanon).* Chicago: University of Chicago Press.

Gairdner, W. (1925). *The phonetics of Arabic.* London: Oxford University Press.

Giannini, A., and Pettorino, M. (1982). *The emphatic consonants in Arabic.* Speech Laboratory Report IV, Salerno: Istituto Universitario Orientale di Napoli.

Gordon, R.G., Jr. (Ed.). (2005). *Ethnologue: Languages of the world* (15th ed.). Dallas, TX: SIL International. Online version: http://www.ethnologue.com/.

Gueunier, N., and Haddad, K. (1993). *Le français du Liban, cent portraits linguistiques.* Paris: ACCT, Didier-Erudition.

Haddad, G. F. (1984). *Problems and issues in the phonology of Lebanese Arabic.* Unpublished Ph.D. dissertation, University of Illinois, Urbana.

Hage, G. (2002). *Arab-Australians today: Citizenship and belonging.* South Victoria: Melbourne University Press.

Hourani, A. (1992). Introduction. In A. Hourani and N. Shehadi (Eds.), *The Lebanese in the world: A century of emigration* (pp. 3–11). London: Centre for Lebanese Studies.

Jamous, R. M., (1981). *Linguistic deviations in the acquisition of colloquial Lebanese Arabic as a first language.* Unpublished M.A. thesis, American University of Beirut.

Joseph, J. J. (2004). *Language and identity: National, ethnic, religious.* New York: Palgrave Macmillan.

Kenstowicz, M., and Abdul-Karim, K. (1980). Cyclic stress in Levantine Arabic. *Studies in the Linguistic Sciences, 10*(2), 55–76.

Khattab, G. (2002a). /l/ production in English-Arabic bilingual speakers. *International Journal of Bilingualism, 6*(3), 335–353.

Khattab, G. (2002b). VOT in English and Arabic bilingual and monolingual children. In D. Parkinson & and. Benmamoun (Eds.), *Perspectives on Arabic linguistics,* XIII–XIV, (pp. 1–39). Amsterdam Philadelphia: John Benjamins.

Khattab, G. (2002c). /r/ production in English and Arabic bilingual and monolingual speakers. In D. Nelson (Ed.), *Leeds Working Papers in Linguistics & Phonetics, 9*, 1–39.

Khattab, G. (2003). *Sociolinguistic competence and the bilingual's adoption of phonetic variants: Auditory and instrumental data from English-Arabic bilinguals.* Unpublished Ph.D. dissertation, University of Leeds, UK.

Khattab, G. (2004, December). *Acquisition of geminate consonants by Arabic children.* Paper presented at the Department of English Language and Linguistics, University of Sheffield, UK.

Khattab, G. (2006). Phonological acquisition in Arabic–English bilingual children. In Z. Hua and B. Dodd (Eds.), *Phonological development and disorders: A cross-linguistic perspective* (pp. 383–412). Clevedon: Multilingual Matters.

Labaki, B. (1989). Immigration of Lebanese to Australia from the 1970s. *Etudes Migrations, 26*(94), 247–271.

Lakkis, K. M. (1987). *The phonology of the Lebanese dialect of Ba`albeck.* Unpublished M.A. thesis, American University of Beirut.

Laradi, W. J. (1983). *Pharyngealisation in Libyan (Tripoli) Arabic.* Unpublished Ph.D. thesis, University of Edinburgh.

Laufer, A., and Thomas, B. (1988). The emphatic and pharyngeal sounds in Hebrew and Arabic. *Language & Speech, 24*, 39–61.

Leichtman, M. A. (2005). The legacy of transnational lives: Beyond the first generation of Lebanese in Senegal. *Ethnic and Racial Studies, 28*(4), 663–686.

McCarthy, J., and Prince, A. (1990). Prosodic morphology and templatic morphology. In M. Eid and J. McCarthy (Eds.), *Perspectives on Arabic linguistics* (pp. 1–54). Amsterdam: John Benjamins.

Mitchell, T. F. (1990). *Pronouncing Arabic I*. Oxford, UK: Clarendon Press.

Nasr, R.T. (1960). Phonemic length in Lebanese Arabic. *Phonetica, 5,* 209–211.

Nasr, R.T. (1966). *Colloquial Arabic: An oral approach.* Beirut: Librarie du Liban.

Obrecht, D. H. (1968). *Effects of the second formant on the perception of velarization consonants in Arabic.* Mouton: The Hague.

Odisho, E. (1973). *The role of the rear section of the vocal tract in Baghdadi Arabic.* Unpublished M. Phil. thesis, University of Leeds.

Preston, M. S., Yeni-Komshian, G. G., and Stark, R. E. (1967). A study of voicing in initial stops found in the pre-linguistic vocalizations of infants from different language environments. In *Status Report on Speech Research SR-10* (pp. 109–120). New York: Haskins Laboratories.

Saiegh-Haddad, E. (2003). Linguistic distance and initial reading acquisition: The case of Arabic diglossia. *Applied Psycholinguistics, 24,* 431–451.

Salameh, E. K., Nettelbladt, U., and Norlin, K. (2003). Assessing phonologies in bilingual Swedish-Arabic children with and without language impairment. *Child Language Teaching and Therapy, 19*(3), 338–364.

Salibi, K. (1988). *A house of many mansions: The history of Lebanon reconsidered.* Berkeley: University of California Press.

Samore, L.T. (1983). *A sociolinguistic and historical survey of the Lebanese Orthodox-Christian community in Sioux City, Iowa.* Unpublished M.A. thesis, University of Arizona.

Schmidt, E. R. (1970). *A phonological analysis of the speech of a set of four-year-old Arabic-speaking twins.* Unpublished M.A. thesis, American University of Beirut.

Shaaban, K., and Ghaith, G. (2003). Effect of religion, first foreign language, and gender on the perception of the utility of language. *Journal of Language, Identity & Education, 2*(1), 53–77.

Taft, R., and Cahill, D. (1989). Mother tongue maintenance in Lebanese immigrant families in Australia. *Journal of Multilingual and Multicultural Development, 10*(2), 129–143.

Taouk, M., and Coltheart, M. (2004). The cognitive processes involved in learning to read in Arabic. *Reading and Writing, 17,* 27–57.

Thonhauser, I. (2001). Multilingual education in Lebanon: 'Arabinglizi' and other challenges of multilingualism. *Mediterranean Journal of Educational Studies, 6*(1), 49–61.

Versteegh, K. (1997). *The Arabic language.* New York: Columbia University Press.

Watson, J. C. E. (2002). *The phonology and morphology of Arabic.* Oxford, UK: Oxford University Press.

Yeni-Komshian, G. H., Caramazza, A., and Preston, M. S. (1977). A study of voicing in Lebanese Arabic. *Journal of Phonetics, 5,* 35–48.

Zawaydeh, B. (1998). Gradient uvularisation spread in Ammani-Jordanian Arabic. In A. Benmamoun, M. Eid, and N. Haeri (Eds.), *Perspectives on Arabic linguistics XI* (pp. 117–141). Amsterdam/Philadelphia: John Benjamins.

SUMMARY OF STUDIES OF TYPICAL LEBANESE ARABIC SPEECH ACQUISITION

Authors	Year	Country	No. of children	Age of children	Information	Sample type	Data collection
Khattab	2003	UK and Lebanon	6	5, 7, and 10	Bilingual and monolingual acquisition	Single word,+ story telling,+ playing games	Cross-sectional
Preston, Yeni-Komshian, and Stark	1967	USA	2	infants	Bilingual acquisition, VOT	Single word	Cross-sectional

Chapter 36

Cantonese Speech Acquisition

Lydia K. H. So

INTRODUCTION

Cantonese is a dialect of Chinese and is a language with lexical tones. There are 19 consonants, 11 vowels, 11 diphthongs, and 9 tones in Cantonese. The syllable structure is simple with tone and vowel as the obligatory elements and initial and final consonants as optional ones. Research has been undertaken on the acquisition of Cantonese phonology by normally developing Cantonese-speaking children (So and Dodd, 1995; Stokes and To, 2002; Tse, 1978, 1982, 1991). So and Dodd (1995) found that Cantonese-speaking children completed their phonological development before age 6. Cantonese-speaking children have developmental processes similar to children acquiring English and also processes specific for themselves (So and Dodd, 1995). See the Resources section in this chapter for materials pertaining to Cantonese.

Where Cantonese is spoken

Cantonese is spoken in southern China in the Guangdong and Guangxi Provinces (see accompanying map and Appendix D). Over 40 million people, in Hong Kong, Guangdong, and overseas communities in Britain, Canada, Australia, and the USA speak Cantonese.

Components of Cantonese

Consonants

Cantonese has 19 consonants and is most closely related to Putonghua. There are 16 oral phonemes /p, pʰ, t, tʰ, k, kʰ, kʷ, kʷʰ, f, s, h, w, j, l, ts, tsʰ/ and 3 nasal phonemes /m, n, ŋ/ (see Table 36-1). Cantonese stops are contrastive in aspiration, while English is nonconstrastive. Voicing is contrastive in English stops but not in Cantonese (Bauer and Benedict, 1997).

Vowels and diphthongs

There are 11 vowels in Cantonese, seven long vowels /a, i, u, y, ɛ-e, ɔ-o, œ/ and four short vowels /ɐ, ɪ, ɵ, ʊ/. Of the short vowels, ɪ, ɵ and ʊ are allophones of /i/, /œ/ and /u/ respectively. Therefore there are eight contrastive vowels in Cantonese /a, i, u, y, ɛ, ɔ, œ, ɐ/ (Zee, 1999) (see Figure 36-1).

There are 11 diphthongs /ai, ui, ɔi, ei, ɐi, au, iu, ɐu, ou, ɵy, eu/ in Cantonese (see Figure 36-2). Five diphthongs end at the /i/ position while another five diphthongs end at the /u/ position, and one ends in the /y/ position. Table 36-2 lists the Cantonese vowels and compares them to the British English vowels.

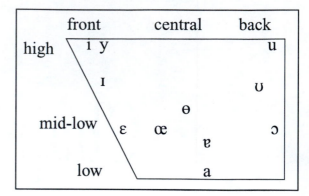

Figure 36-1   Cantonese vowels

Phonotactic restrictions

Syllables

The syllable structure of Cantonese is (C)V(C). The onset and coda are optional while the nucleus is obligatory. There are six possible syllable structures in Cantonese, including V, C, CV, VC, CVV, and CVC. Only two syllables have "C" as the syllable structure. They are the syllabic nasals, namely /m/ and /ŋ/. Syllables with the CV structure can end with any vowels except /ɐ/. For the VC or CVC structures, all

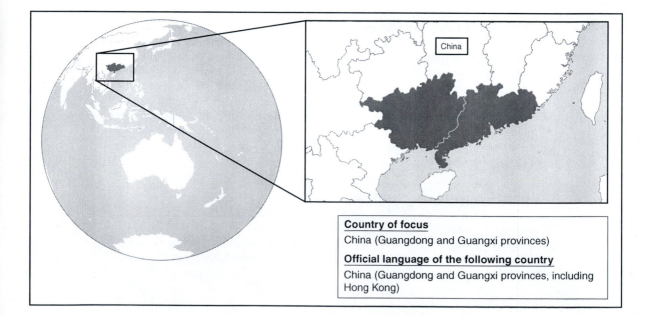

Country of focus
China (Guangdong and Guangxi provinces)

Official language of the following country
China (Guangdong and Guangxi provinces, including Hong Kong)

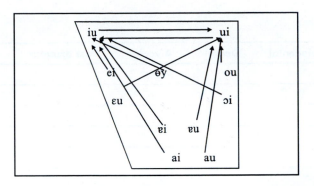

Figure 36-2 Cantonese diphthongs

syllables end with either stops /p, t, k/ or nasals /m, n, ŋ/. For the CVV structure, most syllables end with either the /u/ or /i/ vowels.

The existence of tones within the syllable is a major characteristic of Cantonese syllables. With the tone, the Cantonese syllable can be expressed with the following formula:

$$\frac{\text{Tone}}{(\text{C})\text{V}(\text{C})}$$

Consonants and consonant clusters

Nineteen consonants /p, pʰ, t, tʰ, k, kʰ, f, s, h, m, n, ŋ l, w, j, ts, tsʰ, kʷ, kʷʰ/ can be initial consonants (see Table 36-1). Six consonants /p, t, k, m, n, ŋ/ can act as final consonants. Labialized velars /kʷ, kʷʰ/ are either treated as consonants (e.g., Bauer and Benedict, 1997) or consonant clusters

(e.g., Hashimoto, 1972). If /kʷ, kʷʰ/ are treated as consonants, consonant clusters can be found only in colloquial Cantonese as /kl/ in words such as /kliŋ₅₅ liŋ₅₅ klaŋ₅₅ laŋ₅₅/ 'breaking noise'.

Tones

Cantonese uses tones to differentiate lexical meaning. There are six contrastive tones, namely, high level, high rise, mid level, low fall, low rise, and low level. Including the stopped tones, there are nine tones in Cantonese as described by traditional Chinese phonology. Words with ending in –p, –t, or –k carry the stopped tones. The tone values of the three stopped tones and the three respective level tones are the same. Figure 36-3 provides a summary of the tone values and the pitch graph of the nine tones.

Stress and intonation

Cantonese is a language with syllable-timed rhythm. Each syllable carries a tone, and syllables are nearly equally stressed. Lexical tone contrasts word semantics. Grammatical intonation exists in Cantonese and conveys syntactic information. In Cantonese the end of a declarative sentence is characterized by a falling intonation pattern. Rising intonation helps to indicate questions. Intonation change on the last word of an utterance can convey additional information. For example, a rising intonation on the last word of an utterance turns a declarative sentence into an interrogative one that conveys uncertainty (Kwok and Luke, 1986).

Tones:	high level	high rise	mid level	low fall	low rise	low level	high stopped	mid stopped	low stopped
Pitch graph:	˥	˨	˧	˩	˨	˨	˥	˧	˨
Tone value:	55	25	33	21	23	22	5	3	2

Figure 36-3 Cantonese tonal system

TABLE 36-1 Consonants produced in Cantonese

	Bilabial	Labiodental	Dental	Alveolar	Post alveolar
Plosive	p pʰ			t tʰ	
Nasal	m			n	
Trill					
Tap or flap					
Fricative		f		s	
Lateral fricative	███████████████████████				
Affricate				ts tsʰ	
Approximant					
Lateral approximant	███████████████████████			l	

Black = articulations judged impossible

Based on the International Phonetic Alphabet. Courtesy of the International Phonetic Association (c/o Department of Linguistics, University of Victoria, Victoria, British Columbia, Canada).

Writing system

The writing system of Cantonese consists of characters. Each syllable usually has a corresponding standard Chinese character. Dialectal characters are used when no standard Chinese characters are found. Written Chinese is nonalphabetic and consists of characters that represent lexical morphemes. Chinese words are formed by one or more characters. There are six categories of Chinese characters: pictograph of objects, denotation of events, ideograph, phonetic-logographic compound, figurative extension of meaning, and phonetic loan. The phonetic-logographic compound and phonetic loan characters are connected with speech sound.

Li (1977) estimated that about 80 percent of modern Chinese characters are phonetic-logographic compounds or phonetic compounds. Every Chinese character is presented in a square-shape region, no matter how many strokes there are. Complexity of a character depends on the number of strokes within the character. Although Chinese script is nonalphabetic, it can contain sublexical information for the pronunciation, as most characters contain a "phonetic radical" that indicates how the character is pronounced. For example, the words 'mother' /ma₅₅/, 'horse' /ma₂₃/, and 'scold' /ma₂₂/ have the radical 'horse' in the character and the three words share the same segment /ma/ with a difference in tones only.

Varieties of Cantonese

There are variations in Cantonese due to phonetic variation and change. Bauer and Benedict (1997) listed the major phonetic variations in Hong Kong Cantonese as follows:

Tones

The High Fall tone is changed to the High Level tone, High Falling ˥˨ ⇨ High Level ˥˥, or variation between the two tones, High Falling ˥˨ ~ High Level ˥˥.

Vowels

The high front vowel in a demonstrative pronoun may be diphthongized and there is variation between high front vowel and diphthong or change to diphthong, n/li ~ n/lei or n/li ⇨ n/lei.

Initial consonants

- Variation of nasal and lateral, /l-/ ~ /n-/, or change of nasal to lateral, /n-/ ⇨ /l-/
- Variation of aspirated velar stop and glottal fricative, /kʰɵy/ ~ /hɵy/, or change to fricative, /kʰɵy/ ⇨ /hɵy/, in third person pronoun
- Variation of velar nasal and zero-initial, /ŋ-/ ~ o, or change of velar nasal to zero-initial, /ŋ-/ ⇨ ɔ-

Retroflex	Palatal	Labiovelar	Velar	Uvular	Pharyngeal	Glottal
		kʷ kʷʰ	k kʰ			
			ŋ			
						h
	j	w				

TABLE 36-2 Vowels produced in Cantonese compared with British English (Received Pronunciation)

Received Pronunciation (RP) Location	KEY WORD (Wells, 1982)	RP phonetic/ phonemic symbols (Wells, 1982)	RP examples	Cantonese location	Cantonese symbols	Cantonese examples
High-front	FLEECE	i	b*ea*t	High-front	i	jit₂ 'hot'
	KIT	ɪ	b*i*t	High-front	ɪ	sɪŋ₅₅ 'star'
Mid-low front	DRESS	ɛ	b*e*d	Mid-low front	ɛ	pɛŋ₂₅ 'biscuit'
	TRAP	æ	b*a*d			
High-back, rounded	GOOSE	u	bl*ue*	High-back, rounded	u	fu₃₃ 'trousers'
	FOOT	ʊ	b*oo*k	High-back, rounded	ʊ	jʊk₂₂ 'meat'
Mid-back, rounded	THOUGHT, NORTH, FORCE	ɔ	f*or*m	Mid-low back, rounded	ɔ	tʰɔŋ₂₅ 'candy'
Low back, rounded	LOT	ɒ	dr*o*p			
Low back,	START, BATH, PALM	ɑ	b*ar*d	Low central	a	fa₅₅ 'flower'
Central	COMMA, LETTER	ə	*a*bout, *o*ccur, *u*pon, nev*er*, zebr			
Front-central-mid-open	NURSE	ɜ	b*ir*d	Front-central, mid-low	œ	hœ₅₅ 'boot'
	STRUT	ʌ	b*u*d	Central, mid-low	ɐ	kʰɐm₂₁ 'piano'
				Central, mid	ɵ	sɵn₃₃ 'letter'

Table 36-2 continued

Received Pronunciation (RP) Location	KEY WORD (Wells, 1982)	RP phonetic/ phonemic symbols (Wells, 1982)	RP examples	Cantonese location	Cantonese symbols	Cantonese examples
				High front, rounded	y	jy_{25} 'fish'
Diphthongs	PRICE	ai	*my, b<u>i</u>ke*			t^hai_{55} 'tie'
	MOUTH	aʊ	<u>out</u>, <u>m</u>ouse			au_{55} 'hook'
	CHOICE	ɔi	*b<u>oy</u>*			$ɔi_{33}$ 'love'
	FACE	eɪ	*b<u>ay</u>, b<u>ai</u>t*			fei_{55} 'fly'
	GOAT	oʊ	*b<u>oat</u>, b<u>ow</u>(tie)*			tou_{55} 'knife'
	NEAR	ɪə	*b<u>eer</u>*			
	SQUARE	ɛə	*b<u>ear</u>*			
	CURE	ʊə	*t<u>our</u>*			
					ei	k^wai_{55} 'turtle'
					ey	sey_{25} 'water'
					ui	pui_{55} 'cup'
					eu	iu_{33} 'want'
					eu	keu_{25} 'dog'
					eu	teu_{22} 'throw'

- Variation of labialized and delabialized velars /kw-/ ~ /k-/_ ɔ, or change to delabialized velars, /kw-/ ⇨ /k-/ /_ɔ before back round vowel /ɔ/

Nasal syllabics

Labial assimilation of velar nasal: variation of velar and bilabial nasal syllabics, /ŋ/ ~ /m/, or change to bilabial syllabic before/after labial consonants, /ŋ/ ⇨ /m /_ labial consonant, /labial consonant_.

Final consonants

- Variation between velar nasal final and dental nasal final, /-Vŋ/ ~ /-Vn/, or change to dental nasal final, /-Vŋ/ ⇨ /-Vn/.
- Variation between velar stop final and dental or glottal stop final, /-Vk/ ~ /-Vt/, /-Vʔ/, or change to dental or glottal stop final, /-Vk/ ⇨ /-Vt/, /-Vʔ/.

Typical acquisition of Cantonese

To date there are a few studies of the typical acquisition of Cantonese. J. K. P. Tse (1978) studied his son's tonal development. S. M. Tse (1982), Cheung (1990), A. C. Y. Tse (1991), and So and Dodd (1995) reported Cantonese-speaking children's consonant, vowel, and tonal development considering phonological processes. Stokes and To (2002) studied the feature development of Cantonese-speaking children aged from 0;10 to 4;7. They proposed a three-level (A, B, and C) phonetic implicational hierarchy for Cantonese. Level A includes the contrastive features of consonant, syllabic, and sonorant; Level B includes labial, coronal, and delayed release features; while level C includes continuant and spread glottis features. Stokes and Wong (2002) studied the vowel and diphthong development of 40 children aged 0;10 to 2; 3. The Summary of Studies Table at the end of this chapter contains studies of the acquisition of Cantonese.

Acquired sounds

Consonants

The acquisition of consonants has been studied by several researchers. S. M. Tse (1982) studied three children aged from 1;7 to 2;8 and A. C. Y. Tse (1991) followed a child longitudinally from 1;2 to 3;0. Cheung (1990) studied 155 children whose ages ranged from 2;1 to 6;0 and So and Dodd (1995) studied 268 children aged from 2;0 to 5;11 cross-sectionally. The results of the Cheung (1990) and the So and Dodd (1995) studies were similar, while the four children in the two Tse studies seem to have had a faster acquisition rate. As seen in Table 36-3, the unaspirated bilabial and alveolar stops /p, t/, the alveolar nasal /n/, and the labial-velar and palatal approximant /w, j/ were acquired earliest at the age of 2;0. The bilabial nasal /m/,

and velar nasal /ŋ/ and the labial-velar approximant /w/, were acquired around the age of 2;6. By age 3, the glottal fricative /h/, the lateral /l/, and the unaspirated velar stop /k/ were acquired. Aspirated stops /pʰ, tʰ, kʰ/ and the lateral /l/, were acquired late at about 3;6. Fricatives /s, f/, affricatives /ts, tsʰ/ and the unaspirated labialized velar stop /kʷ/ were acquired later, between 4;0 and 4;6. The aspirated labialized velar stop /kʷʰ/ was the latest to be acquired. Table 36-3 summarizes the age of acquisition of Cantonese consonants from different studies.

In addition, data from the *Cantonese Segmental Phonology Test* (CSPT) (So, 1993) indicate nasals /m, n, ŋ/, semivowels /w, j/, glottal fricative /h/, unaspirated stops /p, t, k/, lateral /l/, and finals /m, n, p/ are acquired early before the age of 3. The fricatives /f, s/, affricates /ts, tsʰ/, aspirated stops /pʰ, tʰ, kʰ/, labialized velars /kʰw, kw/, and final stops

TABLE 36-3   Age of acquisition for Cantonese consonants

Consonant	Tse, S. M. (1982)	Tse, A. C. Y. (1991)	Cheung (1990)	So and Dodd (1995)
			(90% criterion)	(90% criterion)
p	1;7	1;3	2;1	2;0
pʰ	2;5	1;11	3;1	3;6
m	2;0	1;8	2;1	2;6
n	2;0	1;11	2;7	2;0
ŋ	1;7	2;10	3;1	2;6
h	1;7	1;3	2;7	3;0
w	2;5	1;3	2;7	2;6
j	1;7	1;3	2;1	2;0
t	2;0	1;6	2;1	2;0
tʰ	2;5	1;11	3;1	3;6
k	2;0	1;8	3;7	3;0
kʰ	>2;8	>3;0	4;1	3;6
f	2;3	>3;0	3;1	4;0
l	2;3	2;9	2;7	3;6
ts	2	2;10	4;1	4;0
tsʰ	1;7	2;7	4;1	4;6
s	2;3	>3;0	5;7	4;0
kʷ	>2;8	>3;0	3;7	3;9
kʷʰ	>2;8	>3;0	3;7	4;9

Note. NA = not assessed

/-t, -k, -ŋ / are acquired late, around 3;6 to 5;0. Vowels and tones are acquired early and before the age of 2.

Vowels and diphthongs

Vowels and diphthongs were acquired relatively, most by the age of 2. Table 36-4 summarizes age of acquisition of Cantonese vowels from different researchers.

Percent correct

Consonants

The percentage of consonants correct (PCC) increases as age increases. According to So and Dodd (1995), at age 2, the PCC is 85.7 percent and it increases significantly to 91.7 percent and 95.8 percent at ages 2;6 and 3;0 respectively. PCC increases steadily to 99.2 percent by age 5;6 (So and Dodd, 1995). Table 36-5 lists the percentage correct for Cantonese consonants and vowels.

Vowels

Percentage correct for vowels at age 2 is very high (98.8 percent) and it increases steadily to 100 percent by the age of 5;11 (So and Dodd, 1995) (see Table 36-5).

Phonological processes

Speech errors occur during Cantonese phonological acquisition. The common processes used by Cantonese–speaking children (over 10 percent) at age group 2;0 to

TABLE 36-4 Age of acquisition for Cantonese vowels

Vowels	Tse, S. M. (1982)	Tse, A. C. Y. (1991)	Cheung (1990)	So and Dodd (1995)	Stokes and Wong (2002)
a	1;7	1;3	<2;0	<2;0	1;3
i	1;7	1;3	<2;0	<2;0	1;8
u	1;7	1;11	<2;0	<2;0	2;0
y	2;3	1;6	<2;0	<2;0	2;0
ɛe	1;7	1;3	<2;0	<2;0	1;3
ɔo	1;7	1;3	<2;0	<2;0	1;3
œ	1;7	2;2	<2;0	<2;0	2;0
ɐ	1;7	1;3	<2;0	<2;0	2;0
θ	NA	NA	<2;0	<2;0	NA
ɪ	NA	1;6	<2;0	<2;0	NA
ʊ	NA	2;0	<2;0	<2;0	NA
ai	2;8	2;0	<2;0	<2;0	2;0
ui	1;7	2;0	<2;0	<2;0	2;0
ɔi	2;8	2;0	<2;0	<2;0	2;0
ei	2;8	2;0	<2;0	<2;0	1;8
ɐi	1;7	2;0	<2;0	<2;0	2;0
au	1;7	2;0	<2;0	<2;0	2;0
iu	1;7	2;0	<2;0	<2;0	2;0
ɐu	1;7	2;0	<2;0	<2;0	2;0
ou	2;8	2;0	<2;0	<2;0	1;8
θy	1;7	2;0	<2;0	<2;0	2;0
eu	NA	NA	NA	NA	NA

Note. NA = not assessed

TABLE 36-5 Percent correct for Cantonese consonants, consonant clusters, and vowels

Age	Consonants	Vowels
1;0–1;5	NA	NA
1;6–1;11	NA	NA
2;0–2;5	85.6	98.8
2;6–2;11	91.7	99.2
3;0–3;5	95.8	99.7
3;6–3;11	96.4	99.7
4;0–4;5	98.1	99.6
4;6–4;11	97.8	99.6
5;0–5;5	99.5	99.8
5;5–5;11	99.2	100

Note. Data from So and Dodd (1995).

2;5 include assimilation, cluster reduction/delabilization, /h/-deletion, stopping, fronting, deaspiration, affrication, and final consonant deletion. At age group 2;6 to 2;11, the common processes include assimilation, cluster reduction/delabilization, stopping, fronting, deaspiration, affrication, deaffrication, and final consonant deletion.

There are only four common processes for age group 3;0 to 3;5, including cluster reduction/delabilization, stopping, fronting, and deaspiration, and for the age group 3;6 to 3;11, only cluster reduction/delabilization and stopping occur (So and Dodd, 1995). The uncommon processes include initial consonant deletion, frication, aspiration, and backing. Table 36-6 shows examples of the common processes and the oldest age groups when the processes were used.

Intelligibility

To date there are no published studies on intelligibility of Cantonese-speaking children.

Phonetic inventory

A. C. Y. Tse (1991) reported that the child he studied had a wide phonetic inventory before age 2, including 11 consonants, 10 vowels, and 7 tones (see Table 36-7). The phonetic inventories of Cantonese-speaking children increase quickly and are usually complete by the age of 3;6. Tones and vowels are acquired early, usually by the age of 2 (So and Dodd, 1995).

Common mismatches

Mismatches are found in Cantonese-speaking children's phonological acquisition. Common mismatches of different sounds vary and depend on the processes involved. Popular mismatches include deaspiration of aspirated sounds, stopping of fricatives, fronting of back sounds,

TABLE 36-6 Common processes and errors from Cantonese-speaking children

Common processes used	Oldest age groups	Common errors
/h/-deletion	2;0 –2;5	/h/ ⇨ deleted
Assimilation	2;6–2;11	syllable-initial alveolars harmonise with syllable-final velars
Affrication	2;6–2;11	/s/ ⇨ [ts$^{(h)}$]
Deaffrication	2;6–2;11	/ts, ts^h/ ⇨ [s]
Final nasal deletion	2;6–2;11	/-m,-n,-ŋ/ ⇨ deleted
Fronting	3;0–3;5	/f, k, k^h, kw, k^{h}w/ ⇨ [p, f, t$^{(h)}$]
Deaspiration	3;0–3;5	/p^h, t^h, k^h, ts^h, k^{h}w/ ⇨ [p, t, k, ts, kw]
Cluster reduction/delabialization	3;6–3;11	/k^{wh}/ ⇨ [k$^{(h)}$, p$^{(h)}$, f] /k^w/ ⇨ [k, p, f]
Stopping	3;6–3;11	/f, s, ts, ts^h/ ⇨ [t, t^h]

Note. Data from So and Dodd (1995).

TABLE 36-7 Phonetic inventory of Cantonese-speaking children

Age (year;months)	Tse, A. C. Y. (1991)	So and Dodd (1995)
1;6–1;11	m, p, t, tʰ, h, w, j, n, pʰ, tsʰ, k i, e, a, ɔ, e, ɛ, u, y, o, ʊ tones 55, 33, 25, 22, 5, 3, 2	NA
2;0–2;5	l, ŋ, s, f, u tones 21, 23	p, t, m, n, ŋ, h, j, k, l, w, all vowels and tones
2;6–2;11	kʷ, ts, kʰ	f, s, pʰ, ts
3;0–3;5	NA	tʰ, kʰ, tsʰ, kʷ, kʷʰ

deaffrication of affricates, and affrication of fricatives (So and Dodd, 1995). Table 36-8 lists the common mismatches of the more difficult Cantonese sounds.

Syllable structure

Syllable structures are acquired early and before the age of 3. V and CV are acquired at the age of 1;3, before the CVC and VC structures. So and Dodd (1995) reported that 15 percent of children in their 2;0 to 2;6 group and 21 percent of the children in their 2;6 to 2;11 group deleted syllable final consonants, resulting in the CVC structure changing to the CV structure. In the A. C.Y. Tse (1991) study, the CV structure appeared at age 1;3 and the CVC structure appeared around age 1;11.

Tones

Tones were acquired very early, between 1;2 and 2 years old. Tone acquisition is usually complete by the age of 2. Table 36-9 summarizes the data on age of acquisition of Cantonese tones from different researchers.

Phonological awareness

Woo (1993) investigated the phonological awareness of Cantonese-speaking children 4 to 6 years old and concluded that there is a significant progression in phonological awareness between those ages. Syllable awareness comes before rhyme and onset awareness. Syllable awareness was evident in the 5- and 6-year-old children. Rhyme and onset awareness emerged at 5 years and became more evident at 6 years, though not all 6-year-old children have these skills. Chen et al. (2004) studied the phonological awareness of bilingual and monolingual Chinese children and suggested that Cantonese-speaking children developed more advanced onset and rhyme awareness by second grade when they learned Mandarin at school and became bilingual. The first-grade Cantonese-speaking children had more advanced tone awareness than the Mandarin-speaking children, as the Cantonese-speaking children had a more complicated tonal system.

Speech assessment for Cantonese-speaking children

Two speech assessment tools, namely the *Cantonese Segmental Phonology Test* (So, 1993) and the *Hong Kong Cantonese Articulation Test* (Ng and Cheung, 2002), are available for assessment of the speech abilities of Cantonese-speaking children. There is also a *Cantonese Phonological Assessment Guideline* (So, 1992) for assessing Cantonese-speaking children with phonological problems.

TABLE 36-8 Common mismatches of the more difficult Cantonese sounds

Sounds	Common mismatches	Remarks
pʰ	p	
tʰ	t	
k	t	
kʰ	t, k	
kʷ	k, p	
kʷʰ	kʷ, k, t, tʰ	
f	p	
s	t, ts	
l	j	
ts	t	
tsʰ	ts, t	
n	l	Initial /n/ interchanges with /l/
ŋ	ø, n	Initial /ŋ/ may be deleted and replaced by zero initial

Note. Data from So and Dodd (1995).

TABLE 36-9 Age of Cantonese tone acquisition

Tone (Tone value)	Tse, J. K. P. (1978)	Tse, S. M. (1982)	Tse, A. C. Y. (1991)	So and Dodd (1995)	Cheung (1990)
High Level (55)	1;2–1;4	1;9	1;3	1;4	<2;0
High Rise (25)	1;5–1;8	1;9	1;3	1;6	<2;0
Mid Level (33)	1;5–1;8	1;7	1;3	1;4	<2;0
Low Fall (21)	1;2–1;4	1;9	1;8	1;8–1;11	<2;0
Low Rise (23)	1;9	1;7	1;8	1;8–1;11	<2;0
Low Level (22)	1;9	1;7	1;8	1;8–1;10	<2;0
High Stopped (5)	1;5–1;8	1;7	1;3	1;7–1;8	<2;0
Mid Stopped (3)	1;5–1;8	1;7	1;3	1;7–1;8	<2;0
Low Stopped (2)	1;5–1;8	1;7	1;8	1;7–1;8	<2;0

Cantonese Segmental Phonology Test

The CSPT (So, 1993) consists of two parts. There are 31 items in the Part 1 naming test, and Part 2 consists of a story illustrated by five pictures. The CSPT enables speech-language pathologists to check the child's phonetic inventory; analyze the child's contrastive use of phonemes in the inventory; identify the child's performance at single-word level and at discourse level; identify the child who needs further assessment or immediate treatment; and plan further assessment and intervention. The manual of the CSPT provides the age of emergence of the consonants, vowels, and tones in two criteria, 75 percent and 90 percent.

Hong Kong Cantonese Articulation Test

The *Hong Kong Cantonese Articulation Test* (Ng and Cheung, 2002) is a naming test and consists of 46 pictures, including single words and compound words, for testing initial and final consonants, vowels, diphthong, and tones. The test takes about 10 minutes to complete.

Cantonese Phonological Assessment Guideline

In addition, there is a phonological assessment guideline, the *Cantonese Phonological Assessment Guideline* (So, 1992), for assessing the phonological abilities of Cantonese-speaking children. There are six steps in the assessment procedure. The Cantonese phonological system is incorporated in the assessment procedure. The steps include collecting a speech sample of the child (at least 50 utterances); transcribing the child's utterances using narrow phonetic transcription; working out the phonetic inventory of the child's speech (consonants, vowels, tones); identifying the distribution of consonants and vowels in different positions of a syllable; checking the presence of different syllable structure patterns; performing target-error analysis for consonants, vowels, and tones; and identifying any regularities across errors and the phonological processes.

Speech intervention for Cantonese-speaking children

The speech intervention techniques that have been developed for Cantonese-speaking children include:

- Phonological processes method (Hodson and Paden, 1983)
- Nonlinear phonology (Bernhardt and Gilbert, 1992)
- Auditory discrimination training (Berry and Eisenson, 1956)
- Motor approach (Mowrer, 1977)
- Core-vocabulary approach (Dodd and Iacono, 1989)

Working in Hong Kong SAR and Southern China

Job opportunities are favorable in Hong Kong, and speech-language pathologists can work in different settings including government, subsidized, and private settings. There are speech clinics in hospitals where inpatients and outpatients are seen. Speech assessment and therapy services are also available in child assessment centers. Special schools, special child care centers, and early education training centers also provide speech therapy service. Qualified speech-language pathologists can start their own private clinics as well. There are no formal speech-language pathology posts in China yet.

Speech-language pathology work is usually carried out by special education teachers or medical personnel.

The Hong Kong Association of Speech Therapists in Hong Kong, http://www.speechtherapy.org.hk/newastweb/home.html, is the professional association for speech-language pathologists. Interested persons can visit the Web site of the association or contact the committee members for information about speech therapy services, job opportunities, and other related information.

PHONETICALLY SPEAKING

Pronunciation of Cantonese: /k^{w}ɔŋ$_{25}$ tsau$_{55}$ wa$_{25}$/ Relevant words for speech assessment and intervention

Word/Phrase	Formal usage	Pronunciation	Informal usage	Pronunciation
Tongue	舌	/sit$_{33}$/	脷	/lei$_{22}$/
Teeth	牙	/ŋa$_{21}$/	牙	/ŋa$_{21}$/
Lips	嘴唇	/tsœy$_{25}$ sɵn$_{21}$/	嘴唇	/ tsœy$_{25}$ sɵn$_{21}$/
Hard palate	硬顎	/aŋ$_{22}$ ɔk$_{2}$/	硬顎	/aŋ$_{22}$ ɔk$_{52}$/
Soft palate	軟顎	/jyn$_{23}$ ɔk$_{2}$/	軟顎	/jyn$_{23}$ ɔk$_{2}$/
Larynx	喉嚨	/hau$_{21}$ luŋ$_{21}$/	喉嚨	/hau$_{21}$ luŋ$_{21}$/
Lungs	肺	/fɐi$_{33}$/	肺	/ fɐi$_{33}$/
Nose	鼻	/pei$_{22}$/	鼻哥	/pei$_{22}$ kɔ$_{55}$/
Sound	聲音	/siŋ$_{55}$ jem$_{55}$/	聲音	/siŋ$_{55}$ jem$_{55}$/
Word	字	/tsi$_{22}$/	字	/tsi$_{22}$/
Sentence	句子	/kœy$_{33}$ tsi$_{25}$/	句子	/kœy$_{33}$ tsi$_{25}$/
Paragraph	段落	/tsyn$_{22}$ lɔk$_{33}$/	段落	/tsyn$_{22}$ lɔk$_{33}$/

RESOURCES

Books

Bauer, R. S., and Benedict, P. K. (1997). *Modern Cantonese phonology*. Berlin: Mouton de Gruyter.

Cheung, P. (1995). *A speech therapy activity book on Hong Kong Cantonese phonology.* Hong Kong: Transaudio.

Hashimoto, A. O. K. (1972). *Phonology of Cantonese.* Cambridge, UK: Cambridge University Press.

Kao, D. (1971). *Structure of the syllable in Cantonese.* The Hague: Mouton.

Ng, A., and Cheung, P. (2002). *Hong Kong Cantonese articulation test.* Hong Kong: Child Assessment Service.

So, L. K. H. (1993). *Cantonese segmental phonology test.* Hong Kong: Bradford Publishing Company.

Journals, articles, and conference papers

- So, L. K. H., and Dodd, B. (1994). Phonologically disordered Cantonese-speaking children. *Clinical Linguistics and Phonetics, 8*, 235–255.
- So, L. K. H., and Dodd, B. (1995). The acquisition of phonology by Cantonese-speaking children. *Journal of Child Language, 22*, 473–495.
- Stokes, F. S.m and To, C. K. T. (2002). Feature development in Cantonese. *Clinical Linguistics and Phonetics, 16*, 443–459.
- Tse, A. C. Y. (1991). *The acquisition process of Cantonese phonology: A case study.* Unpublished M.Phil. thesis, University of Hong Kong.

- Tse, J. K. P. (1978). Tone acquisition in Cantonese: A longitudinal study. *Journal of Child Language, 5*, 191–204.
- Tse, S. M. (1982). *The acquisition of Cantonese phonology.* Unpublished Ph.D. thesis, University of British Columbia.
- Woo, C. Y. M. (1993). *Phonological awareness in 4–6 year old Cantonese-speaking children.* Unpublished honours dissertation, University of Hong Kong.
- Zee, E. (1999). Chinese (Hong Kong Cantonese). In International Phonetic Association (Ed.), *Handbook of the International Phonetic Association* (pp. 58–60). Cambridge, UK: Cambridge University Press.

Professional associations

The professional association of speech-language pathologists within Hong Kong SAR, China, is Hong Kong Association of Speech Therapists, http://www.speech-therapy.org.hk/newastweb/home.html

Useful Cantonese Web sites

- *Cantonese Language Association,* http://asiane.byu.edu/cla/
- *Jyutping Bat Naan (Cantonese Romanization courseware),* http://www.langcomp.com.hk/english/products/jpbn.html
- *Cantonese phonology and its influence on intervention,* http://www.asha.ucf.edu/so.html

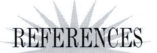

REFERENCES

Bauer, R. S., and Benedict, P. K. (1997). *Modern Cantonese phonology.* Berlin: Mouton de Gruyter.

Bernhardt, B., and Gilbert, J. (1992). Applying linguistic theory to speech-language pathology: The case for nonlinear phonology. *Clinical Linguistics and Phonetics, 6*, 123–145.

Berry, M., and Eisenson, J. (1956). *Speech disorders: Principles and practices of therapy.* London: Peter Owen.

Chen, X., Anderson, R. C., Li, W., Hao, M., Wu, X., and Shu, H. (2004). Phonological awareness of bilingual and monolingual Chinese children. *Journal of Educational Psychology, 96*(1), 142–151.

Cheung, K. H. (1986). *The phonology of present day Cantonese.* Unpublished doctoral thesis, University of London.

Cheung, P. (1990). *The acquisition of Cantonese phonology in Hong Kong: A cross-sectional study.* Unpublished final year B.Sc. project, University College London.

Dodd, B., and Iacono, T. (1989). Phonological disorders in children: Changes in phonological process use during treatment. *British Journal of Disorders of Communication, 24*, 333–351.

Hashimoto, A. (1972). *Studies in the Yue Dialect*. Cambridge, UK: Cambridge University Press.

Hodson, B., and Paden, E. (1983). *Targeting intelligible speech*. San Diego, CA: College-Hill Press.

Kwok, H., and Luke, K. K. (1986). An initial study of intonation in Cantonese. *Language Magazine, 13*, 32–40.

Li, H. T. (1977). *The history of Chinese characters*. Taipei, Taiwan: Lian-Jian.

Mowrer, D. (1977). *Methods of modifying speech behaviors*. Columbus: Charles E. Merrill.

Ng, A., and Cheung P. (2002). *Hong Kong Cantonese articulation test*. Hong Kong: Child Assessment Service.

So, L. K. H. (1992). *Cantonese Phonological Assessment Guideline*. Department of Speech and Hearing Sciences: University of Hong Kong.

So, L. K. H. (1993). *Cantonese Segmental Phonology Test*. Hong Kong: Bradford Publishing.

So, L. K. H., and Dodd, B. (1994). Phonologically disordered Cantonese-speaking children. *Clinical Linguistics and Phonetics, 8*, 235–255.

Stokes, F. S., and To, C. K. T. (2002). Feature development in Cantonese. *Clinical Linguistics and Phonetics, 16*, 443–459.

Stokes, F. S., and Wong, I. M. (2002). Vowel and diphthong development in Cantonese-speaking children. *Clinical Linguistics and Phonetics, 16*, 597–617.

Tse, A. C. Y. (1991). *The acquisition process of Cantonese phonology: A case study*. Unpublished M.Phil. thesis, University of Hong Kong.

Tse, J. K. P. (1978). Tone acquisition in Cantonese: A longitudinal study. *Journal of Child Language, 5*, 191–204.

Tse, S. M. (1982). *The acquisition of Cantonese phonology*. Unpublished Ph.D. thesis, University of British Columbia.

Wells, J. C. (1982). *Accents of English*. Cambridge, UK: Cambridge University Press.

Zee, E. (1999). Chinese (Hong Kong Cantonese). In International Phonetic Association (Ed.), *Handbook of the International Phonetic Association* (pp. 58–60). Cambridge, UK: Cambridge University Press.

SUMMARY OF STUDIES OF TYPICAL CANTONESE SPEECH ACQUISITION

Authors	Year	Country	No. of children	Age of children	Information	Sample type	Data collection
Cheung P.	1990	Hong Kong	155	2;1–6;0	Age of acquisition of consonants, vowels, and tones	Words	Cross-sectional
So and Dodd	1995	Hong Kong	268 4	2;0–5;11 1;2–2;0	Age of acquisition of consonants and vowels Age of acquisition of tone	Single words and connected speech Connected speech	Cross-sectional for consonant and vowels Longitudinal for tones
Stokes and To	2002	Hong Kong	122 10	0;10–4;7 0;11–3;5	Feature development	Connected speech Free speech	Cross-sectional Longitudinal
Stokes and Wong	2002	Hong Kong	40	0;10–2;3	Vowel and diphthong development	Spontaneous speech	Cross-sectional
Tse, A. C. Y.	1991	Hong Kong	1	1;2–3;0	Age of acquisition of consonants, vowels, and tones	Connected speech	Longitudinal
Tse, K. P.	1978	Hong Kong	1	1;2–1;9	Age of acquisition of tones	Spontaneous speech	Longitudinal
Tse, S. M.	1982	Canada	1	1;7–2;8	Age of acquisition of consonants, vowels, and tones	Connected speech	Longitudinal
			2	1;8–2;0			Cross-sectional

Chapter 37

Dutch Speech Acquisition

Ineke Mennen, Clara Levelt, and Ellen Gerrits

INTRODUCTION

Dutch is a West-Germanic language spoken by most inhabitants of the Netherlands (approximately 16 million speakers). It is the official language of the Netherlands, Belgium, Suriname, Aruba, and the Dutch Antilles. It is thought to be spoken by around 24 million people worldwide (Wikipedia, 2005). Dutch has many dialects that differ from Standard Dutch in its vocabulary, syntax, morphology, and phonology. The Netherlands has a heterogeneous population with people from many different nationalities, and as a consequence a wide variety of languages is spoken. The majority of the immigrant population is of Turkish descent, followed by Surinamese and Moroccan descent (Statistics Netherlands, 2005). See the Resources section for materials pertaining to Dutch.

Where Dutch is spoken

Dutch is spoken in the Netherlands (see accompanying map and Appendix D), but also in parts of Belgium (specifically, in the northern part, the provinces of West-Vlaanderen and Oost-Vlaanderen, Antwerpen, Limburg, and Brabant) and in former colonies of the Netherlands (Surinam, Aruba, and the Dutch Antilles, where it is used in education and government; Indonesia, where there are some speakers and it is also used in some law codes). A second official language of the Netherlands is Frisian, which is spoken by approximately 350,000 native speakers in the province of Fryslân (Friesland). Afrikaans, a daughter language of Dutch, is spoken mainly in South Africa and in Botswana, Zimbabwe, and Namibia (Booij, 1995).

Components of Dutch

Consonants

Dutch has 23 consonants (including allophones and marginal consonants) and is most closely related to German (see Table 37-1). The /g/, /ʃ/, and /ʒ/ are put in parentheses because they occur only in loanwords and/or as allophones: [g] as allophone of /k/ before plosives, as in *zakdoek* the Dutch word for 'handkerchief' ['zɑgduk]; [ʃ] as allophone of /s/ before /j/, as in *muisje* ['mœyʃə] 'little mouse'. The alveolars /t, n/ are also palatalized before /j/, so that they are realized as /c, ɲ/ respectively as in *hondje* and *anjer*, the Dutch words for 'doggie' ['hɔncə] and 'carnation' ['ɑɲər]. Unlike English, the /p, t, k/ are voiceless unaspirated, and the /b, d/ are fully voiced (Gussenhoven, 1999). There is considerable variation in the realization of the /r/ phoneme in Dutch (across dialects, sociolinguistic membership, styles, and phonological context). Some speakers use the voiced uvular fricative [ʁ], others the uvular trill [ʀ], alveolar trill [r] or tap [ɾ]. In post-vocalic contexts /r/ in some dialects tends not to be realized (zero-realization, or deletion) or is realized as an approximant [ɹ], and some speakers use an approximant even in initial onset position (Sebregts et al., 2003). Devoicing of voiced fricatives is common in some dialects, so that /v/ is usually realized as [f], /z/ is usually realized as [s], and /ʒ/ is usually realized as [ʃ]. A glottal stop [ʔ] is often inserted before vowel-initial syllables (Gussenhoven, 1999).

Vowels and diphthongs

Dutch has 16 vowel sounds consisting of 14 monophthongs and 3 diphthongs (Booij, 1995). Table 37-2 gives a classification of the 16 Dutch vowels. These vowels can be divided into a set of tense vowels /i, y, u, eː, øː, oː, aː/, a set of lax vowels /ɪ, ɛ, ɔ, ʏ, ɑ/, a reduced vowel /ə/, and diphthongs /ɛi, œy, ʌu/. Some vowels are marginal and occur only in loanwords, specifically [iː] as in *analyse* [anaˈliːzə] 'analysis', [yː] as in *centrifuge* [sɛntriˈfyːʒə] 'spindryer', [uː] as in *rouge* ['ruːʒə] 'rouge', [ɛː] as in *serre* ['sɛːrə] 'conservatory', [œː] as in *freule* ['frœːlə] 'gentlewoman', and [ɔː] as in *zone* ['zɔːnə] 'zone'. These marginal vowels are always long.

Phonotactic restrictions

Syllables

Allowable syllable structures can be described in the formula $C_{0-3}VC_{0-4}$, so that a syllable in Dutch consists of a vowel preceded by zero to three consonants, and followed by zero to four consonants. The smallest allowable syllable consists of a vowel only, usually a diphthong (e.g., *ei* [ɛi] 'egg', *ui* [œy] 'onion'). The Dutch language is known for the fact that it can "glue" words together to form very long words, and there is little restriction as to the number of syllables in a word.

Consonants and consonant clusters

Any consonant except /ŋ/ can occur in syllable-initial position. Similarly, any consonant except /h/ can occur word-finally. There are some language-specific restrictions on the possible combinations of consonants. For example, /h/ never occurs in syllable-initial clusters. Syllable-initial clusters never have two sonorant consonants, that is, combinations of nasals with liquids or glides (e.g., [nl]), or liquids with glides ([lj]), are not allowed in syllable-initial position. There is only a very restricted set of three-element clusters. Where a syllable onset has three consonants, the first consonant is always /s/. Where a syllable ends in more than two consonants, the final consonants are always coronal /t/ and /s/ as in *herfst* [hɛrfst] 'autumn'. Dutch can have many consecutive consonantal phones, as exemplified in *angstschreeuw* ['ɑŋstsxreu] 'cry of fear', which has a total of six consecutive consonantal phonemes. For a full account of phonotactic constraints the reader is referred to Booij (1995).

Tones

Standard Dutch does not use tones to differentiate meaning. However, in some Southern Dutch dialects (many Limburgian dialects) a lexical tone contrast is used alongside intonation. In these dialects two types of tones are used, the so-called *punch tone* and *drag tone*, also referred to as Accent 1 and Accent 2 respectively (cf. Gussenhoven and Aarts, 1999; Gussenhoven and van der Vliet, 1999; Schmidt, 1986). Examples are the words for 'rinse' ['spøːlə] versus 'play' ['⁺spøːlə], and 'territory' [ɣəˈbeːt] versus 'set of teeth' [ɣə⁺beːt], where Accent 2 is marked [ˉ] before the syllable concerned. Some segmentally identical words rely on tones to distinguish singular from plural. These words have Accent 1 in the plural and Accent 2 in the singular. Examples are the words for 'leg' [bɛin], 'horse' [peːʀt], and 'stone' [stɛin].

Stress and intonation

Like most European languages, Dutch is a stress accent language. In Dutch, main stress falls on either the antepenult, penult, or final syllable of a word as long as the penult is open, as in *olifant*, *pyjama*, and *krokodil* the Dutch

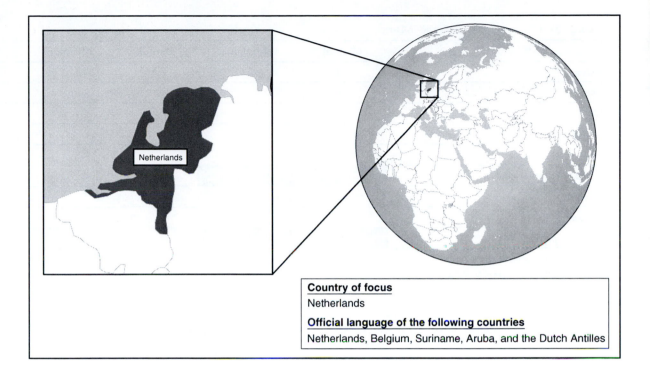

Country of focus
Netherlands
Official language of the following countries
Netherlands, Belgium, Suriname, Aruba, and the Dutch Antilles

words for 'elephant' ['oːliːˌfɑnt], 'pajamas' [piːˈjaːmaː], and 'crocodile' [ˌkroːkoːˈdɪl] respectively. However, if the penult is closed it will fall on the penult or final syllable, as in *oranje* and *framboos* the Dutch words for the color 'orange' [oːˈrɑɲə], and 'raspberry' [ˌfrɑmˈboːs] respectively. In composite words, secondary stress is often present. There are only a few minimal pairs where stress is the only difference between words, for example in the Dutch words for 'canon' ['kaːnɔn] and 'cannon' [kaːˈnɔn] (Gussenhoven, 1999).

The intonation system of Dutch is extremely similar to that of English. Dutch has a total number of eight pitch accents which, when they are combined with boundary tones, generate a total of 24 nuclear intonation contours (Gussenhoven, 2005). The eight pitch accents are H* (high level from the accented syllable), H*L (high fall from the accented syllable), !H*L (low fall from accented syllable, also called downstepped fall), L* (low level from the accented syllable), L*H (rise from low from the accented syllable), L*HL (rise fall from accented syllable) , L*!HL (low rise fall from accented syllable), and H*!H (vocative chant). Gussenhoven, Rietveld, Kerkhoff, and Terken (2003) have developed an interactive training course for the transcription of Dutch intonation, called ToDI (Transciption of

Dutch Intonation), which is available on the Internet (see Resources).

Writing system

Dutch is written in the Latin alphabet. Dutch spelling is not transparent, having no one-to-one correspondence between sounds and letters. This is particularly obvious in the vowels, where there are only five vowel letters (i, u, e, o, and a) for the 14 Dutch vowels (excluding the diphthongs). The spelling of long vowels is particularly complicated. Spelling of consonants is more transparent, with the only complication being the use of double graphemes to indicate single consonants (*ch* for /χ/ and *ng* for /ŋ/) (Booij, 1995).

Varieties of Dutch

There is a large number of regional variants of Dutch, and it is thought that there are as many as 28 different dialects. The most obvious division is that between northern and southern varieties. Particularly, the southern varieties tend to have a full set of voiced fricatives [v, z, ɣ], whereas the northern varieties often have only

TABLE 37-1 Consonants produced in Dutch

	Bilabial	Labiodental	Dental	Alveolar
Plosive	p b			t d
Nasal	m			n
Trill				
Tap or flap				ɾ
Fricative		f v		s z
Lateral fricative	███████	███████		
Affricate				
Approximant		ʋ		
Lateral approximant	███████	███████		l

Black = articulations judged impossible

Based on the International Phonetic Alphabet. Courtesy of the International Phonetic Association (c/o Department of Linguistics, University of Victoria, Victoria, British Columbia, Canada).

[v, z] or only [z] (Gussenhoven, 1999). Furthermore, the southern varieties (i.e., south of the rivers Rhine and Meuse) have the velar fricative contrast [x, ɣ], whereas north of the rivers there is no such contrast, with only a voiceless fricative, which in contrast to the southern varieties is uvular [χ]. The phoneme /r/ is often alveolar in Amsterdam, the northeast of the Netherlands, and parts of Belgium, although there is a lot of individual variation in the pronunciation of /r/. Elsewhere /r/ is often uvular (Gussenhoven, 1999). In the south (including Belgium) the [ʋ] is realized as [w] or [β].

Typical acquisition of Dutch

The Summary of Studies Table at the end of this chapter contains studies of Dutch-speaking children's acquisition of speech.

Acquired sounds

Consonants

Consonants are acquired in a certain order, depending on their position in the syllable (Beers, 1995; Fikkert, 1994). Certain consonants appear early in onsets and late in codas, and vice versa. Table 37-3 contains age of acquisition data for Dutch in initial and final position, according to the >75 percent criterion, from a study by Beers (1995).

Consonant clusters

Table 37-4 contains order of acquisition data for classes of initial consonant clusters from eight children in a study by Fikkert (1994).

Vowels and diphthongs

The place of articulation of vowels appears to present no developmental problems: target front vowels are front and target back vowels are back from the outset (Levelt, 1994). Front rounded vowels are acquired late (Beers, 1995; Levelt, 1994). In terms of vowel height, Levelt (1994) shows that the high and low vowels, /i, u, a, ɑ/, are attempted and acquired first (around the mean age of 1;5), followed by the high-mid vowels /e, ɪ, o, ɔ/. The low-mid vowel /ɛ/ is the most problematic vowel for Dutch children during development. It is attempted relatively late and is error-prone (Levelt, 1994). In terms of vowel length, Fikkert (1994) shows that initially, long and short vowels are used almost interchangeably (e.g., short target /ɑ/ is substituted for long /a/ and vice versa, short /ɔ/ substituted for long /o/ and vice versa, etc.). Even in CV syllables, where short vowels are not allowed in the adult language, children readily produce short vowels. Vowel length is mastered between 2;0 and 2;5 (Fikkert, 1994).

Levelt (2000) shows that the highly frequent schwas in Dutch are often replaced by full vowels in child language, mostly /a/, /ɑ/, or /ɪ/ in phrase-final position, resulting

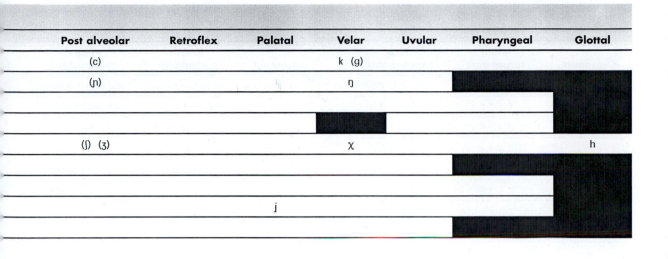

Post alveolar	Retroflex	Palatal	Velar	Uvular	Pharyngeal	Glottal
(c)			k (g)			
(ɲ)			ŋ			
(ʃ) (ʒ)			χ			h
		j				

in forms like ['lopa] for *lopen* the Dutch adult target for 'to walk' /'lopə/, and ['χota] for *grote* 'big' /'χrotə/. Schwa strengthening is persistent and can still be found in the productions of children around the age of 2;5. Table 37-5 lists the order of acquisition of individual vowels as determined by Beers (1995), according to the 75 percent criterion.

Percent correct

Consonants

To date there is no study of percentage of consonants produced correctly.

Consonant clusters

Jongstra (2003) determined the percentages of correct production of 5,562 instances of word-initial consonant clusters (from a total of 23,167 instances) produced by 34 children between the ages of 1;11 and 3;4 (see Table 37-6).

Vowels

Table 37-7 shows the mean percentages correct for Dutch vowels from a study by Levelt (1994) of 6 children between the ages of 1;6 and 2;4. Front rounded vowels and diphthongs were not included in this study:

Phonological processes

The most recent study of phonological processes in Dutch children was conducted by Beers (1995). Simplification processes that are commonly used by Dutch children of 1;3 to 1;11 years of age are cluster reduction, final consonant deletion, devoicing, and weak syllable deletion. Other common processes are reduplication, assimilation, gliding, and stopping. Beers found that

TABLE 37-2   Vowels produced in Dutch

	Front	Central	Back	Diphthongs
close	i(ː), y(ː)		u(ː)	
close-mid	ɪ, e(ː), ʏ, ø(ː)	ə	o(ː)	
open-mid	ɛ(ː)		ɔ(ː)	
open			œː, a(ː), ɑ	ɛi, œy, ʌu

TABLE 37-3 Age of acquisition for Dutch consonants

Consonant	Initial consonants	Final consonants	Consonant	Initial consonants	Final consonants
	Beers (1995)	Beers (1995)	f	2;3–2;5	not determined
p	1;3–1;8	1;3–1;8	l	2;6–2;8	not determined
b	2;3–2;5	NA	ʒ	not determined	NA
m	1;3–1;8	2;3–2;5	ʃ	not determined	not determined
ʊ	2;3–2;5	NA	tʃ	not determined	not determined
n	1;3–1;8	2;3—2;5	dʒ	not determined	not determined
ŋ	not determined	not determined	s	2;0–2;2	2;0–2;2
h	2;0–2;2	NA	z	not determined	not determined
w	NA	NA	r	2;6–2;8	not determined
j	1;3–1;8	NA	v	2;8–3;0	NA
t	1;3–1;8	2;0–2;2	ð	NA	NA
d	2;8–3;0	NA	θ	NA	NA
k	1;9–1;11	1;9–1;11	c	not determined	not determined
g	not determined	not determined	ɲ	not determined	not determined
χ	2;0–2;2	2;0–2;2			

NA = Not applicable, i.e., sound does not occur in Dutch in that position.

final consonant deletion, reduplication, and assimilation showed a sharp decline in their occurrence between 2;0 and 2;5 years, followed by a slower decline up to age 4. The occurrence of cluster reduction and weak syllable deletion increased sharply between 1;3 and 2;6 years, with a sharp decrease between 2;6 and 3;0 years. After age 3;0 these processes show a steady decline. Until age 3;0 years, devoicing was the most frequent substitution process. After that age it rapidly declined, which reflects the acquisition of the voice contrast.

TABLE 37-4 Age of acquisition for Dutch onset cluster types

Onset clusters	child 1	child 2	child 3	child 4	child 5	child 6	child 7	child 8
plosive + liquid	1;8	*	1;6	2;2	2;3	2;0	*	1;10
fricative + liquid	2;4	*	1;7	2;2	*	2;0	*	*
fricative + nasal	*	*	*	*	*	2;1	*	*
plosive + glide	2;2	*	1;11	*	2;0	1;11	*	*
fricative + glide	*	*	*	*	*	2;1	*	*
/s/ + plosive	*	2;9	2;0	2;5	2;4	2;0	2;0	*
/s/ + fricative	*	*	2;1	2;5	*	*	*	*
/s/ + plosive + liquid	*	*	*	*	*	*	*	*

* = age of acquisition could not be determined

TABLE 37-5 Age of acquisition for Dutch vowels

Vowel	Beers (1995)
i	1;3–1;8
u	1;3–1;8
a	1;3–1;8
ɪ	1;3–1;8
ɛ	1;3–1;8
ɔ	1;9–1;11
ɑ	1;9–1;11
e	1;11–2;2
o	1;11–2;2
ʏ	3;0–3;2

TABLE 37-7 Percentage correct for Dutch vowels

Vowel	Percentage correct
i	94
u	91
a	93
ɑ	87
o	81
ɔ	80
ɪ	74
e	68
ɛ	63

TABLE 37-6 Percent correct for Dutch initial consonant clusters

Consonant cluster	Percentage correct
kn	17.51
sχ	21.05
sn	25.58
dr	32.28
sw	33.94
sk	36.07
fr	38.67
tw	38.82
sp	42.15
sm	43.10
xl	45.39
xr	45.44
br	46.99
tr	47.08
kʋ	49.90
pr	54.77
st	55.81
kr	58.46
fl	61.20
sl	62.29
bl	62.77
pl	73.60
kl	73.68
Total	45.86

Note: Data from Jongstra (2003).

Intelligibility

To date there is no study of intelligibility of Dutch children.

Phonetic inventory

Fikkert (1994) presents the phonetic inventory of consonants in terms of classes of sounds for nine children acquiring Dutch (see Table 37-8). Four groups are discerned according to the order in which the different phoneme classes are produced over time in onset position.

For the consonants in coda position a single order of appearance was found. The data presented in Table 37-9 are from five children of Fikkert's (1994) study. The category Glides is not present in the table since there are no glides in this position in the adult language.

Common mismatches

Common mismatches for sounds are sounds with default, unmarked features instead of marked features. For consonants, obstruents are unmarked in comparison to sonorants. Within the obstruents, plosives are unmarked compared to fricatives, and [-voice] is the default value for [voice]. For sonorants, [+voice] is the default value, and nasals are unmarked compared to liquids and glides. In addition, it has been assumed that the default value for place is coronal (Beers, 1995; Fikkert, 1994; Levelt, 1989).

Syllable structure

There are three studies of the acquisition of syllable structure in Dutch (Fikkert, 1994; Levelt, Schiller, and Levelt, 2000; Levelt and van de Vijver, 2004). There is a consistent course of development across children. The

TABLE 37-8 Phonetic inventory in onset position for Dutch

Class	Group I Age				Class	Group II Age		Class	Group III Age		Class	Group IV Age
	child 1	child 2	child 3	child 4		child 5	child 6		child 7	child 8		child 9
Plosives	2;1	1;0	1;6	1;4	Plosives	1;8	1;4	Plosives	1;5	1;9	Plosives	1;10
Nasals	2;1	1;2	1;6	1;4	Nasals	1;8	1;9	Nasals	1;5	1;9	Nasals	1;10
Glides	2;7	1;2	1;7	1;7	Fricatives	1;8	2;0	Fricatives	1;6	1;10	Liquids	1;10
Fricatives	2;8	1;4	1;10	1;8	Liquids	1;10	2;1	Glides	1;11	1;10	Glides	1;11
Liquids	2;11	1;4	2;0	1;10	Glides	2;1	2;3	Liquids	2;3	1;11	Fricatives	2;0

Note. Data from Fikkert (1994).

TABLE 37-9 Phonetic inventory in coda position for Dutch

Class	Age				
	child 1	child 2	child 3	child 6	child 7
Fricatives	2;1	1;3	1;6	1;6	1;7
Plosives	2;2	1;3	1;7	1;7	1;7
Nasals	2;2	1;4	1;8	1;8	1;8
Liquids				2;0	2;0

Note. Data from Fikkert (1994).

TABLE 37-10 Order of acquisition of Dutch syllable structure

	child 1	child 2	child 3	child 4	child 5	child 6	child 7
CV	2;1	1;0	1;6	1;4	1;8	1;4	1;5
CVC	2;1	1;3	1;6	1;4	1;8	1;6	1;7
V(C)	2;1	1;4	1;6	1;4	1;8	1;6	1;7
CCV(C)	2;9	1;6	2;0		2;2	1;8	2;0
(C)VCC		2;4				2;2	1;10

Note. Data from Fikkert (1994).

order of acquisition of the different syllable types is given in Table 37-10. Whether children start out producing complex onsets before complex codas or vice versa might depend on their personal experience with either of the two syllable types.

Prosody

Four studies have discussed the acquisition of Dutch stress (Fikkert, 1994; Nouveau, 1994; Wijnen, Krikhaar, and den Os, 1994; Lohuis-Weber and Zonneveld, 1996), of which

Fikkert (1994) is the most extensive study. There appears to be a trochaic bias in the early stages of acquisition (around 1;6 to 2;0). Bisyllabic words with stress on the initial syllable—trochees—like 'robot' /ˈrobɔt/ and 'kayak' /ˈkajɑk/) remain bisyllabic and show no stress errors. However, bisyllabic iambic words (words with stress on the second syllable, like *ballon* and *gitaar*, the Dutch words for 'balloon' /baˈlɔn/ and 'guitar' /ɣiˈtɑr/), are reduced to a single syllable. The stress pattern of bisyllabic weak Strong (wS) target words is acquired between the ages of 2;0 and 2;5. The stress patterns of longer words are acquired between 3;0 and 3;5 (Fikkert, 1994; Nouveau, 1994).

Phonological awareness

Aarnoutse, van Leeuwe, and Verhoeven (2000) report a longitudinal study of phonemic awareness skills of Dutch children from 4 to 7 years of age. Dutch children begin formal schooling at age 4 (Grade 1). Children at the end of Grade 1 performed relatively poorly on a monosyllabic phoneme segmentation task, with only 29 percent correct. One year later, their performance had increased to 52 percent. A test that included both phoneme blending and word rhyming skills appeared to be much easier: at the end of Grade 2 (ages 5 to 6) children scored 77 percent correct (Aarnoutse et al., 2000). Scheltinga (2002) showed that Dutch 10-year-old children with specific language impairment performed more poorly on a phoneme deletion task than typically developing age-matched children (respectively 17 percent vs. 55 percent correct).

Speech assessment for Dutch children

Dutch SLPs use published tests of articulation and phonology developed and produced in the Netherlands. Some of these tests are based on tests produced in the USA or UK. There has been no survey of the tests that Dutch speech-language pathologists use for assessing children's speech sounds. The tests listed here are mentioned in the Dutch literature:

- *Taaltoets Alle Kinderen, Klankarticulatie* (Verhoeven and Vermeer, 2001)
- *Taaltoets Allochtone Kinderen, Klankarticulatie* (Verhoeven, Vermeer, and van Guchte, 1986)
- *Utrechts Articulatie Onderzoek* (Peddemors-Boon, van der Meulen, and de Vries, 1974)

- *Logo-Art* (Baarda, de Boer-Jongsma, and Haasjes-Jongsma, 2005)
- Conversational speech sampling
- Informal/homemade single-word tests

The following computerized analyses have been designed for analyzing Dutch speech:

- *Fonologische Analyse van het Nederlands* (FAN) documented in Beers (1995).

Speech intervention for Dutch children

Dutch SLPs are familiar with and use intervention techniques from English- and German-speaking countries. In addition, specific intervention programs have been developed for use with Dutch children with speech impairments.

Intervention techniques that have been adapted for use with Dutch children are the following:

- Cycles approach (Hodson and Paden, 1991)
- *Metaphon* (Howell and Dean, 2000)
- *PROMPT* (Hayden, 2003; Raaijmakers and van der Meulen, 2004)
- Traditional articulation therapy (Günther and Kessels-de Beer, 2005; Van Riper and Erickson, 1996)

Speech intervention techniques that have been developed for use with Dutch children include:

- *Behandeling van articulatiestoornissen* (Stess, 2000). An intervention program based on traditional articulation therapy.
- *Dyspraxieprogramma* (Eurlings-Van Deurse et al., 1993). A program for intervention of developmental dyspraxia of speech. It contains auditory, visual, and tactile techniques to elicit speech sounds.
- *Fonologische procesanalyse met oefeningen* (van Borsel, 2003). Intervention in abnormal use of phonological simplification and substitution processes with exercises.
- *Logo-art* (Baarda, de Boer-Jongsma, and Haasjes-Jongsma, 2005). Logo-art contains specific exercises and pictures for each Dutch speech sound.
- *Logopedieklapper* (Paulussen-van Vugt, 1980). A booklet with several stimulus pictures in alphabetic order.
- *Metaphonbox* (Leijdekker-Brinkman, 1998). The Methaphonbox is an adjustment and extension of the Metaphon Resource Pack by Howell and Dean (2000). It contains exercises and suggestions for intervention.

Working in the Netherlands

In the Netherlands the education (bachelor's degree) and the profession of SLP has been regulated and protected by law since 1980. Speech and language therapy is part of the national health system. All SLPs must be registered with the Health Professions Council in order to practice in the Netherlands.

About 4,116 SLPs are organized in the Dutch Association for Logopaedics and Foniatrics, and 97 percent of them are women. Of these 4,116 members, 3,437 speech-language pathologists are working (NVLF administration office, personal communication, July 26, 2005). With 16,313,000 inhabitants, that is an average of 4,746 inhabitants per SLP. The settings in which they work include private practice (37 percent), education settings (31 percent), and health settings (32 percent). The NVLF publishes a clinical journal, *Logopedie en Foniatrie* (see Resources).

PHONETICALLY SPEAKING

Pronunciation of Nederlands 'Dutch' Netherlands: ['neːdərlants]
Relevant words for speech assessment and intervention

Word/Phrase	Formal usage	Pronunciation	Informal usage	Pronunciation
Tongue	*tong*	[tɔŋ]	*tong*	[tɔŋ]
Teeth	*tanden*	['tandə]	*tanden*	['tandə]
Lips	*lippen*	['lipə]	*lippen*	['lipə]
Hard palate	*harde gehemelte*	['hardə χə'heːməltə]	*harde gehemelte*	['hardə χə'heːməltə]
Soft palate	*zachte gehemelte*	['zaχtə χə'heːməltə]	*zachte gehemelte*	['zaχtə χə'heːməltə]
Larynx	*larynx*	['larɪŋks]	*strottehoofd*	['strɔtəhoːft]
Lungs	*longen*	['lɔŋə]	*longen*	['lɔŋə]
Nose	*neus*	[nøs]	*neus*	[nøs]
Sound	*klank*	[klaŋk]	*klank*	[klaŋk]
Word	*woord*	[ʋoːrt]	*woord*	[ʋoːrt]
Sentence	*zin*	[zɪn]	*zin*	[zɪn]
Paragraph	*paragraaf*	[para'χraf]	*paragraaf*	[para'χraf]

RESOURCES

Books

Gillis, S., and Schaerlaekens, A. M. (Eds.) (2000). *Kindertaalverwerving. Een handboek voor het Nederlands*. Groningen: Martinus Nijhoff.

Goorhuis, S. M., and Schaerlaekens, A. M. (2000). *Handboek taalontwikkeling, taalpathologie en taaltherapie bij Nederlandssprekende kinderen*. Utrecht: De Tijdstroom.

Huybrechts, G. (1998). *Articulatie in de praktijk: Consonanten*. Leuven: Acco.

Huybrechts, G. (1999). *Articulatie in de praktijk: Vocalen en diftongen*. Leuven: Acco.

Kooij, J., and Oostendorp, M. van (2003). *Fonologie: Uitnodiging tot de klankleer van het Nederlands*. Amsterdam: Amsterdam University Press.

Journals

- *Logopedie en Foniatrie*
  A clinical journal published in Dutch by Essentials in Rotterdam.
- *Stem-, Spraak- en Taalpathologie*
  A research journal published by Nijmegen University Press in Nijmegen, http://www.sstp.nl

Professional associations

The professional association of SLPs (called *logopedist*) within the Netherlands is *De Nederlandse Vereniging voor Logopedie en Foniatrie*, http://www.nvlf.nl

Colleges offering a bachelor's degree in speech-language pathology

- Chr. Hogeschool Windesheim (Zwolle)
- Fontys Paramedische Hogeschool (Eindhoven)
- Hanzehogeschool Groningen (Groningen)
- Hogeschool Arnhem en Nijmegen (Nijmegen)
- Hogeschool Rotterdam (Rotterdam)
- Hogeschool van Utrecht (Utrecht)
- Hogeschool Zuyd (Heerlen)

Universities offering a master's degree in speech-language pathology

- Radboud University (Nijmegen)
- University of Amsterdam (Amsterdam)
- Universitty of Groningen (Groningen)
- Utrecht University (Utrecht)

Useful Dutch Web sites

- Logopediekrant, http://www.logopediekrant.com
- Logopedie pagina, http://logopedie.pagina.nl
- GGD Kennisnet, http://www.ggdkennisnet.nl
- History of the Dutch language, http://www.ned.univie.ac.at/publicaties/taalgeschiedenis/en
- Dutch language, http://en.wikipedia.org/wiki/Dutch_language
- Transcription of Dutch intonation. ToDI second edition, http://todi.let.kun.nl/ToDI/home.htm

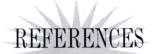

REFERENCES

Aarnoutse, C., Leeuwe, J. van, and Verhoeven, L. (2000). Ontwikkeling van beginnende geletterdheid. *Pedagogische Studiën*, 77, 307–325.

Baarda, D., de Boer-Jongsma, N., and Haasjes-Jongsma, W. (2005). *Logo-art articulatieonderzoek*. Ternat/Axel: Baert.

Beers, M. (1995). *The phonology of normally developing and language impaired children*. Unpublished doctoral dissertation, IFOTT, University of Amsterdam, The Netherlands.

Booij, G. (1995). *The phonology of Dutch*. Oxford, UK: Clarendon Press.

Eurlings-van Deurse, M., Freriks, A., Goudt-Bakker, K., Van der Meulen, Sj., and de Vries, L., (1993). *Dyspraxieprogramma, therapieprogramma voor kinderen met kenmerken van een verbale ontwikkelingsdyspraxie*. Lisse: Swets & Zeitlinger.

Fikkert, P. (1994). *On the acquisition of prosodic structure*. Unpublished doctoral dissertation, University of Leiden. Dordrecht: ICG Printing.

Günther, T., and Kessels-de Beer, A. (2005). De effectiviteit van klassieke articulatietherapie. *Logopedie en Foniatrie, 3*, 84–90.

Gussenhoven, C. (1999). Illustrations of the IPA: Dutch. In *Handbook of the International Phonetic Association* (pp. 74–77). Cambridge, UK: Cambridge University Press.

Gussenhoven, C. (2005). Transcription of Dutch intonation. In S-A. Jun (Ed.), *Prosodic typology: The phonology of intonation and phrasing* (pp. 118–145). Oxford, UK: Oxford University Press.

Gussenhoven, C., and Aarts, F. (1999). The dialect of Maastricht. *Journal of the International Phonetic Association, 29*(2), 155–166.

Gussenhoven, C., Rietveld, T., Kerkhoff, J., and Terken, J. (2003). Transcription of Dutch intonation: ToDI, (2nd ed.) Retrieved from http://www.let.kun.nl/ToDI/home.htm.

Gussenhoven, C., and van der Vliet, P. (1999). The phonology of tone and intonation in the Dutch dialect of Venlo. *Journal of Linguistics, 35*, 99–135.

Hayden, D. (2003). *P.R.O.M.P.T. Introduction to technique: Manual.* Santa Fe, NM: The PROMPT Institute.

Hodson, B. W., and Paden, E. P. (1991). *Targeting intelligible speech: A phonological approach to remediation* (2nd ed.) Austin, TX: Pro-Ed.

Howell, J., and Dean, E. (2000). *Fonologische stoornissen: Behandeling van kinderen volgens de Metaphon therapie.* Amsterdam: Harcourt Assessment B.V.

Jongstra, W. (2003). *Variation in reduction strategies of Dutch word-initial consonant clusters.* Doctoral dissertation, University of Toronto, Canada.

Leijdekker-Brinkman, W. (1998). *Metaphonbox.* Lisse: Swets & Zeitlinger.

Levelt, C. C. (1989) *An essay on child phonology.* Unpublished M.A. thesis, Leiden University, The Netherlands.

Levelt, C. (1994). *On the acquisition of place.* HIL dissertations in Linguistics 8, The Hague: HAG.

Levelt, C. (2000). *Schwa-schma: The development of /ə/ in Dutch child language.* Paper presented at the 16th IATL conference, Tel Aviv, Israel.

Levelt, C., Schiller, N., and Levelt, W. (2000). The acquisition of syllable types. *Language Acquisition, 8*, 237–264.

Levelt, C., and van de Vijver, R. (2004). The acquisition of syllable types in cross-linguistic and developmental grammars. In R. Kager, J. Pater, and W. Zonneveld (Eds.), *Fixing priorities: Constraints in phonological acquisition* (pp. 204–218). Cambridge, UK: Cambridge University Press.

Lohuis-Weber, H., and Zonneveld, W. (1996). Phonological acquisition and Dutch word prosody. *Language Acquisition, 5*(4), 245–284.

Nouveau, D. (1994). *Language acquisition, metrical theory, and optimality: A study of Dutch word stress.* Unpublished doctoral dissertation, University of Utrecht, The Netherlands.

Paulussen-VanVugt, B. (1980). *Logopedieklapper.* Lisse: Swets & Zeitlinger.

Peddemors-Boon, M., Meulen, Sj. van der, and Vries, K. de (1974). *Utrechts Articulatie Onderzoek.* Tilburg: Zwijsen.

Raaijmakers, M., and Meulen, Sj. van der (2005). PROMPT: Articulatietherapie vanuit tactiel-kinestetische input. *Logopedie en Foniatrie, 3*, 76–81.

Scheltinga, F. (2002). *Het belang van fonologische vaardigheden en basale processen bij technisch leren lezen.* Master's thesis, University of Amsterdam, The Netherlands.

Schmidt, J. E. (1986). *Die mittelfränkischen Tonakzente (Rheinische Akzentuierung).* Stuttgart: Franz Steiner.

Sebregts, K., Tops, E., van Bezooijen, R., Van de Velde, H., van Hout, R., Willemyns, R., and Zonneveld, W. (2003). Sociogeografische, fonetische en fonologische variatie in /r/: Een onderzoek in Nederlandse en Vlaamse grote steden. In T. Koole, J. Nortier, and B. Tahitu (Eds.). *Bijdragen aan de 4e Sociolinguistische Conferentie* (pp. 375–385). Delft: Eburon.

Statistics Netherlands (2005). Centraal Bureau voor de Statistiek. Retrieved September 6, 2005, from http://www.cbs.nl

Stess, R. (2000). *Articulatiestoornissen: fenomenen, oorzaken en behandeling.* Leuven: Acco.

van Borsel, J. (2003). *Kinderen met spraakproductieproblemen. Fonologische procesanalyse met oefeningen.* Leuven: Acco.

Van Riper, C., and Erickson, R. (1996). Speech correction: *An introduction to speech pathology and audiology* (9th ed.). New York: Prentice Hall.

Verhoeven, L., and Vermeer, A. (2001). *Taaltoets Alle Kinderen.* Arhem: CITO.

Verhoeven, L., Vermeer, A., and Guchte, C. van (1986). *Taaltoets Allochtone Kinderen.* Tilburg: Zwijsen.

Wijnen, F., Krikhaar, E., and Den Os, E. (1994). The (non)realization of unstressed elements in children's utterances: Evidence for a rhythmic constraint. *Journal of Child Language, 21*, 59–83.

Wikipedia. (2005). Dutch language. Retrieved August 30, 2005, from http://en.wikipedia.org/wiki/Dutch_language.

SUMMARY OF STUDIES OF TYPICAL DUTCH SPEECH ACQUISITION

Authors	Year	Country	No. of children	Age of children	Information	Sample type	Data collection
Beers	1995	Netherlands	90	1;3–4;0	Acquisition of phonological contrasts and occurrence of phonological processes	Connected speech	Cross-sectional
Fikkert	1994	Netherlands	12	1;0–2;11	Acquisition of syllable structure and stress	Connected speech	Longitudinal
Jongstra	2003	Canada/Netherlands	45	1;11–3;4	Acquisition of consonant clusters	Naturalistic speech and elicited speech	Longitudinal
Levelt	1994	Netherlands	12	1;0–2;11	Acquisition of place features and vowel height	Naturalistic speech samples	Longitudinal

Chapter 38

Filipino Speech Acquisition

Valerie Malabonga and Stefka Marinova-Todd

INTRODUCTION

Filipino has been the national language of the Philippines since 1937. There are 180 languages spoken in the Philippines, with 171 indigenous languages (Gordon, 2005), and Filipino is the second language of about 70–90 percent of Filipinos (Himmelmann, 2000). The Philippines has implemented a bilingual Filipino-English educational policy since 1973, and mass media use both Filipino and English (Gonzales, 1999). Filipino is based on Tagalog, a Malayo-Polynesian language. Filipino is mostly Tagalog with borrowed words from foreign languages such as Old Javanese, Malay, Sanskrit, Arabic, Spanish, Chinese, and English. Although foreign words have been introduced, the influence has been mainly on the lexicon and phonology but not the morphosyntax (Himmelmann, 2000). Filipino, as decreed by the 1987 Constitution of the Philippines, is composed of 28 letters, including the 26 letters of the English alphabet plus the velar nasal *ng* (treated as a separate letter) and the Spanish *ñ*. Despite government attempts to "globalize" Filipino, actual use of the language still largely follows the conventions of Tagalog. Compared to English, Tagalog has a very shallow orthography because the relationship between sounds and letters is nearly perfect (Ocampo, 2004). This transparent orthography is reflected in the ancient Tagalog writing system (called *baybayin*). The earliest document with old Tagalog words is dated A.D. 900 (Postma, 1992). When the Spanish colonizers came in 1521, they introduced the Roman alphabet (de Guzman, 2001). While four tribes in the Philippines still use a syllabary writing system very similar to the ancient script, the rest of the country uses the Roman alphabet (Postma, 1971). The *Doctrina Cristiana* (1593) (in Morrow, 2005) demonstrates that Tagalog has changed minimally in the past 400 years (Himmelmann, 2005). See the Resources section of this chapter for other materials pertaining to Filipino.

Where Filipino is spoken

Within the Philippines, Tagalog is spoken in Manila, most of Luzon, and Palawan (see accompanying map and Appendix D). Tagalog is also spoken by Filipinos and those with Philippine ancestry in Canada, Saudi Arabia, United Arab Emirates, United Kingdom, and the USA. People from the Philippines are also represented in the languages of Bahrain, Brunei, Italy, Japan, Jordan, Kuwait, Malaysia, Qatar, and Singapore (Gordon, 2005). In the USA, large populations of Filipino immigrants reside in California, Hawaii, New York, New Jersey, Illinois, Washington, and Texas (Camarota and McArdle, 2003).

Components of Filipino

Consonants

Filipino has 23 consonants and is most closely related to Tagalog (see Table 38-1) (Gomez, 1958; Llamzon, del Rosario, and Sanchez, 1974; Rubino, 2004; Wikipedia. com, 2006). Tagalog has 16 consonant sounds and a glottal stop, none of which are aspirated; /d/ and /r/ are allophones in Tagalog (Nationmaster, 2005). The velar nasal /ŋg/ may occur anywhere in a word, including the beginning (e.g., /ŋg ala ŋgala/ 'palate'). The consonants 'f', 'v', and 'z' do not occur natively in Tagalog, so speakers may substitute Tagalog consonant sounds: [p] for /f/ (*comportabol* for 'comfortable'), [b] for /v/ (*bery* for 'very'), or [s] for /z/ (*sero* for 'zero'). Also, in Tagalog, the glottal stop is important in differentiating the pronunciation of words spelled the same, e.g., *bata* 'bathrobe', *batá* 'child'. The glottal stop occurs where consonants may appear, except in consonant clusters (Ramos and Cena, 1990). In Filipino, the alveolar trill /r/ is pronounced very similarly to the Spanish /r/, i.e., from a flap to a trill. The affricates 'ts' and 'dy' are now more common in Filipino; they represent 'ch' and 'j' in English, respectively (Rubino, 2004). The fricative palatal 'siy' is pronounced similarly to the English 'sh' (Wikipedia, 2006).

Vowels and diphthongs

Tagalog has only five vowel sounds, all of them short: a, e, i, o, u (see Table 38-2). Because long vowels do not exist in Tagalog, speakers may pronounce long vowels as short vowels, (e.g., *bit* for 'beet'). Tagalog has five dipthongs, *iw, iy* or *ey, ay, aw, uy* or *oy*. Two of these, *iw* and *uy*, do not exist in English (Ramos and Cena, 1990).

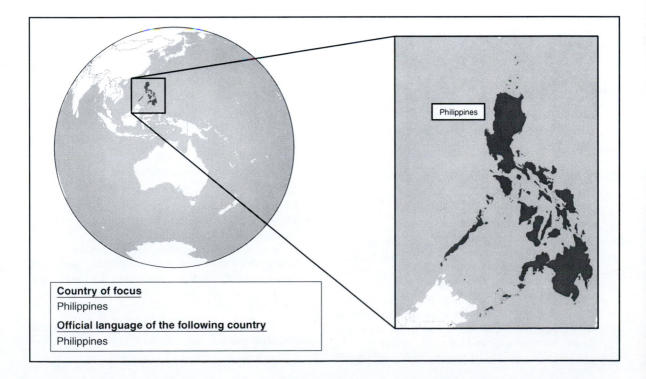

Country of focus
Philippines

Official language of the following country
Philippines

TABLE 38-1 Consonants produced in Filipino

	Bilabial	Labiodental	Dental	Alveolar
Plosive	p b		t̪ d̪	t d
Nasal	m		n	
Trill				r
Tap or flap				
Fricative				s
Lateral fricative	███████████████████████		
Affricate		███████████████	
Approximant	w (labiovelar)			

Black = articulations judged impossible

Based on the International Phonetic Alphabet. Courtesy of the International Phonetic Association (c/o Department of Linguistics, University of Victoria, Victoria, British Columbia, Canada).

Phonotactic restrictions

Syllables

The most common syllable structures in Tagalog are CV and CVC (Himmelmann, 2005). The simplest syllable has a consonant and vowel; the consonant provides the onset. In syllables where the vowel is in the initial position, a glottal stop acts as the onset. Consonant sequences are divided between syllables, except for the *ng*, which cannot be separated (Rubino, 2004). Syllable-internal consonant clusters occur only when unstressed vowels are deleted before glides (e.g., *tuwíd* ⇨ *twíd*) (Himmelmann, 2005). Most affixes in Tagalog can be combined with one another, infixes in verbs are common (Himmelmann, 2000), and reduplication is a frequent morphological tool (Rubino, 2004). Thus, the co-occurrence of multiple affixes with reduplication and stress shifting results in many common polysyllabic words (Himmelmann, 2000) (e.g., *pakíkípagkapwátáo* 'getting along well with people').

Consonants and consonant clusters

Unlike in English, the velar nasal consonant /ŋ/ occurs in all word positions, including word-initial. Consonant clusters frequently occur in derived forms or contractions: *halíkan* ⇨ *hagkan* 'to kiss' (Blake, 1925, in Blust, 1971). There are no native root words with initial consonant clusters (Cena, 1979). Words with initial consonant clusters come from borrowed words that have been integrated into Tagalog vocabulary (e.g., Spanish *prito* 'to fry' or 'fried') (Llamzon, 1975). Also, some Tagalog speakers may find it difficult to pronounce consonant sequences that do not occur natively in Tagalog: *th, ht,* and *ch*. Thus, *th* might be pronounced as [t] (e.g., *tot* for 'thought'); and *ch* as [ts] (e.g., *tsapter* for 'chapter'). Likewise, because of Tagalog's transparency, speakers may have difficulty with words containing silent sounds such as the *b* in 'climb'; the silent *b* might be enunciated (Northern Illinois University, 2005).

Tones

Filipino does not use tones to differentiate meaning.

Stress and intonation

In general, stress is phonemic and is on either of the last two syllables in Tagalog roots (Himmelmann, 2000). Tagalog uses stress to differentiate meaning, for example, *áso* 'dog', *asó* 'smoke'. The glottal stop within words and the final glottal stop within phrases is often dropped when speaking rapidly; for example, *saʔan* in *Saan ka ba nagpunta?* 'Where did you go?', causing *saʔan* to sound like *san* (Ramos and Cena, 1990).

There are five types of accentuation:

- *Mabilís* (fast): stress on last syllable
- *Malumay* (soft): stress on penultimate syllable
- *Malumí* (grave): weak stress on penultimate + grave on last syllable with glottal stop
- *Maragsâ* (strong): strong stress on final syllable + glottal stop; this is shown by the acute glottal accent mark (*kudlít* or vowel-modifying mark) over the vowel, e.g., *â*
- *Mariín* (heavy): two syllables are stressed (Campbell, 2000).

Intonation rises for requests and questions, suspends for nonfinal phrases, and falls for commands, responses, and statements (Ramos and Cena, 1990).

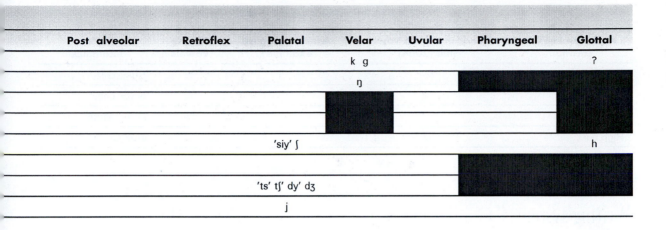

Post alveolar	Retroflex	Palatal	Velar	Uvular	Pharyngeal	Glottal
			k g			?
			ŋ			
		'siy' ʃ				h
		'ts' tʃ dy' dʒ				
		j				

TABLE 38-2 Vowels produced in Filipino compared with General American English

American English Location	American English Vowels Smit (2004)	American English examples	Filipino Vowels	Filipino examples
High-front	i	b*ea*t		N/A
	ɪ	b*i*t	ɪ	b*i*bi 'duck'
	e	r*ai*d		N/A
Mid-low front	ɛ	b*e*d	ɛ	b*e*nta 'sell'
	æ	b*a*d		N/A
High-back, rounded	u	bl*ue*	u	b*u*ntál 'hit'
	ʊ	b*oo*k		búbog 'shard'
Mid-back, rounded	o	b*oa*t		N/A
	ɔ	f*o*rm	ɔ	bólo 'butcher knife'
Low back	ɑ	dr*o*p		N/A
[r]-colored	ɝ			N/A
	ɚ	nev*er*, col*or*		N/A
	ɪr			N/A
	ɛr			N/A
	ʊr			N/A
	ɔr			N/A
	ar			N/A
Central	ə	*a*bout, *o*ccur, *u*pon,		N/A
	ʌ			N/A
Diphthongs	aɪ	m*y*, b*i*ke		baybáy 'spelling'
	aʊ	*ou*t, m*ou*se		N/A
	ɔɪ	b*oy*		apóy 'fire'

Table 38-2 continued

American English Location	American English Vowels Smit (2004)	American English examples	Filipino Vowels	Filipino examples
High-front	iw		iw	*balíw* 'crazy'
Mid-front	ey		ey	*béybi* 'baby'
Low-central	aw		aw	*áyaw* 'refuse'
High back	uy		uy	*arúy* 'Ouch!'

Note. Data from Ramos and Cena (1990).

Writing system

The ancient Philippine script called *baybayin* 'to spell' is syllabic, and had 17 characters representing 14 consonant syllables with an *a*: *ba, ka, da/ra, ga, ha, la, ma, na, nga, pa, sa, ta, wa, ya*, and three vowels: *a, e/i, o/u*. Diacritics differentiated the vowels, i.e., diacritics on top of the consonant represented *e/i*, whereas diacritics at the bottom represented *o/u*. Final consonants were not represented (Rubino, 2004). *D* and *r* had the same character. The transformation rule used up to this day is as follows: letter *d* changes to *r* when in between two vowels, within the same word, or in between two words (e.g., *lákad* 'walk' ⇨ *lákaran* 'path' (Alejandro, 1947). In 2001, the Commission on the Filipino Language (*Komisyon sa Wikang Filipino*) issued revised Filipino spelling guidelines (*Revisyon ng Alfabeto at Patnubay sa Ispeling ng Wikang Filipino*, Catacataca, 2005) which allowed the use of c, f, j, ñ, q, v, x, and z—letters that did not originally exist in the Tagalog alphabet. However, most Filipino dictionaries, books, and media still use the Tagalog spelling and alphabet for foreign or borrowed words (e.g., English *attack*, Spanish *atacar*, Filipino/Tagalog *atáke*). Nevertheless, languages deeply ingrained in Filipino, like Spanish, would retain the original spelling (e.g., *Corazon, Conchita, Quirino, Velasquez)*, but would be pronounced in the Tagalog manner: *Corazon* as *Corason* (de Guzman, 2001). Alejandro (1947, p. 146) provides a guide:

- hard *c* or *ck* ⇨ *k* (*cafe* ⇨ *kapé* 'coffee')
- soft *c* ⇨ *s* (*cepillo* ⇨ *sepílyo* 'toothbrush')
- *q* or *qu* ⇨ *k* (*maquina* ⇨ *mákina* 'machine')
- *ch* ⇨ *ts* (*cuchillo* ⇨ *kutsílyo* 'knife')
- *j* ⇨ *h* (*cajon* ⇨ *kahón* 'box')
- *ll* ⇨ *ly*, (*calle* ⇨ *kálye* 'street')
- *ñ* ⇨ *ny* (*paño* ⇨ *panyó* 'handkerchief')

- *rr* ⇨ *r* (*carro* ⇨ *karo* 'hearse')
- *v* ⇨ *b* (*vaca* ⇨ *báka*, 'beef, cow')
- *x* ⇨ *ks* (*taxi* ⇨ *taksi*, 'taxi')
- *z* ⇨ *s* (*cruz* ⇨ *krus* 'cross').

Today, a Tagalized spelling of English words used more often is the transformation of *j* ⇨ *dy* in juice (*dyús*) (Rubino, 2004).

Varieties of Filipino

McFarland (1983) claims that there is minimal dialectical diversity within Tagalog. On the other hand, Gordon (2005) asserts that there are eight major Tagalog dialects: Lubang, Manila, Marinduque, Bataan, Batangas, Bulacan, Tanay-Paete, and Tayabas-Quezon. The dialects are mutually intelligible although the intonation and lexicon differ. The most unique dialect is Marinduque because it has grammatical features similar to the Visayan languages such as Cebuano, probably because of its proximity to Visayan-speaking provinces (Nationmaster, 2005). Pelaez-Soberano (1977) studied the Tagalog dialects in Marinduque. She found that Tagalog speakers from Manila replace the glottal with vowel lengthening, whereas people from Western Marinduque retain the glottal stop when it is not in the phrase-final position. Manila speakers also have a rising final contour in terms of intonation whereas people from Western Marinduque have a partial fall.

Typical acquisition of Filipino

The Summary of Studies Table at the end of this chapter contains only two studies on the acquisition of Filipino by Filipino children. The first deals with bilingual children while the second involves a trilingual child.

Acquired sounds

To date there is no study of acquired consonants, consonant clusters, vowels, or diphthongs by Filipino children.

Percent correct

To date there is no study of percentage of correct production by Filipino children.

Phonological processes

To date there is no study of phonological processes in Filipino children.

Intelligibility

Montanari (2005) documented the intelligible and unintelligible utterances of a Tagalog-English-Spanish trilingual toddler growing up in the USA. Results show that the trilingual child's utterances were mostly intelligible and predictable from the language of the interlocutor. Her speech errors were also normal for speakers of the language at her age. For example, at age 1;9, she contracted certain words; saying 'ete' instead of 'este' in Spanish; and at age 2;4, she said 'pis', instead of 'please' in English, and 'asen' instead of 'alisin' (remove) in Tagalog. Montanari also found that the percentage of the child's unintelligible words from age 1;9 was about the same at age 2;4.

Phonetic inventory

To date there is no study of phonetic inventory of consonants and vowels produced by Filipino children.

Common mismatches

To date there is no study of common mismatches produced by Filipino children.

Syllable structure

To date there is no study of syllable structure produced by Filipino children.

Prosody

To date there is no study of prosody produced by Filipino children.

Phonological awareness

Everatt, Smythe, Ocampo, and Gyamarthy (2004) assessed third grade, Filipino-English bilingual children in the Philippines. The researchers matched children with low and average English literacy. The low-literacy children scored in the bottom 15 percent on measures of English word reading and spelling, whereas the average-literacy children scored close to the mean on the same measures. However, the two groups had similar scores on general language and nonverbal measures in English. The researchers gave the two groups of children these phonological tests: nonword reading, phoneme tapping, syllable tapping, rapid naming, and auditory short-term memory in English and Filipino. The English test results showed that the two groups of children had significant differences only for nonword reading, rapid naming, and auditory short-term memory. The Filipino tests showed the same differences but also demonstrated significant differences in phoneme tapping. The researchers concluded that testing in the first language (Filipino) should be done to ensure that all the underlying problems of a child are identified. To date, however, there is no longitudinal study of the acquisition of phonological awareness in Filipino children.

Speech assessment for Filipino children

The field of speech-language pathology was established in the Philippines in 1978. Currently, more than 60 percent of practicing speech-language pathologists (SLPs) in the Philippines are in private practice, almost 50 percent work in clinics, hospitals, and special schools, and a small percentage are involved in academe and regular private schools (Cheng, Olea, and Marzan, 2002). There are a myriad of challenges that limit the accessibility to SLP services for the majority of the population: many are of low socioeconomic status (SES), and they use various languages and dialects. Health insurance programs covering SLP services are virtually nonexistent, and there are very few SLP personnel in government-run hospitals (Cheng et al., 2002). Therefore, most SLP services are provided via private practice, which is out of reach for most.

A large portion of the population in the Philippines is bilingual or multilingual. As in North America, SLP service delivery is hindered when there are no SLPs who speak the client's stronger language or dialect. In addition, the multilingual nature of the client pool leads to difficulties in developing standardized assessment tools. (These observations are based on informal interviews with SLPs in the Philippines.) Therefore, SLPs rely on alternative nonstandard methods for assessment and intervention of speech and language skills. Children from families with higher SES tend to be very proficient in English, and thus are tested in English with traditional standardized English measures (e.g., *Peabody Picture Vocabulary Test*), and they tend to do well on them. However, children from low-SES homes tend to be less proficient in English (Williams, 1971), if at all; and so for them, English is not the appropriate language for assessment. Therefore, clinicians develop nonstandardized adaptations or translations of Western-made tests (Cheng et al., 2002), and it is at the clinician's discretion to decide what would be the most appropriate testing method for the particular client.

An additional speech sampling tool that has been developed for use with Filipino children is the *Haló-haló Espesyal* passage, which is used to assess speech sounds in Filipino. It is similar to the Rainbow passage, but much simpler; and thus it is appropriate only for children who can already read. Faculty and students at the University of the Philippines–Manila have undertaken piloting and content validity work, but the *Haló-haló Espesyal* passage is still being revised and updated (Professor F. Ligot, personal communication, January 27, 2006; De la Cruz, Rubite, and Ulan, 2005; Gacer, Mateo, and Santuele, 2004; Lavides, Sotto, Visitacion, and Concepcion, 2003; Pagorogon, De Gorostiza, and Villanueva, 2002; Tolentino, Africa, and Misa, 2002).

Speech intervention for Filipino children

The information provided in the section above is also relevant for this section. To the best of our knowledge, commonly used sets of intervention strategies are nonexistent in the Philippines. It is at the clinician's discretion to decide what intervention approach would be most appropriate with each client, based on the client's SES and the language or dialect with which he or she is most comfortable. Many of the SLPs in private practice are trained abroad (e.g., Australia and the USA; Cheng et al., 2002), and they rely on different assessments and nonuniform intervention strategies in their practice.

Working in the Philippines

The only school offering a four-year bachelor's degree in speech pathology is the University of the Philippines (UP) College of Allied Medical Professions in Manila. This degree is the minimum requirement to practice the profession in the Philippines (Cheng et al., 2002). Although an undergraduate degree, its requirements are similar to the master's-level speech-language pathology programs offered

in countries such as the USA (Cheng et al., 2002). Both UP and the University of Santo Tomas (also in Manila) offer a master's degree in Audiology. In addition, UP offers a master's degree in rehabilitation science on the speech pathology track (UP, 2005). The Philippine Association of Speech Pathologists (PASP) is working with the Philippine legislature to obtain professional licensing, as well as to establish guidelines for practice and standards of professional education (Cheng et al., 2002). A visa is needed from the Philippine government for non-Filipino citizens to work as SLPs in the Philippines.

The increasing number of Filipino immigrants to the USA and Canada contributes to an expansion in the number of Filipino clients in an SLP's workload. Therefore, in order to provide high-quality service delivery to Filipino clients, SLPs in North America need to be aware of the cultural practices and linguistic features of their clients. Ninety percent of Filipino-American students are designated as Fluent English Proficient (Cheng, Nakasato, and Wallace, 1995). In addition, because the literacy rate in the Philippines is high (90 percent), immigrants who come to North America are mostly literate (Roseberry-McKibbin, 1997). However, some of the recent Filipino immigrants to Canada come from rural areas, where their schooling may have been disrupted, so they may have lower literacy and education levels. Accordingly, SLPs in Canada should expect to work with clients with varying degrees of English proficiency and literacy skills (Cheng, et al., 1995). In addition, the great linguistic diversity among the Filipino population makes the task of North American SLPs challenging. If SLPs rely on the services provided by translators and interpreters, they have to ensure that the translators and interpreters speak the particular language of the client being tested (Roseberry-McKibbin, 1997). Whenever possible, the SLP should assess the child's actual oral proficiency in the language which he or she speaks. A Filipino-speaking SLP in Vancouver, Canada, informed us that she uses informal language assessments in Filipino, which may consist of a language sample or a narrative. In addition, she uses dynamic assessment in Filipino, in order to assist her in establishing the child's learning style regardless of language proficiency (M. Courillo, personal communication, September 8, 2005). The oral proficiency in English and Filipino of Filipino-American or Filipino-Canadian students born in North America may be different from the proficiency of Filipino students who have immigrated to North America at later ages because the latter would have been educated in both English and Filipino in the Philippines. Therefore it is crucial that whenever possible, these students' oral proficiency be tested in both languages to obtain a complete representation of their language skills.

PHONETICALLY SPEAKING

Pronunciation of Filipino: /ɤilipinŏ/

Pronunciation of Tagalog: /θagalog/

Relevant words for speech assessment and intervention

Word/ Phrase	Formal usage	Pronunciation	Informal usage	Pronunciation
Tongue	dilá	/dila/		
Teeth	ngipin	/ŋipin/		
Lips	labí	/labi/		
Hard palate	matigás na ngala ngála	/matigas na ŋala ŋala/		
Soft palate	malambót na ngala ngála	/malambot na ŋala ŋala/		
Larynx	gulúng gulungán	/gulung guluŋan/		
Lungs	bagá (S) mga bagá (P)	/baga/		
Nose	ilóng	/ilong/		
Sound	tunóg	/tunog/		
Word	salitâ	/salita/		
Sentence	pangungusap	/paŋguŋgusap/	sentens	/sentens/
Paragraph	tálataán	/talataan/		

- *Pô, hô* - respect particle in Tagalog (Rubino, 2004). Essentially means Sir or Madam, added when addressing an older person or a person superior in rank. Addressing an older or superior person in the third person also shows respect (i.e., *kayo, nila, sila* instead of *ka, ikaw,* you)
- *Kumustá ka? Kumustá pô kayó?* - How are you?
- *Magandáng umága/hápon/gábi.* - Good morning/afternoon/evening.
- *Mabúti.* - I'm fine.
- *Salámat.* - Thank you.
- *Waláng anumán.* - You're welcome. Literally translates as "It is nothing."
- *Oo. Opô. Ohô.* - Yes
- *Hindi.* - No
- *Síge.* - Ok or goodbye
- *Anóng pangálan mo? Anó po ang pangalan nila?* - What is your name?

RESOURCES

Books

Ramos, T., and Cena, R. (1990). *Modern Tagalog: Grammatical explanations and exercises for nonnative speakers.* Honolulu: University of Hawaii Press. Explains how Tagalog sounds are pronounced and provides examples.

Rubino, C. (1998). *Tagalog-English/English-Tagalog Standard Dictionary.* New York: Hippocrene Books. Includes an introduction to grammar, the ancient syllabary, and useful words and phrases.

Journal

• *Philippine Journal of Linguistics* http://www.dlsu.edu.ph/inside/organizations/lsp/journal.asp. The journal of the Linguistic Society of the Philippines, published by De La Salle University Press, Manila, Philippines.

Professional associations

The professional association of speech-language pathologists within the Philippines is the Philippine Association of Speech Pathologists, http://www.ncwdp.gov.ph/drdb/browse_directories.asp?Code2=919

Useful Filipino Web sites

• Horst Ibelgaufts, *Nakalimútan na kíta,* http://www.copewithcytokines.de/TAGALOG/cope.cgi?164, an online Tagalog dictionary.
• Northern Illinois University, http://www.seasite.niu.edu/Tagalog/Tagalog_mainpage.htm. This Web site was the recipient of the Multilingual Learner Award 2002. It provides interactive materials on Tagalog and Filipino culture, including an electronic dictionary, e-mail tutor, and chat room.
• Summer Institute of Linguistics, http://www.sil.org/asia/philippines/plb_download.html. Downloadable articles about the Tagalog language are available

REFERENCES

Alejandro, R. (1947). *A handbook of Tagalog grammar (with exercises).* Manila: University Publishing Co.

Camarota, S. A., and McArdle, N. (2003, September). *Where immigrants live: An examination of state residency of the foreign born by country of origin.* Washington, DC: Center for Immigration Studies. Also available at http://www.cis.org/articles/2003/back1203.html

Campbell, G. L. (2000). *Compendium of the world's languages: Vol. II. Ladakhi to Zuni* (2nd ed.). London: Routledge.

Catacataca, P. D. (2005). *The use of Filipino in official transactions, communication, and correspondence.* Retrieved February 16, 2005, from http://www.ncca.gov.ph/about_cultarts/comarticles.php?artcl_Id=206.

Cena, R. M. (1979). Double representations for some loan words in Tagalog. In C. Edrial-Luzares and A. Hale (Eds.), *Studies in Philippine Linguistics,* 3(1), 125–137. Also available at http://www.sil.org/asia/philippines/sipl/SIPL_3-1_125-137.pdf

Cheng, L., Nakasato, J., and Wallace, G. (1995). The Pacific-Islander population and the challenges they face. In L. L. Cheng, (Ed.), *Integrating language and learning for inclusion: An Asian-Pacific focus* (pp. 63–106). San Diego, CA: Singular.

Cheng, W., Olea, T., and Marzan, J. (2002). Speech-language pathology in the Philippines: Reflections on the past and present, perspectives for the future. *Folia Phoniatrica et Logopaedica, 54,* 79–82.

De la Cruz, M. M. L., Rubite, R. R., and Ulan, C. D. S. (2005). *Pilot testing of the revised "Halo-Halo Espesyal" reading passage for Filipino cleft lip and/or cleft palate speakers.* Unpublished undergraduate thesis, University of the Philippines-Manila.

Everatt, J., Smythe, I., Ocampo, D., and Gyamarthy, E. (2004). Issues in the assessment of literacy-related difficulties across language backgrounds: A cross-linguistic comparison. *Journal of Research in Reading, 27*(2), 141–151.

Gacer, G., Mateo, M. T. R., and Santuele, J. P. (2004). *Revision and pilot testing of "Halo-Halo Espesyal" reading passage as a tool for the assessment of children with cleft lip and palate.* Unpublished undergraduate thesis, University of the Philippines-Manila.

Gomez, L.A. (1958). *An outline of Tagalog phonology.* Unpublished master's thesis, Georgetown University, Washington, DC.

Gonzalez, A. B. (1999). The language planning situation in the Philippines. In R. B. Kaplan and R. B. Baldauf (Eds.), *Language planning in Malawi, Mozambique and the Philippines (pp. 133–171).* Clevedon: Multilingual Matters.

Gordon, R. G. (Ed.) (2005). *Ethnologue: Languages of the world* (15th ed.). Dallas, TX: Summer Institute of Linguistics. Also available at http://www.ethnologue.com/print.asp

Himmelmann, N. P. (2000). Tagalog. In G. Booij, C. Lehmann, J. Mugdan, and S. Skopeteas (Eds.), *Morphology: An International handbook on inflection and word formation* (Vol. 2, pp. 1473–1490). Berlin: de Gruyter.

Himmelmann, N. P. (2005). Tagalog. In K. A. Adelaar and N. P. Himmelmann (Eds.), *The Austronesian Languages of Asia and Madagascar* (pp. 350–376). London: Routledge.

Lavides, E. X. S., Sotto, S. T.Y., Visitacion, N. P., and Concepcion, J. R. (2003). *Content validation of the "Halo-Halo Espesyal" reading passage as a tool for the assessment of children with cleft lip and palate.* Unpublished undergraduate thesis, University of the Philippines-Manila.

Llamzon, T. A. (1975). *Modern Tagalog: A functional-structural approach.* The Hague: Mouton.

Llamzon, T.A., Del Rosario, F. L., and Sanchez, M. (1974). *Makabagong balarila ng wikang Tagalog.* Quezon City, Philippines: Ateneo de Manila University Press.

McFarland, C. D. (1983). *A linguistic atlas of the Philippines.* Manila: Linguistic Society of the Philippines.

Montanari, S. (2005). *Sol!, GANDA, Cute!: A longitudinal study of language choice in a developing trilingual child.* In J. Cohen, K. McAlister, K. Rolstad, and J. MacSwan (Eds.), *Proceedings of the 4th International Symposium on Bilingualism* (pp. 1662–1678). Somerville, MA: Cascadilla Press.

Morrow, P. (2005). *The Lord's Prayer from the Doctrina Cristiana.* Retrieved July 14, 2005, from http://www.mts.net/~pmorrow/lordpray.htm

Nationmaster. (2005). *Encyclopedia: Tagalog language.* Retrieved July 14, 2005, from http://www.nationmaster.com/encyclopedia/Tagalog-language

Northern Illinois University. (2005). Retrieved July 6, 2005 from http://www.seasite.niu.edu/Tagalog/Tagalog_mainpage.htm

Ocampo, D. (2004). Dyslexia in the Philippines. In I. Smythe, J. Everatt, and R. Slater (Eds.), *International book of dyslexia: A guide to practice and resources (pp. 184–189).* West Sussex, UK: John Wiley.

Pagorogon, G., De Gorostiza, A. L., and Villanueva, C. (2002). *The development of a Filipino reading passage of children with cleft lip and palate: Ages 8-11.* Unpublished undergraduate thesis, University of the Philippines-Manila.

Pelaez-Soberano, R. (1977). The dialects of Marinduque Tagalog. In C. Edrial-Luzares and A. Hale (Eds.), *Studies in Philippine Linguistics, 1*(1), (pp. 53–74). Also available at http://www.sil.org/asia/philippines/sipl/SIPL_1-1_053-074.pdf

Postma, A. (1971). Contemporary Mangyan scripts. *Philippine Journal of Linguistics, 2*(1), 1–12.

Postma, A. (1992). The Laguna Copper Plate Inscription: Text and commentary. *Philippines Studies, 40,* 183–203.

Ramos, T., and Cena, R. (1990). *Modern Tagalog: Grammatical explanations and exercises for nonnative speakers.* Honolulu: University of Hawaii Press.

Roseberry-McKibbin, C. (1997). Understanding Filipino families: A foundation for effective service delivery. *American Journal of Speech-Language Pathology, 6,* 5–14.

Rubino, C. (2004). *Tagalog-English/English-Tagalog standard dictionary* (3rd printing). New York: Hippocrene Books.

Tolentino, N., Africa, D., and Misa, J. P. (2002). *The development of a Filipino reading passage of children with cleft lip and palate: Ages 14-17.* Unpublished undergraduate thesis, University of the Philippines-Manila.

University of the Philippines. *University of the Philippines Manila College of Allied Medical Professions.* Retrieved January 27, 2005, from http://www.upm.edu.ph/camp/history.html

Wikipedia (2006). *Tagalog language.* Retrieved February 12, 2006, from http://en.wikipedia.org/wiki/Tagalog_language

Williams, J. D. (1971). Speech and language in the Philippines. *ASHA, 13,* 271-274.

SUMMARY OF STUDIES OF TYPICAL FILIPINO SPEECH ACQUISITION

Authors	Year	Country	No. of children	Age of children	Information	Sample type	Data collection
Everatt, Smythe, Ocampo. and Gyamarthy	2004	Philippines	27	9;0	Phonological awareness and processing	Phonemes, Syllables, Single Words	Cross sectional
Montanari	2005	USA	1	1;9 and 2;4	Intelligibility, discourse, pragmatics	Utterances	Longitudinal

Chapter 39

Finnish Speech Acquisition

Sari Kunnari and Tuula Savinainen-Makkonen

INTRODUCTION

Finland is officially a bilingual country whose national languages are Finnish and Swedish. Finnish is a member of the Finno-Ugrian language family and is most closely related to Estonian. Politically, Finland was a part of Sweden until 1809 and thus greatly influenced by Swedish for a long time. Before becoming an independent republic in 1917, Finland was an autonomous Grand Duchy within the Russian Empire from 1809 to 1917. Currently 5,236,600 people live in Finland and Finnish is the native language of about 92 percent of the population (Statistics Finland, 2004). The population includes a minority group of Swedish-speaking Finns (5.5 percent) and some other smaller minorities too. See the Resources section of this chapter for materials pertaining to Finnish.

Where Finnish is spoken

The vast majority of Finnish-speaking people live in Finland. The biggest Finnish-speaking minority group, outside of Finland, is in Sweden where about 211,000 people speak Finnish as their mother tongue (Statistics Finland, 2004) In addition, there are some Finnish-speaking people in Eastern Karelia, Ingria, and northern Norway. Waves of emigration have also resulted in some other Finnish minorities, too, particularly in North America and Australia (see the accompanying map and Appendix D).

Components of Finnish

Consonants

Disregarding words of recent foreign origin, Finnish has 13 consonants (see Table 39-1). This is the core system, and in addition /b, g, f, ʃ/ may occur in recent loanwords. For many speakers these latter phonemes are not independent and are replaced by the phonetically nearest native phonemes. Although /h/ is usually considered a glottal fricative, it could also be placed near the approximants, due to its great contextual variation in Finnish (Iivonen, 1996a). Finnish /t̪/ is produced as a dental unaspirated plosive. In many languages single rhotics are taps and only geminates are trilled (Ladefoged and Maddieson, 1996), but in Finnish even single rhotics are usually trilled with the tip of the tongue; a tap allophone also occurs. Finnish has a binary quantity opposition in both consonants and vowels, independently of each other, and independently of stress (Suomi, Toivanen, and Ylitalo, 2003). All consonants, with the exception of /d, h, j, ʋ/, can occur in a geminate construction (/d/ occurs double only in loanwords). The need for the control of segment duration is critical, since relative segment durations serve the purpose of distinguishing word meanings (e.g., /t̪ɑkɑ/ 'back', /t̪ɑkkɑ/ 'fireplace').

Vowels and diphthongs

The Finnish vowel system is composed of eight phonemes /i, e, æ, y, ø, ɑ, o, u/ (see Table 39-2), which are unambiguously represented in the orthography by <i, e, ä, y, ö, a, o, u>, respectively. Phonetically there are short and long monophthongs and long diphthongs. Phonologically, the long vowels are analyzed as three kinds of sequences:

• Double vowels (sequences of two identical vowels in the same syllable)
• Diphthongs (sequences of two different vowels in the same syllable)
• Vowel combinations (sequences of two different vowels separated by a syllable boundary)

As in consonants, relative segment durations of vowels serve the purpose of distinguishing words (e.g.,

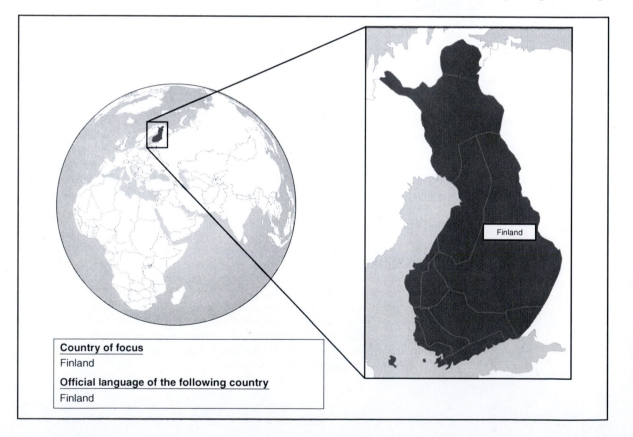

Country of focus
Finland

Official language of the following country
Finland

Finland

/t̪uli/ 'fire', /t̪uuli/ 'wind'). Finnish has 18 diphthongs, which can be divided into two groups according to the final vowel: those ending with a close vowel /i/, /u/, or /y/, and those ending with mid vowels /e/, /ø/, or /o/. Finnish also has about 20 combinations of two vowels where the vowels belong to different syllables. In addition, there can also be sequences of three and even four vowels within a word, these being combinations of the sequences mentioned above and single vowels.

Phonotactic restrictions

Syllables

Finnish has 15 frequently occurring syllable types; about 58 percent of syllable tokens in speech are open, and 42 percent closed (Suomi, Toivanen, and Ylitalo, 2006). The frequent syllable structures can be described by the formula: $C_{(0-2)}V(V/C)C_{(0-1)}$; syllables with a CC onset occur only word-initially, and only in borrowed words, many of which however are very frequent. The shortest syllable consists of a single vowel (e.g., *i*.lo 'joy'), and the longest frequent syllable contains four segments (e.g., *taak*.ka 'burden', *pärs*.ke 'splash'). In more marginal syllable types, the onset of a word-initial syllable can consist of CCC (e.g., *stres*.si 'stress'), or there may be two coda consonants following VV (e.g., *Suort*.ti). In many dialects, Standard Finnish word-initial syllable onsets with more than one consonant are simplified to C onsets.

Consonants and consonant clusters

Of the 13 singleton core consonants, 11 may occur alone in word initial position. /ŋ/ never occurs word-initially and /d/ only in loanwords, many of which however are very frequent. In Standard Finnish, /d/ is an independent phoneme, but in most dialects this phoneme does not exist. Instead, other phonemes (or nothing) occur in its place. For word-initial consonant clusters, see above. All 13 consonants can appear word-medially, while only /t̪, s, n, r, l/ can occur word-finally. Word-medially, heterosyllabic consonant sequences containing up to three consonants are very common (e.g., ka*n*.sa 'people', ka*n*s.sa 'with'), with a syllable boundary always between the last two consonants. As for word-final position, the few clusters that occur are more or less marginal, and a broad generalization is that only single consonants occur word-finally.

Vowels

All Finnish vowels can occur in any word position. However, vowel harmony restricts the vowel combinations. The vowels can be divided into three groups in this respect: front harmonic /y, ø, æ/, back harmonic /ɑ,

o, u/, and harmonically neutral /i, e/ (see Suomi, 1983). The main restriction is that, within an uncompounded word form, vowels from only one of the harmonic groups may occur (e.g., /ystæuæ/ 'friend', /mɑɑlɑus/ 'painting'), whereas the harmonically neutral vowels may be combined with all other vowels (e.g., /puhe/ 'speech'). Vowel harmony rules also apply to the addition of case endings.

Tones

Finnish does not use tones to differentiate meaning.

Stress and intonation

Finnish has fixed stress, as opposed to the moving stress in the Germanic languages. Primary word stress always falls on the first syllable (e.g., ˈkel.lo 'clock'), but because of the great number of polysyllabic and compound words, a secondary stress also occurs frequently (Iivonen, 1998a). In most cases secondary stress falls, in four-syllabic or longer words, either on the third or the fourth syllable, but after that on every second syllable (e.g., ˈap.pel.ˌsii.ni 'orange', ˈeu.roop.pa.ˌlai.nen 'European'). The second and the last syllable of a word are normally unstressed.

Writing system

The Finnish orthography is based on the phonemic principle: with a few clear-cut exceptions, each phoneme in carefully spoken Standard Finnish that closely follows the normative orthography (both of which are taught at school) is represented by one grapheme, and each grapheme represents one phoneme. This presumably facilitates learning to read and write. However, for some Finnish children, marking the phonological quantity distinction orthographically is challenging. Further, there are some phenomena in spoken Finnish that are not marked in the orthography; for example, nasal assimilation (e.g., <pojan pää> [pojɑm pæːæ]) and final reduplication (e.g., <ota lisää> [ot̪ɑllisæːæ]).

Varieties of Finnish

Most speakers of Finnish have command over two varieties: Standard Finnish and the local dialect. Standard Finnish, which is based on the written form of the language, is used in formal situations (e.g., political speeches, sermons, newscasts) while the spoken language is used in everyday communication. Finnish dialects are divided into two main dialect groups, the western dialects and the eastern dialects (Latomaa & Nuolijärvi, 2002). The dialects are almost entirely intelligible to all Finnish-speaking people,

TABLE 39-1 Consonants produced in Finnish

	Bilabial	Labiodental	Dental	Alveolar
Plosive	p (b)		t̪	d
Nasal	m			n
Trill				r
Tap or flap				
Fricative		(f)		s
Lateral fricative	██████	██████		
Affricate				
Approximant		ʋ		
Lateral approximant	██████	██████		l

Black = articulations judged impossible

( ) = marginal consonants

Based on the International Phonetic Alphabet. Courtesy of the International Phonetic Association (c/o Department of Linguistics, University of Victoria, Victoria, British Columbia, Canada).

although there are some phonological and morphological differences between them. During the past few decades, some of these differences in dialects have merged because of rapid changes in society. Karlsson (2004) has listed several omissions (e.g., *punainen* 'red' ⇨ *punanen*), assimilations (e.g., *kauhea* 'terrible' ⇨ *kauhee*), and some other features (e.g., passive forms are used instead of the first person plural ending *me sano/mme* 'we say' ⇨ *me sanotaan*) which are particularly common for the colloquial spoken language when compared to the standard language.

Typical acquisition of Finnish

So far the information on Finnish children's typical speech acquisition has come from case studies. Recently, some larger-scale studies have been published. The Summary of Studies Table at the end of this chapter contains studies of the acquisition of Finnish.

Acquired sounds

Consonants

To date there is no Finnish cross-sectional study of the age of the acquisition of consonants. However, inventory studies (Kunnari, 2000, 2003a, b) and some case studies (e.g., Iivonen, 1998b) show that Finnish children seem to follow the universal tendency of acquiring stops and nasals as their first consonants. Also /s/ is acquired

relatively early (although not necessarily in phonetically correct form) since it is the only fricative consonant in Finnish and its functional load is high (see Warren, 2001). Articulation of Finnish /r/ requires relatively complicated motor performance and this seems to have an effect on its late acquisition. Although /d/ is universally acquired early, Finnish children acquire it very late due to its marginal role in the Finnish consonant system. Further, since the quantity distinction (e.g., /kukɑ/ 'who', /kukkɑ/ 'flower') is crucial in Finnish, children seem to acquire it very early (Aoyama, 2001; Kunnari, Nakai, and Vihman 2001; Richardson, 1998).

Consonant clusters

To date there is no Finnish cross-sectional study of the age of the acquisition of consonant clusters. However, Savinainen-Makkonen (2006) found in her longitudinal study that children did not produce any heterosyllabic medial clusters at age 1;6 but produced already several (mean 6), mainly homorganic clusters /-nt̪-/, /-ŋk-/, and /-mp-/, at age 2;0.

Vowels and diphthongs

Iivonen (2004) reported the vowel acquisition of his two sons and found that by the age of 2;6 both boys had acquired all Finnish vowels, although the quality of some vowels was still variable. Further, in Warren's (2001) multicase study at least 2-year-olds were able to produce some diphthongs. In Turunen's study (2003) of

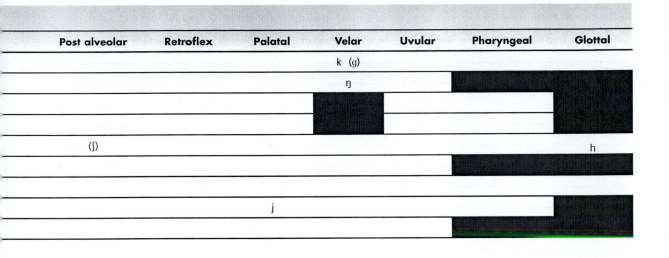

Post alveolar	Retroflex	Palatal	Velar	Uvular	Pharyngeal	Glottal
			k (g)			
			ŋ			
(ʃ)						h
		j				

TABLE 39-2 Vowels produced in Finnish compared with General American English

American English location	American English vowels Smit (2004)	American English examples	Finnish location	Finnish vowels	Finnish examples
High-front	i	_beat_	High-front	i	_ki_ssa 'cat'
	ɪ	_bit_			
	e	_raid_	Mid-front	e*	_ke_llo 'clock'
Mid-low front	ɛ	_bed_			
	æ	_bad_	Mid-low front	æ	_tä_ti 'aunt'
High-back, rounded	u	_blue_	High-back, rounded	u	_ku_kka 'flower'
	ʊ	_book_			
			High-front, rounded	y	_ky_nä 'pencil'
			Mid-front, rounded	ø	_pö_llö 'owl'
Mid-back, rounded	o	_boat_	Mid-back, rounded	o**	_ko_ti 'home'
	ɔ	_form_			
Low back	ɑ	_drop_	Low back	ɑ	_ta_lo 'house'
[r]-colored	ɝ				
	ɚ	_nev_er, col_or_			
	ɪr				
	ɛr				
	ʊr				
	ɔr				
	ar				

Table 39-2 continued

American English location	American English vowels Smit (2004)	American English examples	Finnish location	Finnish vowels	Finnish examples
Central	ə	*about, occur, upon*			
	ʌ				
Diphthongs	aɪ	*my, bike*	Diphthongs	ei	*seinä* 'wall'
	aʊ	*out, mouse*		æi	*äiti* 'mother'
	ɔɪ	*boy*		ui	*kuiva* 'dry'
				ɑi	*laiva* 'ship'
				oi	*poika* 'boy'
				øi	*söin* 'I ate'
				yi	*lyijy* 'lead'
				ɑu	*kaula* 'neck'
				ou	*koulu* 'school'
				eu	*reuna* 'edge'
				iu	*viulu* 'violin'
				æy	*näytös* 'act'
				øy	*pöytä* 'table'
				ey	*leyhytellä* 'to fan'
				iy	*vihkiytynyt* 'dedicated'
				ie	*sieni* 'mushroom'
				yø	*työ* 'work'
				uo	*tuoli* 'chair'

* Finnish [e̞] should be placed between the vowels [e] and [ɛ]

** Finnish [o̞] should be placed between the vowels [o] and [ɔ]

196 children, only 1.5 percent of the children did not produce any diphthongs correctly in a naming task at the age of 2;6, whereas 31 percent of the children produced targetlike diphthongs in all of their productions. The most recent study of the production of vowel harmony, based on a database of nearly 200 children, showed that Finnish vowel harmony is not violated in general at the age of 2;6 (Leiwo, Kulju, and Aoyama, 2006). The proportion of vowel harmony errors in a naming task was approximately 2–4 percent. If violations occurred, they were due to problems with the front vowels /y/, /ø/, and /æ/.

However, these results are based on two target words only. Lieko's (2001) more extensive data revealed that children do produce words that violate vowel harmony until the age of 3;9, especially in complicated test words.

Percent correct
Consonants

To date there is no study of the percentage of consonants produced correctly by Finnish children at early ages. However, some studies focused on articulation skills of

5- to 9-year-olds have shown that children have difficulties almost solely with the consonants /r/ and /s/ (Luotonen, 1998; Pietarinen, 1987). Errors other than with these consonants are rare: /l/ (1.8 percent), /k/ (1.0 percent), /j/ (0.4 percent), and /t̪/ (0.3 percent) (Pietarinen, 1987).

Consonant clusters

To date there is no detailed longitudinal study of percentage of consonant clusters, since the word-initial and word-final clusters are rare in native Finnish words. In Saaristo-Helin, Savinainen-Makkonen, and Kunnari's (2006) cross-sectional study children produced correctly only 16 percent of the targeted medial clusters at the 50-word stage (mean age being 1;8). Savinainen-Makkonen (2006) found that children produced their first adultlike medial clusters at age 2;0. Homorganic clusters /-nt̪-/, /-ŋk-/, and /-mp-/ were correctly produced whenever targeted.

Vowels

To date there are no large-scale studies of the production of vowels by young Finnish children. However, clinical experience has shown that children acquire vowels very early. What we know about older children is that 98.6 percent of the 5-year-olds produce vowels correctly (Pietarinen, 1987).

Phonological processes

Among phonological processes, Finnish researchers have been interested in truncation patterns of long words and wordinitial consonant omissions. Almost 60 percent of the words with three syllables were reduced to disyllabic productions at the 50-word stage (Saaristo-Helin et al., 2006), but only 10 percent of the trisyllabic words were truncated at the age of 2 (Torvelainen, 2005). Since Finnish is a trochaic language and main stress is always on the first syllable, one could assume that children preserve the initial two syllables (SW- template). Indeed, Finnish children usually produce the word-initial foot, but also the sonority of consonants, phonotactics, or geminates later in the word may affect the type of truncated forms (e.g., Laalo, 1994; Savinainen-Makkonen, 2000b; Turunen, 2003; Torvelainen, 2005). Studies have revealed that language-specific features also have effects on phonological processes. For example, word-initial consonant omission, an atypical process among English-speaking children, has been found to be a typical developmental process for Finnish children (Savinainen-Makkonen, 2000a; Kunnari, 2000, 2002; Turunen, 2003).

Intelligibility

Torvelainen (2005) studied the speech intelligibility of 2-year-olds (20 children at-risk for dyslexia and 20 controls). She found that there were 28 percent unintelligible utterances in the speech of the weakest fifth, while in the group of the most advanced fifth the corresponding figure was 4 percent. Luotonen (1998) studied, in her nationwide questionnaire, how intelligible the speech of 3-year-olds was for strangers. She found that 6.9 percent of the boys' speech and only 1.9 percent of the girls' speech was not intelligible at 3 years.

Phonetic inventory

Kunnari (2003a, b) reported that the mean size of the children's word-initial consonant inventories expanded from 0.6 consonants at the 4-word point (mean age 14 months) to 4.5 at the 25-word point (mean age 18 months), whereas the word-medial inventories expanded from 0.8 consonants to 5.1. At the 25-word point, word-initial consonants used by 50 percent of the children typically included the stops [p, t̪, k] as well as the bilabial nasal [m]. Fricatives, liquids, and semivowels were rare and word-final consonants were totally missing. Kunnari, Savinainen-Makkonen, and Paavola (2006) found that the size of the consonant inventory of Finnish 2-year-olds varied greatly: the weakest child produced only one stable consonant, whereas the most advanced children produced almost all Finnish consonants both in word-initial and word-medial position. The trill /r/ was almost totally missing from 2-year-olds' productions. On average, the inventory of word-initial phones was smaller than the word-medial inventory.

The only study to date focusing on vowel inventories revealed that the vowels used by at least 50 percent of Finnish 2-year-olds were /ɑ, e, o/ word-initially, and /ɑ, e, i, o, u, æ/ word-medially (Kunnari et al., 2006). The vowels /y/ and /ø/ were rare in two-year-olds' productions.

Common mismatches

Clinical experience has shown that at early ages, the most common phoneme substitute for /r/ is /l/ (Savinainen-Makkonen and Kunnari, 2004). However, children at a later age try to avoid homonyms, and use some kind of phonetic variant of /r/ (e.g., [ʀ] or [ð]). Young children also generally substitute /s/ with /t̪/, but again at a later age phonetic distortions (e.g., [θ] and [ɬ]) are more common. Among vowels the most challenging are the front vowels /y/, /æ/, and /ø/, which are typically substituted by the corresponding back vowels /u/, /ɑ/, and /o/, respectively. Concerning diphthongs, children who are not able to produce them at age 2;6 produce a long vowel instead (e.g., [pøːt̪æ] <pöytä>, [pøːlæ] <pyörä>) (Turunen, 2003). Using compensatory lengthening, children preserve a heavy stressed syllable, a phenomenon that is also typical in avoiding complex consonant sequences.

Syllable structure

There is only one study of syllable structure produced by Finnish children. This study by Kunnari (2000) concentrated on the period of the first 50 words produced by 10 children. Her analysis indicated that CV was the most common syllable type in early word productions, followed by CVC, CVV, and VV syllables. The proportion of open syllables was much higher (mean 80 percent) than that of closed syllables. The higher proportion of open syllables observed in the children's words than in the adult speech seemed to reflect children's tendency to omit syllable final consonants.

Prosody

To date there is no study of Finnish children's prosody.

Phonological awareness

Silvén, Niemi, and Voeten (2002) found that the detection of alliteration and rhyme by Finnish-speaking children is above chance level already at 3 years of age. By age 5, children are better at detecting larger multiphonemic units in words than single phonemes (Silvén, Poskiparta, and Niemi, 2004). Thus, segmenting words into syllables or detecting alliteration and rhyme units emerge prior to phonemic awareness. Furthermore, detecting single phonemes in words develops earlier in 6- to 7-year-olds compared to blending phonemes into words (Silvén, Poskiparta, Niemi, and Voeten, 2005). Typically, Finnish children commence formal schooling at 7 years of age. The children who could read at school entry recognized, at age 4, alliterations and rhymes in words better than did those children who did not learn to read by school entry. This advanced group could not read at age 5 but was better in all types of phonological awareness tasks compared with their age-mates. At age 6, every third

child appeared to read to a varying extent. The relationship between phonemic awareness and reading emerges earlier in Finnish than in languages with less regular orthographies.

Speech assessment for Finnish children

There are no Finnish standardized tests of articulation and phonology. SLPs use informal/homemade single-word tests, conversational speech sampling, and a few published nonstandardized tests to assess children's articulation skills:

- *Artikulaatiotesti. Äänteenmukainen sanakuvatesti* [Picture naming articulation test] (Remes and Ojanen, 1996)
- *Artikulaation arviointitehtäviä* [Assessment of articulation] (Vainio, 1993)

Speech intervention for Finnish children

Finnish SLPs use traditional articulation and minimal pairs approaches during intervention. Several other methods such as TCM (Touch-Cue Method, Bashir, Grahamjones, and Bostwick, 1984) and MIT (Melodic Intonation Therapy, Albert, Spark, and Helm, 1973; Helfrich-Miller, 1984) have been applied to Finnish and are used in more severe speech impairments.

Working in Finland

The professional and scientific preparation of SLPs takes place at five Finnish universities during a three-year bachelor's-level degree and two-year master's-level degree. The right to engage in the profession of SLP in Finland is certified by the National Authority for Medicolegal Affairs. SLPs work in medical centers, hospitals, family counseling and rehabilitation centers, day care centers, special schools, and institutions for the disabled. They may also run a private practice.

PHONETICALLY SPEAKING

Pronunciation of Finland *Suomi:* /suomi/ and Finnish *suomi:* /suomi/

Word/Phrase	Formal/Informal usage	Pronunciation
Tongue	*kieli*	/kieli/
Teeth	*hampaat*	/hampɑ:t/
Lips	*huulet*	/hu:let/
Hard palate	*kova suulaki*	/kovɑ su:lɑki/
Soft palate	*pehmeä suulaki*	/pehmeæ su:lɑki/
Larynx	*kurkunpää*	/kurkunpæ:/
Lungs	*keuhkot*	/keuhkot/
Nose	*nenä*	/nenæ/
Sound	*äänne*	/æ:n:e/
Word	*sana*	/sanɑ/
Sentence	*lause*	/lause/
Paragraph	*kappale*	/kap:ale/

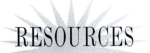

RESOURCES

Books

Sulkala, H., and Karjalainen, M. (1992). *Finnish*. London: Routledge.

Karlsson, F. (2004). *Finnish: An essential grammar*. London: Routledge.

Journals

- *Puhe ja kieli* [Speech and Language], http://www.puhejakieli.fi. A national research journal published by the Finnish Association of Speech and Language Research.

- *SKY Journal of Linguistics,* http://www.ling.helsinki.fi/sky/skyjol.shtml A research journal published by the Linguistic Association of Finland.

- *Virittäjä* [The Journal Virittäjä], http://www.kotikielenseura.fi/virittaja/verkkolehti/index.html A national research journal published by the Society for the Study of Finnish.

- *Puheterapeutti,* [Speech-language pathologists] A clinical journal published by the Finnish Association of Speech Therapists.

Professional associations

The professional association of SLPs in Finland is the Finnish Association of Speech Therapists, http://www.puheterapeuttiliitto.fi. The association was founded in 1966 and has been a member of CPLOL (Comité Permanent de Liaison Orthophonistes – Logopedes – Speech and Language Therapists de l'Union Européenne) since 1995.

Useful Finnish Web sites

• Papunet, http://www.papunet.net/index.php The site on speech impairments and plain language which strives for accessible communication.

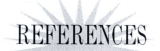

REFERENCES

Albert, M. L., Spark, R., and Helm, N. A. (1973). Melodic intonation therapy for aphasia. *Archives of Neurology, 29*, 130–131.

Aoyama, K. (2001). *A psycholinguistic perspective on Finnish and Japanese prosody: Perception, production and child acquisition of consonantal quantity distinctions.* Boston: Kluwer Academic Publishers.

Bashir, A. S., Grahamjones, F., and Bostwick, R. Y. (1984). A touch-cue method of therapy for developmental verbal apraxia. *Seminars in Speech and Language, 5*, 127–137.

Helfrich-Miller, K. R. (1984). Melodic intonation therapy with developmentally apraxic children. *Seminars in Speech and Language, 5*, 119–126.

Iivonen, A. (1994). Paradigmaattisia ja syntagmaattisia näkökohtia lapsen foneettis-fonologisessa kehityksessä. In A. Iivonen, A. Lieko, and P. Korpilahti (Eds.), *Lapsen normaali ja poikkeava kielen kehitys* (pp. 34–77). (2nd ed.). Helsinki: SKS.

Iivonen, A. (1996a). Phonetic research in progress. In A. Iivonen and A. Klippi (Eds.), *Studies in Logopedics and Phonetics 5* (pp. 11–26). Publications of the Department of Phonetics, University of Helsinki, Series B. Helsinki: Helsinki University Press.

Iivonen, A. (1996b). Syntagmaattisen kompleksisuuden lisääntyminen lapsen fonologiassa. In K. Toivainen (Ed.), *Suomalaiskielten omaksumista tutkimassa* (pp. 69–85). Publications of the Department of Finnish and General Linguistics of the University of Turku 53.

Iivonen, A. (1998a). Intonation in Finnish. In D. Hirst and A. Di Cristo (Eds.), *Intonation systems. A survey of twenty languages.* Cambridge, UK: Cambridge University Press.

Iivonen, A. (1998b). Aspects of the phonotactical acquisition in children. In K. Heinänen and M. Lehtihalmes (Eds.), *Proceedings of the Seventh Nordic Child Language Symposium* (pp. 82–84). Publications of the Department of Finnish, Saami, and Logopedics 13. Oulu: University Press.

Iivonen, A. (2004). Vokaalien kehitys protosanoista kielen mukaiseen järjestelmään. In S. Kunnari and T. Savinainen-Makkonen (Eds.), *Mistä on pienten sanat tehty?* (pp. 74–78). Helsinki: WSOY.

Itkonen, T. (1977). Huomioita lapsen äänteistön kehityksestä. *Virittäjä, 81*, 279–308.

Karlsson, F. (2004). *Finnish: An essential grammar.* London: Routledge.

Kunnari, S. (2000). *Characteristics of early lexical and phonological development in children acquiring Finnish.* Unpublished doctoral dissertation, Acta Universitas Ouluensis, B 34. University of Oulu.

Kunnari, S. (2002). Word length in syllables: Evidence from early word production in Finnish. *First Language, 22*(2), 119–135.

Kunnari, S. (2003a). Consonant inventories: A longitudinal study of Finnish-speaking children. *Journal of Multilingual Communication Disorders, 1*, 124–131.

Kunnari, S. (2003b). Suomea omaksuvien lasten ensisanojen konsonantit. *Puhe ja kieli, 4*, 197–205.

Kunnari, S., Nakai, S., and Vihman, M. M. (2001). Cross-linguistic evidence for acquisition of geminates. *Psychology of Language and Communication, 5*, 13–24.

Kunnari, S., Savinainen-Makkonen, T., and Paavola, L. (2006). Phonological skills of 2-year-old Finnish-speaking children. Manuscript submitted for publication.

Laalo, K. (1994). Kaksitavuvaihe lapsen kielen kehityksessä. *Virittäjä, 98*, 430–448.

Ladefoged, P., and Maddieson, I. (1996). *The sounds of the world's languages.* Oxford, UK: Blackwell.

Latomaa, S., and Nuolijärvi, P. (2002). The language situation in Finland. *Current Issues in Language Planning, 3*, 95–202.

Leiwo, M., Kulju, P., and Aoyama, K. (2006). The acquisition of Finnish vowel harmony. In A. Airola, A. Arppe, O. Heinämäki, M. Miestamo, K. Sinnemäki, U. Määttä, J. Niemi, K. K. Pitkänen & M. Suominen (Eds.), *A man of measure: Festschrift in the Honour of Fred Karlsson on his 60th Birthday. Special Supplement to SKY Journal of Linguistics, 19*, 149–161.

Lieko, A. (2001). Vokaaliharmonian omaksuminen. *Puhe ja kieli, 2* (1), 13–20.

Luotonen, M. (1998). *Factors associated with linguistic development and school performance: The role of early otitis media, gender and day care.* Acta Universitatis Ouluensis, series D Medica, 453. University of Oulu.

Pietarinen, A. (1987). *Vantaalaisten v. 1980 syntyneiden lasten viisivuosisseulalla mitatut kielelliset häiriöt ja niiden yhteydet kehityksen muihin osatekijöihin.* Unpublished master's thesis, University of Helsinki, Department of Phonetics.

Räisänen, A. (1975). Havaintoja lastenkielestä. *Virittäjä, 79,* 251–266.

Remes, K., and Ojanen, A-K. (1996). *Artikulaatiotesti. Äänteenmukainen sanakuvatesti.* Helsinki: Early Learning Oy.

Richardson, U. (1998). *Familial dyslexia and sound duration in the quantity distinctions of Finnish infants and adults.* Unpublished doctoral dissertation, Jyväskylä: Studia Philologica Jyväskyläensia, University of Jyväskylä.

Saaristo-Helin, K., Savinainen-Makkonen, T., and Kunnari, S. (2006). The phonological mean length of utterance: Methodological challenges from a crosslinguistic perspective. *Journal of Child Language, 33,* 179–190.

Savinainen-Makkonen, T. (2000a). Word-initial consonant omissions – a developmental process in children learning Finnish. *First Language, 20,* 161–185.

Savinainen-Makkonen, T. (2000b). Learning long words – a typological perspective. *Language and Speech, 42,* 205–225.

Savinainen-Makkonen, T. (2000c). Learning to produce three-syllable words: A longitudinal study of Finnish twins. In M. Perkins and S. Howard (Eds.), *New directions in language development and disorders* (pp. 223–231). New York: Plenum.

Savinainen-Makkonen, T. (2001). *Suomalainen lapsi fonologiaa omaksumassa.* Unpublished doctoral dissertation. Publications of the Department of Phonetics 42, University of Helsinki.

Savinainen-Makkonen, T. (2006). The early stages of the acquisition of heterosyllabic two-consonant clusters in Finnish. Manuscript submitted for publication.

Savinainen-Makkonen, T., and Kunnari, S. (2004). Artikulaatiovirheet ja viiden kuntoutus. In S. Kunnari and T. Savinainen-Makkonen (Eds.), *Mistä on pienten sanat tehty?* (pp. 155–169). Helsinki: WSOY.

Silvén, M., Niemi, P., and Voeten, M. (2002). Do maternal interaction and early language predict phonological awareness in 3- to 4-year-olds? *Cognitive Development, 17,* 1133–1155.

Silvén, M., Poskiparta, E., and Niemi, P. (2004). The odds of becoming a precocious reader of Finnish. *Journal of Educational Psychology, 96,* 152–164.

Silvén, M., Poskiparta, E., Niemi, P., and Voeten, M. (2005). Language specific precursors of word reading: continuity and change from infancy to first grade in Finnish children. Manuscript submitted for publication.

Statistics Finland. (2004). *Väestörakenne.* Retrieved June 2005 from http://tilastokeskus.fi/til/

Sulkala, H., and Karjalainen, M. (1992). *Finnish.* London: Routledge.

Suomi, K. (1983). Palatal vowel harmony: A perceptually motivated phenomenon? *Nordic Journal of Linguistics, 6,* 1–35.

Suomi, K., Toivanen, J., and Ylitalo, R. (2003). Durational and tonal correlates of accent in Finnish. *Journal of Phonetics, 31,* 113–138.

Suomi, K., Toivanen, J., and Ylitalo, R. (2006). *Fonetiikan ja ääneopin perusteet.* Helsinki: Gaudeamus.

Toivainen, J. (1997). The acquisition of Finnish. In D. I. Slobin (Ed.), *The crosslinguistic study of language acquisition* (Vol. 4., pp. 87–182). Mahwah, NJ: Lawrence Erlbaum.

Torvelainen, P. (2005). *2;0-vuotiaiden lasten fonologisen kehityksen variaatio. Puheen ymmärrettävyyden, sananmuotojen tavoittelun ja tuottamisen sekä sananmuotojen yksikonsonanttisuuden ja -vokaalisuuden tarkastelu.* Unpublished licentiate thesis, University of Jyväskylä, Department of Languages.

Turunen, P. (2003). *Production of word structure: A constraint-based study of 2;6 year old Finnish children at-risk for dyslexia and their controls.* Doctoral dissertation. Jyväskylä Studies in Languages 52. University of Jyväskylä.

Vainio, L. (1993). *Artikulaation arviointitehtäviä.* Helsinki: Early Learning.

Vihman, M. M., and Velleman, S. L. (2000). The construction of a first phonology. *Phonetica, 57,* 255–266.

Warren, S. (2001). *Phonological acquisition and ambient language: A corpus based cross-linguistic exploration.* Unpublished doctoral dissertation. University of Hertfordshire, UK.

SUMMARY OF STUDIES OF TYPICAL FINNISH SPEECH ACQUISITION

Authors	Year	Country	No. of children	Age of children	Information	Sample type	Data collection
Aoyama	2001*	Finland	26	3;0–5;0	Quantity distinction	Single word	Cross-sectional
Iivonen	1986, 1994, 1996b, 2004	Finland	2	0;7–5;7	Variety	Connected speech	Longitudinal
Iivonen	1998b	Finland	3	1;6–3;2	Consonant clusters	Connected speech	Longitudinal
Itkonen	1977	Finland	1	1;6–4;0	Variety	Connected speech	Longitudinal
Kunnari	2000	Finland	10	0;8–1;11	Variety	Connected speech	Longitudinal
Kunnari	2002	Finland	10	0;11–1;11	Word length	Connected speech	Longitudinal
Kunnari	2003a,b	Finland	10	0;11–1;11	Consonant inventory	Connected speech	Longitudinal
Kunnari et al.	2001 *	Finland	5	0;11–1;7	Quantity distinction	Connected speech	Longitudinal
Kunnari et al.	2006	Finland	24	2;0	Consonants and vowels	Connected speech	Cross-sectional
Laalo	1994	Finland	1	0;7–1;9	Long words	Connected speech	Longitudinal
Leiwo et al.	2006	Finland	200	2;6	Vowel harmony	Single word	Cross-sectional
Lieko	2001	Finland	8 & 14	1;3–3;11 and 3;0–7;0	Vowel harmony	Connected speech & Single word	Compilation
Luotonen	1998	Finland	1618	5;0–9;0	Variety	Questionnaire	Cross-sectional
Pietarinen	1987	Finland	1600	5;0	Variety	Connected speech	Cross-sectional
Richardson	1998	Finland	89	0;6–1;6	Quantity distinction	Single word	Longitudinal
Räisänen	1975	Finland	2	1;0–7;4	Variety	Connected speech	Longitudinal

Authors	Year	Country	No. of children	Age of children	Information	Sample type	Data collection
Saaristo-Helin et al.	2006	Finland	17	1;8	Phonological Mean Length of Utterance	Connected speech	Cross-sectional
Savinainen-Makkonen	2000a	Finland	6	1;3–2;5	Word-initial consonant omissions	Connected speech	Longitudinal
Savinainen-Makkonen	2000b	Finland	6	1;3–2;8	Long words	Connected speech	Longitudinal
Savinainen-Makkonen	2000c	Finland	2	1;3–1;8	Long words	Connected speech	Longitudinal
Savinainen-Makkonen	2001	Finland	7	1;2–2;8	Variety	Connected speech	Longitudinal
Savinainen-Makkonen	2003	Finland	1	1;1–1;6	Geminate template	Connected speech	Longitudinal
Savinainen-Makkonen	2006	Finland	12	1;6–2;6	Consonant clusters	Connected speech	Longitudinal
Toivainen	1997	Finland	4	0;8–5;0	Consonants	Connected speech	Longitudinal
Torvelainen	2005	Finland	40	2;0	Variety	Connected speech	Cross-sectional
Turunen	2003	Finland	196	2;6	Variety	Single word	Cross-sectional
Vihman & Velleman	2000*	Finland	5	0;11–1;10	Variety	Connected speech	Longitudinal
Warren	2001*	Finland	15	2;0–5;0	Variety	Connected speech	Cross-sectional

* Cross-linguistic study

Acknowledgement

The preparation of the manuscript was supported by grants from the Academy of Finland and the Emil Aaltonen Foundation. The writers would like to thank Professor Kari Suomi for his helpful comments on an earlier version of this manuscript.

Chapter 40

French Speech Acquisition

Yvan Rose and Sophie Wauquier-Gravelines

INTRODUCTION

French is a member of the Romance language family, which itself is part of the larger Indo-European family. While numbers vary between sources, it is estimated that French is spoken by approximately 87 million people as a mother tongue and by over 190 million people if we include those who speak it as a second language in daily activities. French is an official language in over 30 countries, and an official language of several international organizations including the European Union, the United Nations, and the International Olympic Committee. There are several regional varieties of French spoken in various countries worldwide, which include the varieties spoken in, for example, France, Belgium, Canada, and several African countries (see the accompanying map). Several distinctive dialects of French are also found in a number of these countries. In addition, French provided a basis for the formation of several Creole languages (e.g., Haitian, Mauritanian, Réunionese, and Seychellois creoles). An international project of description and analysis of French phonology, *Phonologie du Français contemporain,* is currently being developed by Durand (ERSS, Toulouse), Lyche (Oslo University), and Laks (Modyco, Paris X) (Durand and Lyche, 2003, see the Resources section below). Many of the French dialects in France and worldwide (e.g., Canadian and Québec French) are under study. This chapter describes the most prominent characteristics of French phonology, with a special emphasis on the dialects spoken in France and Canada. In the next sections, we provide more information on each of these two dialects.

Where French is spoken

Where France French is spoken

France French, as its name indicates, is spoken primarily in France as well as in its overseas territories (see accompanying map and Appendix D), which include the *Départements d'outre-mer* (DOM; Guyane Française, Guadeloupe, Martinique, Réunion), the *Territoires d'outre mer* (TOM; e.g., Polynésie Française, Nouvelle Calédonie, Wallis et Futuna) and the *Collectivités territoriales* (Saint Pierre et Miquelon, Mayotte). It must be noted that each of these territories, despite having linguistic policies aligned with those of France, all have their own linguistic characteristics, which can be reflected either in pronunciations or in lexical items.

The dialect of French that is generally considered to represent the international norm for the language originates from the center of France, in the area around Paris, the country's capital. It shares its most prominent properties with the French dialects spoken in other areas of Northern France. Most of the normative material used in, for example, reference books and manuals of second language instruction, is aligned with this variety of French.

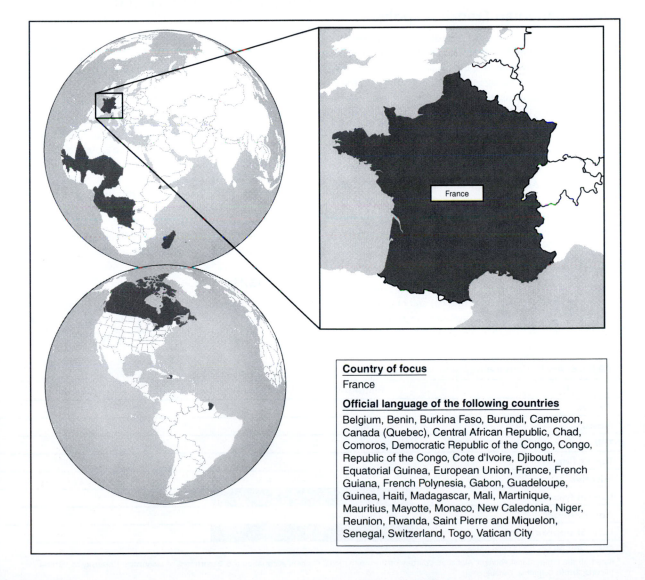

Country of focus

France

Official language of the following countries

Belgium, Benin, Burkina Faso, Burundi, Cameroon, Canada (Quebec), Central African Republic, Chad, Comoros, Democratic Republic of the Congo, Congo, Republic of the Congo, Cote d'Ivoire, Djibouti, Equatorial Guinea, European Union, France, French Guiana, French Polynesia, Gabon, Guadeloupe, Guinea, Haiti, Madagascar, Mali, Martinique, Mauritius, Mayotte, Monaco, New Caledonia, Niger, Reunion, Rwanda, Saint Pierre and Miquelon, Senegal, Switzerland, Togo, Vatican City

It is also noteworthy that within France there are several regional varieties. Some of this variation will be discussed below. In addition, the French spoken in European neighboring countries such as Belgium and Switzerland have their distinctive traits as well. For example, Belgian French is missing the high front rounded glide [ɥ] from its inventory (the bilabial glide [w] is used in places where we find [ɥ] in standard French). References to broad dialects such as European or Continental French must thus be considered as relatively vague. As such, these broad descriptions may or may not be accurate, depending on the situation, and should be used with circumspection.

Where Canadian French is spoken

French is also one of the two official languages of Canada (see accompanying map and Appendix D). Canadian French, which is spoken either as a dominant or as a minority language across the country's provinces and northern territories, must be broken down into several dialects. Among these dialects are Acadian French, spoken primarily in the Atlantic provinces of Canada (New Brunswick, which has the largest population of Acadian French speakers, Nova Scotia, Prince Edward Island, and, to a lesser extent, Newfoundland and Labrador). Acadian French is also spoken in two separate rural areas of Québec (the southern part of the Gaspésie Peninsula and the lower north shore of the St. Lawrence River). Another important dialect of Canadian French is spoken in several areas of Ontario, especially in the more northern cities and communities of the province, as well as the regions bordering the province of Québec. West of Ontario are speakers of Manitoban and Métis French (spoken primarily in Manitoba) and of other, more isolated, French-speaking communities spanning from Manitoba through British Columbia and extending into the Canadian northern territories. Several of these communities also host French speakers hailing from Québec.

Despite this rich diversity of dialects of Canadian French, all of which have distinctive lexical, phonological, and syntactic traits, the portions of this chapter devoted to Canadian French will focus on the dialect spoken by most of the French-speaking Canadians, Québec French. This focus is primarily motivated by the fact that most of the information available on Canadian French comes from the Québec dialect.

Components of France and Québec French

In this section, the phonological systems of France and Québec French are described in parallel, in order to highlight their main similarities and differences. Note that, as we alluded to above, the "France" French denomination stands here for the dialects spoken for the most part in the northern part of the country (especially in and around the Parisian area). This dialect is in fact more closely related to the Québec dialect than the regional varieties of France French spoken in the more southern parts of France. Some differences between the Québec and northern France dialects relative to southern dialects of France French will be highlighted below for clarification purposes. Whenever these dialects share similarities, we will generally refer to them as French without further specification.

Consonants

French has, in its native phonetic inventory, 21 consonants, including three glides (see Table 40-1). However, the France and Québec dialects differ at the level of their

TABLE 40-1   Consonants produced in Filipino

	Bilabial	Labiodental	Dental	Alveolar
Plosive	p b			t d
Nasal	m			n
Trill				
Tap or flap				
Fricative		f v		s z
Lateral fricative				
Approximant	w (labiovelar)			
Lateral approximant				l

Black = articulations judged impossible

Based on the International Phonetic Alphabet. Courtesy of the International Phonetic Association (c/o Department of Linguistics, University of Victoria, Victoria, British Columbia, Canada).

phonotactics, as will be seen below. Note that we include the velar nasal [ŋ] in this inventory. While this consonant is typically not considered to be a native sound in the language, it is used in several English loanwords (e.g., 'camping', 'marketing') that have been well integrated and are commonly used in everyday speech in both dialects. Finally, the phonetic realization of the rhotic consonant varies considerably across dialects of French. While the voiced uvular trill [ʀ] constitutes the norm in Parisian French, the voiced uvular fricative [ʁ] is most commonly found in Québec French; other variants such as the tap [r] and the flap [ɾ] are also attested in various dialects spoken in both France and Québec.

Vowels and diphthongs

While France and Québec French share their consonantal inventories, their vocalic inventories differ significantly, the Québec variety being more conservative from a historical standpoint. Among other details (noted in subsequent sections), the Québec dialect contains four nasal vowels (instead of three in most dialects of France French), and has maintained a phonemic length contrast between some vowels. This is reflected in Table 40-2 through the presence of the low back unrounded vowel [ɑ], a vowel that is generally not found in France French but that represents the contrastive, long counterpart of the low central vowel [a] in Québec French (e.g., *pâte* [pɑt] 'pasta' / *patte* [pat] 'leg'). Other differences lie in the tense/lax allophonic distribution among high vowels that is pervasive in Québec French but absent from the France dialect (see more on this and other phonotactics below). Since the France French vowel inventory represents a subset of the more conservative Québec French inventory, we indicate the Québec French-specific vowels in the table and provide their France French equivalents. Note, finally, that mainly because of the rich regional variation that exists within France, discrepancies exist between

descriptions of the French vowel inventory (e.g., with regard to the distinction between [a] and [ɑ]). We refer the interested reader to works by Walter (1977, 1982), Casagrande (1984), Walker (2001), Coveney (2001), and Durand and Lyche (2004).

French has between three and four nasal vowels /ɛ̃, (œ̃), ɔ̃, ɑ̃/. In most dialects of France French, the opposition between /ɛ̃/ ~ /œ̃/ has been neutralized to /ɛ̃/. Québec French, however, still displays the four vowels, at least in its most prominent dialects. In the southern dialects of France French, a nasal consonantal appendix is often produced after nasal vowels. This nasal resonance is in fact the historical residue of the post-vocalic nasal consonants that triggered a regressive assimilation of the preceding vowel. It is this nasal–assimilated vowel that became a full nasal vowel in later versions of northern dialects of the language. In the southern dialects it is variably nasalized and it could be an oral vowel. For example, the phrase *un grand tapis* [ɛ̃gʀɑ̃tapi] 'a large rug' in the northern and Québec dialects would be produced in southern French as [ɛ̃gʀɑ̃ntapi] and even [ɛ̃gʀɑntapi]. In phrase-final positions, by default, without any assimilation context, this nasal is realized as a velar consonant *bon* [bɔ̃ŋ] 'good' in the southern dialects and [bɔ̃] in the northern and Québec ones.

Phonotactic restrictions in French

In this section, we discuss the most important phonotactic restrictions observed in French and compare, whenever appropriate, the restrictions that are specific to each of the two main dialects under consideration in this chapter.

Depending on a series of phonological contexts, a vowel corresponding to the grapheme <e> in written French may or may not be realized in spoken forms.

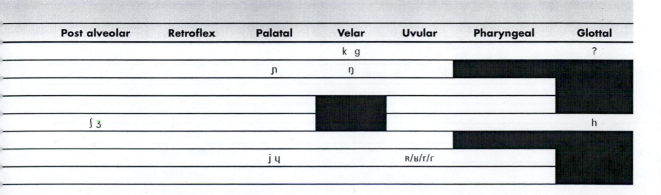

	Post alveolar	Retroflex	Palatal	Velar	Uvular	Pharyngeal	Glottal
				k g			ʔ
			ɲ	ŋ			
	ʃ ʒ						h
			j ɥ		ʀ/ʁ/r/ɾ		

TABLE 40-2   Vowels produced in French compared with General American English

American English location	American English Vowels Smit (2004)	American English examples	French vowels	French examples
High-front	i	_beat_	i	_Riz, si, silence_
	ɪ	b_i_t	ɪ (Québec; [i] in France)	_Rite, site, cil_
High-front rounded	–	–	y	_Mue, but, su, vue_
	–	–	ʏ (Québec; [y] in France)	_Flûte, lutte, futé_
Mid-low front	a	_raid_	a	_Ré, blé, Fée_
	ɛ	b_e_d	ɛ	_Raie, sais, met, têtu_
Mid-low front rounded	–	–	ø	_Peu, lieu, mieux, heureux_
	–	–	œ	_Meule, gueule, seule_
Low-front	æ	b_a_d	–	
Low-central	–	–	a	_Ma, sa, place,_
High-back, rounded	u	_blue_	u	_Roue, sous, poux, cou_
	ʊ	b_oo_k	ʊ (Québec; [u] in France)	_Toute, soupe, coûte_
Mid-back, rounded	o	_boat_	o	_Beau, seau, clos, faux, mot, côte_
	ɔ	f_or_m	ɔ	_Botte, cote, loque_
Low back	ɑ	_drop_	ɑ (Québec; [a] in France)	_Pâte, mâle, châle_
[r]-colored	ɝ		–	
	ɚ	_never, color_	–	
	ɪr		–	
	ɛr		–	
	ʊr		–	
	ør		–	
	ar		–	
Central	ə	_about, occur, upon,_	ə	_Petit, le, faisait, meuble_
	ʌ		–	
Diphthongs	aɪ	_my, bike_	–	
	aʊ	_out, mouse_	–	
	ɪ	b_oy_	–	
Nasal	–		ɑ̃	_Paon, rang, ment_
	–		ɛ̃	_Pain, gain, faim_
	–		ɔ̃	_Bon, taon, rond_
	–		œ̃ (Québec; [ɛ̃] in France)	_Un, aucun_

Depending on the speakers, this lax vowel may be realized anywhere in the articulatory continuum that exists between [œ] and [ə]. The (non-)realization of this schwa depends on segmental and prosodic factors, which together form what is traditionally called the *Règle des trois consonnes* (Delattre, 1966), a general phonotactic against the grouping of three consonants in the speech stream through schwa deletion (Dell, 1978; Tranel, 1987). For example, a phrase such as *je te le donne* /ʒətələdɔn/ 'I give it to you' can be reduced to [ʒətəldɔn] or [ʒtəldɔn] or [ʒətlədɔn] but not to *[ʒtlədɔn][1]; the latter, unattested form contains an illicit sequence of three consonants. In the southern dialects of France French, we typically find much fewer instances of schwa reduction than in the northern or Québec dialects (Durand, Slater, and Wise, 1987; Durand and Eychenne, 2004). Two other factors play a role in schwa deletion: speech rate and speech register (Tranel, 2003). The same distinction exists in word-final position. The northern France and Québec dialects tend to display a general undershooting or deletion of final schwas; as opposed to this, final schwas are typically realized phonetically in the southern dialects of France French.

French also displays a series of segmental alternations at the edge of words in connected speech. The first such phenomenon is that of liaison. This phonotactic is triggered in contexts where a hiatus would be formed at the boundary between two words. Liaison consists of the appearance of a latent consonant between the two words, which gets realized as the onset of the second word. For example, the phrase *un enfant* /ɛ̃ + ɑ̃.fɑ̃/[2] is realized as [ɛ̃.nɑ̃.fɑ̃] 'a child'; similarly, *un petit ami* [ɛ̃ pə.ti a.mi] 'the small friend' is realized as [ɛ̃.pə.ti.ta.mi] (Delattre, 1947; Encrevé, 1988; Tranel, 1995). Liaison is however not found in all contexts where a hiatus could appear between words. Its realization is also variable and subject to various sociolinguistic factors (e.g., speech style and register; Encrevé, 1988; Encrevé and Scheer, 2005). It is also subject to lexical and syntactic restrictions. For example, while liaison is obligatory between clitics and nouns or verbs and obligatory with a preposition, it is either optional (e.g., *des soldats anglais* [dasɔldazɑ̃glɛ] / [dasɔldaɑ̃glɛ] 'English soldiers' or clearly ungrammatical between certain words (e.g., *un soldat anglais* [ɛ̃sɔldaɑ̃glɛ] / *[ɛ̃sɔldataɑ̃glɛ]) and in specific syntactic contexts (e.g., at phrase boundaries, which are governed by prosodic considerations that we briefly explain below).

Another phonotactic phenomenon that occurs at the edge of words is that of enchaînement. In contrast to liaison, enchaînement is well attested in languages other than French. It consists of the realization of a word-final consonant into the onset of the initial syllable of the following word. For example, in dialects where word-final schwa deletion is observed (e.g., northern France, Québec), the phrase *une petite orange* /yn pətit ɔRɑ̃ʒ/ 'a small orange' is syllabified with the word-final consonant of *petite* in the onset of *orange* [yn.pə.ti.to.Rɑ̃ʒ]. Note that as opposed to liaison, enchaînement does not trigger the appearance of a latent consonant; it affects the syllabication of lexical word-final consonants that are systematically produced, no matter the syntactic or phonological context (e.g., Encrevé, 1988, Encrevé and Scheer, 2005).

Another phenomenon taking place at word boundaries is that of elision, a process that consists of the deletion of the vowels of clitics when these clitics appear in front of vowel-initial words. For example, the phrase *le+éléphant* /lə alafɑ̃/ 'the elephant' is realized as *l'éléphant* [lalafɑ̃], not as *[ləalafɑ̃]. Similarly, *il+la+observe* /il la ɔbsɛRV/ 'he observes her' is realized as *il l'observe* [illɔbsɛRV], instead of as *[illaɔbsɛRV].

Interestingly, some words apparently beginning with a vowel do not behave in a regular way: they block the processes of liaison and enchaînement (Delattre, 1966, Cornulier and Dell, 1978; Encrevé, 1988; Pagliano, 2003; Encrevé and Scheer, 2005). For example, words such as *hibou* /ibu/ 'owl' and *onzième* /ɔ̃zjɛm/ 'eleventh' accept neither liaison nor enchaînement (e.g., *le+hibou* [lə.ʔibu], but not *[li.bu] 'the owl'; *les+hiboux* [la.ʔibu], but not *[lazibu] 'the owls'). These words are pronounced with a word-initial glottal stop that has, most of the time, an orthographic correspondence. But, while most of these words are spelled with an initial *h* letter, traditionally called "h-aspiré," some of them do not have initial consonants in written forms (like *onze* 'eleven' or *onzième* 'eleventh'). Also, some h-initial words behave like vowel-initial words in that they allow for both liaison and enchaînement (e.g., *le+hippotame* /lə ipɔpɔtam/ is pronounced [lipɔpɔtam] 'the hippopotamus (sing.)' and *les+hippotames* /la ipɔpɔtam/ is pronounced [lazipɔpɔtam] 'the hippopotamus (pl.)'. This ambiguity is probably one of the reasons why we observe some variation between speakers in the realization of certain words such as *haricot* 'bean', which can display both elision and enchaînement in some speakers and neither of these processes in other speakers.

Moving on to another set of restrictions that affect virtually all varieties of French (including Québec French),

---

1 The asterisk indicates a form that is unattested/impossible.
2 The periods in transcribed forms represent syllable boundaries.

we first discuss the general *Loi de position*, a phonotactic that favors the appearance of tense vowels in open syllables and lax vowels in closed syllables. We can see manifestations of this rule in morphologically related forms such as *céder* [sede] / *cède* [sɛd] 'to give in / gives in'; *lépreux* [laprø] / *lèpre* [lɛpʀ] 'leprous / leprosy'; *léger* [laʒa] / *légère* [laʒɛʀ] 'light (adj. masc.) / light (adj. fem.)'; *fermier* [fɛʀmja] / *fermière* [fɛʀmjɛʀ] 'farmer (masc.) / farmer (fem.)'. In all of these forms, we find the tense vowel [e] in open syllables (first forms) and its lax counterpart [ɛ] in closed syllables (second forms). Similarly, the forms *galop* [galo] / *galope* [gal p] 'gallop (noun) / gallops', and *idiot* [idjo] / *idiote* [idjɔt] 'idiot (masc.) / idiot (fem.)' display an [o]/[ɔ] alternation in open/closed syllables, and the same holds between [ø] and [œ] in front rounded mid vowels (e.g., *peut* [pø] / *peuvent* [pœv] '(he) can / (they) can'; *veut* [vø] / [vœl] *veulent* '(he) wants / (they) want'. As we can see from several of these examples, the [o]/[ɔ] and [ø]/[œ] distinctions are not clearly represented in written forms.

The *Loi de position* is however not found across every French dialect. Its realization depends on factors such as the geographical origins of the speakers (Durand and Lyche, 2004). For example, in the dialects spoken in southern France, the rule applies in a categorical fashion; phonologically mid vowels are realized in closed syllables as mid lax vowels (/e/ ⇨ [ɛ]; /ø/ ⇨ [œ]; /o/ ⇨ [ɔ]). In other dialects (e.g., in the northern dialects of France French and in Québec French), the rule is also governed by stress. For example, in accented open syllables, the distinction between /œ/ and /ø/ is neutralized; only the tense vowel /ø/ can appear in this position. However, in closed accented syllables, both tense and lax front rounded vowels can be found. The /œ/ ~ /ø/ contrast is however maintained in a handful of minimal pairs only (e.g., *jeune* [ʒœn] / *jeûne* [ʒøn] 'young / period of fasting'; *veulent* [vœl] / *veule* [vøl] '(they) want / weak' (Tranel, 1987). The realization of the /œ/ ~ /ø/ contrast is also governed by segmental factors. For example, in a syllable closed by the consonant /ʀ/, only lax /œ/ is attested (e.g., *peur* [pœʀ] 'fear'), while tense /ø/ appears in a syllable closed by the consonant /z/ (e.g., *heureuse* [øʀøʒ] 'happy (fem.)'). Finally, when fluctuation is observed in the realization of this vocalic contrast, we observe a tendency in favor of the lax counterpart. Closed syllables containing /œ/ are much more frequent and the words containing /ø/ in closed syllables typically have lower lexical frequency.

The same patterning generally affects the /ɔ/ ~ /o/ contrast, whose realization is also influenced by factors such as stress and surrounding segmental. However, the number of minimal pairs opposing these vowels in closed accented syllables is much higher (e.g., *hotte* [ɔt] / *haute* [ot] 'chimney hood / high'; *cotte* [kɔt] / *côte* [kot] 'tunic coat / hill'; *pomme* [pɔm] / *paume* [pom] 'apple / palm (of the hand)'; *sol* [sɔl] / *saule* [sol] 'ground / willow'). Note here that the distinction is also generally represented in written forms.

The distribution of /e, ɛ/ is however substantially different. First, in open accented syllables, we observe a contrast between these two vowels (*thé* [te] / *taie* [tɛ] 'tea / pillowcase'; *été* [ete] / *était* [etɛ] 'summer / (he) was'). This distinction is also generally represented in written forms (Wioland, 1991). Note here that while this distinction in open accented syllables is generally maintained in Québec French, it has been disappearing from several dialects of France French. In closed accented syllables, however, we systematically find the lax vowel [ɛ] only (e.g., *mère* [mɛʀ] 'mother', *père* [pɛʀ] 'father', *miel* [mjɛl] 'honey', *sel* [sɛl] 'salt', *épaisse* [epɛs] 'thick'. This holds true of Québec French as well (see below, however, for additional details on this dialect).

Finally, additional factors may play a role in the distributions discussed above. For example, faithfulness to morphological roots may prevent the *Loi de position* from applying in morphologically complex words. For example, in the morphologically related words *cœur* [kœʀ] / *écoeuré* [akœʀa] 'heart / disgusted', one would predict an [œ] / [ø] alternation. The vowel [œ] of the underived form *coeur* is however typically realized in *écoeuré*. Another factor that also intervenes in the realization of these phonotactics is a process of vowel harmony affecting the tense / lax phonological distinctions. For example, in the word pairs *bête* [bɛt] / *bêtise* [betiz] 'stupid / stupidity' and *aimer* [eme] / *aimable* [ɛmabl] '(to) love / lovable', the penultimate vowels in the derived forms often trigger a harmony process whereby a final vowel assimilates the preceding one for tenseness (e.g., *bêtise* [betiz]) or laxness (e.g., *aimable* [ɛmabl]).

Additional differences between France and Québec French

In addition to the details noted in the preceding section, France and Québec French primarily differ in assimilatory behaviors, in the surface realization of certain vowels, and in the shape of word-final clusters. These differences will be discussed in turn.

The *Loi de position* also manifests itself in a peculiar fashion in Québec French high vowels. In addition to the details noted above, high vowels undergo laxing (but no lowering to mid vowels) in surface closed syllables and in word-final position when followed by a single consonant, except if this consonant is one of the four "lengthening" consonants ([v], [z], [ʒ], and [ʀ]); these consonants prevent the occurrence of laxing and instead trigger phonetic lengthening of the vowels. For example, while /i/ is tense in *paniquer* [panike] '(to) panic', it is realized as lax in *panique* [panɪk] 'panic'. However, /i/ remains tense in a word such as *cire* [siʀ] 'wax', where it is followed by a lengthening consonant. This process of vowel laxing is not found in the varieties of France French usually described in the literature (e.g., Casagrande, 1984).

In Québec French, the coronal stops ([t, d]) are affricated (realized as [t͡s, d͡z]) before high front vowels and glides ([i, ɪ, y, ʏ, j, ɥ]; e.g., *petit* /pəti/ ⇨ [pət͡si] 'small'). This allophonic variation does not occur in the France dialects usually described in the literature (e.g., Casagrande, 1984) nor in the general reference works on French (e.g., *Petit Robert* dictionaries).

As described in detail (e.g., Charette, 1991; Dumas, 1981), Québec French vowels tend to be lengthened and, often, diphthongized when they appear in an open syllable, but never when they are followed by a tautosyllabic consonant. (Final consonants can be analyzed as extrasyllabic; see, for example, Charette, 1991, for details.) For example, vowel lengthening / diphthongization is possible in words like *rêve* [ʀɛv]/ [ʀajv] '(a) dream' and *rêver* [ʀɛva] / [ʀajva] '(to) dream', but not in words like *perdu* [pɛʀd͡zy] (* [pɛʀd͡zy] / *[pajʀd͡zy]) 'lost' or *perdre* [pɛʀd] (*[pɛʀd] / *[pajʀd]) '(to) lose'. Notice from this last example that word-final obstruent-liquid clusters tend to be reduced to obstruents in Québec French ([pɛʀd], *[pɛʀdʀ]). The word-final [ʀ] deletion found in this context contrasts with France French, in which these clusters are typically fully realized ([pɛʀdʀ]), especially in the more southern dialects.

Related to the above, and as noted in a preceding section, in southern dialects of France French, word-final consonants as well as falling and rising sonority clusters are regularly followed by schwa (e.g., *raquette* [ʀakɛtə] 'racket'; *ferme* [fɛʀmə] 'farm'; *perdre* [pɛʀdʀə] '(to) lose'). Final schwa is generally not found in Québec French, apart from exceptionally emphatic contexts, for example when each syllable of a word is pronounced in isolation, or when the pronunciation of word-final schwa enables a smoother transition into the next word (e.g., *garde-fou* [gaʀdəfu] 'roadside rail'). This latter context can be related to the *Règle des trois consonnes* discussed above.

Syllables.

While the minimal syllable (and word) in French can contain a single, short vowel only (e.g., *eau* [o] 'water'),

French displays a relatively complex syllable surface structure, namely $C_{(0-3)}VC_{(0-3)}$. It can have as many as three consonants in prevocalic position. These clusters can consist of /s/ followed by an obstruent and a liquid (e.g., *splendide* [splãdid] 'splendid') or of an obstruent-liquid-glide sequence (e.g., *pluie* [plɥi] 'rain'). However, hypothetical sequences consisting of four consonants (s+obstruent+liquid+glide) are not attested in word-initial positions. Such sequences can nonetheless be found word-medially, in words such as *construire* [kõstʀɥiʀ] 'to construct'. However, in such cases, the /s/ is arguably syllabified at the end of the first syllable such that the tautosyllabic cluster contains no more than three consonants. The nucleus (peak) of the syllable consists of single vowels (e.g., *clé* [kla]), rising diphthongs (i.e. glide-vowel sequences; e.g., *puits* [pɥi] '(water) well') and vowel+glide sequences (e.g., *paille* [pɑj] 'straw'). Note that this vowel+glide sequence can be realized as a falling diphthong in Québec French but never in France French, in which [j] always behaves as a consonant (Klein, 1991).

This is due to the diphthongization processes discussed above. Finally, in post-vocalic positions, French allows for up to three consonants (e.g., *arbre* [aʀbʀ] 'tree'). However, as noted above, the final consonant of such clusters is generally not pronounced in everyday speech.

Consonants and consonant clusters

In addition to the facts described in the preceding sections, Québec French also displays a devoicing process affecting approximants in tautosyllabic clusters (e.g., *trop* /tʀo/ ⇨ [tχo] 'too much') as well as a voicing agreement relation in obstruent clusters (e.g., *subconscient* /sybkõsjɑ̃/ ⇨ [sypkõsjɑ̃] 'subconscious'). These assimilatory processes are also attested in several languages, including English (e.g., Harris, 1994).

Tones

France French and Québec French do not use tones to differentiate meaning.

Stress and intonation

French differs from languages such as English that display contrastive stress at the lexical level. Instead, the realization of stress in French is related to the syntactic structure of the utterance (Dell, 1984; Di Cristo, 1999); only vowels that are realized in the last syllable of a phrase receive stress. Note that this is not the case for word-final schwa, a vowel that generally cannot receive stress, unless it is the only vowel in a monosyllabic, phrase-final word. Because of this, stress is located on the penultimate vowel of schwa-final words in the dialects where word-final schwas are pronounced (e.g., southern France French, as noted above).

Intonation is primarily used to convey syntactic information such as the distinction between a declarative and an interrogative sentence. Declarative sentences are characterized by final lowered intonation, while interrogative sentences display a final rising intonation. Other uses of intonation relate to pragmatic purposes or emphasis on part or all of an utterance. For more details concerning prosody and intonation of French, we refer the interested reader to Delais (1994); Di Cristo (1998); Hirst, Di Cristo, and Espesser (2000); Lacheret-Dujour and Beaugendre (2002); and Bessade et al. (2004).

Writing system

The writing system used across all French dialects is the Roman alphabet. Vowels with accents (e.g., "é", "è", "ê") represent different phonetic vowels. Some distinctions that these accents historically represented, which have generally disappeared from contemporary France French, are maintained in Québec French. For example, the difference between "è" and "ê", which historically accounted for the difference between a short and a long /ɛ/, is maintained in Québec French, in which the long /ɛ/ is generally diphthongized, as mentioned above.

Table 40-3 below provides a (nonexhaustive) list of the most frequent sound-to-grapheme associations for consonants. It is followed by Table 40-4, which contains

TABLE 40-3 Sound-grapheme associations for consonants

Consonant	Monographs	Digraphs	Examples
[p]	<p, pp>		*papa, appeler*
[b]	<b, bb>		*bébé, sabbat*
[t]	<t, tt>		*table, attendre*
[d]	<d, dd>		*dire, addition*
[k]	<k>, <c + a, o, u>, <c + L>	<ck>, <ch>, <qu>, <cqu>	*kilo, carotte, côté, cube, clé, craie, rock; orchestre, que, acquisition*
[g]	<g + a, o, u>, <g + L>, <gg>		*gare, golf, figure, glace, aggraver*
[f]	<f, ff>	<ph>	*fête, effort, éléphant*
[v]	<v>		*vie*
[s]	#<s>, <ss>, <ç>, <c + e, i, y>	<sc + e, i>	*sur, tasse, garçon, ciel, cent, cycle, science, scène*
[z]	<VsV>, <z>		*musique, zèbre*
[ʃ]		<ch>, <sh>, <sch>	*chaise, flash, schéma*
[ʒ]	<j>, <g + e, i, y>		*jambon, général, gilet, gym*
[l]	<l, ll>		*lit, belle*
[ʀ]	<r, rr>		*rue, arriver*
[m]	<m, mm>		*manger, homme*
[n]	<n, nn>		*neige, bonne*
[ɲ]		<gn>	*peigne*
[ŋ]		<ng>	loanwords: *meeting, parking*

TABLE 40-4 Sound-grapheme associations for vowels

Vowel	Monographs	Digraphs	Examples
[i]	<i, î, ï, y>		*lit, île, maïs, style*
[a]	<é>	<er, ez, es>#	*bébé, manger, nez, les, des, mes, tes, ses, ces*
[ɛ]	<è, ê>	<et>#, <ai> in southern dialects	*père, tête, poulet, faire*
[a]	<a, à>		*ma, voilà*
[y]	<u, û>		*tu, dû*
[ɔ]		<eu, oeu> in open syllable	*bleu, voeux*
[œ]		<eu, oeu> in close syllable	*peur, soeur*
[ə]	<e>		*9 words: je, me, te, se, ce, le, de, ne, que*
[u]		<ou, où, oû>	*roue, où, goût*
[o]	<ô>, <o>	<eau, au>	*côte, dos, beau, fausse*
[ɔ]	<o>		*porte*
[ɑ]	<â>		*gâteau*
[ɛ̃]		<in>#, <ain>#	*fin, pain*
[œ̃]		<un>#	*brun*
[ɑ̃]		<an>#	*roman*
[ɔ̃]		<on>#	*ballon*

similar associations for vowels. As we can see in both of these tables, there is not always a one-to-one correspondence between sounds and letters. In addition, some sounds can be represented in different ways in orthographic forms.

Varieties of Québec French

Apart from some remote regional varieties (spoken in, e.g., Abitibi, Beauce, Saguenay, Lac-St-Jean, or Gaspésie), Québec French is usually divided into two main dialect areas by a vertical isogloss between the city of Montréal and Québec City. For the sake of discussion, we will refer to these dialects as the western dialect and the eastern dialect, respectively. The distinction between the two dialects is noticeable in the realization of both vowels and consonants. Regarding vowel quality, lexical variation is found in words like *poteau* 'post' and *photo* 'photograph', which are pronounced as [poto] and

[foto] in the western dialect but as [pɔto] and [fɔto] in the eastern dialect. This distinction is specific to some lexical items only, as other words such as *émotion* [amɔʃjɔ̃] 'emotion' are pronounced with [ɔ] in both dialects. In addition, the [o/ɔ] contrast between the two dialects is not observed among in the front counterparts of these vowels [a/ɛ].

Another typical distinction between the western and eastern dialects regards diphthongization. As mentioned above, Québec French vowels tend to be lengthened/diphthongized in specific contexts. Diphthongization is more commonly found in the western dialect than in the eastern dialect (e.g., *arrête* 'stop' is pronounced [aʀajt] / [arajt] in the western dialect and usually as [aʀɛt] in the eastern dialect).

Finally, the [r/ʁ] variation observed above with the example of *arrête* 'stop' in the western dialect constitutes the only distinction between the two dialects in the realization of consonants. While the rhotic is consistently realized as uvular ([ʁ]) in the eastern dialect, it is often realized as apical ([r]) in the western dialect. Note, however, that the use of [ʁ] versus [r] is not determined by geographical factors only; it is also conditioned by sociolinguistic factors such as age, gender, and socioeconomic status, the uvular realization generally enjoying a more prestigious status.

Typical acquisition of French

As alluded to above, and quite surprisingly, there do not exist many studies on the acquisition of French. Most of the observations noted in this section are extracted from research work by both authors of this chapter and also by Vihman (2006). The work by Wauquier-Gravelines focuses essentially on northern varieties of France French, while the work by Rose concentrates on Québec French. Despite the differences in phonetic realizations discussed above, these dialects of French share a great many similarities. We have no a priori reason to think that the vast majority of findings in one of these dialects could not occur in others. However, we do not have data to provide from the southern varieties of France French which, given their peculiarities, could display additional phenomena related, for example, to the realization of nasal vowels or the acquisition of schwa-related processes.

Acquired sounds

Because of the lack of availability of a normative baseline, no age-related figures will be provided for the acquisition of specific sounds in French. Instead, a general discussion of the acquisition of the various classes of sounds is provided below.

Consonants

Stop consonants (either obstruent or nasal), no matter their places of articulation, are attested in early word productions. Labials appear to be the easiest consonants for children, while the acquisition of lingual contrasts, that is, the distinction between alveolar and velar stops as well as the distinction between alveolar and alveo-palatal fricatives, poses more difficulties. As it is the case in other languages, fricatives (especially coronal fricatives) are difficult to produce at early ages; they can be produced as stops or deleted altogether (e.g., Bernhardt and Stemberger, 1998). In addition, the phonetic contrast between alveolar [ʃ, ʒ] and their alveopalatal counterparts [s, z] is typically acquired later than any other distinction on the place dimension. Mastery of this contrast can occur as late as 4 to 6 years of age. Note in this regard that the problems related to the acquisition of lingual contrasts can be related to the physiological shape of the

vocal tract of young children (e.g., Crelin, 1987; Inkelas and Rose, 2003).

Liquids also undergo several processes. While the lateral consonant /l/ is often produced as [j] by young children (with some children sometimes producing it as stop [d]), the uvular rhotic /ʀ/ appears as the most difficult consonant for most children. When it does not undergo deletion altogether, this consonant can be produced in several different forms, as a stop, a fricative, or an approximant (Wauquier-Gravelines, 2005b), and at various places of articulation. The place substitutions, however, appear to be systematic and driven by the child's phonological system (Rose, 2000). This observation calls for the need of a global assessment of the phonology of the child's system before conclusions can be drawn on the nature of consonant harmony–related substitutions.

Because of a lack of large-scale studies on the acquisition of French, especially from a longitudinal perspective, it is impossible to provide a normative baseline for the acquisition of the sound system. This gap clearly indicates a need for further studies in this area.

Consonant clusters

Despite the lack of a large-scale empirical database for the development of the French sound system, it is possible to make preliminary observations on the acquisition of consonant clusters, again based on the evidence provided by Rose (2000). The most important finding in this study is that onset clusters appear to develop in a positionally determined way: they were acquired by both children in (final) stressed syllables before being aquired in (nonfinal) unstressed syllables. Note, however, that Kehoe and Hilaire-Debove (2004), in their study of the development of France French, did not find such an effect; it is possible that the discrepancy between the two studies comes from the fact that the methodologies employed were different—the Kehoe and Hilaire-Debove study was based on cross-sectional, rather than longitudinal, data.

Vowels and diphthongs

As it is the case in other languages (e.g., Dutch; see Fikkert, 1994), the vocalic system appears to develop before the consonantal system is acquired, if one bases observations on impressionistic phonetic transcriptions. This also seems to be the case in French, where most vowel contrasts appear to be acquired in early word productions. However, this claim cannot be fully supported because of empirical and methodological issues. First, very few studies on the acquisition of vowels and diphthongs based on acoustic measurements are currently available, for any target languages, and no such study was found for the acquisition of French. Second, conducting such studies is inherently challenging, primarily because of the physiological differences that exist between adult and child vocal tracts, which make the acoustic correlates of children's vocalic productions difficult to compare with those of adults. Consequently, building a reliable model of vocalic development remains a difficult task requiring further investigation.

Percent correct

Due to the lack of empirical evidence for speech development in French learners mentioned above, it would be premature to provide a normative baseline with percentages. This point is further reinforced by observations made by Rose (2000). Indeed, both children in that study displayed very similar developmental patterns, if considered from a phonological perspective only. However, if we consider age only, the children were approximately one year apart, even though they were both developing normally on all counts. This observation alone provides clear evidence that tremendous variation can take place between children acquiring the same language/dialect. It also strongly suggests that normative baselines should be produced from very large sets of data only, and should include standard deviation data, which could provide indications of what should be considered normal variation between language learners.

Phonological processes

Similar to the above, no exhaustive inventory of phonological processes can be made for children acquiring French. The Rose (2000) study provides evidence for processes such as the following: consonant cluster reduction, both pre-vocalically and post-vocalically; word-final vowel epenthesis after target final consonants; syllable truncation, which generally affects nonfinal (unstressed) syllables; syllable reduplication, stressed syllables being prime targets of reduplication; consonant harmony (found to be systematic in one of the two children's productions); gliding of the target lateral approximant /l/; and several sound substitution processes also observed in other languages (see Bernhardt and Stemberger, 1998, for a cross-linguistic survey). While processes such as velar fronting (e.g., Brett, Chiat, and Pilcher, 1987; Inkelas and Rose, 2003; Stoel-Gammon, 1996) and coronal backing (e.g., Morrisette, Dinnsen, and Gierut, 2003) were not observed in the Rose study, these processes are to be expected in Québec French acquisition as well.

The issue of liaison has been recently documented in a series of works by Wauquier-Gravelines (2005a and

for a review of all the data and analyses, 2005b) and Chevrot (2005). Two distinct stages have been identified by Wauquier-Gravelines. First, between the ages of 2 and 4, most children make mistakes with latent consonants. For example, *les éléphants* [lazalafɑ̃] ⇨ *[lanalafɑ̃] 'the elephants' (Marie; 3); *Blanche-Neige et les sept nains* [blɑ̃ʃnaʒalasɛtnɛ̃] ⇨ *[blɑ̃ʃnaʒalasetɛ̃] 'Snow White and the seven dwarfs' (Lélia, 3,5). The errors appear to be systematic in nominal contexts where liaison is obligatory. Children exhibit word segmentation difficulties, which manifest themselves through mistakes in determining whether the liaison consonant belongs to the first or the second word. Their most common mistake consists of associating the liaison consonant with the second word and using this consonant in an inappropriate context. For example, drawing on phrases such as *un éléphant* [ɛ̃nalafɑ̃] 'an elephant', in which the [n] acts as the liaison consonant, they analyze *éléphant* as an [n]-initial word and produce target phrases such as *l'éléphant* [lalafɑ̃] 'the elephant' as *[lənalafɑ̃]. Another, less frequent, error pattern also occurs, according to which they end up analyzing an actual consonant as a liaison consonant, which yields a deletion of this consonant in contexts where liaison is not required. For example, in *Blanche-Neige et les sept nains* [blɑ̃ʃnaʒalasɛtnɛ̃] 'Snow White and the seven dwarfs', produced as *[blɑ̃ʃnaʒalasɛtnɛ̃], the child wrongly analyzes the initial [n] as a liaison consonant and deletes it from the phrase, and realizes the final [t] of *sept* in lieu of the word-initial [n] of *nain*. These types of errors, which seem to occur most predominantly during the vocabulary burst, are typically not attested in the speech of adult speakers.

The second stage identified affects relatively older speakers who no longer have problems with obligatory liaison contexts but are still struggling with contexts in which liaison is optional. For example, the phrase *ce n'est pas à moi* /sə na pa a mwa/ 'it is not mine' can optionally be realized with liaison as [sənapaʒamwa]. In such contexts, it is possible to find speakers who select the wrong liaison consonant (e.g., *[sənapaṯamwa]). Such mistakes are also found among adult speakers.

These mistakes, in both young and older speakers, are also observed in French-based Creoles (Alain Kihm, personal communication; Tranel, 2003). The error patterns observed are generally related to the fact that several of the phenomena described in preceding sections (liaison, enchaînement, schwa deletion) make word boundaries more opaque at times, yielding a certain degree of abstractness that negatively affects word learning and production in connected speech.

Finally, anecdotal evidence suggests that the process of syllable reduplication, often observed in early speech, and reported for French adults in colloquial speech (Plénat, 1984, 1999), is more prominent in French than in languages such as English (Wauquier-Gravelines, 2003). While this observation may be related to the status of French as syllable-timed, as opposed to English, a stress-timed language (Abercrombie, 1967; Dauer, 1983), more research is needed in this area to determine with more certainty the relative prominence of this pattern and its underlying causes.

Last, Braud (2003) documented patterns of syllable truncation. She demonstrated that French-learning children tend to delete word-medial syllables while preserving initial and final syllables. For example, *un rhinoceros*, 'a rhinoceros' [ɛ̃rinosaʀɔs] ⇨ *[ɛ̃risaʀɔs]. The data also showed that the determiner is available at a very earlier stage for French children. Wauquier-Gravelines (2005) supports this assumption.

Intelligibility

To date there is no study of intelligibility for children who speak French.

Phonetic inventory

To date there is no study of phonetic inventories for children who speak French.

Common mismatches

To date there is no study of common mismatches for children who speak French.

Syllable structure

Very few studies are available on children who speak French. A comparative longitudinal study can be found in Rose (2000). Moreover, the acquisition of onsets (empty onsets and branching onsets) have been studied by Wauquier-Gravelines in a cross-linguistic project (Fikkert et al., 2004), comparing Romance languages (French and Portuguese) and Germanic languages (Dutch and English). From the earliest stage onsetless syllables are observed in French and European Portuguese child data, while in English and Dutch onsetless syllables appear later, although still relatively early. Furthermore, syllables with codas are present early in Germanic languages but appear later in French and Portuguese. To account for this pertinent difference between Romance and Germanic languages Fikkert et al. (2004) follow the proposal of Frota, Vigário, and Freitas (2003), who suggest that rhythm helps the bootstrapping of syllable structure constraints. Germanic and Romance languages differ in basic rhythmic structure (Abercrombie, 1967; Dauer, 1983; Ramus et al., 1999). Germanic languages are stress timed, with often just one full vowel per word, and a complex syllable structure. Hence, consonants may play a more prominent role than vowels, also in acquisition. French and Portuguese are syllable-timed languages, with a relatively simple syllable structure. Here, vowels are more prominent than in Germanic languages, also in acquisition.

Prosody

To date there is no study of prosody for children who speak French. Prosodic factors are, however, considered in several of the analyses proposed in Rose (2000). Following Vihman's proposals, Wauquier-Gravelines (2005) also argues in favor of a prosodic template that could be for French children the domain of phonological generalizations.

Phonological awareness

To date there is no study of phonological awareness for children who speak French.

Speech assessment and speech re-education in France

A very important number of published tests of oral and written language and speech impairment and related disorders are available and used by French speech pathologists. Some of them are available on the Web site of the main editor of such tests in France, http://www. ecpa.fr under the 'ECPA-ortho' reference. All the tests commonly used in France are detailed in Belot and Tricot (2001). The most popular and most frequently used by the speech pathologists can be divided into three main trends.

The first trend is based on a constructivist approach established during the 1960s following the Piagetian tradition. Borel-Maisonny, who initiated the development of speech therapy in France, developed a reading method for nondisordered children as well as assessment and reeducation methods in oral and written French for disordered children, which can be found in Borel-Maisonny (1985, 1986). Additional tests following the same method include *L'alouette* (Lefavrais, 1967) and the *Test de langage* (Sadek-Khalil, 1968).

The second trend follows a psycholinguistic approach based on a global conception of language competence and evaluating the children's performances for oral and written language and for different language components (e.g., phonology, morpho-syntax, pragmatics, and the lexicon) both in production and comprehension. This approach includes evaluations of general attention, working memory, information's treatment strategies that children are able to use for linguistic tasks in production, perception, and comprehension. Tests based on this approach include, for example, EEL (1981), O52 (1987), LMC (1990), LMCR (1999), BEPL-A (1997), BEPL-B (1997), L2MA (1997), ELO (2001), N-EEL (2001), Lexique vivant (2004), and BLI (2002) (see Resources for more information on these tests).

The third trend is based on an approach evaluating neuropsychological disorders that have linguistic consequences but that could be reflected in other modalities and tasks. Very few tests designed under this approach concern children, except for NEPSY (2003).

While the descriptions of these approaches outlined above may suggest that they are mutually exclusive, this is definitely not the case. They all influence each other to some degree, and are all generally considered, to some degree, by speech-language pathologists working in France. Diagnosis and intervention tools and methods deriving from these approaches are clearly set out on the Web site http://www.orthoedition.com/, which is connected to the main association of speech-language pathologists in France (FNO; see Resources). Data are however not available to establish a detailed report of the proportion of the different intervention techniques used. In their practice, speech-language pathologists generally use personal combinations of the different tools available and, at times, also design their own tools and methods.

Speech intervention in French

For the 2004–2005 year, approximately a quarter million speech-related interventions took place in France. The majority of these interventions (48 percent) concern written language impairment (e.g., dysorthography and dyslexia), 32 percent concern speech-language impairments (e.g., stuttering, speech delays, motor delays, mental delays, autism, deafness, genetic diseases), 10 percent of the interventions focus on speech and articulatory re-education, both for children and for adults affected by developmental or acquired speech disorders, and 6 percent concern SLI children. These percentages were based on information declared to the public health insurance, http://www.ameli.fr.

There are approximately 15,000 speech-language pathologists working in France and overseas territories, about 95 percent of whom are female, with a mean age of approximately 40 years. Most of these professionals run their own private practice (about 80 percent). The remaining 20 percent work in public institutions, mainly in medico-social centers and education settings as well as in public general or psychiatric hospitals, schools, and other health centers. Most of the interventions are performed on an individual basis, with a small proportion performed with groups, the latter being concentrated in educational settings. These data and more detailed information concerning interventions in France are available on the Web sites of the speech-pathology associations FOF and FNO (see below).

Working in France

All advertised jobs require a four-year undergraduate degree provided by one of the 13 speech-language pathology schools (see list below) affiliated with the health faculties of French universities. Admission to these schools is limited, with approximately 680 positions available every year. People hailing from other European countries in which they received training in SLP can get equivalences in France. People originating from non-European countries, even if they receive training in SLP, have to obtain a four-year undergraduate degree in one of the 13 French schools in order to obtain the right to practice in France. A visa issued by the French government is also needed. More detailed information is also available on the Web sites of FOF and FNO.

Speech-language pathologists are grouped within two associations: the *Fédération Nationale des Orthophonistes* (FNO) and the *Fédération des Orthophonistes de France* (FOF) (see Resources for more details). FNO is linked with UNADREO, a scientific society oriented toward research on speech disorders and neurolinguistics. Annual national and European congresses are organized by these associations. Finally, three publications are available to speech-language pathologists: *L'orthophoniste*, *Glossa*, and *Ortho magazine*.

Speech assessment for Québec French children

Speech and language assessments in Québec French are primarily based on translations of assessment tools initially developed for the English language. Other assessment tools have been adapted from materials developed in France, such as the *Échelle de communication verbale de Bordeaux* (Darrigrand and Mazaux, 2000). An important source of documentation on this topic can be found on the Web site of the École d'orthophonie et d'audiologie at Université de Montréal: http://132.204.140.194/accueilmthqueOrthov2.htm/.

Speech intervention for Québec French children

No systematic information could be collected with regard to speech intervention in Québec French. However, as it is the case above for assessment techniques, most methods of intervention are based on the current theoretical and applied trends observed in North America and France.

Additional information can be found by contacting the Ordre des Orthophonistes et Audiologistes du Québec (http://www.ooaq.qc.ca/), or each of the three schools in speech and language pathology offering training in French. These schools are located at:

- Université Laval: http://machaon.fmed.ulaval.ca/readaptation/default.asp
- Université de Montréal: http://www.eoa.umontreal.ca/
- University of Ottawa: http://www.health.uottawa.ca/sr/index.htm

Working in Québec

Since June 2003, all advertised positions in Québec require membership with the *Ordre des orthophonistes et audiologistes du Québec*. These professionals can work in schools, hospitals, readaptation centers, long-term housing or treatment centers, community health centers, or private offices. They are also entitled to teach and conduct research activities. One interesting ramification of the legislation regulating these professions is the fact that speech and language pathologists cannot establish audiology diagnoses, nor can audiologists issue diagnoses over the specifics of speech and language pathology, even if the training required for both professions significantly overlaps.

PHONETICALLY SPEAKING

Pronunciation of Québec French: [kabɛk fʁɛnʃ]
Pronunciation of France French: [fʁɑ̃ʃ fʁɛnʃ]

Relevant words for speech assessment and intervention

Word/Phrase	Formal usage	Pronunciation	Informal usage	Pronunciation
Tongue	*langue*	[lɑ̃g]	*langue*	[lɑ̃g]
Teeth	*dents*	[dɑ̃]	*dents*	[dɑ̃]
Lips	*lèvres*	[lɛvʀ]	*lèvres*	[lɛv]
Hard palate	*palais dur*	[palɛ dyʀ]	*palais*	[palɛ]
Soft palate	*voile du palais*	[vwal dy palɛ]	*palais mou*	[palɛ mu]
Larynx	*larynx*	[laʀɛ̃ks]	*gorge*	[gɔʀʒ]
Lungs	*poumons*	[pumɔ̃]	*poumons*	[pumɔ̃]
Nose	*nez*	[na]	*nez*	[na]
Sound	*son*	[sɔ̃]	*son*	[sɔ̃]
Word	*mot*	[mo]	*mot*	[mo]
Sentence	*phrase*	[fʀɑz]	*phrase*	[fʀɑz]
Paragraph	*paragraphe*	[paʀagʀaf]	*paragraphe*	[paʀagʀaf]

Note. These words are transcribed according to France French pronunciations; see above for Québec French derivatives.

RESOURCES

Books about France French

The linguistic properties of French are described in a number of works. A description of the relevant facts can be found in the following books:

Argod–Dutard, F. (1996), *Eléments de phonétique appliquée*, Armand Colin.

Benveniste, C. B. (1997). *Le français parlé, études grammaticales*, Paris: CNRS éditions.

Encrevé, P. (1988), *La liaison, avec et sans enchaînement*, Paris: Le Seuil.

Lacheret-Dujour, A., and Beaugendre, F. (2002), *La prosodie du français*, Paris: CNRS éditions.

Léon, P. (1992). *Phonétisme et prononciation du français*, Nathan Université.

Tranel, B. (1987). *The sounds of French: An introduction.* Cambridge, UK: Cambridge University Press.

Yaguello, M. (2003), *Le grand livre de la langue française*, Paris: Seuil.

The phonetic and lexical peculiarities of French are also documented from a historical perspective, in the following books:

Chaurand, J. (1999), *Nouvelle histoire de la langue française*, Paris: Le Seuil.

Picoche, J., and Marchello-Nizia, C. (1996), *Histoire de la langue française*, Nathan Université.

Resources in speech pathology and neurolinguistics in French

Brin, F., Courrier, C., Lederlé, E., and Masy, V. (1997), *Dictionnaire d'orthophonie*, Paris: Ortho édition.

Chevrie-Muller, C., and Narbona, J (1999), *Le langage de l'enfant, aspects normaux et pathologiques,* Masson.

Mazeau M. (2005), *Neuropsychologie et troubles des apprentissages,* Masson.

Nespoulous, J. L. (1994), Le langage, Introduction. Linguistique, neurolinguistique et neuropsycholinguistique. Un parcours en quatre étapes... In X. Séron and M. Jeannerod (Eds), *Neuropsychologie humaine*. Bruxelles: Mardaga.

Rondal, J.A., and Séron, X. (1999), *Troubles du Langage, bases théoriques et rééducation*. Bruxelles: Mardaga.

Books about Québec French

The linguistic properties of Québec French are described in a number of works. A description of the relevant facts can be found in the following two books. The first one provides a good description of the phonetic properties of Québec French. The second one discusses these properties in relation with the issue of linguistic norms:

Dumas, D. (1987). *Nos façons de parler: les prononciations en français québécois*. Québec: Presses de l'Université du Québec.

Ostiguy, Luc et Claude Tousignant (1993). *Le français québécois: normes et usages*. Montréal: Guérin.

More recently, a sociolinguistic study addressing the situation of the Québec French-speaking community vis à vis factors such as the international norm (which is mostly influenced by Parisian French) and the English-dominant North American context was also published:

Razafimandimbimanana, E. (2005). *FRANÇAIS, FRANGLAIS, QUÉBÉ-QUOI? Les jeunes Québécois et la langue française: enquête sociolinguistique*. Paris: L'Harmattan.

The phonetic and lexical peculiarities of Québec French are also documented from a historical perspective, in the following two books:

Mougeon, R., and Béniak, E. (1994), *Les origines du français québécois*. Québec: Presses de l'Université Laval.

Leclerc, J. (1989), *Qu'est-ce que la langue?* (2nd ed). Laval: Mondia.

Finally, the issue of lexical frequency is documented in the following book:

Beauchemin, N., Martel, P., and Théoret, T. (1992). *Dictionnaire de fréquence des mots du français parlé au Québec: fréquence, dispersion, usage, écart réduit*. New York: Peter Lang.

CD-ROMs about Québec French

While Québec French represents the norm in first language instruction, the teaching of French as a second language is typically done using materials that follow a more international norm centred on the Parisian dialect of French. For this reason, very few language teaching tools are based on the Québec variety. One exception to this is KitQC2, a Windows-only free software program, which can be downloaded through the following Web link:
http://www.alpha.cdeacf.ca/les_ressources/kitqc1/

Journals about France French

While French and acquisition of French has been documented in virtually all major linguistic journals, these journals are of special interest because they publish special issues containing articles documenting linguistic aspects of French, from either theoretical or applied perspectives.

- *Corpus*, http://revel.unice.fr/corpus/
- *Glossa*, www.unadreo.org
- *L'orthophoniste*, www.orthoedition.com
- *Langages*, http://www.editions-sedes.com/langages_larousse/langages.html
- *Langue française*, http://www.editionssedes.com
- *Lidil,*http://fr.isbn.pl/A-LIDIL-revue-de-linguistique-et-de-didactique-des-langues-universit-Stendhal-de-Grenoble
- *Marges linguistiques*, http://www.marges-linguistiques.com/
- *Ortho-magazine*,www.info-presse.fr/fiches/ortho-magazine_2022_pro.htm
- *Recherches Linguistiques de Vincennes*, http://rlv.revues.org
- *Revue française de linguistique appliquée*, http://perso.wanadoo.fr/rfla/

Journals about Québec French

While Québec French has been documented in virtually all major linguistic journals, these journals are of special interest because they contain several articles documenting linguistic aspects of Québec French, from either theoretical or applied perspectives:

- *Revue Québécoise de Linguistique*, http://www.erudit.org/revue/rql/
- *Langue et Linguistique*, http://www.fl.ulaval.ca/lli/
- *La revue canadienne de linguistique / Canadian Journal of Linguistics*, http://www.chass.utoronto.ca/~cla-acl/
- *La revue canadienne de linguistique appliquée / Canadian Journal of Applied Linguistics*, http://www.aclacaal.org/

Useful information on France French variation and dialects

An international project of description and analysis of French dialects, *La phonologie du français contemporain: usages, variétés et structure* (PFC) is directed by J. Durand (ERSS, Toulouse), C. Lyche (Universités d'Oslo et Tromso) et B. Laks (Modyco, Paris X), http://www.projet-pfc.net/

Walter, H. (1982). *Enquête phonologique et variétés régionales du français*, Paris: PUF.

Professional associations relevant to speakers of France French

- Fédération Nationale des orthophonistes (FNO): http://www.orthophonistes.fr
- Fédération des orthophonistes de France (FOF): http://www.perso.wanadoo.fr/f.o.f/
- Union Nationale pour le Développement de la Recherche et de l'Evaluation en Orthophonie (UNADREO): http://www.unadreo.org
- Comité permanent des orthophonistes logopèdes de l'Union européenne: http://www. cplol.org
- Orthophonistes du monde which is a benevole care association connected with Médecins du Monde, Handicap International http://www.orthophonistes.fr/Theme.php?NumTheme=99

Professional associations relevant to speakers of Québec French

The professional association of speech-language pathologists within Québec is Ordre des Orthophonistes et Audiologistes du Québec (http://www.ooaq.qc.ca/).

This association works in close collaboration with its national counterpart, the Association canadienne des orthophonistes et audiologists/Canadian Association of Speech-Language Pathologists and Audiologists: http://www.caslpa.ca/.

Schools of speech pathology in France

Ecole d'Orthophonie Service ORL Audio Phonologie Place St Jacques 25030 BESANCON Cedex 19 étudiant(e)s

Faculté de Médecine Av. de la Forêt de la Haye BP 184 54505 VANDOEUVRE LES NANCY 41 étudiant(e)s

Faculté de Médecine Avenue de Vallombrose 06034 NICE Cedex 27 étudiant(e)s

UER de Médecine 1 rue Gaston Veil 44035 NANTES Cedex 01 39 étudiant(e)s

UER de Médecine 2 bis Bd Tonnelé 37032 TOURS Cedex 39 étudiant(e)s

UER de Médecine d'Aix Marseille II 27 Bd Jean Moulin 13385 MARSEILLE Cedex 5 27 étudiant(e)s

UER de Médecine PARIS VI CHU Pitié Salpetrière 47 Bd de l'Hôpital 75013 PARIS 100 étudiant(e)s

UER Sciences Médicales 4 rue Kirschleger 67085 STRASBOURG CEDEX 21 étudiant(e)s

UFR de Médecine 2 rue Ecole de Médecine 34060 MONTPELLIER Cedex 1 34 étudiant(e)s

Université Claude Bernard Techniques de réadaptation 8 rue Rockefeller 69373 LYON Cedex 08 91 étudiant(e)s

Université de Bordeaux II 146 rue Léo Saignat 33076 BORDEAUX Cedex 28 étudiant(e)s

Université de Lille II 42 rue Paul Duez 59800 LILLE 107 étudiant(e)s

Université Paul Sabatier Toulouse III Ens. Techniques de réadaptation CHU de Rangueil Chemin de Vallon Bat L2 31054 TOULOUSE Cedex 27 étudiant(e)s

Tests which are commonly used in France

Oral Speech tests

Borel-Maisonny, S. (1985, 8ème édition), *Langage oral et écrit, tome 1*, Delachaux & Niestlé, Neufchâtel, Paris

Borel-Maisonny, S. (1986, 8ème édition), *Langage oral et écrit, tome 2*, Delachaux & Niestlé, Neufchâtel, Paris

Chevrie-Muller, C. Simon, A.M., Fournier, S. (1981). L2MA: *Batterie Langage oral, Langage écrit, Mémoire, Attention*. Paris: ECPA.

Chevrie-Muller, C., Simon, A.M., Le Normand, M.T., Fournier, S. (1988). BEPL-A: *Batterie d'évaluation psycholinguistique* A. Paris: ECPA.

Chevrie-Muller, C., Simon, A.M., Le Normand, M.T., Fournier, S. (1988). BEPL-B: *Batterie d'évaluation psycholinguistique* B. Paris: ECPA.

Chevrie-Muller, C., Simon, A. M., Le Normand, M. T., Fournier, S., (1981). EEL: *Epreuve pour l'Examen du Langage*. Paris: ECPA.

Chevrie-Muller, M. Plaza, S. Fournier, (2001). N-EEL: *Nouvelles Epreuves pour l'Examen du Langage*. Paris: ECPA.

Khomsi A. & Bourg, E. (2004), *Lexique vivant*. Paris: ECPA.

Khomsi, A. (1987), O52: *Evaluation des stratégies de compréhension en situation orale*. Paris: ECPA.

Khomsi, A. (2001), ELO: *Evaluation du Langage Oral*. Paris: ECPA.

P. Lecocq, (1996), E. CO.S.SE: *Epreuve de COmpréhension Syntaxico-Semantique*, Psychologie Cognitive, Presse Universitaire du Septentrion, Villeneuve d'Ascq

Sadek-Khalil (1968). *Test de langage*: Delachaux et Niestlé, Paris/ Neufchâtel

Written language tests

Khomsi, A. & Khomsi, J., (2002). BLI: *Bilan de Lecture Informatisé*. Paris: ECPA.

Khomsi, A. (1999), LMC-R: Lecture de Mots et Compréhension Révisé, A. Paris: ECPA.

Lefavrais, P. (1967), *L'alouette*. Paris: ECPA.

P. Lecocq, (1996), E. CO.S.SE: *Epreuve de COmpréhension Syntaxico-Semantique*, Psychologie Cognitive, Presse Universitaire du Septentrion, Villeneuve d'Ascq

Neuropsychological tests

Korkman, M., Kirk, U. & Kemp, S. (2003), NEPSY: *Bilan neuropsychologique de l'enfant*. Paris: ECPA.

Useful Web sites about Québec French

Finally, a number of Web sites contain interesting information about Québec French. Four such site are listed below:

- Le français québécois, http://www.republiquelibre. org/cousture/FRANC2.HTM
- Phonétique du français québécois, http://www.ciral. ulaval.ca/phonetique/
- Lexilogos, http://www.lexilogos.com/quebecois_ langue_dictionnaires.htm
- Phono, http://www.ciral.ulaval.ca/phonetique/ phono/debutph.htm

Additional information can be found online, using terms such as "français québécois" or "Québec French" with Internet search engines.

REFERENCES

Abercrombie, D. (1967). *Elements of general phonetics*, Edinburgh: Edinburgh University.

Belot, C., and Tricot, M. (2001). *Les tests en orthophonie, tome 1: Langage oral, langage écrit, enfants et adolescents*, Ortho edition, Paris.

Bernhardt, B. H., and Stemberger, J. P. (1998). *Handbook of phonological development from the perspective of constraint-based nonlinear phonology*. San Diego, CA: Academic Press.

Beyssade, C., Delais-Roussarie, E., Doetjes, J., Marandin J.-M., and Rialland, A. (2004). Prosody and information in French. In F.

Corblin and H. de Swärts (Eds.), *Handbook of French semantics* (pp. 477–500). Chicago: CSLI.

Braud, V. (2003). *Acquisition de la prosodie chez les enfants francophones. Les phénomènes de troncations*. Unpublished Ph.D. dissertation, Université de Nantes.

Brett, L., Chiat, S., and Pilcher, C. (1987). Stages and units in output processing: Some evidence from voicing and fronting processes in children. *Language and Cognitive Processes, 14*, 275–300.

Casagrande, J. (1984). *The sound system of French*. Washington, DC: Georgetown University Press.

Charette, M. (1991). *Conditions on phonological government.* Cambridge, MA: Cambridge University Press.

Chevrot, J-P., Dugua, C., and Fayol, M. (2005). Liaison et formation des mots, un scénario développemental, In J-P. Chevrot, M. Fayol, and B. Laks (Eds). *Langages, Nouvelles approches de la liaison,*158, (pp. 38–53), Paris: Larousse.

Cornulier, B. de, and Dell, F. (Eds.) (1978). *Etudes de phonologie du français.* Paris: CNRS.

Coveney, A. (2001). *The sounds of contemporary French: Articulation and diversity.* Exeter: Elm Bank Publications.

Crelin, E. S. (1987). *The human vocal tract: Anatomy, function, development, and evolution.* New York: Vantage Press.

Darrigrand, B., and Mazaux, J-M. (2000). L'échelle de communication verbale de Bordeaux: une évaluation des compétences communicatives des personnes aphasiques. *Glossa: Les Cahiers de l'UNADREO,* 73, 4–14.

Dauer, R. M. (1983). Stress-timing and syllable-timing reanalysed, *Journal of Phonetics,* 11, 51–69.

Delais, E. (1994). Structure rythmique et prosodique du français: Pour une approche psychocognitive, *Linx,* 29, Université Paris X Nanterre.

Delattre, P. (1947). La liaison en français, tendances et classification, *The French Review, XXI,* 148–157.

Delattre, P. (1966), *Studies in French and comparative phonetics,* Mouton: La Haye.

Dell, F. (1978). Epenthèse et effacement de schwa dans des syllabes contiguës en français. In B. de Cornulier and F. Dell (Eds.), *Etudes de phonologie française,* (pp. 75–81). Paris: Editions du CNRS.

Dell, F. (1984). L'accentuation dans les phrases en français, In F. Dell, D. Hirst, and J.-R. Vergnaud, (Eds), *Forme sonore du langage; structure des représentations en phonologie,* (pp. 65–122). Paris: Hermann.

Di Cristo, A. (1998). Intonation in French. In D. Hirst and A. Di Cristo, (Eds), *Intonation systems: A survey of twenty languages.* Cambridge, UK: Cambridge University Press.

Di Cristo, A., (1999). Le cadre accentuel du français contemporain: essai de modélisation partie 1, *Langues,* 2(3), 184–205.

Dumas, D. (1981). Structure de la diphtongaison québécoise. *Canadian Journal of Linguistics,* 26(1), 1–61.

Durand, J., and Eychenne, J. (2004). Le schwa en français: pourquoi des corpus? In T. Scheer (Ed.), *Usage des corpus en phonologie, Corpus 3,* (pp. 311–356). Paris: CNRS & Université de Nice - Sophia Antipolis.

Durand, J., and Lyche, C. (2003) Le projet 'Phonologie du Français Contemporain' (PFC) et sa méthodologie. In E. Delais and J. Durand (Eds), *Corpus et variation en phonologie du français: méthodes et analyses* (pp. 213–276). Toulouse: Presses Universitaires du Mirail.

Durand, J., and Lyche, C. (2004). Structure et variation dans quelques systèmes vocaliques du français, l'enquête « Phonologie du français contemporain », In A. Coveney and C. Sanders (Eds.) *Variation et francophonie,* Paris: L'Harmattan.

Durand, J., Slater, C., and Wise, H. (1987). Observations on schwa in Southern French. *Linguistics* 25(2), 983–1004.

Encrevé, P. (1988). *La liaison avec et sans enchaînement, phonologie tridimensionnelle et usages du français.* Paris: Le Seuil.

Encrevé, P., and Scheer T. (2005, May), *Association is not automatic.* Paper presented at the 13th Manchester Phonology Meeting.

Fikkert, P. (1994). *On the acquisition of prosodic structure.* Dordrecht: ICG Printing.

Fikkert, P., Freitas, M. J., Grijzenhout, J., Levelt, C., and Wauquier S. (2004, April). Syllabic markedness, segmental markedness, rhythm and acquisition, *GLOW Phonology Workshop.*

Harris, J. (1994). *English sound structure.* Cambridge, MA: Blackwell.

Hirst, D.J., Di Cristo, A., and Espesser, R. (2000), Levels of representation and levels of analysis for intonation. In M. Horne (Ed) *Prosody: Theory and experiment.* Dordrecht: Kluwer.

Inkelas, S., and Rose, Y. (2003). Velar fronting revisited. In A. Brown and F. Conlin (Eds.), *Proceedings of the 27th Annual Boston University conference on language development* (pp. 334–345). Somerville, MA: Cascadilla Press.

Kehoe, M., and Hilaire-Debove, G. (2004). *The structure of branching onsets and rising diphthongs: Evidence from the acquisition of French.* Paper presented at the 28th Annual Boston University Conference on Language Development, Somerville, MA.

Klein, M. (1991). *Vers une approche substantielle et dynamique de la constituance syllabique: le cas des semi-voyelles et des voyelles hautes dans les usages parisiens,* Unpublished dissertation, University of Paris 8.

Lacheret-Dujour, A., and Beaugendre, F. (2002). *La prosodie du français,* Paris: CNRS éditions.

Morrisette, M. L., Dinnsen, D. A., and Gierut, J. A. (2003). Markedness and context effects in the acquisition of place features. *Canadian Journal of Linguistics,* 48(3/4), 329–355.

Pagliano, C. (2003). *L'épenthèse consonantique en français. Ce que la syntaxe, la sémantique et la morphologie peuvent faire à la phonologie: parles-en ta numérotation ?impossible.* Unpublished Ph.D. dissertation, Université de Nice.

Petit Robert 1. (1990). *Dictionnaire alphabétique et analogique de la langue Française.* Paris: Dictionnaire Le Robert.

Plénat, M. (1984). Toto, Fanfa, Totor et même guiguite sont des anars. In F. Dell, D. Hirst, and J.R. Vergnaud (Eds.), *Forme sonore du langage* (pp. 161-183). Paris: Hermann.

Plénat, M. (1999). Prolégomènes à une étude variationniste des hypocoristiques à redoublement en français, *Cahiers de grammaire, 24*, 183–219.

Ramus, F., Nespor, M., and Mehler, J. (1999). Correlates of linguistic rhythm in the speech signal. *Cognition, 73*(3), 265–292.

Rose, Y. (2000). *Headedness and prosodic licensing in the L1 acquisition of phonology.* Unpublished Ph.D. dissertation, McGill University.

Smit, A. B. (2004). *Articulation and phonology: Resource guide for school-age children and adults.* Clifton Park, NY: Thomson Delmar Learning.

Stoel-Gammon, C. (1996). On the acquisition of velars in English. In B. H. Bernhardt, J. Gilbert, and D. Ingram (Eds.), *Proceedings of the UBC international conference on phonological acquisition* (pp. 201–214). Somerville, MA: Cascadilla Press.

Tranel, B. (1987). *The sounds of French. An introduction.* Cambridge, UK: Cambridge University Press.

Tranel, B. (1995). Current issues in French phonology: Liaison and position theories. In J. A. Goldsmith (Ed.), *The handbook of phonological theory* (pp. 798–817). Oxford: Blackwell.

Tranel, B. (2003). Les sons du français. In M. Yaguello (Ed.) *Le grand livre de la langue française*, Paris: Le Seuil.

Vigario, M., Frota, S., and Freitas, M. J. (2003). In B. Beachley, A. Brown, and F. Colin (Eds), *Proceedings of the 27th Annual Boston University Conference on Language Development* (pp. 809–821). Sommerville, MA: Cascadilla Press.

Vihman M., and Kunnari, S. (in press). The source of phonological knowledge: A cross linguistic perspective. In S. Wauquier-Gravelines (Ed), « Du traitement précoce aux représentations, l'acquisition phonologique », *Recherches Linguistiques Vincennes*, 34, St Denis: Presses Universitaires de Vincennes.

Walker, D. C. (2001). *French sound structure.* Calgary: University of Calgary Press.

Walter, H. (1977). *La phonologie du français*, Paris: Presses Universitaires de France.

Walter, H. (1982). *Enquête phonologique et variétés régionales du français*, Paris: PUF.

Wauquier-Gravelines, S. (2003). Troncation et reduplication. Peut-on parler de gabarits morphologiques dans le lexique précoce? In B. Fradin, G. Dal, M. Hathout, F. Kerleroux, M. Roché, and M. Plénat (Eds), *Les unités morphologiques. Silexicales* 3, Université de Lille III.

Wauquier-Gravelines, S. (2005b). *Statut des représentations phonologiques en acquisition, traitement de la parole continue et dysphasie développementale.* Paris: EHESS.

Wauquier-Gravelines, S., and Braud, V. (2005a). Proto-déterminant et acquisition de la liaison obligatoire en français. In J-P. Chevrot, M. Fayol, and B. Laks (Eds.) *Langages, Nouvelles approches de la liaison*, 158, (pp. 53–66) Paris: Larousse.

Wauquier-Gravelines, S., Encrevé, P., and Scheer, T. (2005). Liaison in French, towards an unified explanation of variation, *colloque PFC, Phonological variation, the case of French* (pp. 25–27). Tromso, Norway: CASTL.

Wioland, F. (1991). *Prononcer les mots du français. Des sons et des rythmes.* Paris: Hachette.

SUMMARY OF STUDIES OF TYPICAL FRENCH SPEECH ACQUISITION

Authors	Year	Country	No. of children	Age of children	Information	Sample type	Data collection
Rose	2000	Canada	2	Child 1 (Clara): 1;00.28–2;07.19 Child 2 (Théo): 1;10.27–4;00.00	Development of syllable structure; Emergent processes	Connected speech, mostly spontaneous; some imitated productions	Longitudinal
Wauquier-Gravelines	2003	France	1	Child 1 (Claire) 1;9–2;3	Development of syllables structure; Emergent processes Gliding Liaison	Connected speech, mostly spontaneous; some imitated productions	Longitudinal
Wauquier-Gravelines	2004	France	4	1;3–1;8	Syllable onset	Repetition Directed speech	Transversal
Wauquier-Gravelines	1997	France	23 23	2;6–3;6 4;0–5;0	Liaison	Picture naming	Experimental
Wauquier-Gravelines	1997	France	18 SLI children	3;0 to 16;0	Liaison	Picture naming	Experimental
Wauquier-Gravelines and Sauzet	1997	France	18 SLI children	3;0 to 16;0	Morphological derivation	Derivation test	Experimental
Wauquier-Gravelines Braud	1999	France	24	4;0–5;0	Morphological derivation	Derivation test speech	Experimental

Acknowledgements

The authors have contributed equally to this publication. Since neither of us is a specialist in SLP, we also had to rely on the help of other people, who generously provided significant help and support. Elisabeth Peuvrel from the École d'orthophonie de Nantes, Centre Universitaire de Nantes, and Suzanne Calvarin, speech-language pathologist and instructor at the École d'orthophonie de Nantes, provided information on current SLP-related documents and practices in France. Joël Macoir and Audette Sylvestre, both assistant professors in the Department of Rehabilitation of Laval University (Québec City, Canada) were instrumental in our quest for information about SLP-related issues in Québec. Jacques Durand provided help with some of the characterization of the southern dialects of France French, and Alain Kihm provided useful information on French-based creoles. Many thanks to Éliane Lebel, who contributed compilations of sound-spelling correspondences in French from which Tables 40-3 and 40-4 were adapted. We are immensely grateful to all these people for their useful assistance. Of course, all errors or omissions are our own. Finally, we would like to express special thanks to Sharynne McLeod for her patient work in assembling this much anticipated volume.

Chapter 41

German Speech Acquisition

Annette V. Fox

INTRODUCTION

German is a member of the West Germanic branch of Indo-European languages and is the first language of approximately 123 million people in 15 countries, the largest communities being in Western and Central Europe. There are regional variations in pronunciation, from accents to dialects, of the official language *Hochdeutsch* (Standard German), which is based on a North German pronunciation of the written language. *Hochdeutsch* is the medium of instruction in kindergarten, school, and university. The spelling of standard German generally gives a clear guide to pronunciation. The majority of people of Germany and Austria are monolingual German-speakers (from an acquisition point of view). About 10 percent of residents in Germany have a nationality other than German, Turkish immigrants forming the biggest group of bilingual speakers. In recent years, however, the number of immigrants from central and eastern European countries, such as Poland, Russia, and so forth, has increased significantly. For the majority of immigrant children a successive bilingualism is the norm, with an L2 (German) onset age of 3 years, when children enter German kindergarten. In these children, language competence at school entry (age 6) is often far from sufficient. See the Resources section in this chapter for materials pertaining to German.

Where German is spoken

German is the official state language in Germany, Austria, and parts of Switzerland, Liechtenstein, Luxembourg, and South Tyrol in Northern Italy (Crystal, 1997). See the accompanying map and Appendix D.

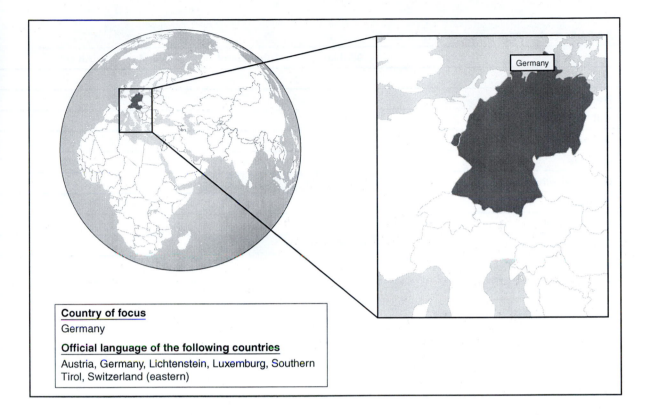

Country of focus
Germany

Official language of the following countries
Austria, Germany, Lichtenstein, Luxemburg, Southern
Tirol, Switzerland (eastern)

Components of German

Consonants

Hochdeutsch contains 23 consonant phonemes /p, b, t, d, k, g, f, v, s, z, ʃ, ç, x, h, m, n, ŋ, ʁ, l, ʔ, j, ts, pf/ (see also Table 41-1). The glottal stop /ʔ/ appears before syllable-initial vowels and is compulsory. The sounds /pf/ and /ts/ will be treated as affricates, following Ternes (1987), and not two-element clusters, despite disagreement in the literature (Kohler, 1995; Ternes, 1987; Wiese, 1996). Whether /ç/ and /x/ should be considered as two phonemes or as allophones is also controversial (Kohler, 1995; Wiese, 1996) but for ease of presentation they will be classified as phonemes. In word-final position the contrast between voiced and voiceless consonants is neutralized, with all fricatives and plosives being voiceless.

Vowels and diphthongs

The vowel system of *Hochdeutsch* contains 15 monophthongs and 3 diphthongs (see Table 41-2). In general, the vowel quality varies depending on the location in Germany, Austria, or other areas. Vowel quality length is important to differentiating meaning. Long vowels are always produced more closed while short vowels are produced more openly. A number of minimal pairs exist (e.g., *Beet* [beːt] – *Bett* [bɛt]).

Phonotactic restrictions

Syllables

The smallest possible syllable is V, for example, /aɪ/ = *Ei* 'egg'. Structures of the combinations $C_{0-3}VC_{0-3}$ in monosyllabic nouns are possible: Onset C_{0-3}, e.g., /ʃpʁ/ in *Sprung* 'jump'; Coda C_{0-4}, e.g., /rpst/ in *Herbst* 'autumn'. Inflection of verbs can even result in codas such as C_{0-5} e.g., /mpfst/ in *du schrumpfst* 'you shrink.' German is an agglutinating language where, by addition of nouns, words can be made up to about eight syllables or more, like *Hallenhandballweltmeisterschaft* 'indoor handball world championship' (Meinhold and Stock, 1980). Commonly used words contain one to four syllables, with the majority containing two to three syllables.

TABLE 41-1 Consonants produced in German

	Bilabial	Labiodental	Dental	Alveolar
Plosive	p b			t d
Nasal	m			n
Trill				r
Tap or flap				
Fricative		f v		s z
Lateral fricative	■■■■■■			
Affricate	pf			ts
Approximant				
Lateral approximant	■■■■■■			l

Black = articulations judged impossible

Based on the International Phonetic Alphabet. Courtesy of the International Phonetic Association (c/o Department of Linguistics, University of Victoria, Victoria, British Columbia, Canada).

Consonants and consonant clusters

In word-initial position in Standard German there are 22 two-element clusters and two three-element clusters. There are also many word-medial and word-final clusters. Assimilation processes in word-final unstressed syllables /ən/ and /əl/ can lead to further syllable-final clusters: [geːbn] instead of /geːbən/ *geben* 'to give,' [foːgl] instead of /foːgəl/ *Vogel* 'bird.' Further, similar assimilation patterns can be observed for all word positions in a number of regional variations or dialects, for example, /ksaːkt/ *gsagt* in southern German, Swiss, or Austrian German, instead of *gesagt* 'said.'

Tones

German does not use tones to differentiate meaning.

Stress and intonation

The arguments of Jassem (1952) and others about the basic rhythmic structure of English apply, with some modifications, to German. In contemporary analyses, the basic unit is the *foot* consisting of an accented syllable followed by one or more unaccented syllables; in addition to the basic trochaic or dactylic structure of these units, Jassem (1952) introduces an additional iambic element, the *anacrusis*, of unaccented syllables before the accented syllable creating a *Total Rhythm Unit* (see also Jassem and Gibbon, 1980).

Writing system

German uses the 26 letters of the modern English alphabet. The name of almost every letter in German contains the sound ordinarily represented by that letter.

Varieties of German

While *Hochdeutsch* is the official language, a number of different dialects are reported for German; estimates on the number of dialects vary from 50 to 250 (see König, 1994). The number of people who still speak a dialect is falling in most regions of Germany, even though some efforts are being made to keep dialects alive. Distinct accents nonetheless indicate people's origins. Some distinct regional changes of the consonant system should be mentioned. In a number of regions, the affricate /pf/ is realized as /f/ only in word-initial position. Voicing and devoicing patterns of consonants are highly dependent on the region where German is spoken, with extremes such as Swabia, where nearly all fricatives and plosives are devoiced, and Saxony, where all consonants are voiced. Also dependent on the region is the realization of /r/, which is realized as an uvular /ʁ/ in Middle, East, and North Germany or as alveolar /r/ in some regions in southern Germany. Whenever /r/ is realized as [ʁ] or [ʀ], in all positions other than before vowels /ʁ/ is realized as a vocalic

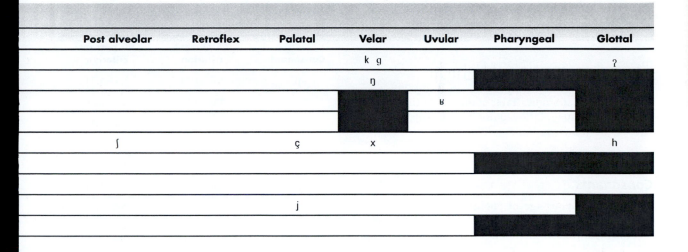

TABLE 41-2 Vowels produced in German

German Location	Standard-German vowels	Example words	English Translation
High front	i:	_Biene_	'bee'
	ɪ	_Bild_	'picture'
High front rounded	y:	_Bühne_	'stage'
	ʏ	_Mücke_	'midge'
Mid-low front	e:	_Besen_	'broom'
	ɛ	_Bäcker_	'baker'
	ɛ:	_Käse_	'cheese'
Mid-low front rounded	ø:	_Söhne_	'sons'
	œ	_Köpfe_	'heads'
High back	a:	_Sahne_	'cream'
	a	_Bank_	'bank'
High back rounded	u:	_Buch_	'book'
	ʊ	_Butter_	'butter'
Mid-back rounded	o:	_Sohn_	'son'
	ɔ	_Kopf_	'head'
Central*	ə	_Biene_	'bee'
Diphthongs	aɪ	_Bein_	'leg'
	au	_Auto_	'car'
	ɔɪ	_Leute_	'people'

* Unclear phoneme status, occurring only in unstressed syllables

Ersatzlaut (substitution sound) [ɐ]. This fact creates several additional long or short diphthongs as in *Wurst* [vuːɐst] 'sausage' or *Berg* [beːɐk] 'mountain.'

Typical acquisition of German

The Summary of Studies Table at the end of this chapter contains studies of the acquisition of German. They have been summarized in Fox (2005).

Acquired sounds
Consonants

Table 41-3 contains age of phoneme acquisition data from the study by Fox and Dodd (1999). In this cross-sectional study 178 monolingual German-speaking children aged 1;6 to 5;11 were assessed for their speech abilities. No differences between boys and girls were observed.

Consonant clusters

The same cross-sectional study (Fox and Dodd, 1999) also investigated the acquisition of word-initial clusters. Even though German-speaking children were observed producing a range of clusters as early as age 2;0 to 2;5 (Fox and Schäfer, 2006), clusters started to be acquired by the age of 3;0 to 3;11 (Fox and Dodd, 1999). Clusters containing /ʃ/ + other were observed to be produced correctly between 3;6 and 4;6 years of age, the three-element clusters /ʃtʁ/ and /ʃpʁ/ being acquired last around the age of 4;5 (Fox and Dodd, 1999).

Vowels and diphthongs

To date no study has investigated vowel acquisition in detail. However, Fox and Dodd (1999) and Fox and Schäfer (2006) found that very young children aged 1;6 to 2;11 already make hardly any vowel errors.

Percent correct
Consonants

Percentage of consonants produced correctly has been studied by Fox and Dodd (1999). The overall error rate of phonemes for each age group is given in Table 41-4. In row 1 the means for incorrect production across all children (PPI = Percentage Phonemes Incorrect) for each age group are shown, with standard deviation values shown in row 2. Rows 3 and 4 present the mean error percentage for single consonants compared to the total number of consonant (PCI) occurrences per word position.

TABLE 41-3 Age of acquisition for German consonants

Consonant	75 percent criterion	90 percent criterion
p	1;6 – 1;11	1;6 – 1;11
b	1;6 – 1;11	2;0 – 2;5
m	1;6 – 1;11	1;6 – 1;11
n	1;6 – 1;11	2;0 – 2;5
ŋ	2;6 – 2;11	2;6 – 2;11
h	2;0 – 2;5	2;6 – 2;11
j	2;6 – 2;11	3;0 – 3;5
t	1;6 – 1;11	2;6 – 2;11
d	1;6 – 1;11	1;6 – 1;11
k	2;6 – 2;11	2;6 – 2;11
g	2;6 – 2;11	3;0 – 3;5
f	2;6 – 2;11	2;6 – 2;11
l	2;6 – 2;11	2;6 – 2;11
ʃ	3;6 – 3;11	4;6 – 4;11
s	2;0 – 2;5	2;6 – 2;11
z	2;0 – 2;5	2;6 – 2;11
v	2;0 – 2;5	2;6 – 2;11
x	2;6 – 2;11	2;6 – 2;11
ʁ	2;6 – 2;11	3;0 – 3;5
ç	3;0 – 3;5	4;0 – 4;5
pf	2;6 – 2;11	3;0 – 3;5
ts	3;0 – 3;5	3;6 – 3;11

Note. Data from Fox and Dodd (1999).

Consonant clusters

No study has yet explicitly investigated the percentage of consonant clusters produced correctly.

Vowels

Fox and Dodd (1999) also assessed vowel production. The overall vowel error percentage for vowels found within the first three age groups was less then 3 percent, which was confirmed by Fox and Schäfer (2006). In the later age groups the error percentage was about

TABLE 41-4   Percent phoneme/consonants incorrect (PPI/PCI) depending on age

Age	1;6–1;11	2;0–2;5	2;6–2;11	3;0–3;5	3;6–3;11	4;0–4;5	4;6–4;11	5;0–5;5	5;6–5;11
$\bar{X}$PPI	26.05	21.19	12.59	9.011	5.75	4.86	3.80	2.57	1.92
+/– SD	11.1	10.5	8.1	5.1	4.1	3.5	4.0	2.4	2.3
PCI WI	28.05	26.14	15.40	9.93	5.98	5.56	3.85	2.77	2.31
PCI WF	25.71	31.73	14.93	11.39	7.51	10.06	6.55	4.67	4.88

Note. WI/ WF = word-initial and word- final percentage incorrect consonant production

1 percent. Diphthong errors were more common, the first element being retained in 67 percent of error examples.

Phonological processes

The most recent studies of developmental phonological processes in German were conducted by Fox and Schäfer (2006). The data replicated the data from Fox and Dodd (1999, reanalyzed 2003; see Fox 2005), indicating the following processes to be developmental for German:

- Overcome by the age of 2;5: glottal replacement /ʁ/ and fronting /ŋ/
- Overcome by the age of 2;11: weak-syllable deletion; final-consonant deletion, especially /l/; stopping; deaffrication
- Overcome by the age of 3;5: fronting /k, ɡ/, backing /ʃ, s/
- Overcome by the age of 3;11: cluster reduction, assimilation; voicing/devoicing;
- Overcome by the age of 4;5/ 4;11: fronting /ʃ, ç/

A study looking at the acquisition of word production consistency (i.e., children reaching a level of inconsistency in word production below 40 percent; see also Dodd, 1995, for criterion definition) in 2-year-olds by Schäfer and Fox (in press) showed that children in the age group 2;6 to 2;11 were highly consistent, but that distinct phonological process patterns were observable already in the younger age group, 2;0 to 2;5.

Intelligibility

No studies have yet assessed intelligibility in German-speaking children.

Phonetic inventory

The study by Fox and Dodd (1999) assessed the phonetic inventory of German-speaking children. Results indicated that very young children aged 1;6 to 2;5 already produce the majority of phones correctly. By the age of 3;0 to 3;5 all phones should be viewed as acquired, apart from /ʃ/ and /ç/, which were acquired between 3;6 and 4;11. The phones /s/ and /z/ present a special case, since none of the age groups reached the acquisition criterion. Even until the age of 10 years (children older than that were not assessed), 30–40 percent of all children showed an interdental or addental lisp, suggesting that the interdental realization is slowly becoming a variation of the norm, rather than a speech impairment (Fox, 2005).

Common mismatches

There is as yet no study on common mismatches produced by German-speaking children.

Syllable structure

There is as yet no study on syllable structure produced by German-speaking children.

Prosody

An investigation of the acquisition of prosody revealed that the trochaic foot—typical for German—can be observed already in the babbling of children aged 13 weeks (Penner, 2002; Penner and Fischer, submitted, cited in Penner 2003).

Phonological awareness

No study has yet adequately investigated the acquisition of phonological awareness in German-speaking children. A pattern similar to that for English-speaking children is assumed (Hartmann, 2002). Two pilot studies were able to support this hypothesis (Fricke, 2005; Stenzel, 1999). However, Stenzel (1999) was able to show, in contrast to English-speaking children, the ability of syllable segmentation prior to rime detection in 3-year-old German-speaking children.

Speech assessment for German-speaking children

Two groups of assessment tools are currently used in clinics, and they differ only in analysis. The first group contains assessments that are segment orientated: every item targets one phoneme, and only the realization of that one phoneme is noted. Most of these materials were designed by colleges of SLP or therapists in clinics. They are usually not published and have never been evaluated. For the second group the interpretation of the test results is based on a phonological process analysis. However, most of these are not linguistically balanced and naming reliability has not been assessed. Most assessment materials consist of picture-naming tasks. Table 41-5 provides an overview on materials available.

There is currently one assessment tool available for bilingual German-Turkish-speaking children, the WIELAU-T (Lammer and Kalmàr, 2004).

Speech intervention for German-speaking children

Until recently, the dominant intervention approach used in all German-speaking countries was articulation therapy (van Riper, 1963). Since the late 1990s, a change from articulation to phonological intervention has been observed following the introduction of classification systems such as that by Dodd (1995). The following phonological approaches are now used in addition: *Methaphon* (Howell and Dean, 1995; translated by Jahn, 2000), Minimal Pair Therapy (Saben and Ingham, 1991; translated by Hacker and Wilgermein, 1999) and *P.O.P.T. – Psycholinguistic-Orientated Phonological Therapy* (Fox, 2005). Moreover, the Inconsistency Approach (Fox, 2005) is slowly gaining ground.

Working in Germany

There are currently a number of different professions working in the field of SLP in Germany. The main

TABLE 41-5   Most popular tests for assessing German-speaking children's speech sounds

Tool	Author(s)	SO	PO	IT	Norms
Ravensburger Stammler Prüfbogen	Frank and Grziwotz (1974)	+	–	–	–
Werscherberger Lautprüfbogen	Gey (1976)	+	–	–	–
Stammler Prüfbogen	Metzger (1967)	+	–	–	–
Logo Ausspracheprüfung	Wagner (1994)	–	+	–	–
AVAK – Analyseverfahren zu Aussprachestörungen bei Kindern	Hacker and Wilgermein (2002)	–	+	–	–
ADD – Aachener Dyslalie Diagnostik	Stiller and Tockuss (2000)	–	+	–	–
Patholinguistische Diagnostik von Sprachentwicklungsstörungen	Kauschke and Siegmüller (2002)	–	+	–	–
PAP Pyrmonter Ausspracheprüfung	Babbe (2003)	–	+	–	–
PLAKSS – Psycholinguistische Analyse kindlicher Aussprachestörungen	Fox (2005)	–	+	+	+
Bilderbuch zur Ausspracheprüfung bei Kindern	Hild (2002)	–	+	–	–

*Note. SO = Segment-orientated; PO = Process-orientated; IT = Inconsistency Test

group, *Logopäden* (equivalent to SLP), treat people with all kinds of communication impairments. Their training at colleges or polytechnics is vocational and they do not gain a university degree. As yet, only one university of applied sciences for SLP offers a BSc degree in SLP. All referrals to *Logopäden* come from pediatricians, ear-nose-and-throat specialists, phoniatrists, or neurologists. *Logopäden* mostly work freelance or are employed in private surgeries but also in hospitals and rehabilitation or special language centers. The second group, *Sprachheilpädagogen*, are university trained and may be either be trained for working in language units, nurseries, and schools for speech- and language-impaired children, or also work in clinics as *Logopäden* do. Additional professionals are *Atem-, Sprech- und Stimmlehrer, Patho- or Clinical Linguists,* or *Klinische Sprechwissenschaftler.* Speech therapy costs are covered by the national and private medical insurances. For information about Austria, Switzerland, Liechtenstein, and South Tyrol, see the list of Web sites in the Resources section.

In order to work in Germany as an SLP, it is necessary to apply for a certificate that proves one's qualification as a *Staatlich anerkannter Logopäde.* Depending on the *Bundesland* 'federal state' one wants to work in, a different institution is responsible for issuing the certificate. It can be the *Amt für Gesundheit und Soziales* (e.g., in Hamburg) or the *Regierungspräsident* (e.g., in North-Rhine Westphalia or Hesse). Membership in a professional body such as the *dbl (Deutscher Bundesverband für Logopädie e.V.)* is not compulsory. An annual conference is held by both professional bodies of speech and language therapy, the *dbl* and the *dbs (Deutscher Bundeverband der akademischen Sprachtherapeuten e.V.).* Both also publish a journal: the dbl, the *Forum Logopädie* and the dbs, *Die Sprachheilarbeit.* The dbl is a member of the CPLOL (http://www.cplol.org), the *Standing Liaison Committee of Speech and Language Therapists/Logopedists in the European Union,* which also hosts a conference every two years.

PHONETICALLY SPEAKING

Pronunciation of German: Deutsch: [dɔɪtʃ]
Relevant words for speech assessment and intervention

Word/Phrase	Formal usage	Pronunciation	Informal usage	Pronunciation
Tongue	*Zunge*	/tsʊŋə/	*Zunge*	/tsʊŋə/
Teeth	*Zähne*	/tsæːnə/	*Zähne*	/tsæːnə/
Lips	*Lippen*	/lɪpən/	*Lippen*	/lɪpən/
Hard palate	*Harten Gaumen*	/haːtɐ gaumən/	*Harten Gaumen*	/haːtɐ gaumən/
Soft palate	*Velum*	/veːlʊm/	*Weicher Gaumen*	/vaɪçɐ gaumən/
Larynx	*Larynx*	/laːʁɪŋks/	*Kehlkopf*	/keːlkɔpf/
Lungs	*Lunge*	/lʊŋə/		/lʊŋə/
Nose	*Nase*	/naːzə/		/naːzə/
Sound	*Laut*	/laut/		/laut/
Word	*Wort*	/vɔɐt/		/vɔɐt/
Sentence	*Satz*	/zats/		/zats/
Paragraph	*Absatz*	/apzats/		/apzats/

RESOURCES

Books

König, W. (1994). *dtv-Atlas zur deutschen Sprache.* München: Deutscher Taschenbuch Verlag.

Journals

- *Forum Logopädie,* http://www.dbl-ev.de/service/forum_logopaedie.shtml A clinical journal published by the *dbl.*
- *Die Sprachheilarbeit,* http://www.dbs-ev.de/index2.htm A clinical journal published by *dbs* and *dgs.*
- *Sprache-Stimme-Gehör,* http://www.thieme.de/fz/ssg/ An international research journal published by Thieme in conjunction with the DGPP, the German Society of Phoniatrics and Pedaudiology.
- *L.O.G.O.S Interdisziplinär,* http://www.elsevier-deutschland.de/artikel/647568 A clinical journal published by Elsevier Publishers in cooperation with researchers in the field.

Professional associations

The **German** professional association of speech and language pathologists 'Logopäden' is the *dbl*, the *Deutsche Bundesverband für Logopädie e.V.,* http://www.dbl-ev.de.

The **German** professional association of speech and language therapists 'Sprachheilpädagogen' is the *dbs*, the *Deutscher Bundeverband der akademischen Sprachtherapeuten-e.V.,* http://www.dbs-ev.de.

The **Austrian** professional association of speech and language therapists is the *Bundesverband Diplomierte LogopädInnen Österreich,* http://www.dla.at.

The **German-speaking Swiss** professional association of speech and language therapists is the *DLV Deutschschweizer Logopädinnen- und Logopäden-Verband,* http://www.logopaedie.ch.

The professional association of speech and language therapists in **Liechtenstein** is the *Berufsverband der Logopädinnen und Logopäden Liechtensteins,* e-mail: isabelle.kratochwil@powersurf.li.

Universities offering courses in Speech-Language Pathology/Logopädie in Germany

So far in Germany and Austria, the majority of courses leading to a degree in SLT are nonuniversity degrees. They are gained from *Berufsfachschulen* offering a three-year college degree (a list of colleges can be found at http://www.logo-ausbildung.de/schulen). Currently, only one private university in Germany offers a four-year Bachelor of Health in Speech Therapy in accordance with the Bologna Agreement and international standards (University of Applied Sciences Fresenius, Idstein, http://www.fh-fresenius.de). College-trained speech therapists can continue their education currently at four different universities and gain a BSc or BA in Speech Therapy (University of Applied Sciences Hildesheim/Holzminden/Göttingen, http://www.fh-hildesheim.de, University of Applied Sciences Europa Fachhochschule Fresenius, http://www.fh-fresenius.de, University of Applied Sciences Oldenburg/Ostfriesland/ Wilhelmshafen, http://www.fh-oow.de), or a *Diplom* (equivalent to MA) in Lehr- und Forschungslogopädie at Aachen University, http://www.rwth-aachen.de/zentral/sul_logopaedie.htm.

Useful German Web sites

- *About: German language Essential German,* http://www.german.about.com/library/blessent.htm
- *Startseite des IDS Mannheim,:* http://www.ids-mannheim.de
- *Languages online: German,* http://eleaston.com/german.html

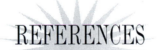

REFERENCES

Ament, W. (1899). *Entwicklung von Sprechen und Denken.* Leipzig: Verlag von Ernst Wunderlich.

Babbe. T. (2003). *PAP—Pyrmonter Aussprache Prüfung.* Köln: Prolog.

Berg, T. (1992). Phonological harmony as a processing problem? *Journal of Child Language, 19,* 225–257.

Brunner, E. (1994). *Phonologische Prozesse bei sprachunauffälligen Vorschulkindern.* Unpublished MA thesis, Karl-Franzens Universität, Graz.

Crystal, D. (1997). *Encyclopedia of language.* Cambridge, UK: Cambridge University Press.

Dodd, B. (1995). *Differential diagnosis and treatment of children with speech disorder.* London: Whurr.

Elsen, H. (1991). *Erstspracherwerb—Der Erwerb des deutschen Lautsystems.* Wiesbaden: Deutscher Universitäts Verlag.

Fongaro-Leverin, S. (1992). *Der Erwerb des Lautsystems und die Phonologischen Prozesse sich normal entwickelnder Kinder: Ein Interlinguistischer Vergleich Deutsch/Portugiesisch.* Unpublished PhD thesis, Ludwig-Maximilian-Universität, München.

Fox, A. V. (2005). *Kindliche Aussprachestörungen—Phonologische Entwicklung, Differentialdiagnostik und Therapie* (3rd ed.). Idstein: Schultz Kirchner Verlag.

Fox, A. V., and Schäfer, B. (2006). Phonologieerwerb deutschsprachiger Kinder- ergänzende Daten. Manuscript submitted for publication.

Fox, A. V., and Dodd, B. J. (1999). Der Erwerb des phonologischen Systems in der deutschen Sprache. *Sprache - Stimme - Gehör, 23,* 183–191.

Frank, G., and Grziwotz, P. (1974). *Lautprüfbogen.* Ravensburg: Ravensburger Sprachheilzentrum Selbstverlag.

Fricke, S. (2005). *Average phonological awareness skills of German preschool children.* Unpublished master's dissertation, Sheffield University, Sheffield, UK.

Gey, M. (1976). *Werscherberger Lautprüfbogen.* Oldenburg: Prull.

Grijzenhout, J., and Joppen, S. (1998). *First steps in the acquisition of German phonology: A case study.* Düsseldorf: Heinrich-Heine-Universität.

Grohnfeldt, M. (1980). Erhebung zum altersspezifischen Lautbestand bei drei- bis sechsjährigen Kindern. *Die Sprachheilarbeit, 5,* 169–177.

Hacker, D., and Wilgermein, H. (2002). *AVAK-Test: Analyseverfahren zu Aussprachestörungen bei Kindern.* (2nd. ed.) München: Ernst Reihnhardt Verlag.

Hacker, D., and Wilgermein, H. (1999). *Aussprachestörungen bei Kindern.* München - Basel: Ernst Reinhardt Verlag.

Hartmann, E. (2002). *Möglichkeiten und Grenzen einer präventiven Intervention zur phonologischen Bewusstheit von lautsprachgestörten Kindergartenkindern.* Fribourg: Sprachimpuls.

Hild, U. (2002). *Bilderbuch zur Ausspracheprüfung bei Kindern.* Kassel: Orca.

Howell, J., and Dean, E. (1995). *Treating phonological disorders in children - Metaphon - theory to practice* (2nd ed.). London: Whurr.

Jahn, T. (2000). *Phonologische Störungen bei Kindern - Diagnostik und Therapie.* Stuttgart: Thieme Verlag.

Jassem, W. (1952). *Intonation of conversational English.* Wroklaw: Nakl Wroclawskiego Tow.

Jassem, W., and Gibbon, D. (1980). Re-defining English stress. *Journal of the International Phonetic Association, 10,* 2–16.

Kauschke, C., and Siegmüller, J. (2002). *Psycholinguistische Diagnostik von Sprachentwicklungsstörungen.* München: Urban & Springer.

Kohler, K. (1995). *Einführung in die Phonetik* (2nd ed.): Berlin: Erich Schmidt Verlag.

König, W. (1994). *dtv-Atlas zur deutschen Sprache.* München: Deutscher Taschenbuch Verlag.

Krüger, B. (1998). *Produktionsvariabilität im frühen Lauterwerb: Eine Typologie kindlicher Abweichungen von Modellwörtern.* Unpublished PhD thesis, Christian-Albrechts-Universität, Kiel.

Lammer, V., and Kalmar, M. (2004). *WIELAU-T, Wiener Lautprüfverfahren für Türkisch sprechende Kinder.* Wien: Lernen mit Pfiff.

Lleò, C., and Prinz, M. (1996). Consonant clusters in child phonology and the directionality of syllable structure assignment. *Journal of Child Language, 23,* 31–56.

Meinhold, G., and Stock, E. (1980). *Phonologie der deutschen Gegenwartssprache.* Leipzig: VEB Bibliographisches Institut.

Metzker, H. (1967). Stammler-Prüfbogen. *Die Sprachheilarbeit, 3,* 89–95.

Möhring, H. (1938). Lautbildungsschwierigkeit im Deutschen. *Zeitschrift für Kinderforschung, 47,* 186–235.

Penner, Z. (2003, January). *Zwischen Forschung und Praxis. Die Grundlagen eine bereichsspezifischen Frühintervention.* Paper presented at the 4. Wissenschaftliches Symposion des dbs e.V.: Früh genug, zu früh, zu spät?, Fulda.

Penner, Z., and Fischer, A. (submitted). Very early babbling and the emergence of the trochaic feet.

Piske, T. (1998). *Artikulatorische Muster und ihre Entwicklung im L1-Lautwerwerb.* Kiel: Christian-Albrechts-Universität.

Romonath, R. (1991). *Phonologische Prozesse an sprachauffälligen Kindern, eine vergleichende Untersuchung an sprachauffälligen und nichtsprachauffälligen Vorschulkindern.* Berlin: Edition Marhold.

Saben, C. B., and Ingham, J. C. (1991). The effects of minimal pairs treatment on the speech sound production of two children with phonologic disorders. *Journal of Speech and Hearing Research, 34,* 1023–1040.

Schäfer, B., and Fox, A. V. (in press). The acquisition of word production consistency in German-speaking two-year olds. *Sprache-Stimme-Gehör*

Stenzel, S. (1999). *The development of phonological awareness skills in German-speaking children (aged 3-6 years) and cross-linguistic comparisons with normative Australian data.* Unpublished MSc thesis, Department of Speech, Newcastle University, Newcastle upon Tyne, UK.

Stern, C., and Stern, W. (1928). *Die Kindersprache.* Darmstadt: Wissenschaftliche Buchgesellschaft.

Stiller, U., and Tockuss, C. (2000). *ADD - Aachener Dyslalie Diagnostik - Artikulationsprüfung mit 98 Photos auf CD-Rom.* Braunschweig: Schubi.

Ternes, E. (1987). *Einführung in die Phonologie.* Darmstadt: Wissenschaftliche Buchgesellschaft.

van Riper, C. (1963). *Speech correction: Principles and methods* (4th ed.). New York: Prentice Hall.

Wagner, I. (1994). *Logo-Ausspracheprüfung.* Oldenburg: Logo Verlag für Sprachtherapie GbR.

Wiese, R. (1996). *The phonology of German.* Oxford, UK: Claredon Press.

SUMMARY OF STUDIES OF TYPICAL GERMAN SPEECH ACQUISITION

Authors	Year	Country	No. of children	Age of children	Information	Sample type	Data collection
Ament	1899	Germany	1	0;6–2;2	Phonological processes	Connected Speech	Longitudinal
Berg	1992	Germany	1	2;7–2;11	Assimilation processes	Connected speech	Longitudinal
Brunner	1994	Austria	20	5;2–6;3	Phonological processes	Picture naming	Cross-sectional
Elsen	1991	Germany	1	0;0–3;0	Consonants Vowels Phonological Processes	Connected speech	Longitudinal
Fongaro-Leverin	1992	Germany	24	2;1–5;0	Consonants Phonological Processes	Single word	Cross-sectional
Fox and Schäfer	2006	Germany	96	3;0–4;5	Phonological processes	Single word	Cross-sectional
Fox and Schäfer	2006	Germany	327	3;0–6;11	Phonological processes	Single word	Cross-sectional
Fox and Schäfer	2006	Germany	29	2;0–2;11	Phonological processes Phoneme inventory	Single word	Cross-sectional
Fox and Dodd	1999	Germany	178	1;6–5;11	Consonants Vowels Clusters Phonological Processes	Single word	Cross-sectional
Grijzenhout and Joppen	1989	Germany	1	1;2–1;8	Optimality theory syllable structure	Connected speech	Longitudinal
Grohnfeld	1980	Germany	319	3;0–6;0	Consonants	Single word	Cross-sectional
Krüger	1998	Germany	8	1;0–2;0	Consonants Articulation pattern	Connected speech	Longitudinal
Lleo and Prinz	1996	Germany	5	0;9–2;1	Clusters	Single word	Longitudinal
Möhring	1938	Germany	2102	6–11 yrs	Consonants	Single word	Cross-sectional
Piske	1998	Germany	8	0;7–1;1	Consonants Articulation pattern	Connected speech	Longitudinal
Romonath	1991	Germany	34	5;3–7;2	Phonological processes	Connected speech	Cross-sectional

Chapter 42

Greek Speech Acquisition

Ineke Mennen and Areti Okalidou

INTRODUCTION

Modern Greek (henceforth Greek) is the descendent of Ancient Greek. It is spoken by most inhabitants of Greece (approximately 11 million speakers) and is the official language of Greece. The linguistic situation in Greece has been characterized by diglossia from the middle of the nineteenth century until 1976. The two varieties of Greek diglossia are called *Katharevousa* and *Dhimotiki*. Katharevousa was created during the early nineteenth century and was the midpoint between Ancient and Modern Greek. It had many archaized forms of modern words and an archaic grammar. Dhimotiki was the variety spoken by Greeks in their daily lives and it became the official language in 1976 when Katharevousa was officially abolished. However, remnants of Katharevousa have remained in the Greek language, particularly in its written form.

Where Greek is spoken

Greek is mainly spoken in Greece and Cyprus (see accompanying map and Appendix D). It is also spoken in some parts of Italy—Southern, east of Reggio; Salento (Colimera, Sternatía, Zollino); and Aspromonte (Bova, Condofuri, Palizzi, Roccoforte, Roghudi)—where dialects of Greek (Salento, Aspromonte) are spoken. It is also spoken in southern Albania, Egypt (Alexandria), Romania, Bulgaria (Sarakatsanika), southern Syria (Hamidye), Lebanon (Tripoli), Turkey (Istanbul city), and in the Ukraine (around Marioupolis—also called Zdanov—and in the Zaporozye district). In addition, it is spoken in Greek immigrant communities in North America (about 1.1 million Americans are of Greek origin), Canada, and Australia.

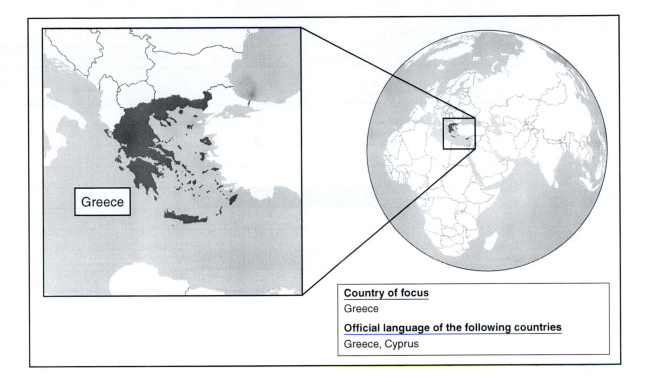

Country of focus
Greece

Official language of the following countries
Greece, Cyprus

Components of Greek

Consonants

Greek has 31 consonants including allophones and affricates and is most closely related to Ancient Greek (see Table 42-1). The voiceless plosives [p, t, k] are unaspirated, and the voiced plosives [b, d, g] are fully prevoiced and sometimes prenasalized [ᵐb, ⁿd, ᵑg] in formal speech depending on personal speaking style and dialect (Arvaniti and Joseph, 2000; Botinis, Fourakis, and Prinou, 2000). The following allophones (bracketed in Table 42-1) appear in Greek: [c, ɟ, ç, ʝ] occur as palatal allophones of /k, g, x, ɣ/ before the front vowels /i/ and /ε/, as in χέρι, κάγγελο, χιόνι, and γιαγιά the Greek words for 'hand' [ˈçeɾi], 'fence' [ˈkɐɟelo], 'snow' [ˈçoni], and 'granny' [jɐˈjɐ] respectively; /ʎ/ and /ɲ/ occur as palatal allophones of /l/ and n/ before a sequence of /i/ and another vowel *within* a single syllable, as in λιοντάρι and μπάνιο the Greek words for 'lion' [ʎoˈdɐɾi] and 'bath' [ˈbɐɲo]; /ɱ, ŋ/ occur as allophones of the nasals /m, n/, which adopt the place of articulation of following fricatives, as in αμφιθέατρο and άγχος, the Greek words for 'amphitheatre' [ɐɱfiˈθeɐtɾo], and 'stress' [ˈɐŋ.xos];

and finally [ᵐb, ⁿd, ᵑg] sometimes occur as allophones of /b, d, g/, as in αμπέλι, πάντα, or αγγούρι the Greek words for 'vineyard' [ɐˈᵐbɛli], 'always' [ˈpɐⁿdɐ], or 'cucumber' [ɐˈᵑguɾi]. The use of prenasalization appears to be in decline, however, as it was found that younger Athenian speakers produce it only rarely (Arvaniti and Joseph, 2000).

Nicolaidis (2001; 2003) has documented the maximum point of contact for productions of lingual consonants by Greek adults using electropalatography (EPG). The frames in Figure 42-1 were selected as representative ones from the Nicolaidis compilation of EPG studies.

Vowels and diphthongs

Greek has five vowels: /i, ε, ɐ, o, u/ (Jongman, Fourakis, and Sereno, 1989) as shown in Table 42-2. Unstressed /i/ and /u/ may be devoiced or elided in casual speech (Dauer, 1980). Furthermore, vowel sequences can sometimes be pronounced as a short diphthong (Arvaniti, 1999a). Examples of such short diphthongs are κλαίει, σκιουράκι, and φράουλα the Greek words for 'cries' (second person singular) [ˈklɛi], 'little squirrel' [sçiuˈɾɐci], and 'strawberry' [ˈfɾɐulɐ].

TABLE 42-1 Consonants produced in Greek

	Bilabial	Labiodental	Dental	Alveolar
Plosive	p b (ᵐp) (ᵐb)		t d	
Nasal	m	(ɱ)	n	
Trill				
Tap or flap				ɾ
Fricative		f v	θ ð	s z
Lateral fricative	■	■		
Affricate				ts dz
Approximant				
Lateral approximant	■	■		l
Consonants (non-pulmonic)				

Black = articulations judged impossible

Based on the International Phonetic Alphabet. Courtesy of the International Phonetic Association (c/o Department of Linguistics, University of Victoria, Victoria, British Columbia, Canada).

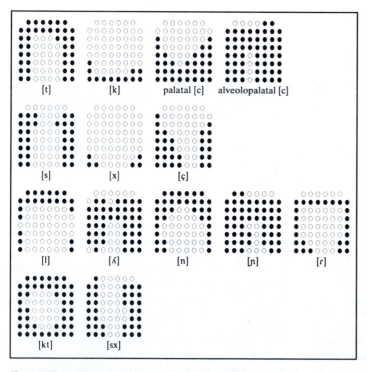

Figure 42-1 Representative sample of EPG studies.
Note: Data from Nilcolaidis (2001).

Phonotactic restrictions

Syllables

The syllable structure of Greek can be described in the formula $C_{(0-3)}VC_{(0-1)}$. Greek, however, has a tendency to have open syllables (Holton, Mackridge, and Philippaki-Warburton, 1998), and most words tend to be bisyllabic or multisyllabic (Setatos, 1974). The vowel /i/ is realized differently depending on its position in the syllable. When /i/ is followed by another vowel *within* the same syllable, the /i/ is pronounced as a voiced (after voiced consonants) or voiceless (after voiceless consonants) palatal fricative, so that the underlying /i/ in κλειδιά the Greek word for 'keys' /kli.ˈðje/ becomes [kli.ˈðjɐ] and the underlying /i/ in αφτιά the Greek word for 'ears' /ɐ.ˈftiɐ/ becomes [ɐ.ˈftçɐ] (e.g., Charalambopoulos, Alvanoudi, Didaskalou, Lambropoulou, and Poulli, 2003). Finally, the /i/ in /m/+/i/+vowel sequences forming one syllable is pronounced as /ɲ/, as in μυαλό the Greek word for 'mind' [mɲɐ.ˈlo] (e.g., Arvaniti, 1999a).

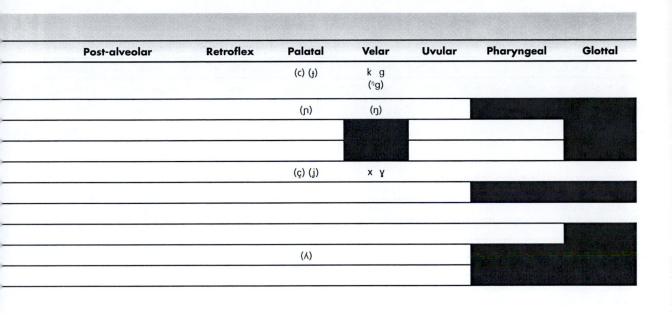

Post-alveolar	Retroflex	Palatal	Velar	Uvular	Pharyngeal	Glottal
		(c) (ɟ)	k g (ᵑg)			
		(ɲ)	(ŋ)			
		(ç) (ʝ)	x ɣ			
		(ʎ)				

Consonants and consonant clusters

Any consonant can occur in syllable-initial position. Consonants in syllable-final word-final position are restricted to /s/ and /n/, except in loanwords (Setatos, 1974) or in remnant words from Katharevousa (Holton et al., 1998) where other final consonants (or clusters) can occur. As a result, many Greek words end in a vowel. Consonants that occur in syllable-final word-within position are mainly /ɾ/, /l/, and /n/ (PAL, 1995). Greek has a number of juncture phenomena, including /n/ deletion, voicing of /s/, and assimilation in certain well-defined contexts. The reader is referred to Arvaniti (1999a) for an overview.

TABLE 42-2	Vowels produced in Greek		
	Front	Central	Back
Close	i		u
Close-mid			o
Open-mid	ɛ		
Open		ɐ	

Setatos (1974) recognizes as many as 65 clusters in syllable-initial and word-initial position. Clusters can appear in word-initial and word-medial position, but are not allowed in word-final position (except in borrowings from Katharevousa and some loanwords). Table 42-3 contains the most common Greek clusters in syllable-initial position. Homorganic sequences are not permissible in Greek (Malikouti-Drachman, 1984), and there is a tendency to convert a sequence of two voiceless fricatives or stops into a fricative plus stop sequence (Newton, 1972; Holton et al., 1998). In /s/-clusters, the /s/ assimilates to the following consonant and becomes voiced before a voiced consonant, as in σβήνω the Greek word for 'erase' /'zvino/. There are also many hetero-syllabic clusters in Greek that can consist of up to four consonant phonemes (Setatos, 1974), such as in εκστρατεία the Greek word for 'crusade' [ɛkstɾɐ'tiɐ].

Tones

Greek does not use tones to differentiate meaning.

Stress and intonation

Greek is a syllable-timed language (Dauer, 1980; Arvaniti, 1994), and its rhythmic characteristics are very similar to

TABLE 42-3 Consonant clusters in syllable-initial position in the word

Syllable-initial		Example	Example	Syllable-initial	Example	Example
/p, b, k, f, v, θ, x, ɣ/	+ /l/	'book'	[vi'vlio]	/z/ + /m, ɣ/	'curly'	[zɣu'rɐ]
/p, b, t, d, k, g, f, v, θ, ð, x, ɣ/	+ /r/	'train'	['trɛno]	/tm/	'department'	['tmimɐ]
/p, k, m, x, ɣ/	+ /n/	'opinion'	['ɣnomi]	/skn/	'midge'	['sknipɐ]
/p, k, f, x/	+ /t/	'money'	[lɛ'ftɐ]	/sc/	'dog'	['scilos]
/p, k/	+ /s/	'fish', 'wood'	[psɐ'ri], ['ksilo]	/pç/	'duck'	['pɐpçɐ]
/s/ + /p, t, k, f, x/		'house'	['spiti]	/bj/	'buttons'	[ku'bjɐ]
/s/ + /p, k/ + /l/		'hard'	[skli'ros]	/tç/, /fç/	'eyes'	['mɐtçɐ]
/s/ + /p, t, f/ + /r/		'eraser'	['ksistrɐ]	/ðj/	'apron'	[po'ðjɐ]

those reported for Italian (Arvaniti, 1994). Main stress falls on one of the last three syllables of a word, and stress placement is mostly determined by morphology. Secondary stress occurs only when words with stress on the antepenult (or penult) are followed by one (or two) enclitic(s) and the additional stress is placed on the penultimate syllable of the word+enclitic group. An enclitic is an unstressed word that is incapable of standing on its own and is phonologically joined at the end of a preceding word to form a single unit. An example of a word with stress on the antepenult is δάχτυλο the Greek word for *finger* ['ðɐxtilo], which when an enclitic such as *my* [mu] is added receives additional stress, as in *my finger* [ˌðɐxti'lomu]. There are several minimal pairs where stress is the only difference between words, for example in κύμα and κιμά the Greek words for 'wave' ['cimɐ] and 'minced meat' (accusative case) [ci'mɐ], or πόδια and ποδιά 'legs' ['poðjɐ] and 'apron' [po'ðjɐ] (Arvaniti, 1999a).

Greek has five pitch accents:

- L*+H (rise from low from the accented syllable to high after the accented syllable; frequently used in nuclear position in calls, imperatives, negative declaratives, and wh-questions)
- L+H* (rise from low to the accented syllable, which is high; often used to signal narrow focus)
- H* (high level from the accented syllable; often used as the nucleus in broad focus declaratives)
- H*+L (a fall from high pitch in the accented syllable, indicating a more nonchalant attitude on the part of the speaker than H*)
- L* (low level from the accented syllable; it appears as the nuclear accent before a continuation rise, in yes/no questions, and in suspicious calls)

The most common of these is the L*+H pitch accent. The pitch accents can be combined with three types of phrase accents and three types of boundary tones to form intonation contours (Arvaniti and Baltazani, 2005). The same authors have developed a transcription system for Greek intonation called GRToBI (Greek Tones and Break Indices), which can be found on the Internet (see the Resources section). For further readings on Greek intonation see Botinis (1989), Mennen and den Os (1993), and Mennen, (1999, 2004).

Writing system

Greek is written in the Greek alphabet, which developed in classical times (ca. ninth century BC). The Greek alphabet has 24 letters as well as an accent mark to indicate stressed vowels in bisyllabic or multisyllabic words and to disambiguate meaning among homorganic monosyllabic words (Holton et al., 1998). Greek spelling is fairly transparent, as in Greek orthography most letters consistently represent the same sound. However, the same sound can be represented by different letters or pairs of letters. For example, there are five different spellings for the sound [i], two different spellings for the sound [o], and two different spellings for the sound [s]. This should make spelling more difficult than reading.

Varieties of Greek

There is consensus (Kontos, 1997; Newton, 1972) that northern dialects are distinguished from southern dialects of Greek, with the exception of the two major cities

(Athens and Thessaloniki), which hardly differ from one another with respect to their phonological features (Newton, 1972). In particular, northern varieties tend to drop unstressed high vowels /i/ and /u/, and to raise the unstressed mid vowels /ɔ/, /ɛ/ to high vowels /i/, /u/ respectively. In southern varieties there is a strong tendency for fronting before the front vowels /i/ and /ɛ/ or before a glide, so that /k/, /x/, /ɣ/ are produced as /c/, /ʃ/, /ʒ/ or sometimes they are produced further forward to become /tʲ/, /s/, /z/ in some dialects.

Cypriot-Greek dialect

Cypriot-Greek (CYG) is a southeastern dialect of Greek and it is spoken on the island of Cyprus. Cypriot-Greek is considered a closer variety to ancient Greek and therefore bears several phonological, lexical, and syntactic differences as compared to Greek (Petinou and Terzi, 2002). The phonological phenomena of the CYG dialect are similar to the ones described above for the southeastern dialect. Note that as in Greek, velar plosives and velar fricatives as well as the glide [l] have palatalized variants when preceding a front high vowel. In sum, the special phonetic characteristics of CYG include:

- All sonorants and voiceless obstruents can geminate in word-initial and word-medial positions (Arvaniti, 1999b; Charalambopoulos, 1982; Tserdanelis and Arvaniti, 2001).

- Consistently prenasalized voiced plosives (Arvaniti, 1999b)
- Both aspirated and unaspirated plosives (Arvaniti, 1999b)
- Post-alveolar sibilants: voiced /ʒ/ and unvoiced /ʃ/ (Newton, 1972)
- Palato-alveolar affricates: voiced /dʒ/ and unvoiced /tʃ/ (Newton, 1972)
- Five vowels: /i, ɛ, ɐ, ɔ, u/. The back mid vowel /ɔ/ is more open than the Greek one, and the /u/ is slightly more peripheral (Arvaniti, 1999b).

Typical acquisition of Greek

The Summary of Studies Table at the end of this chapter contains studies of the acquisition of Greek.

Acquired sounds

Consonants

Table 42-4 contains age of acquisition data for Greek from studies by Magoula (2000), PAL (1995), Papadopoulou (2000), and Thomadaki and Magoula (1998), all of which used the criterion of 75 percent correct production in word-initial, -medial, and -final positions. (Papadopoulou also used the 90 percent criterion.) It should be noted that voicing distinctions are acquired by 2;6 to 3;0 years

TABLE 42-4 Age of acquisition for Greek consonants

Consonant	Magoula (2000)	Thomadaki and Magoula (1998)	PAL (1995)	Papadopoulou (2000)	Papadopoulou (2000)
Criterion	75% criterion	75% criterion	75% criterion	75% criterion	90% criterion
p	1;9–2;2	–	2;6–3;0	3;7–4;0	3;7–4;0
b	2;1–2;2	–	2;6–3;0	3;7–4;0	3;7–4;0
m	1;6–1;8	–	2;6–3;0	3;7–4;0	3;7–4;0
n	1;6–1;8	–	3;0–3;6	3;7–4;0	3;7–4;0
ᵑg	–	–	–	* (4;6)	* (4;6)
j	NA	NA	NA	NA	NA
t	1;5–2;0	–	2;6–3;0	3;7–4;0	3;7–4;0
d	1;6–2;2	–	3;0–3;6	3;7–4;0	3;7–4;0
k	–	–	2;6–3;0	3;7–4;0	3;7–4;0
g	–	–	2;6–3;0	3;7–4;0	3;7–4;0

Table 42-4 continued

x	–	–	3;0–3;6	3;7–4;0	3;7–4;0
f	–	–	3;6–4;0	3;7–4;0	3;7–4;0
l	1;6–1;11	–	3;6–4;0	3;7–4;0	3;7–4;0
ʒ	NA	NA	NA	NA	NA
ʃ	NA	NA	NA	NA	NA
ts	–	–	4;6–5;0	3;7–4;0	4;1–4;6
dz	–	–	4;6–5;0	4;1–4;6	* (4;6)
s	–	–	3;6–4;0	3;7–4;0	* (4;6)
z	–	–	3;6–4;0	3;7–4;0	* (4;6)
r	–	–	5;6–6;0	* (4;6)	* (4;6)
v	2;1–2;6	–	3;0–3;6	3;7–4;0	3;7–4;0
ð	–	–	4;0–4;6	3;7–4;0	4;1–4;6
θ	–	–	4;0–4;6	3;7–4;0	* (4;6)
c	–	–	2;6–3;0	3;7–4;0	* (4;6)
ɟ	–	–	2;6–3;0	4;1–4;6	* (4;6)
ç	–	–	3;0–3;6	4;1–4;6	4;1–4;6
j	–	–	3;0–3;6	3;7–4;0	3;7–4;0
ʎ	–	2;6	4;0–4;6	4;1–4;6	4;1–4;6
ɲ	–	2;6	2;6–3;0	3;7–4;0	3;7–4;0

* = Sound was not acquired at age in parentheses

– = Sound was not tested

NA = Not applicable, i.e., sound does not occur in Greek

old (Magoula, 2000; Okalidou, Petinou, Theodorou, and Karasimou,, 2002). Interestingly, palatal allophones /ʎ/, /ɲ/ attain proper use (that is, as allophonic variations in certain contexts) only after the alveolar consonants /l/ and /n/ are acquired, even though /ʎ/ and /ɲ/ appear earlier in children's phonetic repertoire (Magoula, 2000). Also note that for some consonants the reported ages of acquisition differ between the different studies, most notably for the phonemes of /n/, /d/, /l/, /ts/, /v/, /ʎ/, and /ɲ/. This may be due to the differences in sample size and/or sample task.

Consonant clusters

Table 42-5 contains data for age of consonant cluster acquisition from studies by PAL (1995) and Papadopoulou (2000). Both of these studies used the criterion of 75 percent correct production regardless of the position in the word. Due to the high number of clusters in Greek, both studies had tested only a restricted number of clusters. The most active period of cluster acquisition was between 3;6 and 4;6, when most of the two-element clusters with /s/, the clusters consisting of plosive/fricative + /l/, most of the nasal clusters, and clusters with /r/ were acquired. Interestingly, PAL observed that children often acquire two-element clusters with /r/ before they have acquired /ɾ/ as a singleton. This finding was corroborated by Papadopoulou (2000). Cluster acquisition was not complete by the age of 6;0, when most three-element clusters and clusters with palatal fricatives have not been acquired yet. Tzakosta (2001)—not represented in the table—reported a longitudinal case study on the development of consonant clusters in a 2;1- to 2;9-year-old boy. At age 2;9, the acquired clusters consisted of less marked

TABLE 42-5 Age of acquisition for Greek consonant clusters

Consonant cluster	PAL (2000)	Papadopoulou (2000)	Consonant cluster	PAL (1995)	Papadopoulou (2000)
sp	3;6–4;0	–	fr	–	4;1–4;6
st	4;0–4;6	–	vr	4;6–5;0	4;1–4;6
sk	4;0–4;6	–	ɣr	5;0–5;6	* (4;6)
sc	4;0–4;6	3;7–4;0	θr	5;6–6;0	* (4;6)
sf	4;6–5;0	4;1–4;6	ðr	5;6–6;0	* (4;6)
sx	* (6;0)	4;1–4;6	pç	3;6–4;0	–
pl	3;6–4;0	3;7–4;0	bj	* (6;0)	–
kl	3;6–4;0	3;7–4;0	tç	* (6;0)	–
fl	4;0–4;6	3;7–4;0	ðj	4;0–4;6	–
vl	3;6–4;0	3;7–4;0	zm	4;0–4;6	–
ɣl	5;0–5;6	4;1–4;6	zɣ	4;6–5;0	–
ft	4;6–5;0	3;7–4;0	pn	3;6–4;0	–
st	–	3;7–4;0	kn	3;6–4;0	–
xt	4;0–4;6	3;7–4;0	mn	4;0–4;6	–
ps	4;0–4;6	4;1–4;6	xn	4;6–5; 0	4;1–4;6
ks	4;0–4;6	4;1–4;6	vɣ	3;6–4;0	3;7–4;0
pr	–	4;1–4;6	spr	–	* (4;6)
br	–	4;1–4;6	str	5;0–5;6	* (4;6)
tr	4;0–4;6	* (4;6)	sfr	–	* (4;6)
dr	4;6–5;0	* (4;6)	xtr	5;6–6;0	–
kr	4;0–4;6	4;1–4;6	ftç	* (6;0)	–

* = Sound was not acquired at age in parentheses

– = Sound was not tested

consonant elements in both word-initial and word-medial positions. Three-element consonant clusters were reduced to two-element consonant clusters. Some easy consonant clusters were /ft/, /vɣ/, /fç/, /vl/, /ðj/, /xt/, /ɣm/. In case of multisyllabic words containing more than one cluster, the child first began to retain the one that occurred word-medially unless the word-initial cluster had fewer consonants. Also, clusters were retained more easily in stressed than unstressed syllables.

Vowels and diphthongs

Papadopoulou (2000) found that by the age of 4;0, 90 percent of children had acquired all five Greek vowels.

Percent correct

Consonants

To date there is no study of percentage of consonants produced correctly.

Consonant clusters

To date there is no study of percentage of consonant clusters produced correctly.

Vowels

To date there is no study of percentage of vowels produced correctly.

Phonological processes

Magoula (2000) reported the following processes between 1;6 and 2;0 years of age: reduplication, consonant harmony, final consonant deletion, and cluster reduction. PAL (1995) reports the following processes. Between 2;6 and 3;0 years of age cluster reduction, consonant deletion, final consonant deletion, consonant harmony, metathesis/migration, fronting, backing, and stopping were common. Between 3;0 and 3;6 consonant deletion, fronting, and backing were declining, and between 3;6 and 4;0 consonant harmony and stopping were declining while some clusters were appearing (except /r/ clusters). Between 4;0 and 5;0 syllable reduction, metathesis/migration, and final consonant deletion were declining, and /r/ clusters were appearing. Between 5;0 and 5;6 three-element clusters were appearing. Between 5;6 and 6;0 all three-element clusters except /ftç/ were acquired in syllable-initial word-initial position.

With respect to the process of consonant harmony, partly different findings were obtained by another study (Papadopoulou, 2000), which found that it was still present in 83 percent of children between 3;7 and 4;0, and in 63 percent of children between 4;1 and 4;6.

Intelligibility

To date there is no study of intelligibility of Greek-speaking children.

Phonetic inventory

Table 42-6 shows the phonetic inventory of Greek children from the ages of 1;5 to 2;6 (Magoula, 2000) and 3;7 to 4;6 (Papadopoulou, 2000), presenting sounds that were produced by at least 75 percent of the children in the sample. The highlighted sounds represent the newly acquired sounds at each age level. In general, it appears that the first sounds produced by Greek children are plosives, nasals, and glides at bilabial and alveolar places of articulation. Then, velar plosives, their palatal allophones, and labiodental fricatives are produced, which subsequently are followed by dental fricatives and the liquid /ɹ/. By the age of 4;6 the majority of sounds have emerged, with the exception of [ɟ].

Common mismatches

During the period between 1;6 and 2;0 years of age, Magoula (2000) indicates that /j/ acts as a "default," substituting for a variety of other consonants. Later on, between 3;7 and 4;6 years of age, Papadopoulou (2000) reports on some other common mismatches. Greek children frequently substituted /ɾ/ with [l]. This particular mismatch is also frequently observed in children speaking Italian, Hindi, Igbo, Portuguese, Quiche, and Spanish (Bortoloni and Leonard, 1991). Another common mismatch was the substitution of /ɟ/ by [g]. The affricates /ts/ and /dz/ were mainly substituted by the alveolar fricatives /s/ and /z/ respectively. Substitutions of fricatives were common; /s/ was mostly substituted by [ɬ], /z/ mostly by [ʐ], /s/ and /ð/ by [z]. Finally, the lateral approximant /ʎ/ was mostly substituted by [j].

Syllable structure

A few studies have investigated the development of syllable structure in Greek (e.g., Kappa 2002; Tzakosta, 2005). Kappa (2002) reported a case study of a girl aging from 1;7 to 3;0 years old. Her first word productions attempted to preserve a minimum prosodic form of words and were usually bisyllabic (CVCV) but often also trisyllabic with reduplicated syllables. She used exclusively open syllables (CV) with simple consonant onsets and avoided onsetless

TABLE 42-6 Phonetic inventory of Greek children

Ages 1;5–1;8	Ages 1;9–2;0	Ages 2;1–2;2	Ages 2;3–2;6	Ages 3;7–4;0	Ages 4;1–4;6
p, d, t	p, d, t	p, d, t	p, d, t	p, d, t	p, d, t
m, n, l, j	m, n, l, j	m, n, l, j	m, n, l, j	m, n, l	m, n, l
	b, k, c, v	b, k, c, v	b, k, c, v	b, k, c, v	b, k, c, v
		f	f, ð, ɹ	f, ð, r, g	f, ð, r, g
				θ, s, z, ç, x, ɣ, ɲ, ʎ, ts	θ, s, z, ç, x, ɣ, j, ɲ, ʎ, ts
					dz

Key Note. Data from Magoula (2000) and Papadopoulou (2000). The highlighted sounds represent the newly acquired sounds at each age level.

syllables (V) either by inserting an initial consonant (CVCV) or by deleting the onsetless syllable. For words containing clusters she simplified her output by retaining the less sonorous element. Syllable reductions in multisyllabic words were made by preserving the trochaic two-syllable pattern (first syllable stressed and a final unstressed syllable). However, Tzakosta (2005) provided evidence that despite the multisyllabic nature of Greek, children aged from 1;7 to 3;6 years old also produce monosyllabic truncations with 0.4–16.8 percent occurrence.

Prosody

To date there is no study of Greek children's prosody.

Phonological awareness

Longitudinal studies by Porpodas and colleagues provided evidence for the significance of syllable and phoneme awareness in Greek literacy acquisition (e.g., Porpodas, 1993). Generally, it is affirmed that, in contrast with English, a substantial degree of phonological awareness is gained as early as 7 years, and accounts posit the orthographic transparency of the Greek language (e.g., Nikolopoulos and Goulandris, 2000). Aidinis and Nunes (2001) have shown that syllable awareness precedes phoneme awareness, with performance in both tasks varying as a function of word length, stress, and position for ages 5;2 to 5;11, 6;1 to 6;11 and 7;1 to 7;11. Indicatively, syllable awareness at initial position was 73 percent for 5-year-olds, 92 percent for 6-year-olds, and 100 percent for 7-year-olds. Consonants yielded better results than vowels. Nikolopoulos, Goulandris, and Snowling (2003) demonstrated that performance for 7-year-olds (grade 2) decays for more cognitively elaborate tasks such as phoneme counting (87 percent), phoneme substitution (80 percent), consonant segmentation (65 percent), and spoonerisms (48 percent).[1]

Speech assessment for Greek children

To date the only available test for speech assessment is the *Assessment of Phonetic and Phonological Development* (PAL, 1995), which is an adaptation of Grunwell's (1985) *Phonological Assessment of Child Speech* (PACS). However, SLPs in Greece also use informal/homemade single-word tests and conversational speech sampling during assessment. No studies have so far documented professional practices on speech assessment. Also, no additional speech sampling tools have been developed for use with Greek children. However, some standardized tests contain sections for speech (PAL, 2005; Paraskevopoulos, Kalatzi-Azizi, and Giannitsas, 1999).

Speech intervention for Greek children

No studies have so far investigated the speech intervention practices in Greece. However, these are some commonly used intervention approaches:

- Traditional articulation therapy (Van Riper and Erickson, 1996)
- Minimal pair therapy (Weiner, 1981)
- Core vocabulary (Bradford and Dodd, 1997)

Working in Greece

It is estimated that over 700 SLPs currently practice in Greece, of whom only 55 to 75 are employed in the public sector, in either health or education facilities. Yet, the legislation for professional licensing is pending. Many SLPs were educated abroad, mainly in Europe or the USA. At an undergraduate level, there are two accredited speech therapy courses in Greece, at the Technological Institute (ATEI) of Patras and at the ATEI of Ioannina (the former established earlier, in 1996). There are no accredited undergraduate courses at any of the Greek universities or in any of the major cities (e.g., Athens, Thessaloniki). At a graduate level, two master's programs have recently been developed with a focus on special education issues. Finally, speech pathology courses are currently being taught in other university departments, an education and a medical department. There are three independent professional organizations. SLPs are employed in hospitals, semi-public health institutions (i.e. PIPKA), psychiatric health centers, school centers for diagnosis, assessment, and support (KDAY), and special schools, but the majority engage in private practice. PAL publishes a clinical journal and holds an annual conference and several professional workshops. (See the Resources section for more on the foregoing).

---

1 Higher performance for spoonerisms (70 percent) was obtained by Nikolopoulos and Goulandris (2000) testing a larger sample of 7-year-olds.

PHONETICALLY SPEAKING

Pronunciation of Greek ελληνικά: [ɛliniˈke]

Relevant words for speech assessment and intervention

Word/Phrase	Greek word	Pronunciation
Tongue	γλώσσα	[ˈɣlose]
Teeth	δόντια	[ˈðondje]
Lips	χείλια	[ˈxiʎe]
Hard palate	σκληρή υπερώα	[skliˈri ipeˈroe]
Soft palate	μαλθακή υπερώα	[melθeˈki ipeˈroe]
Larynx	λάρυγγας	[ˈleriⁿges]
Lungs	πνευμόνια	[pnevˈmoɲe]
Nose	μύτι	[ˈmiti]
Sound	ήχος	[ˈixos]
Word	λέξη	[ˈleksi]
Sentence	πρόταση	[ˈprotesi]
Paragraph	παράγραφος	[peˈreɣrefos]

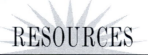

RESOURCES

Books

Botinis, A. (1989). *Stress and prosodic structure in Greek.* Lund: Lund University Press.

Holton, D., Mackridge, P., and Philippaki-Warburton, I. (1997). *Greek: A comprehensive grammar of the modern language.* London: Routledge.

Joseph, B., and Philippaki-Warburton, I. (1986). *Modern Greek.* London: Croom Helm.

Journals

• *Glossologia.* http://www.leaderbooks.com/. Glossologia focuses on synchronic and diachronic studies of the Greek language (on any research domain: phonetics-phonology, morphology, syntax, semantics, pragmatics, etc.).

• *Epikoinonia* (language, speech, voice). http://www. logopedists.gr. Epikoinonia is a clinical journal where professionals publish current information, ideas, and research updates from international literature.

Professional associations

The most established professional association of speech-language pathologists within Greece is the Panhellenic Association of Logopedists. There is also a smaller organization of Special Educators-Logotherapists educated in Germany and an organization by graduates of the technological institutions of Greece.

Universities offering courses in speech pathology in Greece

Department of Psychiatry, Neurology and Social Medicine, Athens Medical School, University of Athens, Athens.

Department of Educational and Social Policy, University of Macedonia, Thessaloniki.

Graduate Program in Special Education-Logotherapy-Counseling, Department of Primary Education, University of Athens, Athens.

Graduate Program in Logotherapy: Intervention in disorders of oral and written language of learning-disabled children. Department of Primary Education, University of Ioannina.

Useful Greek Web sites

- GRToBI (Greek Tones and Break Indices), http://ling.ucsd.edu/~arvaniti/grtobi.html for an overview of Greek intonation and how to transcribe it.
- Πανελλήνιος Σύλλογος Λογοπεδικών (ΠΣΛ), http://logopedists.gr for an overview of speech pathology information
- Pedagogical Institute of the Ministry of Education and Religious Affairs of Greece, http://pi-school.gr for an overview of research and educational programs of the Institute of Education, Ministry of National Education and Religion.

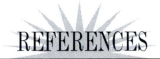

REFERENCES

Aidinis, A., and Nunes, T. (2001). The role of different levels of phonological awareness in the development of reading and spelling in Greek. *Reading and Writing: An Interdisciplinary Journal, 14*, 145–177.

Arvaniti, A. (1994). Acoustic features of Greek rhythmic structure. *Journal of Phonetics, 22*, 239–268.

Arvaniti, A. (1999a). Standard Modern Greek. *Journal of the International Phonetic Association, 29*(2), 167–172.

Arvaniti, A. (1999b). Cypriot Greek. *Journal of the International Phonetic Association, 29*(2), 173–178.

Arvaniti, A., and Baltazani, M. (2005). Intonational analysis and prosodic annotation of Greek spoken corpora. In S-A. Jun (Ed.), *Prosodic typology: The phonology of intonation and phrasing* (pp. 84–117). Oxford, UK: Oxford University Press.

Arvaniti, A., and Joseph, B. (2000). Variation in voiced stop prenasalization in Greek. *Glossologia, 11-12*, 113–166.

Bortoloni, U., and Leonard, L. (1991). The speech of phonologically-disordered children acquiring Italian. *Clinical Linguistics and Phonetics, 5*, 1–12.

Botinis, A. (1989). Stress and prosodic structure in Greek: A phonological, acoustic, physiological and perceptual study. Unpublished Ph.D. dissertation. Lund University.

Botinis, A., Fourakis, M., and Prinou, I. (2000). Acoustic structure of the Greek stop consonants. *Glossologia, 11-12,* 167–199.

Bradford, A., and Dodd, B. (1997). A treatment case study of inconsistent speech disorder. *Australian Communication Quarterly* (Autumn), 24–28.

Charalambopoulos, A. (1982). Consonant "doubling" and aspiration in Cypriot [in Greek]. *Studies in Greek Linguistics, 3,* 237–255.

Charalambopoulos, A., Alvanoudi, A., Didaskalou, M., Lambropoulou, A., and Poulli, A. (2003). Realization in the pronounciation of unstressed /i/ of the phonological sequence C+i+V and influencing parameters [in Greek]. *Studies in Greek Linguistics, 23*(2), 943–952.

Dauer, R. M. (1980). The reduction of unstressed high vowels in Modern Greek. *Journal of the International Phonetic Asscociation, 10,* 17–27.

Grunwell, P. (1985). *Phonological assessment of child speech* (PACS). Windsor: N.F.E.R.- Nelson.

Hatzis, A., Green, P. D., and Howard, S (1997). Optical Logo-Therapy (OLT): A computer based real time visual feedback application for speech training. Proceedings of European conference on speech communication and technology (Eurospeech). Rhodes: ISCA.

Holton, D., Mackridge, P., and Philippaki-Warburton, I. (1998). *Grammar of Greek language* [in Greek]. Athens: Pataki.

Jongman, A., Fourakis, M., and Sereno, J. A. (1989). The acoustic vowels space of Modern Greek and German. *Language and Speech, 32*, 221–248.

Kappa, I. (2002). On the acquisition of syllabic structure in Greek. *Journal of Greek Linguistics, 3*, 1–52.

Kontos, P. (1997). *The phonological analysis of the Etolian dialect.* Athens: National and Kapodistrian University of Athens.

Magoula, E. (2000). *The acquisition of phonological system in Modern Greek: The case of consonants* [in Greek]. Unpublished Ph.D. thesis, University of Athens.

Malikouti-Drachman, A. (1984). Syllables in Modern Greek. In W. Dressler, W. U. Dressler, H. C. Luschützky, O. E. Pfeiffer, and J. R. Rennison, *Phonologica* (pp. 181–186).Cambridge, UK: Cambridge University Press.

Mennen, I. (1999). *Second language acquisition of intonation: The case of Dutch near-native speakers of Greek.* Unpublished Ph.D. thesis, University of Edinburgh, UK.

Mennen, I. (2004). Bi-directional interference in the intonation of Dutch speakers of Modern Greek. *Journal of Phonetics 32*, 543–563.

Mennen, I., and den Os, E. (1993). On the intonation of several Modern Greek sentences. In I. Philippaki-Warburton, K. Nicolaidis, and M. Sifianou (Eds.), *Themes in Greek Linguistics* (pp. 233–239). Amsterdam: John Benjamins.

Newton, B. (1972). *The generative interpretation of dialect.* Cambridge, UK: Cambridge University Press.

Nicolaidis, K. (1994). Aspects of lingual articulation in Greek: An electropalatographic study. In I. Philippaki-Warburton, K. Nicolaidis, and M. Sifianou (Eds.) *Themes in Greek linguistics* (pp. 225–232). Amsterdam: John Benjamins.

Nicolaidis, K. (2001). An electropalatographic study of Greek spontaneous speech, *Journal of the International Phonetic Association, 31*(1), 67–85.

Nicolaidis, K. (2003). An electropalatographic study of palatals in Greek [in Greek]. In D. Theophanopoulou-Kontou, C. Lascaratou, M. Sifianou, M. Georgiafentis, and V. Spyropoulos.

Current trends in Greek linguistics [in Greek]. (pp. 108–127). Athens: Patakis.

Nikolopoulos, D., and Goulandris, N. (2000). The cognitive determinants of literacy skills in a regular orthography. In M. Perkins and S. Howard (Eds), *New directions in language development and disorders* (pp. 261–269). New York: Plenum.

Nikolopoulos, D., Goulandris, N., and Snowling, M. (2003). Developmental dyslexia in Greek. In N. Goulandris (Ed.), *Dyslexia in different languages: Cross-linguistic comparison* (pp. 53–57). London: Whurr.

Okalidou, A., Petinou, K., Theodorou, E., and Karasimou, E. (2002). Development of voicing contrasts in stop sounds in Modern Greek and Cypriot Greek children. In C. Clairis (Ed.), *Proceedings of the 5th Colloque International De Linguistique Grecque* (pp. 127–130) Paris: L' Harmattan.

PAL [Panhellenic Association of Logopaedics] (1995). *Assessment of phonetic and phonological development.* Athens: PAL.

PAL [Panhellenic Association of Logopaedics] (2005). *Anomilo 4. Screening test for speech and language disorders for 4 year old children* [in Greek]. Athens: Ellinika Grammata.

Papadopoulou, K. (2000). *Phonological acquisition of Modern Greek.* Unpublished BSc Honours dissertation. University of Newcastle upon Tyne, UK.

Paraskevopoulos, I., Kalatzi-Azizi, A., and Giannitsas, N. (1999). *Athena Test for Assessing Learning Disabilities* [in Greek]. Athens: Ellinika Grammata.

Petinou, K., and Terzi, A. (2002). Clitic misplacement in normally developing and language impaired Cypriot-Greek children. *Language Acquisition, 10,* 1–29.

Porpodas, C. (1993). The relation between phonemic awareness and reading and spelling of Greek words in the first school years. In M. Caretero, M. Pope, R. Simmons, and J. Pozo (Eds.), *Learning and instruction* (Vol. 3, pp. 203–217). Oxford: Pergamon Press.

Setatos, M. (1974). *Phonology of Modern Greek* [in Greek]. Athens: Editions Papazisis.

Thomadaki, E., and Magoula, E. (1998). The acquisition of palatals /ʎ/ and /ɲ/ in Modern Greek. *Studies in Greek Linguistics, 18,* 211–221.

Tserdanelis, G., and Arvaniti, A. (2001). The acoustic characteristics of geminate consonants in Cypriot-Greek. In Y. Aggouraki, A. Arvaniti, J. I. M. Davy, D. Goutsos, M. Karyolaimou, A. Panayotou, A. Papapavlou, P. Pavlou, and A. Roussou (Eds.), *Proceedings of the 4th International Conference on Greek Linguistics* (pp. 29–36). Thessaloniki: University Studio Press.

Tzakosta, M. (2001). The realization of consonant clusters in child speech. *Studies in Greek Linguistics, 21,* 736–746.

Tzakosta, M. (2005). What do truncations consist of? Segmental selection in onosyllabic truncated forms. *Studies in Greek Linguistics, 25,* 595–606.

Van Riper, C., and Erickson, R. L. (1996). *Speech correction: An introduction to speech pathology and audiology* (9th ed.). Boston, MA: Allyn & Bacon.

Weiner, F. (1981). Treatment of phonological disability using the method of meaningful minimal contrast. Two case studies. *Journal of Speech and Hearing Research, 46,* 97–103.

SUMMARY OF STUDIES OF TYPICAL GREEK SPEECH ACQUISITION

Authors	Year	Country	No. of children	Age of children	Information	Sample type	Data collection
Kappa	2003	Cretan	1	1;7–3;0	Development of syllables	Connected speech (spontaneous)	Longitudinal
Magoula	2000	Athenian Greek	4	1;6–2;6	Age of acquisition of consonants	Connected speech (spontaneous + single word)	Longitudinal
Okalidou, Petinou, Theodorou, and Karasimou	2002	Standard Greek (northern and southern) and Cypriot Greek	12	2;0–4;0	Development of voicing	Elicited non-sense words	Cross-sectional
PAL	1995	Athenian Greek	300	2;6–6;0	Age of acquisition of consonants, clusters; phonological process analysis	Single word	Cross-sectional
Papadopoulou	2000	Katerini (northern Greece) Greek	34	3;7–4;6	Age of acquisition of consonants, vowels, clusters; phonological process analysis; error forms	Single word	Cross-sectional
Tzakosta	2005	Athenian Greek	11	1;7–3;0	Segmental selection in monosyllabic truncation forms	Connected speech (spontaneous)	Cross-sectional and Longitudinal
Tzakosta	2001	Cretan Greek	1	2;1–2;9	Consonant clusters	Connected speech (spontaneous)	Longitudinal

Chapter 43

Hungarian Speech Acquisition

Krisztina Zajdó

INTRODUCTION

Hungarian is a Uralic language. It belongs to the Ugric subbranch of the Finno-Ugric language family. Thus, it is one of the few languages of Europe that does not belong to the Indo-European language family. Languages that are most closely related to Hungarian are Vogul (inner name Mansi) and Khanti (also called Hanty, Xanty; inner name Ostyak) spoken in Russia. Other related languages include Finnish and Estonian (for data on the Uralic language family, see Bárczi, Benkő, and Berrár, 1987; for data on Finno-Ugric languages, see Hajdú, 1975).

Other languages spoken in Hungary include Standard German (250,000 speakers in 1988), Bavarian (also called Bayerisch or Bavarian-Austrian; with an estimated 170,000 speakers), Romanian (also called Rumanian, Daco-Romanian, Moldavian; with 100,000 speakers), Slovakian (with 11,000 speakers in 2000), and Slovenian (with 5,000 speakers in 2000). Further, 48,000 speakers use one of the dialects of Romani (also called *Cigány* meaning 'Gypsy'). The four major Romani dialects used include Balkan Romani, Carpathian Romani, Sinte Romani, and Vlah Romani. According to the 2001 Hungarian census data, populations living in Hungary also include native speakers of Bulgarian, Greek, Polish, Croatian, Serbian, Ukrainian, Rusyn (Ruthenian), and Wendic (dialectal Slovenian of the Mura area). Further, an increasing number of Chinese immigrants who have been settling in the country, particularly in the Budapest area, speak various dialects of Chinese as their native language.

Unless noted otherwise, the general descriptions below are of Standard Hungarian, a somewhat idealized form that developed from the Eastern Hungarian dialect when, from the last third of the sixteenth century, Eastern Hungarian became a "high prestige" literary language that shaped Standard Hungarian. Hungarian dialects are characterized by regional variations in pronunciation (and in grammar and vocabulary items, too). Standard Hungarian is the medium of instruction in kindergarten, school, and university. The spelling of Standard Hungarian gives a relatively clear guide to pronunciation. See the Resources section in this chapter for materials pertaining to Hungarian.

Where Standard Hungarian is spoken

The Republic of Hungary is situated in Central Europe. Hungarian is the official language of Hungary (and thus one of the official languages of the European Union). Additionally, in the areas close to the Hungarian borders, it is one of the six official languages in the Vojvodina region of Serbia, one of the two official regional languages in Slovenia, and a regional language in Austria. Hungarian is the first language of an estimated 14–15 million speakers around the world. The largest community of its speakers live in Hungary (9.5 million; 2001 Hungarian census data). Hungarian is called *Magyar* /ˈmɔɟɔr/ by native speakers.

Larger communities of Hungarian speakers are also present in Australia (25,000; Australian census 2001 data; estimated population 65,000), Austria (approximately 22,000; 2001 census data, although there are estimates of 70,000 speakers), Canada (75,000; 2001 Canadian census data), Croatia (17,000), Israel (estimates vary between 10,000 and 70,000), Romania (1.44 million; 2002 Romanian census data), Serbia (284,000; 2002 Serbian census data), Montenegro (Serbia and Montenegro together have an estimated 450,000 speakers), Slovakia (approximately 550,000 to 600,000), Slovenia (approximately 10,000), Ukraine (150,000 according to the 2001 Ukrainian census data), and the USA (118,000 speakers, according to the 2000 U.S. census data). Hungarian speakers are also found in Argentina, Brazil, Venezuela, and other South American countries (population estimates for this region vary between 70,000 and 160,000) Belgium, the Czech Republic, Finland, France, Germany, the United Kingdom, the Netherlands, Italy, Switzerland (population estimate for Western European countries is 260,000 to 270,000), South Africa (estimated population 10,000), and in other parts of the world, living mostly in immigrant groups (see accompanying map and Appendix D).

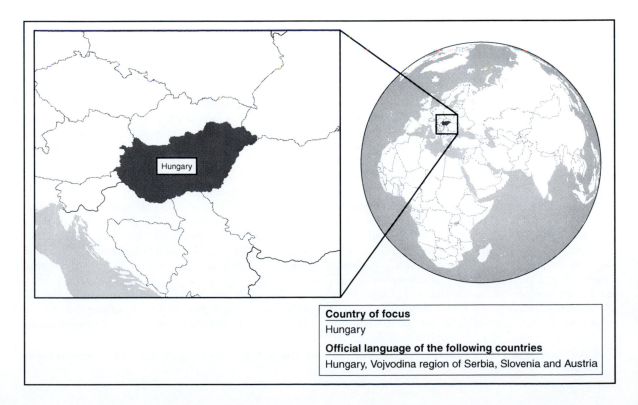

Country of focus
Hungary

Official language of the following countries
Hungary, Vojvodina region of Serbia, Slovenia and Austria

Components of Standard Hungarian

Consonants

According to Szende's analysis (1999), Standard Hungarian has 25 consonant qualities: /p, b, t, d, k, g, m, n, ɲ, r, f, v, s, z, ʃ, ʒ, h, ts, dz, tʃ, dʒ, cç, ɟʝ, j, l/. It is important to note that Szende (1999) does not include allophones in his phonological (rather than phonetically oriented) analysis of the consonant inventory. Each of these 25 sounds may appear as either a phonemically short or long consonant. Difference in phoneme length typically signals a difference in meaning (e.g., consider the difference in pronunciation and meaning between *megy* /ˈmɛɟɟ/ (3ʳᵈ sing. 'go') vs. *meggy* /ˈmɛɟɟ/ 'sour cherry'; *hal* /ˈhɔl/ 'fish' vs. *hall* /ˈhɔlː/ (3ʳᵈ sing. 'hear'). Taking into account the difference between the short and long versions of consonants, Szende (1992) concluded that the number of consonants in Standard Hungarian is 50.

However, some linguists (e.g., É Kiss and Papp, 1984; Siptár, 1989, 2003; Siptár and Törkenczy, 2000) argued that the consonant /dz/ appears only in the phonological surface structure but not in the underlying structure. Thus, following this argument, /dz/ does not constitute an individual consonant, at least from a phonological perspective. Accordingly, some would argue that the number of consonant qualities in Standard Hungarian is 24 and the number of all consonants (adding up the number of phonemically short and long consonants) is therefore 48.

Others, however, also include allophones in their phonetically rather than phonologically based analyses. Allophones occur only in certain (rather restricted) sound environments. These elements of the consonant inventory that are considered "combinatorial variants," (Kassai, 1998; p. 117) include the sounds /ɱ, ŋ, ç, x́, x, ɦ/ (Kassai, 1998). The voiced labiodental nasal /ɱ/ is realized as an allophone of /m/ and /n/ before labiodentals (e.g., *dámvad* /ˈdãːɱvɔd/ 'fallow-deer'; *szenvedés* /ˈsɛ̃ɱvɛdeːʃ/ 'suffering'). The voiced velar nasal /ŋ/ is produced before velar plosives (e.g., *rönk* /ˈrõŋk/ 'log'; *hang* /ˈhõŋg/ 'voice'. The voiceless palatal fricative /ç/ is produced in syllable-final position after voiceless consonants (e.g., *lökj* /ˈløkç/ ('push', 2ⁿᵈ sing. present imperative, indefinite verb conjugation). The voiceless palatovelar fricative /x́/ is produced before high vowels (e.g., *düh* /ˈdyx́/ 'fury'). The voiceless velar fricative /x/ is produced in two positions: (a) in

word-medial position when followed by a consonant (e.g., *ihlet* /ˈixlɛt/ 'inspiration') and (b) in a word-final position when realized after a non-high back vowel (e.g., *potroh* /ˈpotrox/ 'abdomen of insects'). Note that a word-final /h/ may be completely deleted (e.g., méh /mẽː/ 'bee'). The voiced glottal fricative /ɦ/ shows up in two positions: (a) occasionally, word-initially (e.g., *harang* /ˈɦɔrõŋg/ 'bell') and (b) in an intervocalic position (e.g., *suhogás* /ˈʃuɦogaːʃ/ 'rustling').

Gósy (2004) also lists the consonants /ɣ, ʝ/ as members of the inventory (while she does not postulate the existence of /x́/ as an allophone). The voiced velar fricative /ɣ/ is produced in intervocal position (e.g., *mohos* /ˈmoɣoʃ/ 'moss-grown' (adj.)). The voiced palatal fricative shows up in interconsonantal position when the surrounding consonants are voiced (e.g., *szabj bele* /ˈsɔbʝbɛlɛ/ 'tailor' 2ⁿᵈ sing. present imperative, indefinite verb conjugation + in). Validly, Gósy points out that the allophones /ɱ, ŋ, ʝ, ç, ɣ, ɦ/ occur only as phonemically short (but not long) consonant variations (p. 82).

The status of the affricates /cç/ and /ɟʝ/ within the consonant inventory has been debated. When constructing the IPA chart showing the Standard Hungarian consonant inventory, Szende (1999) used the symbols /cç/ and /ɟʝ/ for the voiceless and voiced palatal affricates, respectively, thereby emphasizing the properties of these complex speech sounds that validate the argument to enlist them as affricates. However, other linguists (e.g., Nádasdy and Siptár, 1989; Siptár, 1989) have argued that these affricates are closer with respect to their production characteristics to plosives and therefore should be considered as such. Following this argument, Gósy (2004; p. 83) lists the symbols /c/ and /ɟ/ among plosives. Szende (1999), while arguing for the affricate nature of /cç/ and /ɟʝ/, noted that formal style is characterized by producing the plosive rather than the affricate consonants. The consonant inventory is shown in Table 43-1.

Hungarian voiceless plosives are unaspirated and characterized by a positive voice onset time (VOT), while the voiced ones are prevoiced with a negative VOT (for measures of VOT in Hungarian voiceless plosives in adult speech, see Gósy, 2001; see Figure 43-1 for the bilabial plosives).[1]

The consonant /r/ is realized as a trill. According to Gósy (2004), /r/ is produced by generating only one to two trills in everyday running speech. When generating

---

1 For VOT acquisition data from Hungarian children, see Zajdó (2005) and Stout, Rath, Nickerson, and Zajdó (2006) and the Acquired sounds: Consonants section in this chapter.

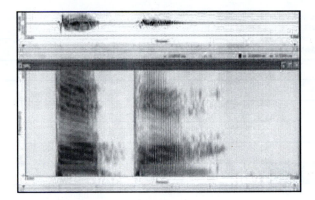

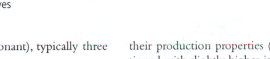

Figure 43-1 Hungarian bilabial plosives

its long counterpart (the /rː/ consonant), typically three trills are realized.

Often, nasals nasalize either the preceding or the following vowel, or both (Gósy, 2004). The dentoalveolar nasal may be deleted before a consonant (Szende, 1999, p. 106) (e.g, vándor /ˈvãːdor/ 'migrant').

Vowels

Hungarian vowels are differentiated along four dimensions: (1) tongue advancement (front, central and back), (2) jaw position (high, half-closed, half-open, or open), (3) rounded or unrounded lip position, and (4) short or long duration (which signals phonological vowel length). Phonological vowel length differentiates meaning (e.g., consider the phonetic, phonological, and semantic difference between *bor* /ˈbor/ 'wine' vs. *bór* /ˈboːr/ 'boron'; *tör* /ˈtør/ 'break' (3ʳᵈ sing.) vs. *tőr* /ˈtøːr/ 'small-sword'; *szint* /ˈsint/ 'level' vs. *szính* /ˈsĩːnt/ 'color' (+ accusative).

The vowel inventory of Standard Hungarian includes 14 monophthongs with nine vowel qualities. The pairs are perceived by native speakers as seven phonological vowel pairs.[2] Since Standard Hungarian does not have lexical diphthongs (although many dialects of Hungarian do), only monophthongs are included in the vowel inventory.[3]

With the exception of duration, the members of five vowel pairs (/i/ vs. /iː/; /y/ vs. /yː/; /u/ vs. /uː/; /ø/ vs. /øː/; and /o/ vs. /oː/) are fairly similar to each other in

their production properties (although long ones are positioned with slightly higher jaw positions and the tenseness in the muscles may be stronger). The remaining two vowel pairs differ both in their quality and quantity: /ɔ/ vs. /aː/ and /ɛ/ vs. /eː/. These vowels are considered pairs from the phonological but not from a phonetic perspective.

In terms of tongue advancement, /i/, /iː/, /y/, /yː/, /ɛ/, /eː/, /ø/, and /øː/ are front vowels, while /u/, /uː/, /o/, /oː/, /ɔ/, and /aː/ are back vowels.

In terms of jaw position, high vowels include /i/, /iː/, /y/, /yː/, /u/, and /uː/. The half-closed vowels are /eː/, /ø/, /øː/, /o/, and /oː/. The half-open vowels include /ɛ/ and /ɔ/. The only open vowel is /aː/.

In terms of lip configuration, front rounded vowels include the vowel pairs /y/ vs. /yː/ and /ø/ vs. /øː/. Back rounded vowels include /u/ vs. /uː/, /o/ vs. /oː/, and /ɔ/ (/ɔ/ is considered slightly rounded by many). Thus, unlike English, Hungarian has both front and back rounded vowels. Implicitly, the vowels /i/, /iː/, /ɛ/, /eː/, and /aː/ are unrounded. In comparison to English, Hungarian rounded vowels are produced with a much more pronounced lip rounding (with the exception of /ɔ/).

In terms of duration, short vowels include /i/, /y/, /u/, /ɛ/, /ø/, /o/, and /ɔ/. Long vowels are /iː/, /yː/, /uː/, /eː/, /øː/, /oː/, and /aː/. The average duration difference between short and long vowels is quite pronounced: it has been reported to be around 1:2 (e.g., Kassai, 1979; Tarnóczy, 1974). For a summary of factors

---

2 The vowel system also includes three marginal vowels: /eː, a, ɔː/ that are extremely rare. Thus, these vowels are not included in the vowel inventory.

3 V+V structures do exist, but these vowels constitute separate syllables, e.g., Európa /ˈɛ.u.roː.pɔ/ (Europe). From a phonetic perspective, some of these clusters might be similar to diphthongs, but this question requires further investigation.

TABLE 43-1 Consonants produced in Standard Hungarian

	Bilabial	Labiodental	Dento-alveolar	Alveolar-Post-alveolar
Plosive	p b		t d	
Nasal	m	(ɱ)	n	
Trill			r	
Tap or flap				
Fricative		f v	s z	ʃ ʒ
Lateral fricative	■■■			
Affricate			ts dz*	tʃ dʒ
Approximant				
Lateral approximant	■■■		l	

Based on the International Phonetic Alphabet. Acknowledgement is made to the International Phonetic Association (c/o Department of Linguistics, University of Victoria, Victoria, British Columbia, Canada).

Black = articulations judged impossible

Note. Symbols embedded in parentheses indicate speech sounds (allophones) that are considered by some, but not all, to be members of the consonant inventory.

* Some phonologists do not consider the consonant /dz/ to be an independent phoneme (see Kiss and Papp, 1984; Siptár, 1989).

ᵗ Some argue that /h/ is not a glottal but rather a pharyngeal consonant /ħ/ (see Kassai, 1998, p. 116; Gósy, 2004, p. 79).

affecting vowel length differences, see Zajdó (2002c). See Figure 43-2 and Table 43-2 for vowel properties.

In Hungarian, /ə/ is not an independent phoneme. However, it does appear in cases when physiological constraints are at play. For example, in the word *mágnás* /maːgənaːʃ/ 'magnate' a schwa is produced between the voiced velar plosive and the voiced dentoalveolar nasal as a result of reorganizing tongue configuration while producing voicing.

In terms of vowel reduction, Hungarian is quite resistant to centralization processes. In unstressed position, vowels are somewhat centralized but, in comparison with English, the extent of vowel reduction is small.

Phonotactic restrictions
Syllables

The syllable structure of Standard Hungarian is C0-3VC0-3. That is, the only compulsory element of a syllable is a single vowel (V), for example, 'ő' /øː/ (3rd sing. personal pronoun); filling of the onset is not compulsory. The most complex onset is thus #CCC, such as in the word *strázsa* /ˈʃtraːʒɔ/ 'sentinel'; the most complex coda is CCC# *mihelyst* /ˈmiɦɛjʃt/ 'as soon as'. Common syllable structures include V, VC, CV, CVC, CVV, VV, VVC, CVVC, and VCCV.

Hungarian is an agglutinating language where, by addition of nouns, verbs, prefixes, and suffixes, words can be made up to 10 syllables or more. Commonly used words contain one to four syllables, with the majority (~ 60 percent) containing two syllables. Only 0.2 percent of words have five or more syllables (without prefixes and suffixes; Tompa, 1961).

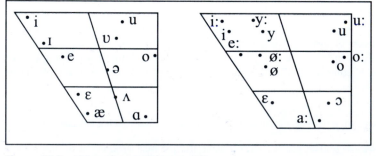

Figure 43-2 Hungarian vowel properties

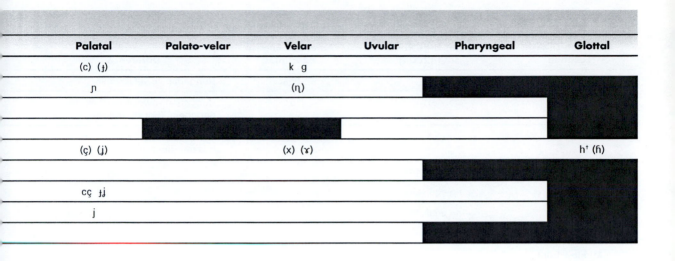

Consonant clusters

Standard Hungarian has a rich inventory of consonant clusters. As many as 50 types of word-initial CC clusters have been identified. Word-initial CCC clusters include /str-/, /skl-/, /ʃpr-/, /ʃtr-/, and /ʃkr-/. Standard Hungarian has 150 types of word-final CC clusters and 18 types of word-final CCC clusters. The number of intervocalic CC clusters well exceeds 200. Twelve types of CCCC clusters appear in monomorphemic items; there is only one word with a word-medial CCCCC cluster (e.g., *angstrom* /ˈɔŋkʃtrøm/ 'Angström').

VV clusters that appear within the same word stem include 40 different types.[4] An additional 100 types of VV clusters that are separated by morpheme boundaries have been identified. For a review on phonotactics, see Siptár and Törkenczy (2000).

Tones

Standard Hungarian does not use tones to differentiate meaning.

Stress and intonation

Hungarian typically uses first-syllable stress on words pronounced in citation form. In special cases (e.g., in some, but not all, compound words), secondary stress can also be used on other syllables (e.g., *kilenc-százkilencven* 'nine hundred and ninety') pronounced /ˈkilentsaːsˌkilentsvẽ/ (see Siptár and Törkenczy, 2000; p. 21). For a detailed analysis of stress patterns, see Varga (2002).

In terms of language-specific intonation patterns, Varga (2002) identified 12 meaningful intonation contours: 11 character contours and one appended contour in Hungarian. He showed that, through a detailed analysis, these 12 basic contour patterns can be reduced to three more basic ones. These basic patterns contain only three tones. In all three patterns, two adjacent tones are identical: the structure of the half falling contour is H*.L.L.§, the high monotone contour contains the elements H*.H.§, and the monotone falling contour is built as H*.H.L.§.

4 Note that, in Standard Hungarian, each vowel constitutes a separate syllable. Thus, VV structures are not diphthongs. See the section on vowels in this chapter.

TABLE 43-2 Vowels produced in Hungarian compared with General American English

American English Location	American English Vowels Smit (2004)	American English examples	Difference
High-front	i	b<u>ea</u>t	Hungarian vowel is similar
	ɪ	b<u>i</u>t	Hungarian vowel is much more peripheral (not centralized)
	e	r<u>ai</u>d	Hungarian vowel is a mid vowel; it is not diphthongized
no equivalent			
no equivalent			
no equivalent			
no equivalent			
Mid-low front	ɛ	b<u>e</u>d	Hungarian vowel is similar
High-back, rounded	u	bl<u>ue</u>	Hungarian vowel is more rounded and more dorsal
	ʊ	b<u>oo</u>k	Hungarian vowel is more rounded and more peripheral
Mid-back, rounded	o	b<u>oa</u>t	Hungarian vowel is more rounded and is not diphthongized
no equivalent			
	ɔ	f<u>or</u>m	Hungarian vowel is produced with a lower jaw position
Low back	ɑ	dr<u>o</u>p	
no equivalent			
[r]-colored	ɝ		
	ɚ	nev<u>er</u>, col<u>or</u>	
	ɪr		
	ɛr		
	ʊr		
	ɔr		
	ar		
Central	ə	<u>a</u>bout, <u>o</u>ccur, <u>u</u>pon,	In Hungarian, /ə/ is not an independent phoneme; it is produced only as a result of physiological constraints (see the text)
	ʌ		
Diphthongs	aɪ	m<u>y</u>, b<u>i</u>ke	
	aʊ	<u>ou</u>t, m<u>ou</u>se	
	ɔɪ	b<u>oy</u>	

Standard Hungarian Location	Standard Hungarian	Standard Hungarian examples	English translation
High-front	iː	gyík /ˈɟjiːk/	lizard
	i	kint /ˈkɪnt/	outside
Mid-low front	eː	lé /ˈleː/	juice
High-front	yː	tű /ˈtyː/	needle
	y	füst /ˈfyʃt/	smoke
Mid-front	øː	őz /øːz/	deer
	ø	pötty /ˈpøcç/	dot
Mid-low front	ɛ	nyelv /ˈɲɛlv/	Tongue/language
High-back, rounded	uː	lúd	goose
	u	juh /ˈju/	sheep
Mid-back, rounded	oː	ló /ˈloː/	horse
	o	bot /ˈbot/	stick
Mid-low back rounded	ɔ	bal /ˈbɔl/	left
	no equivalent		
Low-central, unrounded	aː	ág /ˈaːg/	branch
	no equivalent		
	no equivalent		
	no equivalent		
	no equivalent		
	no equivalent		
	no equivalent		
	no equivalent		
	no equivalent		
	no diphthong in Standard Hungarian		
	no diphthong in Standard Hungarian		
	no diphthong in Standard Hungarian		

For example, the structure of a finished statement is HL̲L̲.§. (The underlined characters indicate a tone that is high or low relative to the preceding one.) Building a yes/no question requires the intonation structure HHL.§. An interrogative question is built up by using the tone elements HH̲L̲.§. The structure of an unfinished statement is HLH.§ (see Chapter 3).

Writing system

The Hungarian writing system, which contains 42 letters, is nearly completely phonemic; thus it is relatively easy to predict pronunciation on the basis of written language. The system is based on the Latin alphabet; however, additional letters such as letters with acute accents (e.g., *á* /aː/, *é* /eː/, *í* /iː/, *ó* /oː/, *ő* /øː/, *ú* /uː/, and *ű* /yː/ [5]) and letters with umlauts (e.g., (ö /ø/ and ü /y/ [6]) are also used. Letter pairs with 'y' as a second element indicate palatalized consonants (e.g., *ny* /ɲ/, *ty* /cç/). However, *ly* is pronounced as /j/. The letter *gy* /ɟ/ is confusing since it is not a palatalized version of the voiced velar plosive; rather, it is a palatalized version of /d/. The letter *s* stands for /ʃ/, the letter pair *sz* represents /s/. *Cs* stands for /tʃ/. The letter pair *zs* should be produced as /ʒ/. Two rarely used letters are *dz* /dz/ and *dzs* /dʒ/. When a long consonant is produced, only the first element of a consonant pair is doubled (e.g., *ssz* should be produced as /sː/).

Varieties of Hungarian

This chapter introduces the reader to the properties of Standard Hungarian. There are 10 major dialects of Hungarian. Seven of these are spoken within the current borders of Hungary and in the areas surrounding the borders, while the other three are spoken in Transylvania, the Hungarian-populated area of Romania (Juhász, 2003). Dialects differ from Standard Hungarian and each other primarily in their vowel (rather than consonant) inventories (Fodor, 2003). Many dialects have several types of diphthongs; some have triphthongs. For the most part, dialects are mutually understandable.

Typical acquisition of Standard Hungarian

To date, very few studies have investigated speech acquisition patterns in children acquiring Standard Hungarian. The Summary of Studies Table at the end of this chapter contains some studies of the acquisition of Standard Hungarian.

Acquired sounds
Consonants

Table 43-3 contains age of acquisition data for Standard Hungarian. Nagy's (1980) data allow us to determine the time when 90 percent of the children he examined (N[3;0] = 155; N[4;0] = 170; N[5;0] = 3,495; N[6;0] = 3,491; N[7;0] = 145; N[8;0] = 146) produce a given consonant correctly. Correct production means that the child produces a consonant correctly, with 100 percent accuracy, in all positions (word-initial, word-medial, and word-final). The study used 23 consonants from the consonant inventory. All consonants were examined as a phonemically short consonant with the

TABLE 43-3   Age of acquisition for Standard Hungarian consonants

Consonant	Age when 90 percent of children produce the sound correctly in all positions	
p	Prior to 3;0 years	At 3;0 years, 93.5 percent of children produce the consonant correctly
b	At around 4;0 years	At 4;0 years, 90.4 percent of children produce the consonant correctly
t	Prior to 3;0 years	At 3;0 years, 92.9 percent of children produce the consonant correctly
d	Prior to 3;0 years	At 3;0 years, 92.8 percent of children produce the consonant correctly
k	At around 3;0 years	At 3;0 years, 90.3 percent of children produce the consonant correctly
g	Between 3;0 and 4;0 years	At 4;0 years, 91.4 percent of children produce the consonant correctly (at 3;0 only 87.1 percent)

5 Accents indicate long vowels, independently of whether one or two accents are used.
6 Umlauts are used in the letters ö /ø/ and ü /y/.

Table 43-3 continued

Consonant	Age when 90 percent of children produce the sound correctly in all positions	
m	At around 3;0 years	At 3;0 years, 90.3 percent of children produce the consonant correctly
n	At around 3;0 years	At 3;0 years, 89.7 percent of children produce the consonant correctly
ɲ	Between 3;0 and 4;0 years	At 4;0 years, 91.9 percent of children produce the consonant correctly (at 3;0 only 81.3 percent)
l	Between 3;0 and 4;0 years	At 4;0 years, 94.5 percent of children produce the consonant correctly (at 3;0 only 84.5 percent)
r	Between 5;0 and 6;0 years	At 6;0 years, 91.2 percent of children produce the consonant correctly (at 5;0 only 84.6 percent)
f	Prior to 3;0 years	At 3;0 years, 91.6 percent of children produce the consonant correctly
v	Between 3;0 and 4;0 years	At 4;0 years, 94.5 percent of children produce the consonant correctly (at 3;0 only 88.4 percent)
s	At around 5;0 years	At 5;0 years, 90.2 percent of children produce the consonant correctly
z	Between 5;0 and 6;0 years	At 6;0 years, 92.1 percent of children produce the consonant correctly (at 5;0 only 87.2 percent)
ʃ	At around 5;0 years	At 5;0 years, 90.1 percent of children produce the consonant correctly
ʒ	Between 5;0 and 6;0 years	At 6;0 years, 91.3 percent of children produce the consonant correctly (at 5;0 only 86.4 percent)
j	Between 3;0 and 4;0 years	At 4;0 years, 93.6 percent of children produce the consonant correctly (at 3;0 only 89.0 percent)
h	Prior to 3;0 years	At 3;0 years, 92.3 percent of children produce the consonant correctly
ts	At around 5;0 years	At 5;0 years, 90.0 percent of children produce the consonant correctly
tʃ	Between 4;0 and 5;0 years	At 5;0 years, 91.2 percent of children produce the consonant correctly (at 4;0 only 88.8 percent)
cç	Between 4;0 and 5;0 years	At 5;0 years, 91.0 percent of children produce the consonant correctly (at 4;0 only 89.4 percent)
ɟj	At around 4;0 years	At 4;0 years, 90.5 percent of children produce the consonant correctly

Note. Data are from Nagy (1980).

exception of /f/, /l/, /r/, /cç/, and /n/, which sounds were also tested as long consonants (/fː/, /lː/, /rː/, /cçː/, and /nː/). No data are available on the accuracy of the other phonemically long consonants. Results are based on perceptual analysis.

Table 43-4 shows data about the acquisition of voice onset time (VOT) in 2;0- to 4;0-year-old children (see Stout et al., 2006; Zajdó, 2005). Results indicate that children are producing increasingly adultlike VOT in their voiceless consonants (no data are available about adult VOT values in voiced plosives). Overall, the acquisition of language-specific VOT is not yet complete in 4;0-year-old children.

TABLE 43-4 Voice onset time measures in Standard Hungarian (msec)

	Plosives					
	Voiceless			Voiced		
Age	p	t	k	b	d	g
2;0	40	48	63	-58	-76	-65
3;0	44	61	49	-57	-42	-61
4;0	38	30	53	-31	-33	-34
Adult speech	21	28	43	No data	No data	No data

Consonant clusters

To date, no systematic study has been carried out to examine acquisition patterns of consonant clusters in children acquiring Standard Hungarian.

Vowels

Nagy (1980) investigated the production of the front rounded vowels /øː/ and /y(ː)/ in 3;0- to 8;0-year-old children. Of the members of the vowel inventory, these two vowels were investigated because their production is reported by speech-language pathologists to remain a challenge for some 6;0-year-old children starting school. Nagy's results are based on perceptual examination.

Zajdó (2002a, b, c; Zajdó and Stoel-Gammon, 2003) investigated the acquisition of all nonmarginal vowels of the vowel inventory. The results of perceptual examination indicate that, in general, (a) unrounded vowels are acquired earliest, (b) back rounded vowels are acquired next, and (c) front rounded vowels are acquired last during development (see Table 43-5).

Cross-linguistic comparison of acoustic data from Hungarian and Dutch vowel acquisition in 2;0-year-old children (e.g., Zajdó, van der Stelt, and Wempe, 2004; Zajdó, van der Stelt, Wempe, and Pols, 2005) revealed that difficulties with lip rounding affect how vowel categories are formulated. That is, in Hungarian, where the vowel quality /u/ is produced with considerable lip rounding, the correct realization of this vowel is not yet possible for many children at this age. Thus, children produce less peripheral and somewhat centralized and lowered high vowels. Surprisingly, Hungarian-speaking children's production of the vowel quality /i/ shows that many of these vowels are produced in a high central position, possibly indicating the effect of the two vowel categories on each other, which results in a considerable overlap between the acoustic spaces utilized for the two vowel categories. However, in Dutch, where the /u/ vowel is produced with much less lip rounding, there is no overlap between the acoustic spaces of these two high vowels.[7]

Nagy's (1980) results show that the youngest age group where all children produce the examined front vowels correctly (in word-initial, word-medial, and word-final positions) is the group of 8;0-year-old children, as attested by the results of perceptual analysis. Thus, one may argue that it is by the age of 8;0 years when children acquire the Standard Hungarian vowel inventory (see Figure 43-3).

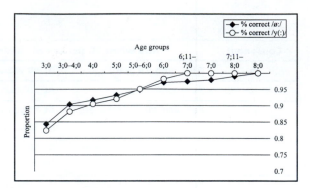

Figure 43-3 Age comparison of when children produce the front vowels correctly (from Nagy, 1980)

Percent correct
Consonants

Table 43-6 shows the percentage of children in six age groups (from 3;0 to 8;0 years) who produce a given consonant correctly, with 100 percent accuracy, in all positions (word-initial, word-medial, and word-final), as shown by the results of perceptual analysis (Nagy, 1980).

Consonant clusters

To date, no study has investigated the acquisition of consonant clusters in children acquiring Standard Hungarian.

Vowels

In a cross-sectional study, Zajdó (2002a, c; Zajdó and Stoel-Gammon, 2003) examined percentage correct data for Standard Hungarian vowels in children 2;0, 2;6, 3;0, 3;6, and 4;0 years old. Vowel accuracy was investigated by eliciting the production of $C^1V^1(ː)C^1V^1(ː)$ structured tokens during a conversation in a play situation. See Table 43-7 for results.

Nagy (1980) published data on the acquisition of the vowel qualities /ø/ and /y/ (see Table 43-8).

Data that are available on the proportion of correctly produced speech sounds in Hungarian-speaking children are shown in Table 43-9.

Phonological processes
Devoicing

Nagy (1980) examined devoicing processes by having 3;0- to 8;0-year-old children repeat a sentence that contained

---

7 Similar results were obtained when comparing Russian (which is similar to Hungarian in terms of having rounded vowels with strong lip protrusion) and Dutch (Pols, Lyakso, van der Stelt, Wempe, and Zajdó, 2006).

the consonants /ɟɟ, d, b, ʒ, b, v, z/. Table 43–10 contains data on the percentage of children in each age group who did not exhibit devoicing of the voiced consonants.

Vowel harmony

According to Gósy (1992), rules of Hungarian vowel harmony are hardly ever broken by Hungarian-speaking

TABLE 43-5   Age of acquisition for Standard Hungarian vowels

Vowel	Age when 90 percent of children produce the vowel correctly in all (word-initial, word-medial and word-final) positions; perceptual analysis (Nagy, 1980)	Age at which the production of children is 90 percent correct (in word-medial and word-final positions); perceptual analysis (Zajdó, 2002c)
ɔ	No data	**Prior to 2;0 years** at 2;0 years, 94.0 percent of production is correct
aː	No data	**Prior to 2;0 years** at 2;0 years, 92.0 percent of production is correct
ɛ	No data	**Prior to 2;0 years** at 2;0 years, 92.5 percent of production is correct
eː	No data	**At around 3;0 years** at 3;0 years, 89.5 percent of production is correct
i	No data	**Prior to 2;0 years** at 2;0 years, 93.0 percent of production is correct
iː	No data	**Prior to 2;0 years** at 2;0 years, 95.5 percent of production is correct
o	No data	**Prior to 2;0 years** at 2;0 years, 95.5 percent of production is correct
oː	No data	**Prior to 2;0 years** at 2;0 years, 92.0 percent of production is correct
ø	No data	**Between 3;0 and 3;6 years** at 3;0 years, 83.5 percent of production is correct at 3;6 years, 95.5 percent of production is correct
øː	**Between 3;0 and 4;0 years** at 4;0 years, 91.9 percent of children produce the vowel correctly (at 3;0 only 84.5 percent)	**Between 3;0 and 3;6 years** at 3;0 years, 80.5 percent of production is correct at 3;6 years, 93.0 percent of production is correct
u	No data	**Between 3;0 and 3;6 years** at 3;0 years, 86.0 percent of production is correct at 3;6 years, 98.0 percent of production is correct
uː	No data	**Between 2;0 and 2;6 years** at 2;0 years, 86.0 percent of production is correct at 2;6 years, 94.0 percent of production is correct
y	**At around 4;0 years** at 4;0 years, 90.5 percent of children produce the vowel correctly (at 3;0 only 82.6 percent) (Note: Phonemically short and long vowels were grouped together)	**After 4;0 years** at 4;0 years, 86.0 percent of production is correct
yː	**At around 4;0 years** at 4;0 years, 90.5 percent of children produce the vowel correctly (at 3;0 only 82.6 percent) (Note: Phonemically short and long vowels were grouped together)	**At around 4;0 years** at 4;0 years, 89.5 percent of production is correct

TABLE 43-6   Percent of children between 3;0 and 8;0 years of age who produce consonants with 100 percent accuracy

Consonant	3;0	4;0	5;0	6;0	7;0	8;0
			years			
p	93.5	96.4	97.2	99.5	100.0	100.0
b	88.4	92.1	94.3	97.0	99.3	100.0
t	92.9	95.9	96.5	98.0	99.3	100.0
d	92.8	94.0	95.0	98.0	99.3	100.0
k	90.3	94.5	95.3	97.7	99.3	100.0
g	87.1	91.7	92.1	96.0	100.0	100.0
m	90.3	95.5	97.0	98.0	100.0	100.0
n*	89.7	95.1	97.0	98.1	100.0	100.0
ɲ	81.3	91.9	94.2	97.3	100.0	100.0
l*	84.5	94.5	95.0	97.0	100.0	100.0
r*	52.9	79.2	84.1	91.2	98.3	98.9
f*	91.6	95.2	96.5	98.0	100.0	100.0
v	88.4	94.5	95.5	98.1	100.0	100.0
s	74.2	84.1	90.2	93.6	99.3	99.3
ʃ	71.0	88.0	90.1	93.5	99.5	99.8
z	74.2	80.0	87.2	91.2	99.3	99.3
ʒ	67.1	80.9	86.4	91.3	100.0	100.0
j	89.0	93.6	96.5	98.0	100.0	100.0
h	92.3	96.2	97.1	98.2	100.0	100.0
ts	73.5	86.1	90.0	95.4	100.0	100.0
tʃ	75.5	88.8	91.2	96.0	100.0	100.0
cç*	71.6	89.4	91.0	95.0	100.0	100.0
ɟj	76.1	90.5	93.0	96.4	100.0	100.0

* These consonants were tested as both phonemically short and long sounds

children, even in the earliest phases of development.[8] Her results indicate that even the babbling data gathered from her two children reflects the application of vowel harmony rules. It should be noted that the speech of Hungarian-speaking children sometimes contains data that seem to indicate otherwise; for example, S. Meggyes (1971) cites the word csücsülök /'tʃytʃylok/ ('I am sitting'; correct production would be csücsülök /'tʃytʃyløk/) produced by a 2 year old; however, in light of the finding that many children struggle with the production of front rounded vowels (see Zajdó, 2002c), one might argue that the child is not breaking the rules of vowel harmony but rather is having difficulty with articulating (formulating the lip rounding necessary for) the required front rounded vowel /ø/.

Syllabification

Kassai (1999) studied syllabification skills in kindergarteners (n = 180; average age 6;1). Results indicated that this population already represents and applies implicitly the major rules of Hungarian phonotactics, as they apply to syllable types and positions. However, the children's knowledge of frequency distribution of syllable types is inadequate. According to the author, this lack of knowledge is a major source of syllabification errors.

Intelligibility

No systematic study has been carried out on intelligibility in children acquiring Standard Hungarian.

Phoneme inventory

A. Molnár (1978) reported the following phonetic inventory for a child between 1;6 and 1;9 years: consonants include /p, b, t, d, k, g, m, n, ɲ, f, v, s, z, ʃ, ʒ, j, ts, dʒ, tʃ/, vowels include all phonemes of the inventory.

Gósy (1984) reports the following phoneme inventory at 3;0 years of age: /p, b, t, d, k, g, m, n, ɲ, l, r, f, v, s, z, ʃ, ʒ, j, h, ts, dʒ, tʃ, c (cç), ɟ (ɟj)/. Vowels include all phonemes of the inventory.

Common mismatches

Mismatches of consonants that can be identified from the literature are shown in Table 43–11.

Vowel mismatches

Table 43-12 shows the most common mismatches available in the literature for children acquiring Standard Hungarian:

Zajdó (2002c, 2003) reported the quality and quantity of vowel errors in 2;0 to 4;0 year old boys vs. girls (see Table 43-13 for results).

8 Vowel harmony rules regulate which vowels can show up within the same word stem and which vowels should be used when determining the appropriate version of a suffix that has several forms with different vowels. Hungarian is characterized by front-back and rounding harmonies. That is, a word stem that contains front rounded vowels should be matched up with a suffix with front rounded vowel(s). For a full description of the rules of Hungarian vowel harmony, see Siptár and Törkenczy (2000).

TABLE 43-7 Percent correct for vowel production in boys and girls acquiring Standard Hungarian

Vowel	Age	Boys (n=8 in all age groups)	Girls (n=8 in all age groups)	Average
ɔ	2;0	94	94	94
	2;6	97	98	97.5
	3;0	99	97	98
	3;6	99	99	99
	4;0	98	100	99
aː	2;0	86	98	92
	2;6	88	96	92
	3;0	95	97	96
	3;6	100	99	99.5
	4;0	98	98	98
ɛ	2;0	90	95	92.5
	2;6	84	95	89.5
	3;0	95	94	94.5
	3;6	99	95	97
	4;0	99	98	98.5
eː	2;0	87	78	82.5
	2;6	83	92	87.5
	3;0	85	94	89.5
	3;6	99	97	98
	4;0	97	97	97
i	2;0	93	93	93
	2;6	94	99	96.5
	3;0	99	99	99
	3;6	99	100	99.5
	4;0	99	100	99.5
iː	2;0	94	97	95.5
	2;6	93	98	95.5
	3;0	97	95	96
	3;6	99	98	98.5
	4;0	96	98	97
o	2;0	89	92	90.5
	2;6	90	97	93.5
	3;0	92	98	95
	3;6	96	97	96.5
	4;0	97	95	96
oː	2;0	86	98	92
	2;6	97	98	97.5
	3;0	98	97	97.5
	3;6	98	99	98.5
	4;0	98	98	98

Table 43-7 continued

Vowel	Age	Boys (n=8 in all age groups)	Girls (n=8 in all age groups)	Average
ø	2;0	70	70	70
	2;6	73	79	76
	3;0	83	84	83.5
	3;6	93	97	95
	4;0	95	85	90
ø:	2;0	72	77	74.5
	2;6	94	83	88.5
	3;0	78	83	80.5
	3;6	89	97	93
	4;0	98	92	95
u	2;0	78	85	81.5
	2;6	89	95	92
	3;0	86	86	86
	3;6	99	97	98
	4;0	97	93	95
u:	2;0	82	90	86
	2;6	90	98	94
	3;0	93	87	90
	3;6	98	98	98
	4;0	94	94	94
y	2;0	73	81	77
	2;6	88	71	79.5
	3;0	83	81	82
	3;6	88	96	92
	4;0	93	79	85.5
y:	2;0	68	75	71.5
	2;6	88	77	82.5
	3;0	75	80	77.5
	3;6	89	96	92.5
	4;0	93	86	89.5

Syllable structure

No systematic studies have been carried out on syllable structure acquisition. Gósy (1997) reported on a child's production of syllables between the ages of 1;6 and 1;9. Data analysis indicated the child's inability to produce words with more than two syllables. Even the production of some of the bisyllabic target words appeared challenging. Results are shown in Table 43-14.

Prosody

Kassai (1988) investigated the acquisition of intonation contours in a child between 1;0 and 1;7 (see Table 43-15). Results indicate that the child's performance reflects relatively high-level capabilities of using the correct language-specific intonation patterns that signal different modalities. In contrast, the child's stress production is not similar to patterns commonly used in the language community (e.g., using two stresses in a word).

TABLE 43-8 Percentage of children with 100 percent accuracy of vowel production

Vowel	3;0	4;0	5;0	6;0	7;0	8;0
ø	84.5	91.9	93.3	97.1	98.0	100.0
y	82.6	90.5	92.0	98.3	100.0	100.0

TABLE 43-9 Percent correct for Standard Hungarian consonants, consonant clusters, and vowels

Age	Consonants (Nagy, 1980)	Consonant clusters	Vowels (Zajdó, 2002c)
2;0	N/A	No data	85.2 percent
2;6	N/A	No data	90.1 percent
3;0	82.1 percent	No data	90.4 percent
3;6	N/A	No data	96.8 percent
4;0	90.8 percent	No data	95.1 percent
4;6	N/A	No data	N/A
5;0	93.2 percent	No data	N/A
6;0	96.2 percent	No data	N/A
7;0	99.7 percent	No data	N/A
8;0	99.9 percent	No data	N/A

TABLE 43-10 Percentage of children in each age group who exhibit normal production of voiced consonants while producing a sentence

	Age groups					
	3;0	4;0	5;0	6;0	7;0	8;0
percent	67.1	80.9	84.0	90.0	98.3	98.6

Phonological awareness

No systematic study has been carried out about phonological awareness skills in children acquiring Standard Hungarian. However, Nagy (1980) examined phonemic differentiation skills in children between 3;0 and 8;0 years of age by having an adult produce one member of minimal pairs that included voiceless vs. voiced consonants in a

word-initial position and instructing the child to show the corresponding picture. Analysis of the data showed that the differentiation of the plosive pair /t-d/ is most challenging, followed by the differentiation of the fricative pairs /f-v/ and /ʃ-s/, respectively. Results are included in Table 43-16.

Speech assessment for children who speak Standard Hungarian

No specific tests have been developed for assessing speech sound production in Hungarian-speaking children. For the purposes of assessing speech sound awareness, minimal pairs (e.g., *toboz-doboz*) have been used. Most recently, the GMP assessment test (Gósy, 1995), which has a subtest on speech sound awareness, is gaining ground. No additional speech sampling tools have been developed for use with children acquiring Standard Hungarian. No assessment test has been designed for analyzing Standard Hungarian speech.

Speech intervention for children who speak Standard Hungarian

The speech intervention techniques that have been used for Standard Hungarian include two traditional methods:

- Articulation therapy
- Phonological treatment (this method has been gaining ground since the 1980s)

Working in Hungary

Currently, the minimal degree requirement for working as an SLP in a government-funded position in Hungary is a bachelor's degree (or an equivalent) in special education with a specialization in speech-language pathology. Two types of bachelor's degrees can be conferred: one gives the degree holder a special education teacher certificate; the other is a *terapeuta* (specialist) degree without a teaching certificate. SLPs work either in school settings and hospital/clinic settings or in private practices.

The first master's program in speech-language pathology started in Budapest, Hungary, in 2005. However, in the near future it is not anticipated that the state will increase the minimal degree requirements for practice.

Other professionals who participate in speech therapy include individuals with a teachers' certificate who obtain an additional certification called "speech development specialist." However, these individuals can participate in (continued on page 433)

TABLE 43-11 Most commonly reported mismatches for Hungarian-speaking children

Consonant to be substituted	Substitution(s)	Age	Author
k	t	1;9	Viktor, 1917
		Between 2;0 and 3;0	Keresztes, 1940
		3;0	Gósy, 1984
	c	1;10	Viktor, 1917
g	d	3;0	Gósy, 1984
n	ŋ	3;0	Gósy, 1984
ɲ	n	1;6–1;9	A.Molnár, 1978
ŋ	g	Not given	Keresztes, 1940
r	ɟ	1;10	Viktor, 1917
	l, j	Not given	Keresztes, 1940
		3;0	Gósy, 1984
f	ts	Not given	Vértes, 1905
	p	Not given	Keresztes, 1940
	p, pf, t	1;6–1;9	A.Molnár, 1978
	h	3;2	Jablonkay, 1935
v	b	1;10	Viktor, 1917
	b, m, l	1;6–1;9	A.Molnár, 1978
	h	2;1	Jablonkay, 1935
s	c	1;9	Viktor, 1917
	ts	1;10	Viktor, 1917
	t	1;6–1;9	A.Molnár, 1978
z	s	Not given	Keresztes, 1940
	ts	1;10	Viktor, 1917
	d	1;6–1;9	A.Molnár, 1978
ʃ	s, h	Not given	Keresztes, 1940
	c	1;10	Viktor, 1917
	s	3;0	Gósy, 1984
ʒ	z	Not given	Keresztes, 1940
		3;0	Gósy, 1984
j	l	1;8	A.Molnár, 1978
h	c, ts	1;10	Viktor, 1917
ts	pf	1;9	Viktor, 1917
tʃ	t, ts	2;1	Jablonkay, 1935
c (cç)	t	3;0()	Gósy, 1984
ɟ ɟʲ	d	1;9	Viktor, 1917
		3;0	Gósy, 1984

TABLE 43-12 Vowel error patterns for Hungarian-speaking children

Vowel that is substituted	Substitution	Frequency of pattern	Age (if identified)	Author
a:	ɔ	occasionally	At 2;0	S. Meggyes, 1971
		occasionally	At 3;0	Gósy, 1984
ɛ	a:	occasionally	At 1;10	Viktor, 1917
e:	i	occasionally	At 2;0	S. Meggyes, 1971
e:	ɛ	occasionally	At 2;0	S. Meggyes, 1971
i	ɔ	occasionally	At 1;7	Kenyeres, 1924
o	ɔ	systematically	At 2;2	Jablonkay, 1935
o:	u:	occasionally	At 1;9	Jablonkay, 1935
o:	y:	occasionally	At 1;10	Viktor, 1917
ø	o	systematically	Not identified	Csapodi, 1905
		occasionally	at 2;0	S. Meggyes, 1971
		systematically	in some 25 percent of children at 3;0 years	Gósy, 1984
ø	ë*	systematically	Not identified	Csapodi, 1905
ø:	o:	systematically	Until 1;4	Balassa, 1893
		Less frequently	After 1;4	Balassa, 1893
		occasionally	At 3;0	S. Meggyes, 1971
		systematically	in some 25 percent of children at 3;0 years	Gósy, 1984
ø:	e:	less frequently	Not identified	Balassa, 1893
y	u	systematically	Not identified	Csapodi, 1905
		systematically	in some 25 percent of children at 3;0 years	Gósy, 1984
y	i	systematically	Not identified	Csapodi, 1905
y:	ɛ	occasionally	At 2;0	S. Meggyes, 1971
y:	u:	systematically	Until 1;3	Balassa, 1893
		less frequently	After 1;3	Balassa, 1893
		systematically	in some 25 percent of children at 3;0 years	Gósy, 1984
y:	i:	less frequently	Not identified	Balassa, 1893

* /ë/ stands for ɛ.

TABLE 43-13 Vowel error patterns in Hungarian-speaking children aged 2;0–4;0

Age groups	Error types	# of error types	percent error	BOYS percent correct	Target vowel	GIRLS percent correct	percent error	# of error types	Error types
2;0	o, ɛ	2	6	94		94	6	1	i
2;6	u	1	3	97		98	2	2	o, del
3;0		0	1	99	ɑ	97	3	1	a:
3;6		0	1	99		99	1	1	del
4;0		0	2	98		100	0	0	
2;0	ɑ, ø, del	3	10	90		95	5	2	del, ɑ
2;6	ɑ, ø	2	16	84		95	5	2	ø, i
3;0	ø	1	5	95	ɛ	94	6	3	ɑ, i, del
3;6		0	1	99		95	5	2	ɑ, ø
4;0		0	1	99		98	2	0	
2;0	ɛ, del	2	7	93		93	7	2	ɛ, del
2;6	y,u	2	6	94		99	1	0	
3;0		0	1	99	i	99	1	0	
3;6		0	1	99		100	0	0	
4;0		0	1	99		100	0	0	
2;0	ɑ, u, ø, del	4	11	89		92	8	3	ɑ, ø, i
2;6	ø, ɑ, u, del	4	10	90		97	3	1	ɑ
3;0	u, ɑ	2	8	92	o	98	2	1	del
3;6	ɑ, del	2	4	96		97	3	1	u
4;0	u	1	3	97		95	5	2	u, ɑ
2;0	o, ɛ, ɑ, u, y, del	6	30	70		70	30	6	ɛ, o, i, del, u, e:
2;6	ɑ, o, ɛ, u	4	27	73		79	21	2	o, ɛ
3;0	ɑ, ɛ, y, i, o	5	17	83	ø	84	16	3	ɛ, o, del
3;6	o, ɑ, ɛ	3	7	93		97	3	1	o
4;0	ɛ	1	5	95		85	15	3	o, u, ɛ
2;0	o, ɑ, del, ɛ, i, ø, y	7	22	78		85	15	5	o, ɑ, a:, ɛ, del
2;6	ɑ, ø, o	3	11	89		95	5	2	o, i
3;0	o, del	2	14	86	u	86	14	4	o, ɑ, y, ɛ
3;6		0	1	99		97	3	1	ø
4;0	del	1	3	97		93	7	1	o
2;0	i, u, ɑ, ɛ, del, o	6	27	73		81	19	6	i, del, ɛ, ɑ, o, u
2;6	i, del, ɑ, u	4	12	88		71	29	5	i, u, o, ɑ, del
3;0	u, ɛ, del	3	17	83	y	81	19	5	i, ɛ, del, ɑ, u

Table 43-13 continued

Age groups	Error types	# of error types	percent error	BOYS percent correct	Target vowel	GIRLS percent correct	percent error	# of error types	Error types
3;6	u, o, i	3	12	88		96	4	3	i, ɑ, del
4;0	del, i	2	7	93		79	21	4	u, i, o, del
2;0	ɑ, del, ø	3	14	86		98	2	1	ɑ
2;6	ɑ, del, o	3	12	88		96	4	2	y, u
3;0	ɑ	1	5	95	a:	97	3	1	ɑ
3;6		0	0	100		99	1	0	
4;0	ɑ	1	2	98		98	2	1	ɑ
2;0	del, i, ɛ, o, u	5	13	87		78	22	4	i, ɑ, a:, ɛ
2;6	i, ɛ, del	3	17	83		92	8	2	i, u
3;0	i, ɛ, del	3	15	85	e:	94	6	3	i, del, ɛ
3;6	i	1	1	99		97	3	2	i, del
4;0	i, ɛ	2	3	97		97	3	1	o
2;0	u	1	6	94		97	3	1	ɛ
2;6	y, del, u	3	7	93		98	2	1	y
3;0	y	1	3	97	i:	95	5	3	u, ø, ɛ
3;6		0	1	99		98	2	0	
4;0	y, e:	2	4	96		98	2	0	
2;0	ɑ, ø, ɛ, del, e:, y	6	14	86		98	2	0	
2;6		0	3	97		98	2	1	del
3;0	ɑ	1	2	98	o:	97	3	2	del, ɑ
3;6	u	1	2	98		99	1	0	
4;0	del	1	2	98		98	2	1	del
2;0	o, ɑ, ɛ, del, u	5	28	72		77	23	6	o, ɛ, u, e:, y, i
2;6	o, ɛ	2	6	94		83	17	4	o, e, u, e:
3;0	o, del, ɛ	3	22	78	ø:	83	17	4	ɛ, e:, o, i
3;6	o	1	11	89		97	3	2	o, del
4;0	del	1	2	98		92	8	2	ɛ, o
2;0	o, del, ø, ɑ, a:, ɛ	6	18	82		90	10	4	o, i, del, y
2;6	y, ø, a:, del	4	10	90		98	2	1	del
3;0	o, del	2	7	93	u:	87	13	3	o, ɑ, y
3;6	y	1	2	98		98	2	0	
4;0	e:, del, o	3	6	94		94	6	1	o

Table 43-13 continued

Age groups	Error types	# of error types	percent error	BOYS percent correct	Target vowel	GIRLS percent correct	percent error	# of error types	Error types
2;0	ø, ɑ, ɛ, u, del, eː, i, o	8	32	68		75	25	5	u, ø, o, del, i
2;6	del, i, ø, u	4	12	88		77	23	7	u, o, del, ø, ɑ, i, eː
3;0	u, ø, del	3	25	75	y:	80	20	6	i, ɑ, ø, eː, u, ɛ
3;6	u	1	11	89		96	4	2	u, i
4;0	del, ø, i	3	7	93		86	14	4	o, u, del, ø

*Note. del indicates vowel deletion.

TABLE 43-14 The number of syllables in words produced between the ages of 1;6 and 1;9

Number of syllables in target word	Number of syllables in the child's production	
	Identical with number of syllables in the target word	Decreases
1-2	64 percent	23 percent >> to 1 syllable
3	none	7 percent >> to 2 syllables
		5 percent >> to 1 syllable
4	none	N/A

TABLE 43-15 Contour patterns identified in a child (1;0–1;7)

Utterance type/Modality	Contour patterns identified
Monosyllabic declaratives	Level contour
Disyllabic declaratives (n=69)	Overall rising contour (n=8)
	Level contour (n=19)
	Falling contour (n=36)
Interrogatives	Sharp rise of about a large fourth up to the end of the phonation from mid to high tone
Imperatives	Steep fall from high to low
Calls	Level contour, kept in the mid tone

TABLE 43-16 Percentage of children with 100 percent accuracy of identifying corresponding picture

Consonant pairs	3;0	4;0	5;0	6;0	7;0	8;0
			years			
/t-d/ *toboz* /toboz/ 'cone' vs. *doboz* /doboz/ 'box'	49.7	71.2	77.0	87.4	92.4	95.9
/f-v/ *fonal* /fonal/ 'yarn' vs. *vonal* /vonal/ 'line'	60.0	79.2	83.0	91.3	94.5	96.6
/ʃ-s/ *sál* /ʃaːl/ 'scarf' vs. *szál* /saːl/ 'strand'	65.2	80.3	87.1	93.0	94.3	97.7

speech treatment only in a very limited capacity (e.g., helping the child with speech practice as prescribed by a speech-language pathologist).

Schools conferring degrees

Two schools are conferring degrees:

- Bárczi Gusztáv Faculty of Special Education, Eötvös Loránd University, Budapest (B.A., M.A., Speech Development Specialist Certificate): http://www.barczi.hu
- Csokonai Vitéz Mihály Faculty of Pedagogy, University of Kaposvár, Kaposvár (B.A.): http://www.u-kaposvar.hu/eng/pedagogy.htm

See Resources for materials pertaining to Standard Hungarian.

PHONETICALLY SPEAKING

Pronunciation of Hungarian (Magyar): /ˈmɔɟɔr/ (alternatively, /ˈmɔɟ̠ɔr/)

Relevant words for speech assessment and intervention

Word/Phrase	Formal usage	Pronunciation	Informal usage	Pronunciation
Tongue	nyelv	/ˈɲɛlv/		
Teeth	fogak	/ˈfogɔk/		
Lips	ajkak	/ˈɔjkɔk/	száj (mouth)	/ˈsaːj/
Hard palate	kemény szájpad	ˈkɛmẽːɲ ˈsaːjpɔd/		
Soft palate	lágy szájpad	/ˈlaːɟ̟ɟ ˈsaːjpɔd/		
Larynx	gégefő	/ˈgeːgɛføː/	gége	/ˈgeːgɛ/
Lungs	tüdő	/ˈtydøː/		
Nose	orr	/ˈorː/		
Sound	hang	/ˈhõŋg/		
Word	szó	/ˈsoː/		
Sentence	mondat	/ˈmõndɔt/		
Paragraph	bekezdés	/ˈbɛkɛzdeːʃ/		

RESOURCES

Books

Bolla, K. (1995). *Magyar fonetikai atlasz* [Atlas of Hungarian phonetics]. Budapest: Nemzeti Tankönyvkiadó.

Molnár, J. (1970). *A magyar beszédhangok atlasza* [Atlas of Hungarian speech sounds]. Budapest: Tankönyvkiadó.

Siptár, P., and Törkenczy, M. (2000). *The phonology of Hungarian*. Oxford, UK: Oxford University Press.

Varga, L. (2002). *Intonation and stress: Evidence from Hungarian*. Basingstoke, Hampshire, UK: Palgrave Macmillan.

Book series

Approaches to Hungarian

Hungarian Papers in Phonetics

CD-ROMs

By Original Language / Hungarian. DVD

Journals

- *Beszédgyógyítás*,
  http://mfflt.freeweb.hu/beszgyogyitas.html
  The journal of the Hungarian Association of Phonetics, Phoniatrics and Logopedics

- *Gyógypedagógiai szemle*, no Web site.
  The journal of the Hungarian Association of Special Education Teachers
- *Magyar Nyelv* (Hungarian Language),
  http://www.c3.hu/~magyarnyelv/
  Journal of the Society for Hungarian Linguistics (in Hungarian and English)

Professional associations

Hungarian Association of Phonetics, Phoniatrics and Logopedics (Major professional association of speech-language pathologists in Hungary)

Hungarian Association of Special Education Teachers (with a subsection of logopedics)

Hungarian Association of Special Education Teachers in Romania, http://www.gyogypedagogia.ro/page.php?page=rolunk

Useful Hungarian Web sites

- http://szotar.sztaki.hu/index.hu.jhtml English-Hungarian-English; German-Hungarian-German, French-Hungarian-French, Italian-Hungarian-Italian, Dutch-Hungarian-Dutch and Polish-Hungarian-Polish dictionary, with pronunciation models, and with manual signs.
- http://www.ectaco.com Hungarian Electronic talking dictionaries

REFERENCES

A. Molnár, I. (1978). A hanghelyettesítések típusai a gyermeknyelvben 18–21 hónapos kor között [The types of sound substitutions in child language between the ages of 18–21 months]. *Hungarian Papers in Phonetics*, 1, 44–52.

Balassa, J. (1893). A gyermek nyelvének fejlődése [The development of the child's language] I–II. *Nyelvtudományi Közlemények*, 23, 60–73 and 129–144.

Bárczi, G., Benkő, L., and Berrár, J. (1987). *A magyar nyelv története* [The history of the Hungarian language] (5th ed.). Budapest: Tankönyvkiadó.

Csapodi, I. (1905). Gyermekek nyelvtudománya [Linguistic knowledge of children]. *Magyar Nyelvőr*, 34, 464–467.

É. Kiss, K., and Papp, F. (1984). A *dz* és a *dzs* státuszához a mai magyar fonémarendszerben [On the status of /dz/ and /dʒ/ in the phoneme system of present day Hungarian]. *Általános Nyelvészeti Tanulmányok*, 15, 151–160.

Fodor, K. (2003). A nyelvjárási hangtani jelenségek [Phonetic properties of dialects]. In J. Kiss (Ed.), *Magyar dialektológia* [Hungarian dialectology] (pp. 325–350). Budapest: Osiris Kiadó.

Gósy, M. (1984). *Hangtani és szótani vizsgálatok hároméves gyermekek nyelvében* [Phonetic and semantic studies in the language of three-year-olds]. Budapest: Akadémiai Kiadó.

Gósy, M. (1992). Magánhangzó harmónia a gyermeknyelvben [Vowel harmony in child language]. *Magyar Nyelvőr*, 116, 424–437.

Gósy, M. (1995). *GMP Diagnosztika* [GMP diagnostics]. Budapest: Nikol.

Gósy, M. (1997). A szavak hangalakjának változása a gyermeknyelvben [Changing of the phonetics of words in child language]. *Beszédkutatás* '97, 1–38.

Gósy, M. (2001). The VOT of the Hungarian voiceless plosives in words and in spontaneous speech. *International Journal of Speech Technology*, *4*, 75–85.

Gósy, M. (2004). *Fonetika, a beszéd tudománya* [Phonetics, the science of speech]. Budapest: Osiris Kiadó.

Hajdú, P. (1975). *Finno-Ugrian languages and peoples*. London: Deutsch.

Jablonkay, G. (1935). *Gyermeknapló: Gyermekmegfigyelési feljegyzések* [Child diary: Notes on examining children]. Budapest: Dunántúl Pécsi Egyetemi Könyvkiadó és Nyomda.

Juhász, D. (2003). A magyar nyelvjárások területi egységei [Regional units of Hungarian dialects]. In J. Kiss (Ed.), *Magyar dialektológia* [Hungarian dialectology] (pp. 262–324). Budapest: Osiris Kiadó.

Kassai, I. (1979). *Időtartam és kvantitás a magyar nyelvben* [Duration and quantity in the Hungarian language]. *Nyelvtudományi Értekezések*, 102. Budapest: Akadémiai Kiadó.

Kassai, I. (1988). Prosodic development of a Hungarian child: The one word utterance stage. *Hungarian Papers in Phonetics*, *19*, 72–81.

Kassai, I. (1998). *Fonetika* [Phonetics]. Budapest: Nemzeti Tankönyvkiadó.

Kassai, I. (1999). Szótaghatárok és fonológiai jólformáltság nagycsoportos óvodások intuitív szótagolásában [Syllable boundaries and phonological well-roundedness in the intuitive syllabification of kindergarteners]. In I. Kassai (Ed.), *Szótagfogalom – szótagrealizációk* [The concept and realization of syllables] (pp. 131–142). Budapest: MTA Nyelvtudományi Intézet.

Kenyeres, E. (1924). A *gyermek beszédének fejlődése* [The development of the child's speech]. Budapest: Studium.

Keresztes, M. (1940). *A gyermeknyelv* [Child language]. Pécs: Taizs József Könyvnyomda.

Nagy, J. (1980). *5-6 éves gyermekeink iskolakészültsége* [Preparedness for school of five to six years old children]. Budapest: Akadémiai Kiadó.

Nádasdy, Á., and Siptár, P. (1989). Issues in Hungarian phonology: Preliminary queries to a new project. *Acta Linguistica Hungarica*, *39*, 3–27.

Pols, L.C.W., Lyakso, E., van der Stelt, J. M., Wempe, T., and Zajdó, K. (2006, April). *Vowel data of early speech development in several languages*. Paper presented at Multiling 2006, Stellenbosch University, South Africa.

S. Meggyes, K. (1971). *Egy két éves gyermek nyelvi rendszere* [The linguistic system of a two years old child]. Nyelvtudományi Értekezések, 73.

Siptár, P. (1989). How many affricates are there in Hungarian? In T. Szende (Ed.), *Proceedings of the Speech Research '89 International Conference. Hungarian Papers in Phonetics*, 20, 123–126.

Siptár, P. (2003). Phonology. In K. É. Kiss, F. Kiefer and P. Siptár, *Új magyar nyelvtan* [New Hungarian Grammar]. (pp. 287–381). Budapest: Osiris Kiadó.

Siptár, P., and Törkenczy, M. (2000). *The Phonology of Hungarian*. Oxford: Oxford University Press.

Stout, G., Rath, E., Nickerson, L., and Zajdó, K. (2006, April). *Voice onset time acquisition: Data from 2;0 and 4;0 years old Hungarian speaking boys*. Poster presented at the 12th Grand Rounds & Annual Research Day of the College of Health Sciences, University of Wyoming, Laramie, Wyoming.

Szende, T. (1992). Phonological representation and lenition processes. *Hungarian Papers in Phonetics*, *24*.

Szende, T. (1999). Hungarian. In *Handbook of the International Phonetic Association: A guide to the use of the International Phonetic Alphabet* (pp. 104–107). Cambridge, UK: International Phonetic Association.

Tarnóczy, T. (1974). A magánhangzók akusztikai vizsgálatának problémái [Problems encountered during the acoustic examination of vowels]. *Általános Nyelvészeti Tanulmányok, X.* (10), 181–196.

Tompa, J. (Ed.) (1961). *A mai magyar nyelv rendszere* [The system of present-day Hungarian]. Budapest: Akadémiai Kiadó.

U.S. Census (2000). U.S. Census Bureau, Population Division, Education and Social Stratification Branch.

Van der Stelt, J. M., Zajdó, K., and Wempe, T.G. (2005). Investigating the acoustic vowel space in two-year-old children: Results for Dutch and Hungarian. *Speech Communication*, *47*, 143–159.

Varga, L. (2002). *Intonation and stress: Evidence from Hungarian*. Basingstoke, Hampshire, UK: Palgrave Macmillan.

Vértes, J. (1905). *A gyermeknyelv hangtana* [The phonetics of child language]. Nyelvészeti Füzetek, 22.

Viktor, G. (1917). *A gyermek nyelve* [The language of the child]. Nagyvárad: Béres és Held Könyvnyomdája.

Zajdó, K. (2002a). Vowel acquisition in Hungarian: A first look at the data. In J. Larson and M. Paster (Eds.), *Proceedings of the Twenty-Eighth Annual Meeting of the Berkeley Linguistics Society*, (pp. 363–374). Berkeley, CA: Berkeley Linguistics Society.

Zajdó, K. (2002b, June). *Vowel acquisition in Hungarian: Unrounded vs. rounded vowels*. Poster presented at the EURESCO Conference on Human Brain Development and Cognition, Acquafredda di Maratea, BZ, Italy.

Zajdó, K. (2002c). *The acquisition of vowels by Hungarian-speaking children aged two to four years: A cross-sectional study*. Unpublished doctoral dissertation, University of Washington, Seattle.

Zajdó, K. (2003, July). *Vowel error patterns in Hungarian-speaking children*. Poster presented at the UBC Child Phonology Conference, Vancouver, British Columbia, Canada.

Zajdó, K. (2005, November). *Developmental processes in speech timing: Voice onset time acquisition in Hungarian-speaking children*. Poster presented at the 2005 Annual Convention of the American Speech-Language-Hearing Association, San Diego, CA.

Zajdó, K., and Stoel-Gammon, C. (2003). The acquisition of vowels in Hungarian: Developmental data. In M. J. Solé, D. Rescasens, and J. Romero (Eds.), *Proceedings of the 15th International Congress of Phonetic Sciences*, Barcelona, 3-9 August, 2003

(Vol. 3., pp. 2229–2232). Barcelona: Universitat Autònoma de Barcelona.

Zajdó, K., Van der Stelt, J. M., and Wempe, T. G. (2004, November). *The organization of the acoustic vowel space in 2;0 year-old children: Results from Dutch and Hungarian*. Poster presented at the American Speech and Hearing Association Annual Convention, Philadelphia, PA.

Zajdó, K., Van der Stelt, J. M., Wempe, T., and Pols, L.C.W. (2005). Cross-linguistic comparison of two-year-old children's acoustic vowel spaces: Contrasting Hungarian with Dutch. *Proceedings of InterSpeech 2005: The 9th European Conference on Speech Communication and Technology* (pp. 1173–1176). Lisbon, Portugal, September 4–8, 2005. Bonn, Germany: ISCA.

SUMMARY OF STUDIES OF TYPICAL STANDARD HUNGARIAN SPEECH ACQUISITION

Authors	Year	Country	No. of children	Age of children	Information	Sample type	Data collection
A. Molnár	1978	Hungary	1	1;6–1;9	Sound and Phoneme inventory	Speech sample	Cross-sectional
Gósy	1984	Hungary	29	3;0	Sound and Phoneme inventory	Speech sample	Cross-sectional
Gósy	1992	Hungary	30 / 20 / 30	5;0–5;4 / 6;2–6;6 / 9;2–9;6	Vowel harmony rules	Oral production and written work	Cross-sectional
Kassai	1988	Hungary	1	1;0–1;7	Prosody	One word utterances	Cross-sectional
Kassai	1999	Hungary	180	Average age 6;1	Syllabification	Words	Cross-sectional
Kenyeres	1924	Hungary	1	0;0–2;0	Sound inventory	Words and phrases	Developmental
Nagy	1980	Hungary	7602	3;0–8;0	Sound production accuracy; devoicing; phonological awareness	Words; Sentences	Cross-sectional
Zajdó	2002	Hungary	80	2;0–4;0	Age of acquisition of vowels	Words and nonwords produced during conversation	Cross-sectional

Note: This table is not exhaustive, but is representative of studies of Hungarian speech acquisition.

Chapter 44

Israeli Hebrew Speech Acquisition

Avivit Ben-David and Ruth A. Berman

INTRODUCTION

Hebrew is described as belonging to the Canaanite branch of West Semitic (Faber, 1998), but in fact Modern Hebrew is a typologically mixed language, due to the sociohistorical circumstances of its development (Berman, 1978, 1998; Ravid, 1995). The major periods in the documented history of Hebrew range from the classical Biblical period (circa 1300 to 200 BC) via Mishnaic or Rabbinical Hebrew (until about 800 AD) and Medieval Hebrew, lasting until modern times (Berman, 1992; Eytan, 1971; Kutscher, 1982).[1] The variety of Modern Hebrew described in this chapter is what Blanc (1964) described as "General Israeli," with occasional mention of an "Arabicized Israeli" pronunciation used by people of Near Eastern background.

Israeli Hebrew evolved from the nationalist movement of Zionist resettlement in Palestine in the late nineteenth century and has served as the majority language of the state of Israel since its establishment in 1948 (Blanc, 1957). Hebrew did not function as a first or native language or even a major means of communication for any speech community for nearly two thousand years. From around 200 AD until the late nineteenth century, Hebrew served mainly for ritual and liturgical purposes along with local vernaculars in the countries of the Jewish diaspora. This hiatus in Hebrew as an everyday spoken language compared with its continuity as a written means of expression (Harshav, 1990) has affected the language to this day. On the one hand, as a language used in a small country, with a centralized system of government, education, and media, Israeli Hebrew shows almost no regional variation or rural versus urban dialects. Yet it is subject to multiple other sources

---

1 The bibliography is not entirely representative, since in the interests of general accessibility, we have favored studies written in English rather than in Hebrew.

of variation. First, lack of continuity in the evolution of spoken Hebrew has led to a situation where the language makes concurrent use of words and constructions from different periods in its history (Bendavid, 1967; Rubinstein, 1980). Second, there is considerable tension and wide disparity along a continuum from the conservative norms of usage—in pronunciation as well as lexicon and grammar—that are prescribed by the Hebrew language establishment, through the intermediate level of usage adopted by the mass media, to the rapidly shifting everyday speech of adolescents and young adults (Berman, 1987; Ravid, 1995; Schwarzwald, 1981). Third, the population of Israel started out as (and to some extent still is) largely immigrant in makeup, and Hebrew is influenced by numerous contact languages, originally mainly Yiddish and Slavic, subsequently mainly Arabic and English (Blau, 1981; Fellman, 1971; Schwarzwald, 1998; Shohamy, 2004).

The peculiar circumstances of the revival of Hebrew as a spoken vernacular among the Jewish population of Palestine around the turn of the twentieth century had a marked impact on its phonology. Thus, the pronunciation that came into general use and has been maintained across four to five generations of native speakers was taken over both from the so-called *Sfardi* accent of Jews of Spanish-Portuguese descendancy and from the Yiddishized *Ashkenazi* accent of European Jewry.[2] In essence, vowels of General Israeli Hebrew are Sfardi-based, and consonants are Ashkenazi-based. This has involved several levelings of phonological distinctions. For example, current Hebrew has only two mid-vowels /e/ and /o/, whereas Ashkenazi speech distinguishes between the vowel and diphthong /e/ and /ej/ for the front vowel and between /o/ and something like /aw/ for the back-vowel, depending on the particular substratum dialect of Yiddish. Another such leveling is the historical distinction between a set of six stops /p, b, t, d, k, g/ and their allophonic fricative versions /f, v, θ, ð, x, ɣ/ respectively (Ashkenazi Hebrew also distinguishes the pair /t-s/.) Today, only three of these alternations still apply, the three stops /p, b, k/ and the three fricatives /f, v, x/, generally analyzed as distinct phonemes (see Adam, 1993, 2002; Schwarzwald, 1976; Tobin, 1997).

These neutralizations are accompanied by other levelings of pronunciations that are still found in the "Arabicized Hebrew" of Israelis of different Arabic-speaking origins. Speakers whose families originate from Iraq, North Africa, or the Yemen still often pronounce the pharyngeal /ʕ/ and /ħ/ as such; in "General Israeli Hebrew," in contrast, the /ʕ/ has been neutralized to zero in most contexts (or is pronounced as a glottal stop /ʔ/ before a stressed vowel), and the /ħ/ is pronounced /x/, the same as the spirant alternant of the velar stop /k/. Furthermore, the emphatics of Arabicized pronunciation are not distinguished in General Israeli Hebrew, so that emphatic /q/ is pronounced the same as the velar stop /k/, the emphatic /tˤ/ is neutralized to the same as the voiceless alveolar stop /t/, and the emphatic /sˤ/ is pronounced the same as the ordinary alveolar sibilant /s/. Loss of consonant gemination and of the distinction between long vowels and short vowels are further causes of opacity.[3]

Many of these distinctions are still reflected in the orthography of current Hebrew (as described below and detailed in Berman, 1992; Bolozky, 1978; Ravid, 2005). These levelings have led to considerable opacity in the morphophonemics of Israeli Hebrew, since many distinctions that lack any phonetic motivation in contemporary speech continue to affect a wide range of morpho-phonological processes. For example, historical pharyngeals attract the low vowel /a/, in contrast to their currently homophonous counterparts the glottal stop /ʔ/ and the velar fricative /x/ respectively. This makes acquisition of these alternations a formidable task for young children acquiring Hebrew as their first language (Berman, 1981, 1985; Ravid, 1995).

The fact that current Hebrew favored Sfardi over Ashkenazi forms of pronunciation also had a marked effect in the domain of word stress, since Ashkenazi word stress was typically penultimate, whereas Israeli Hebrew has predominantly word-final stress (see below, on Stress).

In general, the preschool children who have been the subjects of most research on language development in Hebrew are raised by parents who are speakers of a sociolect that can be termed "standard," the language of native-born Israelis of educated, Hebrew-speaking backgrounds (Berman, 1985; Berman and Neeman, 1994; Ravid, 1995). The children discussed in this chapter are typically at least second-generation speakers of non-Arabicized "General

---

2 The term *Sfardi*—from the word *Sfarad* 'Spain'—refers to Jews originally from the Iberian peninsula, mainly native speakers of Ladino (Judeo-Spanish); the term *Ashkenazi* comes from the Hebrew name for Germany, and refers to mainly Yiddish-speaking Jews from Eastern as well as Western Europe.

3 The specific source of any given effect due to these situations of languages in contact is not always clear—for example, whether the impact is of Yiddish or Russian. Besides, certain changes may be attributed to a language-internal shift toward less marked forms rather than to external influences.

Israeli Hebrew," the native language of the first author of this chapter. Unless otherwise noted, this is the dialect referred to throughout this chapter, and this is what is labeled here "Hebrew." (See the Resources section for relevant background materials).

Where Hebrew is spoken

Hebrew as a first and official language is spoken only in Israel (see accompanying map and **Appendix D**). It also serves as the liturgical language used for prayer, Bible study, and other religious purposes in Jewish communities throughout the diaspora (e.g., in Europe and North and South America) and as a means of spoken intercourse among emigrants from Israel across the world.

Components of Hebrew

This section describes "General Israeli Hebrew," characterized above as what is referred to under the label "Hebrew" throughout the chapter.

Consonants

Hebrew speech consists of 23 consonants, as shown in Table 44-1 (based on Laufer, 1992).

Three of these consonants are borrowed from other languages: the fricative /ʒ/ as in the loan word /ʒaˈket/ 'jacket' and two affricates /tʃ/ as in the word /tʃips/ 'chips = French fries', and /dʒ/ as in /dʒip/ 'jeep.' These sounds are of low frequency, occurring mainly in loan words, but they can be taken to function as phonemes (Ornan, 1982; Laufer, 1998). Scholars disagree on the pronunciation of the phoneme /ʁ/ (representing orthographic resh)—as the uvular fricative /ʁ/, as a velar fricative /ɣ/, or as a uvular trill /ʀ/—even in the usage of the same speaker (Chayen, 1973; Ornan, 1996; Schwarzwald, 1985). As against these views, Laufer (1984, 1992) claims that the phoneme /ʁ/ is generally pronounced as a sonorant approximant and sometimes as a uvular trill. Bolozky (1972) also views this phoneme as often behaving like a liquid consonant, a proposal supported by the fact that in clusters, /ʁ/ displays the phonological features of a sonorant consonant. These different analyses might reflect inter- and intraspeaker variation, although as far as we know, there is no detailed research on this phoneme in current Hebrew.

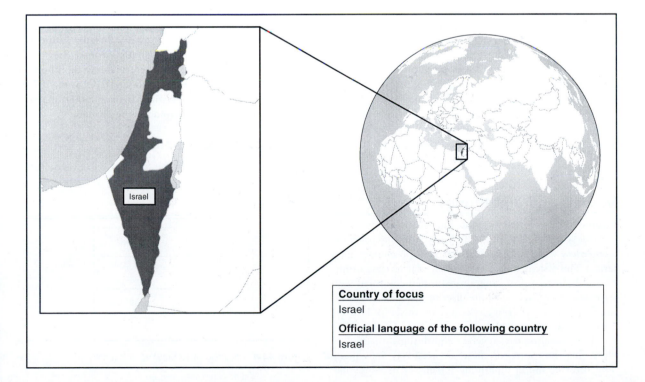

Country of focus
Israel

Official language of the following country
Israel

TABLE 44-1   Consonants produced in Hebrew

	Bilabial	Labiodental	Dental	Alveolar
Plosive	p b			t d
Nasal	m			n
Trill				
Tap or flap				
Fricative		f v		s z
Lateral fricative	■			
Affricate				ts
Approximant				
Lateral approximant	■			l

Black = articulations judged impossible

Based on the International Phonetic Alphabet. Courtesy of the International Phonetic Association (c/o Department of Linguistics, University of Victoria, Victoria, British Columbia, Canada).

The phoneme /x/ is articulated between the velum and the uvula, and it, too, differs in pronunciation from speaker to speaker and even within the same person, with its place of articulation often changing in keeping with the phonetic environment in which it occurs (Bolozky, 1997; Laufer, 1986; Schwarzwald, 1981). The glottal consonants /h, ʔ/ are often deleted, especially in unstressed syllables and intervocalically, and are generally pronounced only utterance initially. Further, the consonant /ʔ/ is often pronounced in place of /h/, mainly in word-initial position or at the beginning of a stressed syllable (Bolozky, 1978; Chayen, 1973; Laufer, 1990; Rabin, 1973; Weinberg, 1966).

In sum, the consonantal system of Hebrew shows a certain amount of variability in pronunciation, reflecting the impact of borrowed sounds and neutralization of historical distinctions.

Vowels and diphthongs

Hebrew has five vowels, articulated in a manner close to the cardinal vowels: high front and back, mid front and back, and a single low vowel (the least marked in morphophonological terms). This system, too, reveals considerable leveling of historical distinctions (e.g., long or geminated compared with short vowels attested to in the diacritic system of vocalization; see below on Writing system). The vowels of Hebrew are depicted in Figure 44-1.

Hebrew also has several diphthongs, mainly in word-final position, but these are relatively infrequent. The most common diphthong is /ei/, as in words like /lifˈnei/ 'before', /heiˈxan/ 'where' —although in some cases, and with some speakers, this is pronounced as the vowel /e/ (Plada, 1959). Other diphthongs are /ai/ as in /dai/ 'enough', /oi/ as in /noi/ 'beauty', and /ui/ as in /tsaˈfui/ 'likely.' There is only one morphological pattern that regularly entails the diphthong /ui/—the passive participial or resultative pattern CaCuC in roots ending with phonological /j/, as in /ʁaˈtsui/ 'wanted', 'desirable', /kaˈnui/ 'bought', /ʃaˈtui/ 'drunk' (Berman, 1994). Some scholars analyze these Hebrew diphthongs as strings of vowel plus the off-glide /j/ (Chayen, 1973; Laufer, 1990), indicating that their status is rather unclear and that they appear to be undergoing change.

Phonotactic restrictions

Under this heading, address the topics of syllable structure and consonant clusters.

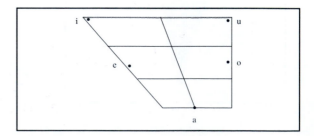

Figure 44-1   Position of Hebrew vowels (based on Laufer, 1990)

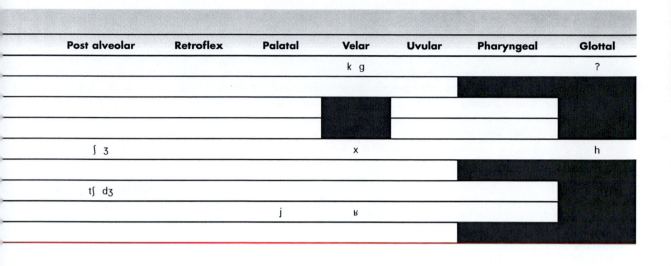

	Post alveolar	Retroflex	Palatal	Velar	Uvular	Pharyngeal	Glottal
				k g			ʔ
	ʃ ʒ			x			h
	tʃ dʒ						
			j		ʁ		

Syllables

The most common types of syllables in Hebrew are CV and CVC, for example /lo/ 'no', 'not', /kis/ 'pocket', although up to three consonants can appear in onset or coda position. There can also be syllables with no consonant at all in either the onset or coda position (Laufer, 1991), even though the writing system invariably indicates both onset and coda as having a consonant. (For example, the feminine ending –a is rendered orthographically by the letter *heh* /h/, is pronounced with a vowel coda, e.g., PRH /pa'ʁa/ 'cow', YLDH /jal'da/ 'girl').[4] Speakers of Hebrew typically pronounce words without any onset consonant when these take the shape of the glottal consonants /ʔ, h/—orthographic *alef, heh*—and the voiced pharyngeal fricative /ʕ/—orthographic *ayin*—both word-initially and word-medially. For example, the word for 'Daddy' is written as ʔBʔ and pronounced /'aba/ while orthographic MHR 'quick' is pronounced /ma.'eʁ/. The same is true for syllables that lack a consonantal coda, yielding so-called open syllables in word-final position (Ravid, 1995), for example, /po/ 'here', /pa.'ʁa/ 'cow', in contrast to the more typical CVC syllabic structure of words like /kiʁ/ 'wall', /kis/ 'pocket', /ʃul'xan/ 'table'. Syllables that contain a coda in word-final position are commoner than their "final open-syllable" counterparts (Cohen-Gross, 1997).

Hebrew words are most typically two syllables in length, although trisyllabics are quite common, especially in morphologically complex words (e.g., /jela'dim/ 'children', /xave'ʁim/ 'friends', or /jaldu'ti/ 'childish', /xave'ʁut/ 'friendship'). Words of more than three syllables are either derivationally complex or else borrowed (e.g., /samxuti'jut/ 'authoritarianism' and the loan words /kleman'tina/ 'tangerine', /melafe'fon/ 'cucumber'). Hebrew has no long vowels and does not distinguish phonologically between light and heavy syllables.

Consonants and consonant clusters

All the consonants in Table 44-1 can appear in word-initial position in current Hebrew, although historically, and also in normative usage, the fricatives /f, v, x/ were disallowed in syllable-initial position, which required their stop alternants /p, b, k/ (Adam, 1993, Bolozky, 1978; Schwarzwald, 1976). The fricatives /f, v/ are relatively infrequent in onset position even today.

Hebrew allows numerous biconsonantal clusters in onset position (e.g., /gvi'na/ 'cheese', /tmu'na/ 'picture'), and these are subject to far fewer restrictions than in English (Schwarzwald, 2004).[5] A wide variety of clusters is possible in onset position, in all cases that do not violate the sonority scale (Bat-El, 1994; Bolozky, 1972, 1978; Laufer 1991; Rosén, 1973; Tene, 1973). Words with more than two initial consonants are rare, mainly in borrowings (e.g., /sprei/ 'spray'), where the first consonant is typically a sibilant (Laufer, 1992).

---

4 We adopt the convention of rendering Hebrew (consonant) letters by upper case Roman symbols.
5 In fact, normative usage disallows initial consonant clusters and requires that these be separated by a *schwa*.

Occurrence of consonants in coda position is unconstrained in Hebrew, but due to traditional rules of spirantization, the stops /p, b/ rarely occur at the end of words, except for borrowed words (e.g., /dʒip/ 'jeep', /pab/ 'pub'). Final consonant clusters are confined mainly to the second person feminine past tense (2FemSg) suffix /t/, as in /heˈramt/ 'lifted-2FemSg = you lifted', /aˈxalt/ 'ate-2FemSg = you ate' or to loan words (e.g., /paʁk/ 'park', /faks/ 'fax', /ˈambulans/ 'ambulance'). Words ending in three consonants are even rarer, and are invariably borrowed (e.g., /tekst/ 'text') (Laufer, 1992).

Tones

Tones are not a distinctive feature of the sound system of Hebrew.

Stress and Intonation

Stress

Hebrew has mainly word-final stress (e.g., /paˈʁa/ 'cow', /ʃulˈxan/ 'table') but for sociolinguistic as well as grammatical reasons, numerous words have nonfinal stress, including: (1) penultimate stress in morphological categories such as the so-called segolates (i.e., words in the pattern CéCeC),[6] (e.g., /ˈjeled/ 'boy', /ˈsefeʁ/ 'book')—or with medial historical pharyngeals like, /ˈlaxan/ 'tune'; (2) words with certain grammatical suffixes—e.g., /haˈlaxʕti/ 'walked-1st = I walked', /jaˈʃavʕnu/ 'sat+1stPlural = we sat'; (3) loan words like /ˈketʃop/ 'ketchup', /baˈnana/ 'banana', and /ˈʃokolad/ 'chocolate', /ˈotobus/ 'bus', with antepenultimate stress; (4) nicknames or pet names, e.g., /ˈsigi/ for /siˈɡal/, /ˈkobi/ for /jaˈakov/; and (5) words that have word-final stress when pronounced normatively, but penultimate stress when used as names of people, places, or children's games; for example, the word /bʁaˈxa/ 'blessing' has final stress, but the girl's name 'Bracha' typically has penultimate stress /ˈbʁaxa/; the word /ʁexoˈvot/ 'streets' contrasts with the name of the city 'Rehovot' /ʁeˈxovot/ and the noun /klaˈfim/ 'cards' is stressed on the final syllable, but any game played with cards has penultimate stress /ˈklafim/, as is true for the ordinal numbers like /ʁiˈʃon/, /ʃeˈni/ 'first', 'second', and so forth in normal counting compared with children's games (Bahat, 1991; Bat-El, in press; Berman, 1985; Bolozky, 1978; Chayen, 1973; Cohen-Gross, 1997; Rosén, 1973; Schwarzwald, 1991).

According to Bat-El (1989, 1993), some Hebrew words (mainly nouns) are lexically accented, and the rest are phonologically specified as having word-final stress. Thus, when a suffix is added to the base word (e.g., the plural suffix masculine /im/ or feminine /ot/), in words with phonological stress, the stress shifts to word-final position (to the suffix, e.g., /mitˈbax/ 'kitchen'-/mitbaˈxim/ 'kitchens', /ʃulˈxan/ 'table' - /ʃulxaˈnot/ 'tables'). In words that have lexical accent, this shift either does not occur or is not to the final position (e.g., /ˈtʁaktoʁ/ 'tractor'- /ˈtʁaktoʁim/ 'tractors', /ˈtelefon/ 'telephone' - /teleˈfonim/ 'telephones'. This dual system of stress may yield minimal pairs distinguished only by stress, e.g., /ˈtxina/ 'tehini' (the food) versus /txiˈna/ 'plea', or /ˈbiʁa/ 'beer' versus /biˈʁa/ 'capital' (city). Moreover, some bisyllabic words constitute grammatically determined minimal pairs, distinguished by word-final stress on the verb compared with initial, penultimate stress on the noun, e.g., /paˈxad/ was 'afraid' - /ˈpaxad/ 'fear', /taˈam/ 'tasted' - /ˈtaam/ (a) 'taste'.

Hebrew thus constitutes an interesting case for acquisition, since its stress patterns cannot be clearly identified as either word-final or penultimate. Note, finally, that Hebrew does not have relative stress, so that a syllable is either stressed or unstressed, and any syllable can take word stress irrespective of its internal composition (Bolozky, 1982). Secondary stress is virtually automatic, and most of the time every syllable that is once removed from the stressed syllables receives secondary stress (Bolozky, 1997).

Intonation

The most common intonation pattern in declarative utterances is high, with a falling intonation at the end (Laufer, 1987). Wh-questions typically have a similar pattern as declaratives, falling at the end, but typically with a rather sharper decline. In contrast, yes/no questions are generally marked by utterance-final rising intonation, often the only marker of these constructions in Hebrew, since speakers tend to delete the question word and simply mark the question by a rising intonation. These major intonation patterns fall into numerous tone groups based on factors like communicative intent, emphasis, and affect. Lefkowitz (2004) describes a rise-fall contour at the end of phrases as more typical of speakers with a Sfardi accent, and as used by speakers with an Ashkenazi accent only to express and evoke affect. Other features of a Sfardi accent are a wide pitch range, relatively short prosodic phrases, and common use of high-pitched accents in stressed syllables.

---

6 Throughout the chapter, we follow the Semitic convention of indicating root consonants by C with the vowels represented by their phonemic value. Where non-word-final, stress is indicated by an accent aigu on the relevant prefinal vowel.

Writing system

The Hebrew orthography used to this day is that of classical Biblical Hebrew, derived from the ancient Phoenician script in the form of what is called an *abjad*[7] (Daniels, 1998; Tolchinsky, 2003). This means that only consonant letters are represented, 22 in all, written from right to left. These 22 consonant letters include a graphemic representation of several phonemes that, as noted earlier, are neutralized in the pronunciation of Israeli Hebrew—for example, different letters represent the velar stop /k/ and the emphatic /q/, the alveolar stop /t/ and the emphatic /tˤ/, as well as both the spirant /x/ and the pharyngeal /ħ/, and the pharyngeal /ʕ/, the glottal stop /ʔ/, and the glottal spirant /h/ are represented by three distinct letters.

In addition to the 22 consonant letters, a system of diacritics, so-called *nikud* 'pointing', was introduced around a thousand years ago to indicate vowel values by means of dots placed underneath and to the side of the consonantal letter, with dots inside certain letters distinguishing stops from spirants or representing historical doubling (Coulmas, 2003; Shimron, 1993; Tolchinsky, 2003, p. 66, fn). For example, the word pronounced /baʁˈzel/ 'iron' is written בַּרְזֶל (BRZL) without any vowels.

Vowel pointing is used to this day in school primers, in children's storybooks, in materials for (second) language learners, and in poetry, while the Hebrew Bible, studied throughout the school years in Israel, is also vowel-pointed. However, by second or third grade, Israeli children typically read without the aid of these markers, and this is the normal way Israelis read and write everything—newspapers, advertisements, novels, and scientific research (Ravid, 1996).

Hebrew speakers are aided by the fact that the current orthography is fleshed out by so-called *matres lectionis*-'mothers of reading', the letters *yod* and *waw* standing for the high vowels /i/ and /u/, historical /j/ and /w/, but today pronounced as consonants as /j/ and /v/ respectively. Thus, for example, the multiply ambiguous series of consonants SPR can be partially disambiguated in so-called lenis or full script as SYPR, SPYR and also as SWPR or SPWR— standing for /siˈpeʁ/ 'told' and /saˈfiʁ/ 'countable' and for /soˈfeʁ/ 'writer' and /siˈpuʁ/ 'story' respectively.[8] But even this is not fully transparent, since the letter *waw* (ו) can stand for both the back vowels /o/ and /u/ as well as for the consonant sound

/v/. Besides, even the "full," nonvocalized script with the letters *yod* (י) and *waw* (ו) provides only a partial representation of phonemically relevant distinctions. Thus, the string SPYR could stand for both the adjective /saˈfiʁ/ 'countable' and the noun /saˈpiʁ/ 'sapphire', and the string SWPR could stand for both /soˈfeʁ/ 'writer' and also /suˈpaʁ/ 'was-told'. Moreover, the three letters SPR can be read and pronounced as any of the following: /saˈpaʁ/ 'barber', /saˈfaʁ/ 'counted', /ˈsefeʁ/ 'book', /sfaʁ/ 'border'. In other words, Hebrew—while basically an alphabetic script—represents a "deep" orthography (Gillis and Ravid, 2001; Pacton and Fayol, 2004). That is, there is no way to go from letters to sounds directly in the nonvocalized script of normal usage, and people need to know the language in order to be able to read it. Reading Hebrew requires taking into account the syntactic and semantic context as well as the morphological structure of words, and research on early literacy shows that morphological analysis is essential to children's success in reading and writing Hebrew (Levin and Korat, 1993; Levin, Ravid, and Rappoport, 2001; Ravid, 2001, 2005; Share and Levin, 1999).

Varieties of Modern Hebrew

Israeli Hebrew is spoken in a relatively small country with a centralized system of education and the same radio, television, and newspaper media used across the country. There is thus almost nothing in the way of regional variation, except for local versions of the names of children's games such as "marbles" and also some very minor alternations in, say, the pronunciation of the number "two hundred" as /maaˈtaim/, with a long vowel, in Jerusalem, and as /maˈtaim/ in other places in the country.

The major variation in the pronunciation of Modern Hebrew as a first language—ignoring immigrant and other second language learners—derives from the country of origin of speakers rather than from geographical area or social status. The main dialect other than the General Israeli Hebrew described in this chapter is "Arabicized Hebrew" (Blanc, 1964) or the "Oriental dialect" (Laufer, 1990), the variety spoken mainly by Israelis whose families are of Arabic-speaking extraction. This differs from General Israeli mainly in pronunciation of the so-called pharyngeals /ħ/ and /ʕ/.

---

7 The writing system is of the kind some refer to as a syllabary, since it represents only consonantal elements. For example, the sentences "The man went home," "The men want him," "The men want ham," and "The man/men won't hum" would all be rendered by the equivalent of TH MN WNT HM in Hebrew orthography. (Thanks to Prof. Yishai Tobin for this example.)

8 Throughout the chapter, we follow the convention of representing orthographic consonants by upper case forms of their phonemic counterparts in English. Thus, the string SPR stands for the letters *samech, peh, resh*.

Speakers of this dialect pronounce the letter *chet* (ח) as /ħ/, whereas most speakers neutralize it to the velar spirant /x/, and they render the letter *ayin* (ע) as /ʕ/, instead of omitting it altogether or else pronouncing it like the glottal stop. Another difference is in realization of the phoneme /ʁ/, pronounced by some speakers of so-called Oriental background as /r/ (Ben-Tulila, 1983; Blanc, 1964; Laufer, 1990).

General Israeli Hebrew represents the mainstream standard usage among Israelis for whom Hebrew is a first language and is the subject of most research on children's language acquisition (Berman, 1985, 2004; Ravid, 1995, 2003), including on phonology (Ben-David, 2001). Consequently, in what follows, Arabicized pronunciations are disregarded.

Typical acquisition of Hebrew

In contrast to relatively rich research on acquisition of lexicon, morphology, syntax, and discourse in Hebrew, there are few studies on acquisition of Hebrew phonology, and these are mostly unpublished seminar papers and a few master's theses. The descriptions that follow thus rely heavily on the first author's doctoral dissertation, the most detailed and as far as we know the only wide-scale longitudinal study of acquisition of Hebrew phonology to date. Ben-David (2001) traced the phonological development of 10 children from the appearance of their first words (average age 1;2, age range from 0;10 to 1;5) to the time when they were judged to be able to correctly produce all segmental sounds (with the exception of producing sibilants as interdentals) and the prosodic units that are common in the repertoire of general Israeli Hebrew in at least some environments (average age 2;10, from 2;5 to 3;6). The naturalistic speech output of three of the children was recorded once a week and these children together with another seven children (six boys and four girls altogether) were tested once a month for the entire three years of the study by means of specially devised production tasks. The description that follows relies on both sources: small-scale cross-sectional studies of specific facets of Hebrew acquisition and Ben-David's longitudinal study (see the Summary of Studies table at the end of this chapter).

Acquired sounds

Consonants

The most extensive study on consonant acquisition is Lavie's (1978) unpublished M.A. thesis, which attempted to establish norms for consonant acquisition. Her cross-sectional

study included 200 preschool children between ages 3;0 and 5;0, using a criterion of 90 percent correct production in word-initial and final position. Girls did better than boys, especially around age 4;0. Table 44-2 describes Lavie's findings for age of consonant acquisition.

Lavie's study showed that acquisition of the sibilant consonants /s, z, ʃ, ts/ was not completed by age 5;0 (the age of the oldest children in her study). Her findings are confirmed by other (likewise unpublished) seminar studies of sibilant acquisition among older children, showing that they are not fully mastered even by age 7 years (Ben Zvi, 1981; Gabay, 1986; Jedwab, 1975). The most frequent misarticulations among 6- and 7-year-olds are substitution of /s/ for /ʃ/ and interdental production of all sibilants, going counter to standard Hebrew pronunciation.

TABLE 44-2   Age of acquisition for Hebrew consonants

Consonants	Age of acquisition
p	3;0
b	3;0
m	3;0
n	3;0
j	3;0
f	3;0
x	3;0
k	3;6
l	3;6
t	4;0
g	4;0
ʁ	4;0
d	5;0
v	after 5;0
h	after 5;0
s	after 5;0
z	after 5;0
ʃ	after 5;0
ts	after 5;0

Note. Data from Lavie (1978).

Ben-David's (2001) longitudinal study defined the notion "acquisition" as the stage when all phonological units considered were produced correctly in at least some words. Thus, a consonant was considered "acquired" when a child produced it at least twice in syllable-initial and syllable-final positions. By this criterion, all 10 children in the study produced all Hebrew consonants before the age of 3;0, although some of them produced the sibilants /s, z, ts/ as interdentals rather than as alveolar or post-alveolar, as required in standard pronunciation (see Table 44-1 above). Table 44-3 shows the order and average ages of acquisition as tracked across the 10 children.

Table 44-3 shows that the non-back stops and nasals are the first to emerge, followed by fricatives and velar stops. Relatively later acquisitions, from age 2 years on, are the sibilants and the sonorants /l, ʁ/, This is similar to what is known for order of acquisition of consonants in other languages.

Consonant clusters

Studies on the acquisition of clusters in Hebrew have focused on three topics: age of acquisition, order of acquisition, and type of errors, all on initial clusters, as the common type in Hebrew. Rosenberg's (1983) cross-sectional study of 33 children aged 2;0 to 4;11 showed that more than half of the clusters (56 percent) were produced correctly by around age 2;6, when the most common

error was reduction of the cluster to a single member. Other types of errors were deleting of the whole cluster and producing a cluster with one of its members replaced by another consonant. At age 3;6, the vast bulk (85 percent) of the clusters were produced correctly, with almost no deletion of an entire cluster. At age 4;6, more then 90 percent of the clusters were produced correctly, leading Rosenberg to conclude that the age of acquisition of clusters by Hebrew-speaking children is around age 4;0.

Forkush's (1997) cross-sectional study of 36 children between ages 1;8 and 4;8 support Rosenberg's findings. The younger subjects (aged 1;8 to 2;11) produced only around one-third (33 percent) of the clusters correctly, increasing to well over half (58 percent) between ages 3;0 and 3;10, and reaching nearly ceiling (87.6 percent) after age 4;0. The most frequent error across the population was reduction of the cluster to one member. Further, across age groups, clusters in CCV syllables were produced more correctly than clusters in CCVC syllables.

Ben-David (2001) found that before the age of 2;6, all 10 children in her study produced at least three or four word-initial consonant clusters, of the form stop + sonorant before, say, stop + fricative or fricative + sonorant. As in the other studies, deletion of one consonant of the cluster was the most frequent error. Other errors were epenthesis of a vowel between the two components of the cluster (e.g., the word /dli/ 'bucket' was produced by the children as [de'li]) and coalescence of features from the two consonants into one consonant (e.g., /tʁu'fa/ ⇨ [ku'fa] 'medicine', /tmu'na/ ⇨ [pu'na] 'picture'). [9]

Ben-David's analysis revealed four stages in the acquisition of cluster production, similar to those described for English by Ingram (1976). In their first attempts to produce a cluster, children delete the entire cluster; next, around age 1;9, they produce a single consonant from the target cluster. A third stage is use of epenthesis or coalescence, a very brief stage that was not noted for all Ben-David's 10 subjects (and for only a few of the children in the other studies). The fourth and last stage is production of both the consonants of the cluster.

The different studies show less agreement as to which consonants children tend to delete. Rosenberg's (1983) younger group (mean age 2;6) showed a slight tendency to delete the second consonant, a year later they showed equal deletions of both components, while in the few deletions by age 4;6, the first consonant was the one deleted. On the other hand, Lavie's (1978) large-scale

TABLE 44-3 Age of first productions of Hebrew consonants

Consonants	Age when all 10 children produced the consonants
p, b, t, d, m, n, j	1;3
s	1;4
f, v, x	1;7
k, g	1;8
l, z	2;0
ʃ, ts	2;6
ʁ	2;8
tʃ	2;9

*Note. Based on Ben-David (2001). The stop consonants /p, b/ were not tested in syllable-final position since processes of spirantization mean they are rare in this position, where they surface typically as /f, v/.

9 From here on, examples from children's productions are given in square brackets [ ] and how the words are pronounced in standard usage is given between slashes / /.

study of 200 children found that deletion of the first consonant in a cluster was common across her population. Neither Rosenberg nor Lavie reports on the phonological features of the consonants that were deleted. Forkush (1997) observed that children deleted mostly stop consonants (in about 40 percent of cases), always the first in the clusters. The consonants that were least often deleted were nasals (9 percent) and laterals (18 percent), always the second consonant of the cluster.

Ben-David's (2001) analysis of the phonological patterns of deleted consonants showed that when the cluster includes liquids (of the type obstruent + liquid), children tended to delete the liquid (the second component of the cluster) and produce the obstruent (e.g., /pʁi/ ⇨ [pi] 'fruit', /ˈglida/ ⇨ [ˈgida] 'ice cream', /ˈfʁida/ ⇨ [ˈfida] (the name) 'Frida', /sliˈxa/ ⇨ [siˈxa] 'sorry'). However, when the cluster did not include a liquid, children tended to delete the first consonants (e.g., /dvaʃ/ ⇨ [vaʃ] 'honey', /ktaˈnim/ ⇨ [taˈnim] 'little' pl., /spaˈgeti/ ⇨ [paˈgeti] 'spaghetti', /zvuv/ ⇨ [vuv] 'fly', /smiˈxa/ ⇨ [miˈxa] 'blanket', /tmuˈna/ ⇨ [muˈna] 'picture'). These findings led her to conclude that in Hebrew, children prefer to produce the second consonant of the cluster, unless it is highly sonorant, like the liquids.

Vowels and diphthongs

The only study known to us on acquisition of vowels in Hebrew is Ben David (2001). She found that the 10 children she studied produced the high vowels /i, u/ and the low vowel /a/ correctly from their first words (average age 1;2) with almost no instances of misarticulation. The mid-back vowel /o/ was acquired a little later, while the mid-front vowel /e/ was the last to be correctly produced (up to three months after children had produced their first 10 words). None of the children produced the vowel /e/ at the first meeting (average age 1;2), when they had productive command of some 10 words each, but typically substituted the unmarked vowel /a/ for /e/ until they were able to produce the latter correctly.

This picture of acquisition of the five Hebrew vowels is supported by findings of the case study of Dromi, Most, and Yehuda (1993) of a child at the one-word stage. The only vowels he produced among his first 10 words (at age 1;4) were the same three as Ben-David found for her 10 subjects /i, a, u/.

Percent correct

None of the available studies specify percentage of consonants, consonant clusters, or vowels that are produced correctly in acquisition of Hebrew.

Phonological processes

The most comprehensive cross-sectional study of phonological processes in acquisition of Hebrew is Shaked (1990). She examined 20 children between ages 1;7 and 2;7, divided into two groups: younger (age 1;7 to 2;1) and older (age 2;2 to 2;7). The most common processes attested in the younger group were cluster reduction, deletion of unstressed syllables, final consonant deletion, sibilant fronting, consonant devoicing, and stopping. The most common processes among the older children were cluster reduction, final consonant deletion, sibilant fronting, /l/ gliding, and final devoicing. Shaked's findings reveal the same general processes as Halpern's (1984) study of the phonological processes of 10 children between ages 1;8 to 2;10.

Phonological processes have also been examined among rather older Hebrew-acquiring children. Izmailov's (1983) study of 10 children aged 3;0 to 4;8 reports that the two youngest children (aged 3;0 and 3;5) manifested processes such as cluster reduction, deletion of unstressed syllable, final consonant deletion, and devoicing. In contrast, nearly all processes of misarticulation among the older children related to the sibilants (e.g., sibilant fronting and depalatalization of /ʃ/ to /s/).

Taken together, these studies indicate that from about the age of 3;6, Hebrew-speaking children reveal a marked decrease in use of immature phonological processes. The most persistent such phenomena concern production of the sibilants which, as noted, are late acquisitions in general.

Intelligibility

To date there is no study of intelligibility of Hebrew-speaking children.

Phonetic inventory

To date there is no study of the inventory of consonants or vowels of Hebrew-speaking children.

Common mismatches

There is to date no research dealing with common mismatches in children's acquisition of Hebrew, but all the studies noted above indicate that the main mismatches on the segmental level are the following: interdental lisp of the sibilants /s, z, ʃ, ts/, substitution of /s/ for /ʃ/ and /ts/, deletion of /ʁ/ or replacing it by a glottal stop, gliding of /l/ and replacing it with /j/, and fronting of the velar consonants /k, g/ and replacing them by /t, d/.

Syllable structure

As in many other languages, children acquiring Hebrew produce CV syllables before other types of syllables like CVC or CCV(C) (Ben-David, 2001; Berman, 1977; Halpern, 1984; Shaked, 1990). Ben-David's (2001) in-depth study of acquisition of syllable structure in Hebrew reveals that in their first words (average age 1;2), the children produced mostly CV syllables, but also V syllables—the latter only at the beginning of disyllabic words (as detailed below). Some weeks later, all 10 subjects produced VC syllables when target words were monosyllabic CV words (e.g., the words /af / *nose* and /od/ *more* were produced by the children as [af] and [od] respectively). Syllables of the type CVC or CCV(C) were acquired later, as described below.

Acquisition of the syllable onset: In their first words, the children often deleted the onset consonants from the first syllable (e.g., /ˈlego/ ⇨ [ˈego] 'Lego', /baˈlon/ ⇨ [aˈlon] 'balloon', /maˈka/ ⇨ [aˈka] (a) 'hit, blow'). This deletion occurred only in this position and not in onsets that were not at the beginning of multisyllabic words. This deletion of consonants cannot be attributed to difficulties in producing these segments, because the same children did produce these same consonants in the onsets of final syllables at this stage of their development. The second stage of acquisition of first syllable onset took the form of full assimilation of the consonants to the one in the next syllable (e.g., /ˈlego/ ⇨ [ˈgego] 'Lego', /tiˈpeʃ/ ⇨ [piˈpes] 'stupid'). Only in the third stage did the children produce the target consonants in the first syllable onset (e.g., /ˈlego/ ⇨ [ˈlego] 'Lego', /baˈlon/ ⇨ [baˈlon] 'balloon'). The first two stages (e.g., deletion and full assimilation) were also found in Berman's (1977) case study of a Hebrew-English bilingual at the one-word stage. Her daughter used many words with deletion of the first consonants (e.g., /ˈjosi/ ⇨ [ˈosi] 'name', /ˈnumi/ ⇨ [ˈumi] 'lullaby', /ˈtali/ ⇨ [ˈali] 'name') as well as with full assimilation of the first consonant (e.g., /ˈsafta/ ⇨ [ˈtata] 'grandma', /ˈdubi/ ⇨ [ˈbubi] 'teddy bear'). The stages noted by Ben-David for consonant deletion and assimilation in initial-syllable onset were found later in the acquisition of three- and four-syllable words as well (e.g., deletion: /maˈgevet/ ⇨ [aˈgevet] 'towel', /baˈnana/ ⇨ [aˈnana] 'banana', /tarneˈgol/ ⇨ [ageˈgol] 'cock'; assimilation: /taʀneˈgol/ ⇨ [gageˈgol] 'cock', /nemaˈla/ ⇨ [memaˈla] 'ant.'

Acquisition of the syllable coda: Coda consonants were deleted from almost all of the children's first words (except for VC words as noted earlier) (e.g., /jad/ ⇨ [ja] 'hand', /ˈozen/ ⇨ [ˈoze] 'ear', /bakˈbuk/ ⇨ [baˈbu] 'bottle'). When they started to produce consonants in

coda position, they did so first in final stressed syllables (e.g., /jad/ ⇨ [ja] 'hand', /bakˈbuk/ ⇨ [baˈbuk] 'bottle', but: /ˈozen/ ⇨ [ˈoze] 'ear', /ˈtiktak/ ⇨ [ˈtita] 'ticktock'), and some weeks later in final nonstressed syllables (e.g., /ˈozen/ ⇨ [ˈozen] 'ear', /ˈtiktak/ ⇨ [ˈtitak] 'ticktock'). Only some months later (around age 2), did they start to produce coda consonants in nonfinal syllables.

The acquisition of nonfinal coda consonants has also been examined in some detail. Thus, Kochva's (1996) study of 3-year-olds reports that at this age, all 15 children still manifested around 20 percent deletions of the nonfinal coda consonant in bisyllabic and trisyllabic words.

Prosody

This section considers the word as a prosodic unit and acquisition of word stress.

Acquisition of the prosodic word

All the studies noted earlier found that deletion of the unstressed syllable is a very common process among children until around age 3 (Amir, 1995; Halpern, 1984; Shaked, 1990). The findings of Amir (1995) show that most deletions of unstressed syllables are of initial syllables, with almost no deletions of final unstressed syllables.

Berman's (1977) case study was the first to consider the production of words as prosodic units in children's Hebrew. She found that her daughter, then at the single-word phase, deleted initial syllables in disyllabic words with final stress (e.g., /toˈda/ ⇨ [da] 'thank you', /maˈka/ ⇨ [ka] 'a hit'), but not in disyllabic words with initial stress.

Ben-David's (2001) longitudinal study revealed several stages in the acquisition of the prosodic word in Hebrew. All 10 children in her study produced monosyllabic as well as disyllabic words in their first 10 words. At the first stage (around age 1;2), when the target word had final stress, the children produced only one syllable of the target word, usually the final stressed one (e.g., /jalˈda/ ⇨ [da] 'girl', /ugiˈja/ ⇨ [ja] 'cookie'). When the target word had penultimate or antepenultimate stress, the children produced both the stressed and the final syllables from the target word (e.g., /ˈima/ ⇨ [ˈima] 'mother', /baˈnana/ ⇨ [ˈnana] 'banana', /ˈtelefon/ ⇨ [ˈtefo] 'telephone'). At the next stage (around age 1;4), the children started to produce two syllables in words with final stress (e.g., /aˈdom/ ⇨ [aˈdom] *red*, /oniˈja/ ⇨ [niˈja] 'ship', /hipoˈtam/ ⇨ [toˈtam] 'hippopotamus'). The syllables selected for production were the final stressed syllable and the one adjacent to it (e.g., /ugiˈja/ ⇨ [giˈja] 'cookie', /melafeˈfon/ ⇨ [feˈfo] 'cucumber'). Two syllables per word was the maximal production for other types of stress patterns as well. At the third stage (around age 1;8), children started to produce three syllables from the target words (e.g., /'otobus/ ⇨ ['otobus] 'bus', /mata'na/ ⇨ [ata'na] 'present/gift'). In the case of target words with four or more syllables (typically loan words), the children produced only three syllables, usually deleting the first one (e.g., /tele'vizja/ ⇨ [a'ziza] 'television', /hipopo'tam/ ⇨ [toto'tam] 'hippopotamus'). In the fourth and final stage (typically around age 2;2), the children would produce all four syllables of the target words.

There is some inconclusive evidence for another stage prior to the first stage described above. At this point, children produce just one syllable from target words, mainly final syllables and some stressed, nonfinal syllables (e.g., /nig'mar/ ⇨ [ma] 'finished', /'kova/ ⇨ [va] 'hat', /'otobus/ ⇨ [bu] 'bus', /lif'toax/ ⇨ [to] 'to open'). Further evidence for this stage comes from Adam's (2002) cross-sectional analysis of phonological acquisition (using published studies of the acquisition of Hebrew combined with databases from Ruth Berman and from Esther Dromi, Tel Aviv University, and supplementary data collected from three children between 1;4 and 2;0). Adam found that in their very first productions, the children's output syllables were not always the final or stressed ones, but those that contain the vowels /a/ or /u/ (e.g., /ba'lon/ ⇨ [ba] 'balloon', /ka'duʁ/ ⇨ [ka] 'ball', /'tutim/ ⇨ [tu] 'strawberries'), leading her to propose that at this initial phase, children's productions are affected by the vowel's segmental features rather than by the prosodic structure of the word. The paucity of relevant empirical data and the different interpretations of findings make it difficult to reach conclusive generalizations on this issue.

In the acquisition of monosyllabic target words, Ben-David found no evidence for processes applied by children at the level of the prosodic word. The only exceptions were deletion of coda consonants or cluster deletions, which—as noted earlier—are attributed to syllable structure simplifications rather than to manipulations of the word as a prosodic unit.

Acquisition of stress

There are no reports of stress mismatches made by children in Hebrew phonological acquisition. Ben-David's analysis of thousands of polysyllabic words produced by the 10 children in her study revealed that only

12 involved errors in stress placement. This negligible rate of error, and the fact that these few errors were both from word-final to penultimate and vice versa, lead to the conclusion that Hebrew-speaking children acquire the patterning of word-stress in their language from the very beginning. As detailed earlier, the Hebrew stress system is highly irregular, due to a range of sociolinguistic and historical as well as structural factors that yield a mixture of both word-final and penultimate or nonfinal word stress. It is thus likely that children acquire stress on a lexical, word-by-word basis—although subsequently they come to recognize the underlying structural or morphological constraints determining where stress is or is not word-final.

Phonological awareness

Research on phonological awareness among Hebrew-speaking children has focused largely on the period of "emergent literacy" in the transition from kindergarten (age 5 to 6 years) to the first years of formal schooling. One such unpublished study (Seidman, 2000) of the same 20 children in kindergarten and first grade showed marked improvement in awareness of syllable structure across these two stages of development. Published studies in this domain have been largely motivated by interest in the relationship between phonological (or, rather, phonemic) awareness and reading abilities, on the one hand, and the effect of learning to read on phonological awareness, on the other (Bentin, 1992; Levin and Korat, 1993; Shimron and Navon, 1982). For example, a large-scale study of the relationship between phonemic awareness and reading skills of Israeli children between the ages of 5 and 7 years (Bentin, Hammer, and Cahan, 1991) showed that school-based experience during the first half of Grade I, when reading is taught, was the "major factor in the dramatic development of phonological awareness typically observed around age 7;6" (Bentin, 1997, p. 195). Another study (Bentin and Leshem, 1993) revealed that kindergarten-age children who had been trained in identifying individual phonemes within or at the beginning or ends of words did significantly better when tested for reading abilities in Grade I than their peers who had not received such training. Table 44-4 specifies norms or at least goals to be aimed at in the domain of phonological awareness in Hebrew. [10]

Clearly, phonological awareness and learning to read and write have a two-way impact. As Gillis and Ravid

---

10 The table is translated from Hebrew, from a report prepared for the Israel Ministry of Education by Iris Levin of Tel Aviv University, entitled "Alphabetical Knowledge: Knowing Letters and Phonological Awareness" [in Hebrew]. The authors are indebted to Dr. Levin for her generosity in making this material available.

TABLE 44-4   Developmental targets in phonological awareness

Age range	Developmental targets
3–4 years	Recognize rhymes and rhyming games
	Recognize repeated strings of sounds in children's stories
4–5 years	Construct rhymes with real or nonsense words
	Segment words into syllables and combine syllables into words
	Identify, isolate, and compare syllables
5–6 years	Divide words into units of sound (combinations of C+V or C+C) and combine units of sound into words
	Identify, isolate, and compare strings of C+V
	Compare, identify, and isolate initial and final consonants in words

Note. Courtesy of Iris Levin, Tel Aviv University.

(in press) note, "There is evidence that [phonological and morphological awareness] … both promote and are promoted by learning to read and write through the establishment of links between phonemes, syllables and morphemes and their written representations" (ms, p. 7). In this connection, note that phonemic awareness is only one facet of phonological awareness in general. Other facets of this cognitive domain, such as recognition of rhyme or the ability to segment words into their component syllables, may develop relatively independently of literacy-related activities, but recognition of phonemes is clearly enhanced by exposure to an alphabetic writing system. In a fascinating cross-linguistic study aimed at exploring the effect of writing systems on word segmentation, Hebrew-speaking and Spanish-speaking children from preschool through second grade were asked to segment similar-sounding words in their native language (e.g., *koka-kola, radyo, shokolad*) both orally and in writing (Tolchinsky and Teberosky, 1997, 1998). When asked to segment such words (the instruction was "say it bit by bit"), the younger children responded similarly in both languages: Their favored strategy was to divide the word up into syllables—evidence of similar awareness of the syllable as a basic phonological unit in Hebrew as in Spanish. In contrast, once children had been exposed to formal instruction in writing, their "script-specific knowledge" exerted a marked impact on their responses at grade-school age: In seeking letter-to-sound correspondences, the Hebrew-speaking children relied very largely on consonants, whereas their Spanish-speaking peers used vowels. This reveals the marked impact of writing (Olson, 1994) and of typological features of particular writing systems—in the case of Hebrew, as a basically consonantal script—on phonological awareness.

Thus, Table 44-4 expects 6-year-olds to identify "word-initial and word-final consonants," although in phonological terms, many of the most common words in Hebrew both begin and end with vowel sounds—although not letters. For example, /ima/ 'Mother', 'Mommy' is written אמא (ʔMʔ) and /aba/ 'Daddy' is written אבא (ʔBʔ), /ani/ 'I', 'me' is written אני (ʔNI), while the name of the game 'Lego' /lego/ is written לגו (LGO). Indeed, for native speakers of Hebrew, the word /ot/ 'letter' is defined by the 22 consonants in the alphabet and, as anyone who has ever taught an introductory linguistics course in Israel knows only too well, it is extremely difficult to get even highly literate native speakers of Hebrew to recognize that not only consonants but also vowels can be assigned the status of (speech) sounds. Their typical reaction is to say "but Hebrew doesn't have any vowels." In this, they differ markedly from preschool speakers of the language, who are just as much at home with vowels as their Spanish-speaking counterparts.

Speech assessment of Hebrew-acquiring children

To date, only a very limited range of instruments is available for assessing articulation and phonology in Hebrew-acquiring children. None of these have been standardized, and there are no established norms.

The only generally quite accepted (although never officially authorized) test for assessing children's speech sounds in the language is a set of pictures for examining articulation and naming. This consists of pictures representing words of one to three syllables and all the consonants of Hebrew in word-initial, medial (onset), and final position (Rosin and Yakir, 2000). An additional instrument for use with Hebrew-acquiring children is the articulation subtest of the *Goralnik Language Screening Test* for preschool children consisting of 15 objects, representing part but not all of the phonemes of Israeli Hebrew in onset and/or coda position (Goralnik, 1995). Based on the author's master's thesis, this test is widely used as an initial means of screening preschool children with possible language or speech impairments. In addition, many speech and language clinicians in Israel use informal, "homemade" tests, mainly constructed out of lists of single words.

A more carefully constructed means of assessing phonological abilities of Hebrew-speaking children is currently being prepared by the first author of this chapter (*Hebrew articulation and phonology test*, Ben-David, 2006a). This consists of photographs of 40 objects representative of the segmental inventory of Hebrew in different positions in the word and syllables as well as common word- and syllable-level structures.

Another method for analyzing the speech of people with communication disorders is based on the approach of "phonology as human behavior" (Tobin, 1997). Children's misarticulations are analyzed in phonetic terms and explained as the consequence of trying to achieve maximum communication with minimum effort (that is, in a trade-off between human physiological factors and the communicative factors of speech).

Speech intervention for Hebrew-acquiring children

Speech intervention techniques that have been developed for Hebrew-speaking children referred to speech-language pathologists include the following.

- *Sound, Shape, and Color (SSC)* (Nachmany, 2004). This is based on visual speech symbolization, combined with kinesthetic and auditory perception, requiring children to produce the precise motions needed for producing speech. The SSC method originated in work with children with cleft-palate disorders and has been in clinical use for nearly 25 years. The SSC method trains children to organize their own movements, improve their body awareness, develop cognitive processes for problem solving, as well as enhancing their metaphonological skills.
- *Phonological Intervention Approach to Articulation Disorders* (Ben-David, 2006b; Ben-David and Peleg, 2005).

This method is based on phonological complexity as revealed by research and fieldwork with phonological acquisition. It takes into account different stages of acquisition, with each successive stage more phonologically complex than the one before.

These two intervention techniques have both been developed only recently, and they are as yet unfamiliar to most speech-language pathologists in the country. Most Israeli clinicians use a traditional approach (based on Van Riper, 1978) with an informal, nonlinguistically sophisticated adaptation to Hebrew. This method is sometimes combined with elements from other approaches such as use of minimal pairs (Weiner, 1981) or oral-motor or metaphonological exercises. To the best of our knowledge, there are yet no accepted, standardized, or otherwise authorized methods for phonological intervention or assessment for Hebrew-acquiring children, whether original to Israel or adapted from methods developed elsewhere for children acquiring other languages (mainly English).

Working in Israel

The following section is based on two decades of clinical experience of the first author, in consultation with colleagues and officers of the Israeli Speech, Hearing, and Language Association (ISHLA). We are grateful to Ms. Frida Korenbrot, chairperson of the Association, for her assistance.

The Israeli Speech, Hearing, and Language Association is a voluntary, nonprofit professional organization that represents most of the speech-language pathologists in Israel, the majority of whom have dual certification in both speech-language pathology and audiology. Details on training and accreditation of speech-language pathologists in Israel are available on the Web (http://www.ishla.org.il/index.html).

There are accredited training programs at three institutions in Israel that grant a B.A. in communication disorders, covering both speech-language pathology and audiology: Tel Aviv University Medical School (since 1969), which also offers graduate level programs for M.A. and Ph.D. Degrees; Haifa University; and the Hadassah Academic College in Jerusalem (the latter two since 2001). Formal training includes both academic studies and clinical fieldwork, and B.A. programs have recently been extended from three to three and a half years. These programs, which require around 220 credit hours, are typically specialized from the start of undergraduate studies.

Recent graduates are expected to work under supervision for the first year, as a requirement for receiving accreditation (granted by the Israel Ministry of Health). In addition, numerous speech-language pathologists and audiologists have immigrated to Israel from other countries (e.g., Argentina, Russia, and the United States), most of whom have been granted recognition by the Ministry of Health.

The Israeli Speech, Hearing, and Language Association hosts a two-day annual conference and publishes a yearly Hebrew-language journal *Dash — Dibur U'shmi'a,* concerned mainly with clinical issues in the country (see the Resources section). The association also conducts regular seminars and workshops in all areas of clinical work in speech-language pathology and audiology.

Most Israeli speech-language pathologists are employed by the Ministry of Education in the area of Special Education (special groups, individual tuition, classes, or schools) or by the Ministry of Health in Child Development clinics and and hospital departments of rehabilitation. In addition, many outpatient and private clinics are under contract to various health funds. Other speech-language pathologists are employed by the Ministry of Social Welfare, the Israel Defence Forces, and other social services (for details, see Korenbrot, Hertzano, and Ben Arroya, 2002; Schwartz, Harris, and Most, 1993).

PHONETICALLY SPEAKING

Pronunciation of Hebrew: /ʔivˈʁit/ or /ivˈʁit/, or in Sfardi accent: /ʕivˈrit/

Word/Phrase	Formal usage	Pronunciation	Informal usage for children	Pronunciation
Tongue	lashon	laˈʃon		
Teeth	shinaim	ʃiˈnaim		
Lips	sfataim	sfaˈtaim		
Hard palate	xex kashe	xex kaˈʃe	ha-gag shel ha-pe	hagag ʃel hape
Soft palate	xex rax/vilon	xex ʁax vilon		
Larynx	garon	gaˈʁon		
Lungs	reot	ʁeˈʔot		
Nose	af	af		
Sound	hege= Speech sound tzlil= Sound	ˈhege tslil		
Word	mila	miˈla		
Sentence	mishpat	miʃˈpat		
Paragraph	piska	pisˈka		

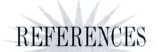

RESOURCES

Books

Berman, R. A. (1978). *Modern Hebrew structure*. Tel Aviv: Universities Publishing.

Glinert, L. (1989). *The grammar of Modern Hebrew*. Cambridge, UK: Cambridge University Press.

Ravid, D. (1995). *Language change in child and adult Hebrew: A psycholinguistic perspective*. Oxford, UK: Oxford University Press.

Ravid, D., and Shyldkrot, H. (Eds.). (2004). *Perspectives on language and language development: Essays in honor of Ruth A. Berman*. Dordrecht: Kluwer.

Shimron, J. (Ed.). (2003). *Language processing and language acquisition in a root-based morphology* (pp. 243–291). Amsterdam: John Benjamins.

Tobin, Y. (1997). *Phonology as human behavior: Theoretical implications and clinical applications*. Durham: Duke University Press.

CD-ROMs

Staiman, M., and Shahar, N. (2000). *Children speak and communicate: The development of communication, language, speech and movement in the first years*. Kineret: Peligon. [in Hebrew]

Journals

* *Balshanut Ivrit*. [Hebrew Linguistics: A journal for Hebrew descriptive, computational, and applied linguistics]: Bar Ilan University, Department of Hebrew Language
* *Dash—Dibur U-Shmi'a*: Journal of the Israel Association of Language, Speech, and Hearing Disorders
* *Leshonenu*: Journal of the Hebrew Language Academy, Hebrew University, Jerusalem
* *Script*: Journal of the Israel Association for Literacy

Professional associations

The professional association of speech-language pathologists within Israel is the Israeli Speech, Hearing, and Language Association (ISHLA): (http://www.ishla.org.il/index.html).

Useful Hebrew Web sites

* Academy of the Hebrew Language: http://hebrew-academy.huji.ac.il
* Language links on Hebrew: http://www.languages-on-the-web.com/links/link-hebrew.htm

REFERENCES

Adam, G. (1993). *Stop-fricative alternation in Modern Hebrew*. Unpublished master's thesis, Tel-Aviv University, Israel. [in Hebrew]

Adam, G. (2002). *From variable to optimal grammar: Evidence from language acquisition and language change*. Unpublished doctoral dissertation, Tel-Aviv University, Israel.

Amir, S. (1995). First language acquisition. *Dash—Dibur U-Shmi'a, 18*, 37–50. [in Hebrew]

Bahat, S. (1991). Stress in foreign words. *Leshonenu la'am, 42*, 32–34. [in Hebrew]

Bat-El, O. (1989). *Phonology and word structure in Modern Hebrew*. Unpublished doctoral dissertation, University of California, Los Angeles.

Bat-El, O. (1993). Parasitic metrification in the Modern Hebrew stress system. *Linguistic Review, 10*, 189–210.

Bat-El, O. (1994). Stem modification and cluster transfer in Modern Hebrew. *Natural Language and Linguistic Theory, 12*, 571–596.

Bat-El, O. (2005). The emergence of trochaic foot in Hebrew hypocoristics. *Phonology, 22*, 115–143.

Ben Zvi, T. (1981). *Production of sibilants among urban compared with kibbutz children*. Seminar paper, Tel Aviv University Department of Communications Disorders. [in Hebrew]

Bendavid, A. (1967). *Biblical and mishnaic Hebrew*. Tel Aviv: Dvir. [in Hebrew]

Ben-David, A. (2001). *Language acquisition and phonological theory: Universal and variable processes across children and across languages.* Unpublished doctoral dissertation, Tel Aviv University, Israel. [in Hebrew]

Ben-David, A. (2006a). *Hebrew articulation and phonology test.* Manuscript in preparation.

Ben-David, A. (2006b). *A phonological intervention approach to articulation disorders.* Tel Aviv University. Manuscript in preparation.

Ben-David, A., and Peleg, S. (2005, February). *Treatment of dyspraxia: A case report.* Paper presented at the 41st annual meeting of the Israeli Association for Speech, Hearing, and Language, Sdom, Israel. [in Hebrew]

Bentin, S. (1992). Phonological awareness, reading and reading acquisition: A survey and appraisal of current knowledge. In R. Frost and L. Katz (Eds.), *Orthography, phonology, morphology, and meaning* (pp. 193–210). Amsterdam: Elsevier.

Bentin, S. (1997). On the connection between phonology, phonemic awareness, and reading processes. In J. Shimron (Ed.), *Research on the psychology of language in Israel: Language acquisition, reading, and writing* (pp. 184–202). Jerusalem: Magnes Press. [in Hebrew]

Bentin, S., Hammer, R., and Cahan, S. (1991). The effects of aging and first-year schooling on the development of phonological awareness. *Psychological Science, 2,* 271–274.

Bentin, S., and Leshem, H. (1993). On the interaction of phonological awareness and reading acquisition: It's a two-way street. *Annals of Dyslexia, 43,* 125–148.

Ben-Tulila, Y. (1983). *Hebrew accents of Israeli villagers of Moroccan descent: A study in social phonology.* Unpublished doctoral dissertation, Hebrew University, Jerusalem. [in Hebrew]

Berman, R. A. (1977). Natural phonological processes at the one-word stage. *Lingua, 43,* 1–21.

Berman, R. A. (1978). *Modern Hebrew structure.* Tel Aviv: Universities Publishing.

Berman, R. A. (1981). Language development and language knowledge: Evidence from acquisition of Hebrew morphophonology. *Journal of Child Language, 8,* 609–626.

Berman, R. A. (1985). Acquisition of Hebrew. In D. I. Slobin (Ed.), *The crosslinguistic study of acquisition* (Vol. 1, pp. 255–371). Hillsdale, NJ: Erlbaum.

Berman, R. A. (1987). Issues and problems in Modern Hebrew research. *Prakim, 7,* 84–96. [in Hebrew]

Berman, R. A. (1992). Modern Hebrew. In W. Bright, B. Comrie, and D. Crystal (Eds.), *Oxford International Encyclopaedia of Linguistics* (pp. 1388–1399). Oxford, UK: Oxford University Press.

Berman, R. A. (1994). Formal, lexical, and semantic factors in the acquisition of Hebrew resultative participles. *Berkeley Linguistic Society, No. 20,* 82–92.

Berman, R. A. (1998). Modern Hebrew. In R. Hetzron (Ed.), *The Semitic languages* (pp. 312–334). London: Routledge.

Berman, R. A. (2004). Between emergence and mastery: The long developmental route of language acquisition. In R. A. Berman (Ed.), *Language development across childhood and adolescence* (pp. 9–34). Amsterdam: John Benjamins.

Berman, R. A., and Neeman, Y. (1994). Development of linguistic forms: Hebrew. In R. A. Berman and D. I. Slobin (Eds.), *Relating events in narrative: A crosslinguistic developmental study* (pp. 285–328). Hillsdale, NJ: Erlbaum.

Blanc, H. (1957). Hebrew in Israel: Trends and problems. *Middle East Journal, 11,* 374–410.

Blanc, H. (1964). Israeli Hebrew texts. In H. B. Rosén (Ed.), *Egyptology and linguistics in honor of H. J. Polotsky* (pp. 132–152). Jerusalem: Israel Exploration Society.

Blau, J. (1981). *The renaissance of Modern Hebrew and Modern Standard Arabic: Parallels and differences in the revival of two Semitic languages.* University of California, Berkeley: Publications in Near Eastern Studies, No. 18.

Bolozky, S. (1972). *Categorical limitations on rules in the phonology of Modern Hebrew.* Unpublished doctoral dissertation, University of Illinois, Urbana.

Bolozky, S. (1978). Some aspects of Modern Hebrew phonology. In R. A. Berman, *Modern Hebrew structure* (pp. 11–67). Tel Aviv: Universities Publishing Projects.

Bolozky, S. (1982). Remarks on rhythmic stress in Modern Hebrew. *Journal of Linguistics, 18,* 275–289.

Bolozky, S. (1997). Israeli Hebrew phonology. In A. S. Kaye (Ed.), *Phonologies of Asia and Africa* (pp. 281–311). Winona Lake, IN: Eisenbrauns.

Chayen, M. J. (1973). *The phonetics of Modern Hebrew.* The Hague: Mouton.

Cohen-Gross, D. (1997). *The morphological-syllabic structure of Modern Hebrew.* Unpublished doctoral dissertation, Bar-Ilan University, Ramat-Gan, Israel. [in Hebrew]

Coulmas, F. (2003). *Writing systems: An introduction to their linguistic analysis.* Cambridge, UK: Cambridge University Press.

Daniels, P. (1998). Scripts of Semitic languages. In R. Hetzron (Ed.), *The Semitic languages* (pp. 16–45). London: Routledge.

Dromi, E., Most, T., and Yehuda, N. (1993, July). *The case of homonymy in early lexical development: Interactional and acoustical analyses.* Paper presented at the 6th International Congress for the Study of Child Language, Trieste, Italy.

Eytan, E. (1971). Hebrew language. *Encyclopaedia Judaica* (Vol, 16, pp. 1560–1662). Jerusalem: Keter.

Faber, A. (1998). Genetic subgrouping of the Semitic languages. In R. Hetzron (Ed.), *The Semitic Languages* (pp. 3–15). London: Routledge.

Fellman, J. (1971). *The revival of a classical tongue: Eliezer Ben Yehuda and the Modern language.* The Hague: Mouton.

Forkush, E. (1997). *The effect of word-stress on acquisition of initial consonant clusters in Hebrew.* Seminar paper, Tel Aviv University Department of Communications Disorders. [in Hebrew]

Gabay, A. (1986). *Acquisition of the sounds /s/ and /ʃ/ in Hebrew in comparison to English.* Seminar paper, Tel Aviv University Department of Communications Disorders. [in Hebrew]

Gillis, S., and Ravid, D. (2001). Language-specific effects on the development of written morphology. In S. Bendjaballah, W. U. Dressler, O. Pfeiffer, and M. Voeikova (Eds.), *Morphology 2000* (pp. 129–136). Amsterdam: John Benjamins.

Gillis, S., and Ravid, D. (in press). Typological effects on spelling development: A crosslinguistic study of Hebrew and Dutch. *Journal of Child Language.*

Goralnik, E. (1995). *Language screening test for Hebrew-speaking preschool children.* Netanya, Israel: Gai agencies.

Halpern, R. (1984). *Phonological processes in the speech of children between ages 1;6–3;0.* Seminar paper, Tel Aviv University Department of Communications Disorders. [in Hebrew]

Harshav, B. (1990). Essay on the revival of the Hebrew language. *Alpayim, 2,* 9–54. [in Hebrew]

Ingram, D. (1976). *Phonological disability in children.* London: Edward Arnold.

Izmailov, L. (1983). *Phonological processes among Hebrew-speaking children aged 3 to 4 years.* Seminar paper, Tel Aviv University Department of Communications Disorders. [in Hebrew]

Jedwab, D. (1975). *An articulation test as a prognostic tool for functional articulation disorders in children aged 6 to 8 years.* Unpublished master's thesis, Tel-Aviv University, Israel.

Kochva, R. (1996). *Medial cluster articulation of 3-year-olds.* Seminar paper, Tel Aviv University Department of Communications Disorders. [in Hebrew]

Korenbrot, F., Hertzano, T., and Ben Aroya, A. (2002). Emerging issues in Israel: Commentaries in a global context. *Folia Phoniatrica et Logopaedica, 54*(2), 72–74.

Kutscher, E. Y. (1982). *A history of the Hebrew language.* Jerusalem: Magnes Press.

Laufer, A. (1984). *The phonetics of Modern Hebrew. Units 5–7.* Tel Aviv: Open University Press. [in Hebrew]

Laufer, A. (1986). A phonetic description of Hebrew consonants. *Mechkarim Be-Fonetika, 7,* 67–107. [in Hebrew]

Laufer, A. (1987). *Intonation.* Jerusalem: Hebrew University Press.

Laufer, A. (1990). Hebrew. *Journal of the International Phonetic Association, 20,* 40–43.

Laufer, A. (1991). Phonemic combinations in Hebrew phonetics. In M. Gottshtein, S., Morag, and S. Kogut (Eds.), Essays on Language in Honor of Chaim Rabin (pp. 179–193). Jerusalem: Hebrew University Press. [in Hebrew]

Laufer, A. (1992). *Introduction to Linguistics, Units 4–5: Phonetics and phonology.* Tel-Aviv: Open University Press. [in Hebrew]

Laufer, A. (1998). On defining the phoneme as the minimal unit of linguistic communication. In S. Sharvit (Ed.), *Studies on Hebrew Language* (pp. 329–344). Ramat-Gan: Bar-Ilan University Press.

Lavie, S. (1978). *Norms for the development of Hebrew consonants between the ages of 3 to 5 years.* Unpublished master's thesis, Tel Aviv University, Israel. [in Hebrew]

Lefkowitz, D. (2004). *Words and stones: The politics of language and identity in Israel.* Oxford, UK: Oxford University Press.

Levin, I., and Korat, O. (1993). Sensitivity to phonological, morphological, and semantic cues in early reading and writing in Hebrew. *Merrill-Palmer Quarterly, 39,* 213–232.

Levin, I., Ravid, D., and Rappaport, S. (2001). Morphology and spelling among Hebrew-speaking children: From kindergarten to first grade. *Journal of Child Language, 28,* 741–769.

Nachmany, A. (2004, February). *Introducing a therapeutic approach to dyspraxia: Sound-Shape-Color, Rational, principles, patterns and treatment processes.* Paper presented at the 40th annual meeting of the Israel Association for Speech, Hearing, and Language, Ashkelon. [in Hebrew]

Olson, D. (1994) *The world on paper: The conceptual and cognitive implications of reading and writing.* Cambridge, UK: Cambridge University Press.

Ornan, U. (1982). *The phonetics of modern Hebrew, Units 1–4.* Tel Aviv: Open University Press. [in Hebrew]

Ornan, U. (1996). The distinctive features method in Hebrew phonology. In M. Bar-Asher (Ed.), *Studies in Hebrew language* (pp. 163–192). Jerusalem: Hebrew University Press. [in Hebrew]

Pacton, S, and Fayol, M. (2004). Learning to spell in a deep orthography: The case of French. In R. A. Berman (Ed.), *Language development across childhood and adolescence* (pp. 163–176). Amsterdam: John Benjamins.

Plada, N. (1959). The frequency of Hebrew sound segments. *Leshonenu, 23,* 237–242. [in Hebrew]

Rabin, C. (1973). Deletion of the glottal stop in spoken Hebrew and the creation of a new vowel group. In U. Ornan (Ed.), *Reader in Phonetics and Phonology* (pp. 230–233). Jerusalem: Hebrew University Press. [in Hebrew]

Ravid, D. D. (1995). *Language change in child and adult Hebrew: Psycholinguistic perspectives.* Oxford, UK: Oxford University Press.

Ravid, D. (1996). Accessing the mental lexicon: Evidence from incompatibility between representation of spoken and written morphology. *Linguistics, 34*, 1219–1246.

Ravid, D. (2001). Learning to spell in Hebrew: Phonological and morphological factors. *Reading and Writing, 14*, 459–485.

Ravid, D. (2003). A developmental perspective on root perception in Hebrew and Palestinian Arabic. In Y. Shimron (Ed.), *Language processing and acquisition in languages of Semitic, root-based morphology* (pp. 293–319). Amsterdam: John Benjamins.

Ravid, D. (2005). Hebrew orthography and literacy. In R. M. Joshi and P. G. Aaron (Eds.), *Handbook of orthography and literacy* (pp. 339 and 363). Mahwah, NJ: Erlbaum.

Rosén, H. (1973). The structure of Israeli Hebrew. In U. Ornan (Ed.), *Reader in Phonetics and Phonology* (pp. 138–153). Jerusalem: Hebrew University Press. [in Hebrew]

Rosenberg, L. (1983). *Developmental stages in acquisition of initial consonant clusters by Hebrew-speaking children.* Seminar paper, Tel Aviv University Department of Communications Disorders. [in Hebrew]

Rosin, D., and Yakir, P. (2000). *Pictures for examining articulation and naming of Hebrew-speaking children in Israel.* Rehovot, Israel.

Rubinstein, E. (1980). *Contemporary and Ancient Hebrew.* Tel Aviv: Israel Defence Forces, University of the Air Publications. [in Hebrew]

Schwartz, R. G., Harris, K. S., and Most, T. M. (1993). Speech, language, and hearing in Israel. *American Journal of Speech-Language Pathology, 2*(3), 5–7.

Schwarzwald, O. (1976). Concrete and abstract approaches in analyzing Hebrew stop-spirant alternation. *Leshonenu, 40*, 211–232. [in Hebrew]

Schwarzwald, O. (1981). *Grammar and reality in the Hebrew verb.* Ramat Gan: Bar Ilan University Press. [in Hebrew]

Schwarzwald, O. (1985). The accent of the younger generation in Israel. *Shevet va'am, 10*, 66–75. [in Hebrew]

Schwarzwald, O. (1991). Stress shifting in Modern Hebrew. In M. Gottshtein, S., Morag, and S. Kogut (Eds.), *Essays on Language in Honor of Chaim Rabin* (pp. 393–414). Jerusalem: Hebrew University Press. [in Hebrew]

Schwarzwald, O. (1998). Word foreignness in Modern Hebrew. *Hebrew Studies, 39*, 115–142.

Schwarzwald, O. (2004). Modern Hebrew consonant clusters. In D. Ravid and H. B.-Z. Shyldkrot (Eds.), *Perspectives on language and language development* (pp. 45–60). Dordrecht: Kluwer.

Seidman, O. (2000). *The connection between phonological awareness, morphological awareness, and writing among kindergarten and first-grade children.* Unpublished master's thesis, Tel Aviv University, Israel. [in Hebrew]

Shaked, G. (1990). *Early phonological acquisition: Phonological processes between ages 1;7–2;7.* M.A. project, Tel Aviv University Department of Communications Disorders. [in Hebrew]

Share, D. L., and Levin, I. (1999). Learning to read and write in Hebrew. In M. Harris and G. Hatano (Eds.), *Learning to read and write* (pp. 89–111). Cambridge, UK: Cambridge University Press.

Shimron, J. (1993). The role of vowels in reading: A review of studies of English and Hebrew. *Psychological Bulletin, 114*, 523–568.

Shimron, J., and Navon, D. (1982). The dependence on graphemes and on their translation to phonemes in reading: A developmental perspective. *Reading Research Quarterly, 17*, 210–228.

Shohamy, E. (2004). Language rights in the multilingual society of Israel. In D. Ravid and H. B.-Z. Shyldkrot (Eds.), *Perspectives on language and language development* (pp. 87–102). Dordrecht: Kluwer.

Tene, D. (1973). Measuring the length of Hebrew vowels. In U. Ornan (Ed.), *Reader in phonetics and phonology* (pp. 204–216). Jerusalem: Hebrew University Press. [in Hebrew]

Tobin, Y. (1997). *Phonology as human behavior. Theoretical implications and clinical applications.* Durham, NC: Duke University Press.

Tolchinsky, L., and Teberosky, A. (1997). Explicit word segmentation and writing in Hebrew and Spanish. In C. Pontecorvo (Ed.), *Writing development: An interdisciplinary view* (pp. 77–98). Amsterdam: John Benjamins

Tolchinsky, L. (2003). *The cradle of culture: What children know about writing and numbers before being taught.* Mahwah, NJ: Erlbaum.

Tolchinsky, L., and Teberosky, A. (1998). The development of word segmentation and writing in two scripts. *Cognitive Development, 13*, 121.

Van Riper, C. (1978). *Speech correction: Principles and methods* (6th ed.). Englewood Cliffs, NJ: Prentice-Hall.

Weinberg, W. (1966). Spoken Israeli Hebrew: Trends in the departures from classical phonology. *Journal of Semitic Studies, 11*, 40–68.

Weiner, F. F. (1981). Treatment of phonological disability using the method of meaningful minimal contrasts: Two case studies. *Journal of Speech and Hearing Disorders, 46*, 97–103.

SUMMARY OF STUDIES OF TYPICAL HEBREW SPEECH ACQUISITION

Author	Year	Country	No. of children	Age of children	Information	Sample type	Data collection
Adam	2002	Israel	23	1;06–3;6	Stages of prosodic acquisition	Naturalistic + Single words + Probes	Longitudinal Cross-sectional
Amir	1996	Israel	4	1;10–3;0	Phonological processes+ processes of "phonology as human behavior"	Single words	
Ben-David	2001	Israel	10	1;2–2;10	Acquisition processes and stages	Naturalistic+ Single words + Connected speech	Longitudinal
Berman	1977	Israel	1	1;6–1;11	Phonological pro-cesses one-word stage (Hebrew-English bilingual)	Naturalistic	Longitudinal
Lavie	1978	Israel	200	3;0–5;0	Age of acquisition of consonants	Single words	Cross-sectional
Shaked	1990	Israel	20	1;7–2;7	Phonological processes	Single words	Cross-sectional

Acknowledgements

We are indebted to Dorit Ravid for her comments on an earlier draft, to Outi Bat-El, Irit Katzenberger, and Yishai Tobin for their careful reading of the entire chapter, and to Bracha Nir–Sagiv for her help in preparing the manuscript. The authors alone are responsible for inadequacies that remain.

Chapter 45

Japanese Speech Acquisition

Mitsuhiko Ota and Isao Ueda

INTRODUCTION

Japanese is the national language of Japan. The genetic affiliation of the language remains unresolved despite countless attempts at establishing its membership in a range of language families including Altaic, Malayo-Polynesian, Tibeto-Burman, and Dravidian. Other languages spoken in Japan include Korean (with an estimated 670,000 speakers in 1988) and Ainu, although the latter, an indigenous language to Japan, is classified as "nearly extinct" by *Ethnologue* (Gordon, 2005). Unless noted otherwise, the general descriptions below are of standard Japanese, a somewhat idealized form of the western Tokyo dialect. See the Resources section in this chapter for materials pertaining to Japanese.

Where Japanese is spoken

Japanese is spoken in Japan by virtually all the native population of 120 million people (see accompanying map and Appendix D). There are also some sizable immigrant groups outside Japan, particularly in Hawaii and Brazil, who speak Japanese as their heritage language.

Components of Japanese

Consonants

Japanese has 15 phonemic consonants. These are given in Table 45-1 along with some important allophones (shown in brackets). All nonlabial consonants are palatalized before

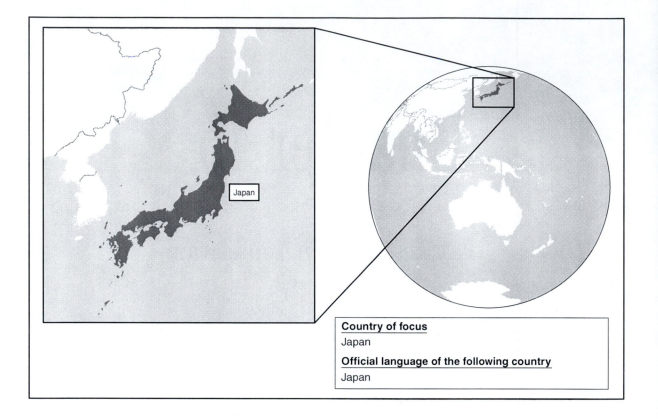

		Country of focus
		Japan
		Official language of the following country
		Japan

TABLE 45-1 Consonants produced in Japanese

	Bilabial	**Labiodental**	**Dental**	**Alveolar**
Plosive	p b			t d
Nasal	m			n
Trill				
Tap or flap				ɾ
Fricative	(ɸ)			s z
Lateral fricative	██████████			
Affricate				(ts)
Approximant	w (labiovelar)			
Lateral approximant	██████████			

Black = articulations judged impossible

Based on the International Phonetic Alphabet. Courtesy of the International Phonetic Association (c/o Department of Linguistics, University of Victoria, Victoria, British Columbia, Canada).

/i/ (e.g., /si/ [ɕi] 'four,' /ni/ [ɲi] 'two,' /hi/ [çi] 'fire'). The alveolar plosive /t/ affricates, as well as palatalizes, before /i/ and /u/ (e.g., /ti/ [cɕi] 'blood,' /tuma/ [tsɯma] 'wife'). A consonant preceding /j/ also palatalizes and, if coronal, absorbs the glide (e.g., /hjaku/ [çjakɯ] 'hundred,' /sja/ [ɕa] 'company,' /tja/ [cɕa] 'tea,' /zjoː/ [ʑoː] 'sympathy'). Syllable-final nasal typically realizes as a nasal stop with a weak uvular contact in word-final position (e.g., /hoN/ [hoɴ] 'book'), as a nasalized vowel before another vowel or an approximant (e.g., /kiNeN/ [kĩ̇eɴ] 'non-smoking'), and as a homorganic nasal stop before other consonants (e.g., /toNbo/ [tombo] 'dragonfly,' /maNga/ [maŋga] 'comics'). Before /u/, /h/ occurs as a bilabial fricative (e.g., /huju/ [ɸɯjɯ] 'winter'). Intervocalically, /g/ is nasalized (e.g., /taga/ [taŋa] 'hoop').

Vowels and diphthongs

Japanese has five short vowels, /a/, /i/, /u/, /e/, and /o/, and five long vowels /aa/, /ii/, /uu/, /ee/, and /oo/. The short-long distinction is primarily that of duration, with little difference in the quality. The high-back vowel /u/ is unrounded: [ɯ]. Any sequence of nonidentical vowels is permitted, but it is not clear whether such a sequence constitutes a diphthong, except possibly /au/ and /ai/ in some contexts (Vance, 1987). The high vowels, /i/ and /u/, are usually devoiced when unaccented

and not contiguous to a voiced sound (e.g., /kutu/ [kɯtsɯ́] 'shoe,' /hasi/ [háɕi] 'chopstick'). Table 45-2 shows the vowels produced in Japanese.

Phonotactic restrictions
Syllables

The syllable structure of Japanese can be described in the formula: (C)(j)VV(C). Canonical syllables can be classified into light syllables, which contain only a short vowel in the rhyme (e.g., /ko/ [ko] 'child'), and heavy syllables, which contain either a long vowel (e.g., /koo/ [koː] 'clause') or a combination of a short vowel and a coda (e.g., /koN/ [koɴ] 'navy blue'). "Superheavy" syllables that contain more rhyme elements, such as a long vowel and a coda, are marked and found only in loanwords (e.g., /kooN/ [koːɴ] 'cone').

Consonants and consonant clusters

Only two types of consonant can occur in the coda position: a nasal (e.g., /hoN/ [hoɴ] 'book,' /reN.ga/ [reŋga] 'brick') and the first half of a geminate, which can be a plosive or a fricative (e.g., /rap.pa/ [ɾapːa] 'horn,' /sak.ka/ [sakːa] 'writer,' /nis.si/ [niɕːi] 'journal'). The only cluster allowed is a two-consonant onset cluster with /j/ in the second position. Any nonapproximant can occur in the

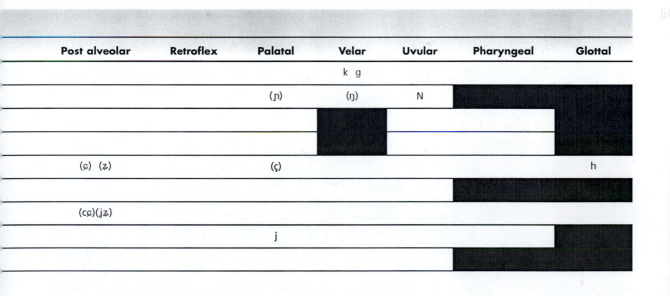

	Post alveolar	Retroflex	Palatal	Velar	Uvular	Pharyngeal	Glottal
				k g			
			(ɲ)	(ŋ)	ɴ		
	(ɕ) (ʑ)		(ç)				h
	(cɕ)(jʑ)						
			j				

TABLE 45-2 Vowels produced in Japanese

	IPA	Examples
High-front, short	i	ʃi̠ 'death'
High-front, long	iː	ʃi̠ː 'chinquapin'
Mid-front, short	e	se̠ɾɯ 'compete'
Mid-front, long	eː	se̠ːɾɯ 'sale'
High-back, short	ɯ	kɯ̠ro 'black'
High-back, long	ɯː	kɯ̠ːro 'airway'
Mid-back, short	o	hodo̠ 'degree'
Mid-back, long	oː	hodo̠ː 'sidewalk'
Low-back, short	a	ka̠do 'corner'
Low back, long	aː	ka̠ːdo 'card'

first position of this cluster (e.g., /kjoo/ [kʲoː] 'today,' /mjoo/ [mʲoː] 'strange,' /rjoo/ [rʲoː] 'quantity').

Tones

Japanese is often cited as a textbook example of a lexical pitch-accent language. All words are either accented or unaccented, and accented words have one accented syllable. The accent consists of a sequence of high and low pitch levels. In an accented syllable that contains a long vowel or a nasal coda, the syllable itself has a high-low pitch contour. In other cases, the accented syllable carries only the high portion of the contour, and the following syllable is low-pitched.

Stress and intonation

Japanese has no lexical stress. Intonation patterns are affected by pitch movements that indicate utterance-level semantics, lexical accent, and phrasal boundaries. A declarative utterance ends in a low pitch and an interrogative utterance in a high pitch. Each utterance consists of one or more accentual phrases, whose beginning is marked by a low pitch except when the first syllable of the phrase is lexically accented. The phrase /akái/ ('it's

red'), for example, has a rise-fall pitch contour due to the low pitch that marks the initial syllable and the high-low pitch sequence on the accented second syllable.

Writing system

Three orthographic systems are used in written Japanese. The first, *kanji*, is a set of ideographic characters borrowed from Chinese. A set of 1,945 characters, designated by the Japanese Ministry of Education as [ʑoːjoː kánʑi] ('daily-use kanji'), are taught in primary and secondary school, but most educated people know a few thousand more characters. Each character represents a semantic concept and also has one or more readings. For example, 犬 means 'dog' and reads /inu/ or /keN/. Kanji characters are usually used to write the roots of nouns, verbs, adjectives, and adverbs. The other two writing systems, *hiragana* and *katakana*, each with 46 symbols, represent sound units that are best described as moraic. Each symbol stands for either the (C)V portion or the remainder of the syllable (i.e., the second half of the long vowel, the first half of the geminate, or the nasal coda). Thus, in hiragana, /toru/ 'to take' is written as とる (to-ru), /tooru/ 'to pass' as とおる (to-o-ru), /totta/ 'took' as とった (to-[geminate]-ta), and /tonda/ 'flew' as とんだ (to-n-da). Hiragana is mainly used to write inflections and various bound morphemes, while katakana is used to transcribe foreign loanwords. A Japanese sentence can be seen with all three characters mixed, as in the following example, where the noun /tomodati/ 'friend' and the stem of the verb /mi/ 'to watch' are written in kanji, the loanword /terebi/ 'TV' in katakana, and the postposition /to/, the accusative marker /o/, and past-tense marker /ta/ in hiragana.

友達と　　テレビを　見た。
/tomodati to terebi o mita/
friend with TV ACC *watch-PAST*
'(I) watched TV with a friend'

Varieties of Japanese

Dialectal variation in Japanese phonology is quite vast. Three important divisions exist between the mainland and Ryukyuan (Okinawan) dialects, between the Western and Eastern dialects, and between the central (around the ancient capital of Kyoto) and peripheral dialects (Shibatani, 1990). Two major characteristics of Ryukyuan are the varied vowel inventories, which range from a three-vowel system (Yonaguni) to seven (Hateruma), and the presence of the glottalized consonants. The "Western" dialect of Kyoto differs from the "Eastern" dialect of Tokyo in several aspects, including (a) the rounding of the high-back vowel /u/; (b) the lack of high vowel devoicing; and (c) the presence of two default phrasal pitch levels (high and low) in addition to the lexical accent, which gives a more complex pitch pattern. In Tohoku, a typical "peripheral" dialect, (a) /s/ palatalizes not only before /i/ but also before /e/, (b) high vowels are centralized, and (c) voiced nonnasal stops are prenasalized.

Typical acquisition of Japanese

The Summary of Studies Table at the end of the chapter contains studies of the acquisition of Japanese.

Acquired sounds

Consonants

Table 45-3 contains age of acquisition data for Japanese from Takagi and Yasuda (1967), Noda, Iwamura, Naito, and Asukai (1969), Nakanishi, Owada, and Fujita (1972), Sakauchi (1967), and Nakanishi (1982). The age range indicates the cross-sectional group that achieved 90 percent correct production of each consonant in syllable-initial position, except for Nakanishi (1982), where the range and mean age of first appearance and complete acquisition are shown based on longitudinal data. Most consonants are acquired by 4;0, but [ɕ], [s], [ts], [z], and [ɾ] are typically mastered later. There is also a noticeable degree of individual variability in the timing of acquisition.

Consonant clusters

Cross-sectional studies by Umebayashi and Takagi (1965), Yasuda (1966), and Sakauchi (1967) show that [Cj] clusters with an initial labial consonant (/mj/, /pj/, /bj/) reach the criterion of 75 percent correct production by 3;0. Velar and palatal clusters (/kj/, /ɡj/, /hj/) reach the criterion slightly later (around 3;0 to 3;6). The /rj/ cluster is the last to be acquired (around 4;0 to 4;5).

Vowels and diphthongs

All five simple vowels emerge fairly early, although the two high vowels, particularly [i], stabilize slightly later than the others (K. Ito, 1990). In a study by Nakajima et al. (1962), 75 percent of the subjects produced [o] correctly at 1;9 to 1;11, [a] at 2;3 to 2;5, [e] and [ɯ] at 2;6 to 2;8, and [i] at 2;9 to 2;11. A longitudinal study by Nakanishi (1982) concludes that most children achieve complete accuracy of simple vowels between 1;10 and 2;3. However, monophthongization of vowel sequences involving /i/ (e.g., [mienai] ⇨ [meːnai], [oide] ⇨ [oːde]) has been reported in some 2-year-olds (K. Ito, 1990; Ota, 2003a).

Percent correct

Most studies collecting percentage correct norms in Japanese have used the syllable as a unit of analysis, for example, [pa], [tsɯ]. Table 45-4 presents the percentage of such syllables produced correctly, reported by Sumio (1978), who used a repetition task with both isolated syllables and words.

Phonological processes

Common segmental processes include stopping of fricatives ([sakana] ⇨ [takana], [ɕɕakana] 'fish'), palatalization ([ɯsagi] ⇨ [ɯɕagi] 'rabbit'), stopping of word-initial /r/ and rhoticization of word-medial /d/ ([ɾapːa] ⇨ [dapːa] 'trumpet'; [kodomo] ⇨ [koɾomo] 'children'), and deletion of /h/ and /r/ ([hana] ⇨ [ana] 'flower'; [koɾe] ⇨ [koe] 'this') (Funayama, 1998; K. Ito, 1990; Okubo, 1977; Owada, Nakanishi, and Oshige, 1969; Ueda, 1996a; Ueda and Davis, 1999, 2001). Also frequently reported are fronting of velars ([eki] ⇨ [eɕi] 'station' (Okubo, 1977; Ueda, 1996b) and backing of alveolars and palatals ([toɾa] ⇨ [koɾa] 'tiger' (Beckman, Yoneyama, and Edwards, 2003; Owada and Nakanishi, 1971). Particularly before 4;0, we also see long-distance segmental processes, such as metathesis (e.g., [teɾebi] ⇨ [teberi] 'TV') and consonant harmony ([happa] ⇨ [pappa] 'leaf'). Cross-sectional and longitudinal examination by Owada et al. (1969) shows that the majority of these segmental processes decline rapidly between 3 and 5. Omission of syllables from long words, in particular those with more than two syllables, is common until 2;6: [hadaka] ⇨ [haka] 'naked'; [banana] ⇨ [bana] 'banana' (Okubo, 1977; Ota, 2003a).

TABLE 45-3 Age of acquisition for Japanese consonants

Consonant	Takagi and Yasuda (1967)	Noda et al. (1969)	Nakanishi et al. (1972)	Sakauchi (1967)	Nakanishi (1982) First appearance (mean)	Nakanishi (1982) Complete acquisition mean
m	3;0–3;5	3;0–3;5	4;0–4;5	2;10–3;3	1;0–1;8 (1;3)	1;10–2;9 (2;2)
j	3;0–3;5	3;0–3;5	4;0–4;5	2;10–3;3	1;1–2;0 (1;5)	1;4–4;0 (2;5)
t	3;0–3;5	3;0–3;5	4;0–4;5	2;10–3;3	1;1–1;10 (1;5)	1;10–2;9 (2;3)
cɕ	3;0–3;5	3;0–3;5	4;0–4;5	2;10–3;3	1;2–1;10 (1;6)	1;8–2;9 (2;5)
p	3;0–3;5	3;6–3;11	4;0–4;5	2;10–3;3	1;2–1;9 (1;5)	1;8–2;6 (2;1)
b	5;0–5;5	3;0–3;5	4;0–4;5	2;10–3;3	1;0–1;6 (1;3)	1;3–2;9 (2;3)
g	3;0–3;5	3;6–3;11	4;0–4;5	2;10–3;3	1;3–2;3 (1;9)	1;7–2;9 (2;3)
d	3;0–3;5	4;6–4;11	4;0–4;5	2;10–3;3	1;2–1;9 (1;5)	1;11–3;0 (2;5)
ɟʑ	3;0–3;5	3;6–3;11	4;0–4;5	3;4–3;8	1;2–2;3 (1;8)	1;11–4;0 (2;8+)
k	4;0–4;5	3;6–3;11	4;0–4;5	2;10–3;3	1;1–1;10 (1;5)	1;1–2;6 (2;2)
w	3;0–3;5	4;6–4;11	4;0–4;5	3;4–3;8	1;1–1;9 (1;5)	1;6–4;0 (2;7)
h	4;0–4;5	4;0–4;5	4;0–4;5	2;10–3;3	1;2–1;8 (1;6)	2;6–4;0 (3;1)
ɸ	3;6–3;11	4;0–4;5	4;0–4;5	2;10–3;3	n/a	n/a
n	3;6–3;11	4;0–4;5	4;0–4;5	3;4–3;8	1;1–1;9 (1;4)	1;10–2;3 (2;0)
ç	4;0–4;5	4;0–4;5	4;0–4;5	after 4;8	n/a	n/a
ɕ	after 6;6	5;6–5;11	4;6–4;11	4;4–4;8	1;1–2;3 (1;8)	2;9–4;0 (3;4+)
z	5;6–5;11	5;6–5;11	5;6–5;11	after 4;8	1;7–3;0 (2;6)	3;0–4;0 (3;6+)
s	after 6;6	5;0–5;5	5;0–5;5	after 4;8	1;5–2;9 (2;3)	3;0–4;0 (4;0+)
ts	after 6;6	5;6–5;11	5;0–5;5	after 4;8	1;6–3;0 (2;8)	3;0–4;0 (3;8+)
ɾ	after 6;6	4;0–4;5	5;6–5;11	after 4;8	1;3–2;3 (1;8)	2;0–4;0 (3;3+)

Intelligibility

Although there are several assessment schema for intelligibility (e.g., Furuya, 1958; Taguchi, 1967), no normative data are available to this date.

Phonetic inventory

Based on previous research, Sakauchi (1967) presents the inventory of consonants and consonant clusters as in Table 45-5.

TABLE 45-4 Percentage of children with correct production of Japanese syllables

Age	Syllable in isolation	Syllable in words
4;0–4;5	95.6 percent	91.7 percent
4;6–4;11	97.0 percent	93.8 percent
5;0–5;5	98.5 percent	95.8 percent
5;6–5;11	98.5 percent	97.9 percent
6;0–6;5	98.5 percent	97.9 percent
6;6–06;11	100.0 percent	97.9 percent

Note. Data from Sumio (1978).

Common mismatches

The most common mismatches involve palatalization of [ts], [s], and [z]. Table 45-6 summarizes mismatches observed in Owada et al. (1969). The unit of comparison was CV.

Syllable structure

Before 2;0, coda nasals in (C)VN.CV contexts are often omitted with concomitant lengthening of the vowel: [panda] ⇨ [paːda] 'panda' (Ota, 2003a). Geminates appear

before 2;0 but the actual duration of closure time in comparison to singletons (e.g., the duration of [kː] vs. [k] in /sakka/ vs. /saka/, [nː] vs. [n] in /hanna/ vs. /hana/) is shorter and does not fully converge on the adult values even at age 5 (Aoyama, 2001).

Prosody

Most children acquiring Tokyo Japanese produce the falling pitch accent contour in correct positions before 1;6 (Hallé, Boysson-Bardies, and Vihman, 1991; Ota, 2003b). The phrase-initial low-pitch may be lacking in some children before 2;0 (Ota, 2003b), but by 3;0, the overall pitch pattern of simple words is in place (Shirose, Kakehi, and Kiritani, 2001). However, the timing of pitch accent acquisition varies across dialects. In Kagoshima Japanese, for example, 4-year-olds tend to overgeneralize penultimate accent to final accent words (Shirose, Kakehi, and Kiritani, 2002).

Phonological awareness

The prominence of the mora as a metaphonological unit in Japanese and its link to the mora-based *kana* writing systems (hiragana and katakana) have been explored extensively. Although there is some limited awareness of moraic units in preliterate 3-year-olds (Ito and Kagawa, 2001; Ito and Tatsumi, 1997), it is subsequent to the learning of kana writing (for most, between 4 and 6) that children become able to fully perform counting and deleting of moras (Inagaki,

TABLE 45-5 Phonetic inventory (consonants and clusters) for Japanese speech acquisition

Age	Inventory
Complete by 3;0	t, ɴ, ŋ, d
Mostly acquired by 3;0	b, p, t, d, k, g, m, n, ɴ, ŋ, ɲ, j, w, ɕ, ʥ, mʲ, bʲ, pʲ
3;5	b, p, t, d, k, g, m, n, ɴ, ŋ, ɲ, j, w, ɕ, ʥ, mʲ, bʲ, pʲ, kʲ, gʲ, çʲ
3;11	b, p, t, d, k, g, m, n, ɴ, ŋ, ɲ, ɸ, ɕ, h, j, w, ɕ, ʥ, mʲ, bʲ, pʲ, kʲ, gʲ, çʲ
4;6	b, p, t, d, k, g, m, n, ɴ, ŋ, ɲ, ɸ, s, z, ɕ, ç, h, j, w, ts, ɕ, ʥ, mʲ, bʲ, pʲ, kʲ, gʲ, çʲ
After 4;6	b, p, t, d, k, g, r, m, n, ɴ, ŋ, ɲ, ɸ, s, z, ɕ, ç, h, j, w, ts, ɕ, ʥ, mʲ, bʲ, pʲ, kʲ, gʲ, çʲ

Note. Data from Sakauchi (1967).

TABLE 45-6 Common mismatches in Japanese speech acquisition

	3;0 (n=47)	3;6 (n=67)	4;0 (n=54)	4;6 (n=35)	5;0 (n=15)	Total
tsɯ⇨ɕɕɯ	39	46	35	13	6	139
zɯ⇨ʝzɯ	36	42	38	15	6	137
sa⇨ɕa	25	28	23	9	4	89
wa⇨ja	6	24	26	19	12	87
sɯ⇨ɕɯ	25	25	23	5	6	84
zo⇨ʑo	20	26	26	7	4	83
ne⇨de	16	29	15	9	6	75
do⇨ro	17	25	13	9	6	70
zo⇨do	18	19	15	7	6	65
çi⇨ɕi	10	19	18	9	7	63
na⇨ra	16	22	15	4	3	62
sa⇨cɕa	16	17	15	3	2	53
All mismatches	502	644	498	210	127	1,981

Note. Data from Owada et al. (1969).

Hatano, and Otake, 2000). Japanese first graders, on the other hand, are generally unaware of phonemes, although fourth graders are able to perform some phoneme manipulation tasks (Goetry, Urbain, Morais, and Kolinsky, 2005; Mann, 1986; Spagnoletti, Morais, Alegria, and Dominicy, 1989).

Speech assessment for Japanese children

A variety of articulation tests have been developed for speech assessment in Japanese. The most widely used test for identification of articulation problems is *Shinteiban Kotoba no Tesuto Ehon* [Word test picture book: New edition] (Taguchi and Ogawaguchi, 1992). *Kōon Hattatsu Yosoku Kensa* [Articulation development prognosis test] (Nagasawa, Fujishima, and Oishi, 1985) is a representative tool used for predicting whether specific problems may persist in individual cases. The most popular diagnostic tool is *Kōon Kensahō* [Articulation test method] developed

collectively by the Japan Association of Speech-Language-Hearing Therapists and the Japan Society of Logopedics and Phoniatrics (see Abe et al., 1981; Funayama, et al., 1989 for documentation). Most articulation tests employ repetition, reading, or naming to collect speech samples of segments, syllables, words, and sentences. In addition, hearing tests, discrimination tests, and examination of speech organs are administered during assessment.

Speech intervention for Japanese children

There are currently approximately 10,000 nationally qualified SLPs in Japan. Satake et al., (2005) surveyed 133 institutions across Japan engaged in treatment of children with speech impairment. The setting in which the surveyed SLPs worked included hospitals (10.7 percent), medical centers (9.0 percent), schools for mentally disabled children (8.2 percent), day care centers for disabled children (7.8 percent), institutions for physically handicapped children (7.4 percent), schools for physically handicapped children (7.4 percent), institutions for the severely mentally and physically handicapped (7.0 percent), and a variety of other welfare facilities. On average, 2.9 full-time and 0.8 part-time SLPs worked for each institution. Nearly half the SLPs (44.8 percent) had more than 11 years of clinical experience, another 18.3 percent had 6 to 10 years, and the remainder (37.0 percent) less than 5 years.

The mainstay of the speech intervention techniques used for Japanese is Van Riper and Erickson's (1996) traditional articulation therapy, in some cases used in combination with minimal pairs therapy (Weiner, 1981). Other proposed techniques are more reliant on medical insights and tend to lack linguistic considerations (Ueda, 1994), but some models incorporating recent advancements in linguistic theory can be found in Imamura and Sakamoto (2002) and Ueda (1994).

Working in Japan

Practicing SLPs in Japan must pass a national qualification examination. Before taking the test, candidates must also have completed training in a three- to four-year speech pathology program or, for those who hold a bachelor's degree, a two-year program in one of the 52 institutes recognized by the Ministry of Health, Labor and Welfare. Those who hold qualifications in other countries can take the national examination with the Ministry's approval, but the examination is given only in Japanese.

PHONETICALLY SPEAKING

Pronunciation of Japanese: [ɲihoŋgo]

Relevant words for speech assessment and intervention

Word	Formal usage	Pronunciation	Informal usage	Pronunciation
Tongue	舌	/ɕita/	舌	/ɕita/
Teeth	歯	/há/	歯	/há/
Lips	唇	/kɯ̥ɕibirɯ/	唇	/kɯ̥ɕibirɯ/
Hard palate	硬口蓋	/koːkóːgai/		
Soft palate	軟口蓋	/naŋkóːgai/		
Larynx	喉頭	/koːtoː/		
Lungs	肺	/hai/	肺	/hai/
Nose	鼻	/hana/	鼻	/hana/
Sound	音	/otó/	音	/otó/
Word	語	/go/	言葉	/kotoba/
Sentence	文	/búɴ/	文	/búɴ/
Paragraph	段落	/danrakɯ/	段落	/danrakɯ/

RESOURCES

Books

Ito, M., and Sasanuma, S. (2002). *Shinpen gengo ryōhō manyuaru* [Manual for speech-language therapy – new edition]. Tokyo: Ishiyaku Publishing.

Kotera, T. (1992). *Gengo chōkaku ryōhō rinshō manyaru* [Clinical manual for speech and hearing therapy]. Tokyo: Kyodo Isho Shuppan.

Shibatani, M. (1990). *The languages of Japan*. Cambridge, UK: Cambridge University Press.

Vance, T. J. (1987). *An introduction to Japanese phonology*. Albany, NY: State University of New York Press.

Recording

Japan Society of Logopedics and Phoniatrics (1989). *Kōgairetsu no kōon shōgai sampuru tēpu* [Tape recorded speech samples of cleft palate patients]. Medical Research Center.

Journals

- *Gengo Chōkaku Kenkyū* [Japanese Journal of Speech, Language, and Hearing Research].
- *Onsei Gengo Igaku* [The Japan Journal of Logopedics and Phoniatrics]

Professional associations

The professional associations of speech-language pathologists and related groups within Japan are the following:

The Association of Japanese Clinical Psychology (http://www.u-netsurf.ne.jp/pajcp/)

Gengo Hattatsu Shōgai Kenkyūkai [authors' translation: Speech development disorder research group] (http://www.lipss.gr.jp/)

Japan Audiology Society (http://www.audiology-japan.jp/)

Japan Society of Developmental Psychology (http://wwwsoc.nii.ac.jp/jsdp/)

Japanese Association of Communication Disorder (http://www.chabashira.co.jp/~communi/)

Japanese Association of Special Education (http://www1.accsnet.ne.jp/~tokkyou)

Japanese Cleft Palate Association (http://square.umin.ac.jp/JCLP/jclp.html)

Neuropsychology Association of Japan (http://www.neuropsychology.gr.jp/)

Institutions offering courses in speech-language pathology

Aso Rehabilitation College (Fukuoka, Fukuoka) (http://www.asojuku.ac.jp/arc/)

Health Sciences University of Hokkaido (Ishikari, Hokkaido) (http://www.hoku-iryo-u.ac.jp)

International University of Health and Welfare (Otawara, Tochigi) (http://www.iuhw.ac.jp)

Kitasato University (Sagamihara, Kanagawa) (http://www.kitasato-u.ac.jp)

National Rehabilitation Center for Persons with Disabilities (Tokorozawa, Saitama) (http://www.rehab.go.jp)

Osaka College of Rehabilitation (Osaka, Osaka) (http://www.ocr.ac.jp)

Tokai College of Health Related Professions (Nagoya, Aichi) (http://www.tokai-med.ac.jp/info/fukushi/)

Prefectural University of Hiroshima (Hiroshima, Hiroshima) (http://www.pu-hiroshima.ac.jp)

REFERENCES

Abe, M., Kato, M., Saito, S., Takeshita, K., Nishimura, B., Funayama, M., Yamashita, S., and Yamashita, Y. (1981). K_onkensah_. *Onsei Gengo Igaku, 22,* 209–217.

Aoyama, K. (2001). *A psycholinguistic perspective on Finnish and Japanese prosody: Perception, production and child acquisition of consonantal quantity distinctions.* Boston: Kluwer.

Beckman, M. E., Yoneyama, K., and Edwards, J. (2003). Language-specific and language-universal aspects of lingual obstruent productions in Japanese-acquiring children. *Journal of the Phonetic Society of Japan, 7,* 18–28.

Funayama, M. (1998). Kodomo no k_onsh_gai. In K. Oishi (Ed.), *Kodomo no komyunik_shon sh_gai* (pp. 99–125) Tokyo: Taishukan Shoten.

Funayama, M., Abe, M., Kato, M., Saito, S., Takeshita, K., Nishimura, B., Yamashita, S., and Yamashita, Y. (1989). K_onkensah_ tsuikah_koku. *Onsei Gengo Igaku, 30,* 285–292.

Furuya, N. (1958). Gengosh_gai no goonmeiry_do kensa (gomeido) ni kansuru kenky_. *Nichijibi, 61,* 1923–1948.

Goetry, V., Urbain, S., Morais, J., and Kolinsky, R. (2005). Paths to phonemic awareness in Japanese: Evidence from a training study. *Applied Psycholinguistics, 26,* 285–309.

Gordon, R. G., Jr. (Ed.). (2005). *Ethnologue: Languages of the world* (15th ed.). Dallas, TX: SIL International.

Hallé, P. A., de Boysson-Bardies, B., and Vihman, M. M. (1991). Beginnings of prosodic organization: Intonation and duration patterns of disyllables produced by Japanese and French infants. *Language and Speech, 34,* 299–318.

Imamura, A., and Sakamoto, T. (2002). *Kin_sei k_onsh_gai ni okeru onseichikan – Ion ni chakumoku shita k_satsu.* Paper presented at the 125th Meeting of the Linguistic Society of Japan, Tohoku Gakuin University.

Inagaki, K., Hatano, G., and Otake, T. (2000). The effect of kana literacy acquisition on the speech segmentation unit used by Japanese young children. *Journal of Experimental Child Psychology, 75,* 70–91.

Ito, K. (1990). *Kodomo no kotoba.* Tokyo: Keiso Shobo.

Ito, T., and Kagawa, A. (2001). Moji kakutoku mae no y_ji ni okeru onritsu tan'i no hattatsu. *Onsei Gengo Igaku, 42,* 235–241.

Ito, T., and Tatsumi, I. (1997). Tokushuhaku ni taisuru metagengo chishiki no hattatsu. *Onsei Gengo Igaku, 38,* 196–203.

Mann, V. A. (1986). Phonological awareness: The role of reading experience. Cognition, 24, 65–92.

Nagasawa, Y., Fujishima, S., and Oishi, M. (1985). *K_onhattatsu yosoku kensa.* Tokyo: Kokuritsu Tokushu Ky_iku S_g_kenky_jo.

Nakajima, S., Okamoto, N., Murai, J., Tanaka, M., Okuno, S., and Maeda, T. (1962). Onsei no kig_ka narabini taiseika katei ni kansuru kenky_ (1). *Sinrigaku Hy_ron, 6,* 1–48.

Nakanishi, Y. (1982). K_on hattatsu. In R. Uchisugawa and Y. Yasuko (Eds.), *K_za gengo sh_gai chiry_ ky_iku 4: K_onsh_gai* (pp. 37–64). Tokyo: Fukumura Shuppan.

Nakanishi, Y., and Owada, K. (1967). Y_ji no k_onsh_gai no hattatsu. *Tokyo Gakugei University Bulletin of the Research Institute for the Education of Exceptional Children, 1,* 1–52.

Nakanishi, Y., Owada, K., and Fujita, N. (1972). K_onkensa to sono kekka ni kansuru k_satsu. *Tokyo Gakugei Daigaku Tokushu Kyoiku Shisetsu Hokoku, 1,* 1–19.

Noda, M, Iwamura, Y., Naito, K., and Asukai, K. (1969). Y_ji no k_onn_ryoku no hattatsu ni kansuru kenky_. *Nihon S_g_ Aiiku Kenky_sho Kiy_, 4,* 153–170.

Okubo, A. (1977). *Y_ji no kotoba to otona.* Tokyo: Sanseido.

Ota, M. (2003a). *The development of prosodic structure in early words.* Amsterdam: John Benjamins.

Ota, M. (2003b). The development of lexical pitch accent systems: An autosegmental analysis. *Canadian Journal of Linguistics, 48,* 357–383.

Owada, K., and Nakanishi, Y. (1971). Y_ji no kotoba no hattatsu (6) – K_on no k_j_sei to kanseijun'i. *Jik_, 43,* 183–192.

Owada, K., Nakanishi, Y., and Oshige, K. (1969). Hoikuenji no k_on no henka nit suite. *Jik_, 41,* 227–231.

Sakauchi, T. (1967). Kodomo no k_on n_ryoku ni tsuite. *Gengo Sh_gai Kenky_, 68,* 13–26.

Satake, T., Iizuka, N., Uchiyama, C., Otomo, T., Takaizumi, Y., and Higashikawa, T. (2005). Gengo hattatsu sh_gai gengo hattatsu chitaiji no genj_ to kadai. *Japanese Journal of Speech, Langauge, and Hearing Research, 2,* 105–113.

Shibatani, M. (1990). *The languages of Japan.* Cambridge, UK: Cambridge University Press.

Shirose, A., Kakehi, K., and Kiritani, S. (2001). Interference of accent system variation with the acquisition of compound accent rule: A cross-dialectal study. *Journal of Cognitive Science, 2,* 33–44.

Shirose, A., Kakehi, K., and Kiritani, S. (2002). *Kagoshima hoogen yooji no tango akusento kakutoku ni kansuru yobiteki kentoo*, Paper presented at the annual meeting of the Acoustic Society of Japan.

Spagnoletti, C., Morais, J., Alegria, J., and Dominicy, M. (1989). Metaphonological abilities of Japanese children. *Reading and Writing: An Interdisciplinary Journal, 2*, 221–244.

Sumio, K. (1978). *Y_jiky_iku sensho. Ry_ikihen: Gengo*. Tokyo: Kawashima Shoten.

Taguchi, T. (1967). *Gengosh_gai chiry_gaku*. Tokyo: Igaku Shoin.

Taguchi, T., and Ogawaguchi, H. (1992). *Shinteiban kotoba no tesuto ehon – Gengo sh_gaiji no senbetsu kensah_*. Tokyo: Nihon Bunkakagakusha.

Takagi, S., and Yasuda, A. (1967). Seij_y_ji no k_onn_ryoku. *Sh_ni Hoken Igaku, 25*, 23–28.

Ueda, I. (1994). A linguistic characterization of 'typical' and 'atypical' in functionally disordered phonologies. *Gengo Kenkyu: Journal of the Linguistic Society of Japan, 106*, 74–94.

Ueda, I. (1995). A consideration of various theoretical and clinical problems pertaining to Natural Process Analysis. *The Japan Journal of Logopedics and Phoniatrics, 36*, 331–337.

Ueda, I. (1996a). Segmental acquisition and feature specification in Japanese. In B. Bernhardt, J. Gilbert, and D. Ingram (Eds.), Proceedings of the UBC International Conference on Phonological Acquisition (pp. 15–27). Somerville, MA: Cascadilla Press.

Ueda, I. (1996b). On the phonology of Japanese "kappacism". In T. W. Powell (Ed.), *Pathologies of speech and language: Contributions of clinical phonetics and linguistics* (pp. 179–186). New Orleans, LA: International Clinical Phonetics and Linguistics Association.

Ueda, I., and Davis, S. (1999). Constraint-based analysis of Japanese rhotacism. In B. Maassen and P. Groenen (Eds.), *Pathologies of speech and language: Advances in clinical and linguistics* (pp. 34–40). London: Whurr Publishers.

Ueda, I., and Davis, S. (2001). Promotion and demotion of phonological constraints in the acquisition of the Japanese liquid. *Clinical Linguistics & Phonetics, 15*, 29–33.

Umebayashi, S., and Takagi, T. (1965). Gakurei mae no kodomo no k_onn_ryoku ni kansuru ichikenky_. *Onsei Gengo Igaku, 6*, 17–18.

Van Riper, C., and Erickson, R. L. (1996). *Speech correction: An introduction to speech pathology and audiology* (9th ed.). Boston, MA: Allyn & Bacon.

Vance, T. (1987). *An introduction to Japanese phonology*. Albany, NY: State University of New York Press.

Weiner, F. (1981). Treatment of phonological disabilty using the method of meaningful minimal contast: Two case studies. *Journal of Speech and Hearing Disorders, 46*, 97–103.

Yasuda, A. (1966). Sansaiji ni okeru k_onn_ryoku. *Onsei Gengo Igaku, 7*, 32–33.

SUMMARY OF STUDIES OF TYPICAL JAPANESE SPEECH ACQUISITION

Authors	Year	Country	No. of children	Age of children	Information	Sample type	Data collection
Aoyama	2001	Japan	22	3–5 yrs	/n/ vs /nn/ contrast	Single word production & perception	Cross-sectional
Goetry, Urbain, Morais, and Kolinsky	2005	Japan and elsewhere	115	5;2–8;11	Phonemic awareness	Phoneme manipulation	Cross-sectional
Ito and Kagawa	2001	Japan	80	3–6 yrs	Segmentation and moras	Single word	Cross-sectional

Authors	Year	Country	No. of children	Age of children	Information	Sample type	Data collection
Ito and Tatsumi	1997	Japan	80	3–6 yrs	Metalinguistic awareness of moras	Single word	Cross-sectional
Kawakami and Ito	1999	Japan	173	1–6 yrs	Segmentation and moras	Single word	Cross-sectional
Nakajima, Okamoto, Murai, Tanaka, Okuno, and Maeda	1962	Japan	550	1;0–2;11	Variety	Single word	Cross-sectional
Nakanishi	1982	Japan	10	1;0–4;0	Age of acquisition of consonants and vowels	Single word	Longitudinal
Nakanishi and Owada	1967	Japan	20	1;0–1;8	Variety	Connected speech	Longitudinal
Nakanishi, Owada, and Fujita	1972	Japan	1,689	4;0–6;11	Age of acquisition	Single word	Cross-sectional
Noda, Iwamura, Naito, and Asukai	1969	Japan	446	2;0–6;6	Age of acquisition	Single word	Cross-sectional
Ota	2003	USA	3	1;0–2;6	Prosodic acquisition	Connected speech	Longitudinal
Owada and Nakanishi	1971	Japan	10	1;0–4;0	Age of acquisition of consonants	Connected speech	Longitudinal
Owada, Nakanishi, and Oshige	1969	Japan	511	3;0–6;0	Processes and mismatches	Single word	Cross-sectional and longitudinal
Sakauchi	1967	Japan	134	2;10–4;8	Age of acquisition of consonants	Single word	Cross-sectional
Shirose, Kakehi, and Kiritani	2001	Japan	191	3–5 yrs	Word accent	Compounds	Cross-sectional and cross-dialectal
Shirose, Kakehi, and Kiritani	2002	Japan	8 children 12 parents	4 yrs	Word accent	Single word	Child-parent comparison
Spagnoletti, Morais, Alegria, and Dominicy	1989	Belgium	23	Means: 6;5, 6;8, and 7;0	Phonological awareness	Phoneme manipulation	Cross-sectional
Sumio	1978	Japan	1600	4;0–6;11	Variety	Isolated syllables and Connected speech	Cross-sectional

Authors	Year	Country	No. of children	Age of children	Information	Sample type	Data collection
Umebayashi and Takagi (also Takagi and Yasuda 1967)	1965	Japan	133	3;6–6;0	Age of acquisition of consonants	Single word	Cross-sectional
Yasuda	1966	Japan	100	3;0–4;0	Age of acquisition of consonants	Single word	Cross-sectional

Acknowledgements

We are indebted to Shinobu Yamaguchi for assistance in collecting valuable information for this chapter.

Chapter 46

Korean Speech Acquisition

Minjung Kim and Soyeong Pae

INTRODUCTION

The Korean language belongs to the Altaic language family, which includes the Turkic, Mongolic, and Tungus-Mauchu language. There are about 75 million people in the world who speak Korean as a first language (48 million in South Korea, 22 million in North Korea, and 5 million outside of Korea) (Korean Overseas Information Service, http://www.korea.net). This chapter is based on the record of South Korea only.

Where Korean is spoken

People in the Korean peninsula in the northeast area of Asia have used the Korean language for a thousand years. Korean is the official language of both North and South Korea (see accompanying map and Appendix D).

Components of Korean

Consonants

Korean has 19 consonants, which are classified as stops, nasals, affricates, fricatives, and a liquid (Lee, 1996; Shin and Cha, 2003). Each category of consonants takes one to three places of articulation (see Table 46-1). There are 9 stop consonants: three bilabial stops /p, p*, pʰ/, three alveolar stops /t, t*, tʰ/, and three velar stops /k, k*, kʰ/. Three nasal sounds take three places, bilabial /m/, alveolar /n/, and velar /ŋ/. Three fricatives occur in two

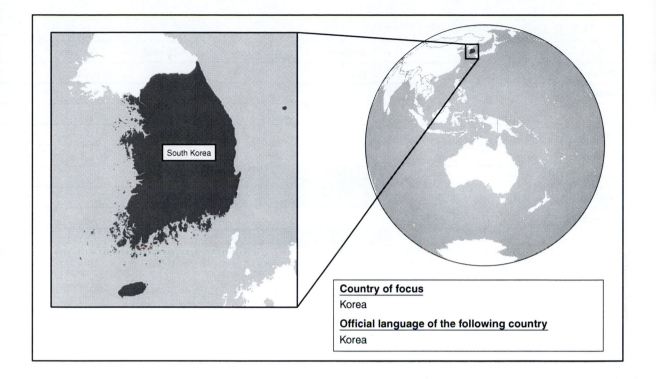

Country of focus
Korea

Official language of the following country
Korea

different places, alveolar /s, s*/ and glottal /h/. Three affricate sounds /tɕ, tɕ*, tɕʰ/ are found in post-alveolar place. Korean affricates are pronounced with no or less lip rounding compared to English (Han et al., 2003; Park, Oh, and Oh, 2004). Liquid sound /l/ occurs in alveolar place. (We follow the Shin and Cha (2003) IPA (International Phonetic Alphabet) with Korean.)

Unlike English, tenseness and aspiration are two important manners of articulation to differentiate word meaning. Korean obstruents are categorized into three major subgroups: voiceless lenis /p, t, k, tɕ, s/, voiceless fortis /p*, t*, k*, tɕ*, s*/, and voiceless aspirated /pʰ, tʰ, kʰ, tɕʰ/. /pul/ 'fire,' /p*ul/ 'horn,' and /pʰul/ 'grass' are three different Korean words.

Some Korean consonants have allophones (Shin and Cha, 2003). For example, lenis stops /p, t, k/ become voiced stops [b, d, g] between the sonorant phonemes and unreleased stops [p˺, t˺, k˺] in the syllable-final position. Liquid is an alveolar flap [ɾ] between vowels, while liquid is a lateral approximant [l] in the syllable-final position. Alveolar fricatives /s, s*/ become prepalatal fricatives [ɕ, ɕ*] when followed by the vowel /i/ or the semivowel /j/. Table 46-1 shows the consonants produced in Korean.

Vowels and diphthongs

Modern Korean has seven monophthongs depending on tongue place, tongue height, and lip rounding (Shin and Cha, 2003) (see Table 46-2). Based on tongue place, there are two front vowels /i, ɛ/, one central vowel /ɑ/, and four back vowels /ɯ, ʌ, u, o/. Three high vowels /i, ɯ, u/ can be categorized based on tongue height, while two rounded vowels /o, u/ are based on the lip rounding (Lee, 1996).

Diphthongs are monophthongs combined with the semivowels /j/, /w/, and /ɥ/. The semivowel /j/ leads five diphthongs /jɑ, jʌ, jo, ju, jɛ/ while the semivowel /w/ produces four diphthongs /wɑ, wʌ, wɛ, wi/. The semivowel /ɥ/ produces one diphthong /ɥi/.

Phonotactic restrictions
Syllables

Korean has a rather distinct syllable boundary in both its speech and writing systems. The syllable structure of Korean is $C_{(0-1)}VC_{(0-1)}$. The smallest allowable syllable of Korean is $V_{(monophthong)}$ and the largest allowable syllable is $CV_{(diphthong)}C$. A rhythmic unit of Korean usually consists

TABLE 46-1 Consonants produced in Korean

	Bilabial	Labiodental	Dental	Alveolar
Plosive	p, p*, pʰ			t, t*, tʰ
Nasal	m			n
Trill				
Tap or flap				(ɾ)
Fricative				s, s*
Lateral fricative	███████			
Affricate	███████			
Approximant				
Lateral approximant	███████			l

Note. The Korean liquid /l/ has two allophones, [l] and [r].

Black = articulations judged impossible

Based on the International Phonetic Alphabet. Courtesy of the International Phonetic Association (c/o Department of Linguistics, University of Victoria, Victoria, British Columbia, Canada).

of three to four syllables in conversational speech (Shin and Cha, 2003).

Consonants and consonant clusters

There are 18 Korean consonants possible for a syllable-initial speech sound. /ŋ/ can occur only as a syllable-final sound. There are only seven syllable-final sounds /p, t, k, m, n, ŋ, l/ in Korean. There is no consonant cluster in syllable-initial and syllable-final position in Korean although intersyllabic consonant clusters are possible (e.g., /taǹkɯn/ 'carrot'). Within intersyllabic consonant clusters, lenis stops cannot succeed lenis stops or sonorants (e.g., /pt/, /tn/) and the alveolar nasal sound /n/ cannot make a consonant cluster with the lateral sound /l/ (e.g., /nl/, /ln/). However, intersyllablic consonant clusters with the same sounds are possible in Korean (e.g., /ʌmmɑ/ 'mommy,' /ʌnni/ 'sister,' /mollɑ/ 'don't know') (Han et al., 2003).

Tones

Korean does not use tones to differentiate word meaning (Han et al., 2003).

Stress and intonation

Korean does not use a stress to differentiate word meaning. Korean words seem to have stress on the first syllable, although this does not change the meaning of a word (Han et al., 2003). /kim tɕʰi/ has its stress on /kim/ although it is acceptable if you put a stress on / tɕʰi/.

Korean uses intonation to differentiate declaratives, questions, and requests without reordering the words of a sentence. The nuclear tone of a sentence seems to be on the final syllable of a sentence. For example, /ʌmmɑkɑ mʌkʌs*ʌ/ 'mommy ate' could be made a declarative, a question, or a request by changing the tone of /s*ʌ/. In conversation between familiar people, Korean uses a rising phrasal tone, unlike English, which uses a high phrasal tone (Han et al., 2003).

Writing system

The Korean language uses the writing system *Hangeul*. There are 10 vowel-related and 14 consonant-related graphemes in Hangeul. (See the Web site of the national academy of the Korean language, http://korean.go.kr/hangeul). Hangeul has a distinct syllable focus and syllable boundary. For example, 장갑 'gloves' has two syllables and the syllable-final graphemes (ㅇ, ㅂ) are located below the consonant + vowel graphemes (ㅈ+ㅏ, ㄱ+ㅏ). Some vowel graphemes (ㅗ, ㅜ, and ㅡ) are placed below a syllable-initial grapheme (e.g., 공부 'study').

Varieties of Korean

Korean has four to six regional dialects (Lee, 2005). People can communicate with each other regardless of their region of birth, although their accents are different from person to person. But the Jeju dialect, which

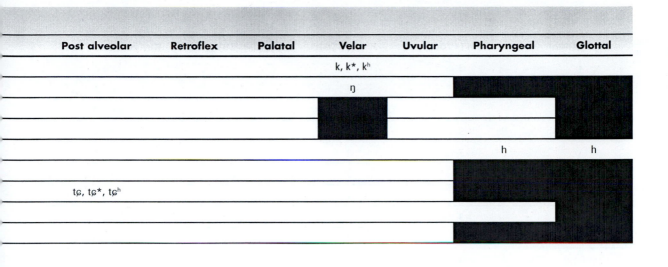

Post alveolar	Retroflex	Palatal	Velar	Uvular	Pharyngeal	Glottal
			k, k*, kʰ			
			ŋ			
					h	h
tɕ, tɕ*, tɕʰ						

includes quite different types of phonological strings for specific words, is hard to understand for many people. Young people seem to prefer a faster speed of speech than older people, and young ladies seem to enjoy the rising intonation for declaratives (Lee, 2005).

Typical acquisition of Korean

There has been a series of research projects on Korean phonological acquisition from the point of view of speech pathologists. The Summary of Studies table at the end of the chapter contains studies of the acquisition of Korean.

Acquired sounds

Consonants

Table 46-3 contains age of acquisition data for Korean based on 75 percent correct production. By around 3 years of age, Korean children have acquired all consonants except liquid /l/ and alveolar fricatives /s, s*/ (Kim 1996; Kim and Pae, 2005; Oum, 1986; Pae, 1995). Among these consonants, bilabials /p, p*, pʰ, m/ and fortis

TABLE 46-2 Vowels produced in Korean

			Vowels
Monophthongs	front vowel	high-front	i
		mid-front	ɛ
	central vowel	low-central	ɑ
	back vowel	high-back	ɯ
		low-back	ʌ
		rounded high-back	u
		rounded mid-back	o
Diphthongs	led by /j/		jɑ, jʌ, jo, ju, jɛ
	led by /w/		wɑ, wʌ, wɛ, wi
	led by /ɰ/		ɰi

TABLE 46-3   Age of acquisition for Korean consonants

Consonant	Oum (1986)	Pae (1995)	Kim (1996)	Kim and Pae (2005)
p*	3	1	2	late 2
t*	3	1	2	late 2
k*	3	1	2	early 3
h	3	2	2	late 2
pʰ	3	2	2	late 2
tʰ	3	2	2	early 3
kʰ	3	2	2	early 4
p	3	4	2	early 3
m	3	4	2	early 3
t	3	4	2	early 3
n	3	4	2	late 3
k	3	4	2	early 4
ŋ	3	4	2	early 4
tɕ*	3	3	3	early 3
tɕʰ	3	3	3	early 3
tɕ	3	3	3	late 3
l	5	5	5	early 5
s	after 5	after 5	4	after late 6
s*	after 5	after 5	3	after late 6

/p*, t*, k*/ were acquired relatively earlier, whereas velars /k, k*, kʰ, ŋ/ and affricates /tɕ, tɕ*, tɕʰ/ were acquired later. Considering syllable position within words, syllable-initial speech sounds were acquired by 2 to 3 years of age while syllable-final speech sounds were acquired by 3 to 4 (Kim and Pae, 2005; Pae, 1995).

Korean children were late in acquiring liquid /l/ and alveolar fricatives /s, s*/. Liquids were acquired by 5 years of age, but alveolar fricatives were not acquired by 5 or 6. However, Kim and Pae (2005) suggested that these consonants were acquired by 4 and 5, taking into account distorted pronunciation.

The late-developing consonants were studied in order to consider allophonic variations. In terms of the liquid /l/, Korean children acquired the approximant liquid [l] of the syllable-final position by 3 years, while they acquired the flap liquid [ɾ] of the syllable-initial position by 5 years (Kim and Pae, 2005; Oum, 1986). In addition, for the alveolar fricatives, Korean children acquired the prepalatal fricatives [ɕ, ɕ*] earlier than the alveolar fricatives [s, s*] (Cheon and Lee, 1999; Oum, 1994).

Consonant clusters

Korean 1-year-olds seem to be very sensitive to the Korean sound structure of a specific word, given that they use intersyllabic consonant clusters with the same speech sounds from early on (e.g., /ʌmma/ 'mommy', /ʌnni/ 'sister') (Pae, 1994). Intersyllabic consonant clusters including syllable-final velars /k, ŋ/ were acquired by 4 years of age (Kim and Pae, 2005).

Vowels and diphthongs

Korean monophthongs are acquired by the age of 3 (Kwon, 1981; Oum, 1994). Korean diphthongs combined with the semivowel /j/ are acquired before the age of 3, although diphthongs combined with the semivowel /w/ don't seem to be acquired by the age of 5. It would be interesting to see whether this phenomenon is related to child-directed speech, since Korean adults tend to simplify diphthongs combined with the semivowel /w/ as monophthongs in daily conversation.

Percent correct

Consonants

Kim and Pae (2005) investigated the percentage of correct consonants (PCC) with the *Korean- Test of Articulation and Phonology for Children* (see Figure 46-1). There was no statistically significant difference between boys and girls. Korean 2- to 3-year-olds seem to be in an active phonological acquisition period.

Cheon and Lee (1999) studied the phonological acquisition of allophonic variation of /s, s*/. The PCCs of [s] and [s*] were 82 percent and 77 percent at the age of 7, while the PCC of [ɕ] was above 90 percent at the age of 5 and the PCC of [ɕ*] was above 90 percent at the age of 6. The following vowel and the tense feature seem to influence the mastery process of /s, s*/.

Consonant clusters

Hong and Pae (2002) suggested that the PCC of intersyllabic consonant clusters ranged from below 50 percent at the age of 2, to about 70 percent at age 3 and above 90 percent at age 4.

Vowels

Kwon (1981) suggested that monophthongs and diphthongs led by /j/ showed above 90 percent accuracy at the age of 3, while diphthongs led by /w/ showed about 20 percent accuracy at age 3 and about 30 percent accuracy at age 4.

Phonological processes

Korean children use rules or phonological processes to acquire Korean phonology (Lee, 1997; Pae, 1994). Kim (2006) investigated phonological processes of Korean children aged 2;6 to 6;5 with a word-based pronunciation test. She focused on phonological processes that a child uses three or more times out of nine or more opportunities. Phonological processes used by more than 10 percent of late 2-year-olds were as follows:

- The whole-word processes, including reduplication or consonant harmony (e.g., [tʰaŋtʰaŋ] for /satʰaŋ/ 'candy,' [mamu] for /namu/ 'tree'), word-final consonant deletion (e.g., [k*o] for /k*ot/ 'flower'), and intersyllabic cluster simplification (e.g., [jampʰa] for /jaŋpʰa/ 'onion').
- The segment-change processes, including tensing or deaspiration (e.g., [ap*a] for /apʰa/ 'sick'), velar fronting (e.g., [patʰi] for /pakʰwi/ 'wheel'), nasalization or stopping of liquid (e.g., [konɛ] or [kodɛ] for /kolɛ/ 'dolphin'), liquid simplification (e.g., [kojɛ] for

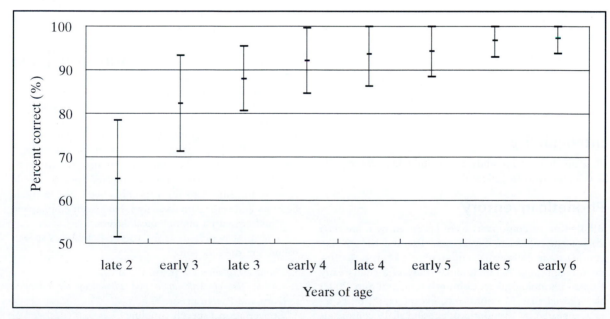

Figure 46-1 The mean of PCC (–) with 1 standard deviation bar (I) in each age (Kim & Pae, 2000)

/kolɛ/ 'dolphin'), affrication or palatalization (e.g., [tɕ*awʌ] for /s*awʌ/ 'fight'), stopping of fricative or affricate (e.g., [t*awʌ] for /s*awʌ/ 'fight'), and inter-dentalization of fricative (e.g., [s̪atʰaŋ] for /satʰaŋ/ 'candy'). Early-disappearing phonological processes were reduplication or consonant harmony, word-final consonant deletion, tensing or deaspiration, velar fronting, and nasalization or stopping of liquid.

Pae (1994) suggested that Korean 1-year-olds showed phonological processes such as syllable deletion (e.g., [pʰo] for /pʰoto/ 'grape'), vowel addition (e.g., [iba] for /pɛ/ 'pear'), syllable-initial consonant deletion (e.g., [o] for /kʰo/ 'nose'), and voicing (e.g., [bwa] for /pwa/ 'see') as well as late-appearing phonological processes.

Regional variation in Korean acquisition was observed in the pronunciation of fortis fricatives. Children in the Daegu area used the untensing phonological process more frequently than children in the Seoul area (Kim, 1992; Kim and Shin, 1992).

Oum (1994) closely investigated substitution in Korean phonological acquisition of /l, s, s*/. The acquisition of the /l/ sound involved the nasalization process (replaced by /n/), then the stopping process (replaced by /t/), and finally gliding (replaced by /j/). The acquisition of the /s, s*/ sound involved stopping (replaced by /t, t*, tʰ/), affrication (replaced by /tɕ, tɕ*, tɕʰ/), and finally interdentalization (replaced by distorted [s̪, s̪*]).

Kim and Pae (2000) indicated error patterns in the acquisition of intersyllabic consonant clusters. A syllable-final consonant of an intersyllabic consonant cluster tends to be deleted or substituted when children are young. When they grow, they seem to assimilate the syllable-final consonant of the intersyllabic consonant cluster with the same place consonant of the following syllable-initial consonant (e.g., [japʰa] ⇨ [jampʰa] for /jaŋpʰa/ 'onion').

Intelligibility

To date there is no study of intelligibility of normally developing Korean children.

Phonetic inventory

All 19 Korean consonants were produced by more than 20 percent of 30 late 1-year-olds (Pae and Kim, 2005). Among these consonants, /m, n, p*, t*, k*, t, k, tɕ/ frequently appeared. A longitudinal study of a child's early Korean phonological acquisition (Hong and Sim, 2002) also proved that 13 consonants, except /s, s*, pʰ, tʰ, kʰ, tɕʰ/, appeared by 13 months of age and all 19 consonants by 20 months.

Common mismatches

To date there is no study of common mismatches produced by Korean children.

Syllable structure

Korean 1-year-olds prefer one- to two-syllable words, while 2-year-olds seem to produce two- to five-syllable strings (Pae, 1994; Pae and Kim, 2005). Among early-appearing syllables, Korean 1-year-olds frequently used one-syllable words such as CV or V (e.g., /nɛ/ or /ʌ/ 'yes') and two-syllable words such as VCCV (e.g., /ʌmma/ 'mommy'), VCV (e.g., /ap*a/ 'daddy'), CVCV (e.g., /k*ak*a/ 'cookie'), or CVV (e.g., /siʌ/ for /siɾʌ/ 'no' or 'don't like').

Prosody

To date there is no study of Korean children's prosody.

Phonological awareness

Korean children's phonological awareness has been researched in relation to reading disorders. Korean 4-year-olds could perform phonological awareness tasks at word level with about 50 percent accuracy (Hong, Jeon, Pae, and Lee, 2002). At syllable level, 4-year-olds and 5-year-olds could perform phonological awareness tasks with about 34 percent and 67 percent correct. At phoneme level, Korean first graders revealed 33 percent accuracy on phonological awareness tasks, second graders 67 percent, and third graders 83 percent accuracy (Yoon, Pae, Kim, and Shin, 2006).

Speech assessment for Korean children

A Korean child's phonological acquisition can be assessed via word-focused standardized tests and/or analysis of connected speech. *The picture articulation test* (Kim, 1994) and the *Korean test of articulation and phonology for children* (Kim and Pae, in press) can be used. A child's phonological development can be observed and analyzed in depth at intra-individual level using connected speech sample analysis. Informal tests for a specific child's speech intelligibility and error pattern analysis have been emphasized for children with a phonological disorder.

The most popular tests for assessing children's speech sounds are the following

- *Picture articulation test* (Kim, 1994)
- *Korean Test of Articulation and Phonology for Children* (Kim and Pae, in press)
- Conversational speech sampling
- Informal single-word tests

Speech intervention for Korean children

Traditional articulation therapy is commonly used when working with Korean children with a phonological disorder. In addition, minimal pairs therapy, the cycle approach, paired stimuli technique, communication-centered approach, metaphonology therapy, whole-word approach, and motor-based programmed approach are being introduced (Seok, 2004). Korean speech pathologists usually prefer individual therapy to group therapy for children who have a phonological disorder. Korean word and/or picture lists for individual speech sounds are available for speech therapy (Kim, 2005; Shin and Kim, 2002).

Working in Korea

Korean speech pathologists work in hospitals and social welfare centers as well as private speech-language clinics. There has been social awareness of the necessity for school-based speech pathologists in Korea. As of 2005, about 1,500 speech pathologists certified by the Korean Association of Speech-Language Pathologists were working for the communication-disordered population. There are two types of certificates for speech pathologists in Korea, one for master's level qualifications and the other for bachelor's level qualifications. Many universities and graduate schools have begun to provide undergraduate and/or graduate level education programs for speech pathology. Refer to the Resources section for Korean graduate level programs, associations, and journals.

PHONETICALLY SPEAKING

Pronunciation of Korean: [haŋ gu gʌ]
Relevant words for speech assessment and intervention

Word/Phrase	Formal usage	Pronunciation
Tongue	혀	[çjʌ]
Teeth	이	[i]
Lips	입술	[ipˀ s*ul]
Hard palate	굳은입천장	[ku dɯn ipˀ tɕʰʌn dʑaŋ]
Soft palate	여린입천장	[jʌ rin ipˀ tɕʰʌn dʑaŋ]
Larynx	후두	[hu du]
Lungs	폐	[pʰ je]
Nose	코	[kʰo]
Sound	소리	[s*o ri]
Word	단어	[ta nʌ]
Sentence	문장	[mun dʑaŋ]
Paragraph	문단	[mun dan]

Note. [b, d, g, dʑ] are allophones of Korean consonants /p, t, k, tɕ/.

[pˀ, tˀ, kˀ] are allophones of Korean consonants /p, t, k/.

[ç] is an allophone of Korean consonant /h/.

[r] is an allophone of Korean consonant /l/.

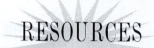

RESOURCES

Books

Sohn, H. (1999). *Korean language*. Cambridge, UK: Cambridge University Press.

The Korea Foundation provides Korea related book lists. http://www.booksonkorea.org

Journals

- *Korean Journal of Communication Disorders*, http://www. kasa1986.or.kr. The Korean Academy of Speech-Language Pathology and Audiology (Issued three times a year by KASA)
- *Korean Journal of Speech & Hearing Disorders*, http:// ksha.taegu.ac.kr Korea Speech-Language and Hearing Association (Issued bi-annually by KSHA)
- *Korean Journal of Speech Science*, The Korean Association of Speech Science (Issued seasonally by KASS)

Professional associations

The professional association of speech-language pathologists within Korea is the Korean Association of Speech-Language Pathologists (KASLA), http:// www.kasla.or.kr

Universities offering courses for the master's degree in speech-language pathology

- The Graduate Schools of Chonbuk National University. Clinical Speech Pathology.

- The Graduate School of Daegu University. Department of Rehabilitation Science.
- The Graduate School of Dankook University. Department of Speech Pathology.
- The Graduate Program of Ewha Woman's University. Interdisciplinary program in communication disorders.
- The Graduate School of Hallym University. Interdisciplinary program in speech pathology and audiology.
- The Graduate School of Social Education of Myongji University. Department of Speech-Language Pathology.
- The Graduate School Rehabilitation Service of Korea Nazarene University. Speech and Language Science.
- The Graduate School of Rehabilitation and Health Science of Yongin University. Department of Language Treatment.
- The Graduate Program of Yonsei University College of Medicine. The graduate program in speech pathology.

Useful Korean Web sites

- The national academy of the Korean language, http://korean.go.kr/hangeul
- Korean Overseas Information Service (KOIS), http://www.korea.net

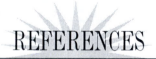

REFERENCES

Cheon, H., and Lee, S. (1999). The development of Korean /s/ and /s*/ in normal children aged 2 to 7 years [in Korean]. *Korean Journal of Communication Disorders, 4*, 37–61.

Han, J., Choe, J., Lee, H., Park, J., Yi, K., Cho, H., Cui, J., and Yi, S. (2003). *Teaching Korean pronunciation* [in Korean]. Seoul: Hollym International Corp.

Hong, G., and Sim H. (2002). A longitudinal study of development of the infant's speech sounds: 18 to 24 months [in Korean]. *Korean Journal of Communication Disorders, 7(2)*, 105–124.

Hong, J., and Pae, S. (2002). Development of final consonants of 2 to 5 year-old children [in Korean]. *Korean Journal of Communication Disorders, 7(2)*, 294–304.

Hong, S., Jeon, S., Pae, S., and Lee, I. (2002). Development of phonological awareness in Korean children [in Korean]. *Korean Journal of Communication Disorders, 7(1)*, 49–64.

Kim, D. (2004). *Exciting speech-language therapy* [in Korean]. Seoul; Paradise Welfare Foundation.

Kim, M. (2006). Phonological error patterns of preschool children for 'Korean Test of Articulation and Phonology for Children' [in Korean]. *Korean Journal of Communication Disorders, 11*(2), 17–31.

Kim, M., and Pae, S. (2000). Phonological error patterns of Korean children with specific phonological disorders [in Korean]. *Korean Journal of Speech Sciences, 7*(2), 7–18.

Kim, M., and Pae, S. (2005). The percentage of consonants correct and the ages of consonantal acquisition for 'Korean Test of Articulation for Children' [in Korean]. *Korean Journal of Speech Sciences, 12*(2), 139–152.

Kim, M., and Pae, S. (in press). *Korean Test of articulation and phonology for children* [in Korean].

Kim, Y. (1992). A study of phonological regression in 2–6 years of Korean children [in Korean]. *Journal of Rehabilitation Science, 10*(1), 49–58.

Kim, Y. (1996). The percentage of consonant correct (PCC) using picture articulation test in preschool children [in Korean]. *Korean Journal of Communication Disorders, 1*, 7–33.

Kim, Y., and Shin, M. (1992). A study of phonological regression in 2–6 years of age (II): In consonant substitution patterns [in Korean]. *Korean Journal of Speech & Hearing Disorders, 2*, 29–52.

Kwon, K. (1981). *Korean language development research: Phonology (II)* [in Korean]. Seoul: Korean Educational Development Institute.

Kwon, K., Lee Y., and Son, M. (1979). *Korean language development research: Phonology (I)* [in Korean]. Seoul: Korean Educational Development Institute.

Lee, H. (1996). *Korean phonetics* [in Korean]. Seoul: Thaehaksa.

Lee, J. (2005). *Understanding of Korean sociolect and regional dialect* [in Korean]. Seoul: Hankookmunhwasa.

Lee, K. (1997). Development of phonetic and phonological rule [in Korean]. *Language Acquisition. Saekukosanghwal, 7* (1), 81–101.

Oum, J. (1986). *Speech-sound development in children aged three to five years in Korean: With special reference to consonants* [in Korean]. Unpublished M.A. thesis, Ewha Women's University, Seoul.

Oum, J. (1994). Speech-sound development (II): Three, four, and five year-old children [in Korean]. In Korean Society of Communication Disorders (Ed.), *The treatment of articulation disorders for children* (pp. 54–66). Seoul: Kunja Inc..

Pae, S. (1994). Speech-sound development (I): 1;4–3;11 year-old children [in Korean]. In Korean Society of Communication Disorders (Ed.), *The treatment of articulation disorders for children* (pp. 54–66). Seoul: Kunja Inc.

Pae, S. (1995). The development of language in Korean children [in Korean]. In Korean Society of Communication Disorders (Ed.), *Training of speech pathologists* (pp. 18–35). Seoul: Hanhaksa.

Pae, S., and Kim, M. (2005, May). *Phonological characteristics in Korean 1-year-old children* [in Korean]. Paper presented at the 16th meeting of KASS, Daegu University (pp., 286–291). Daugu: Korean Association of Speech Sciences.

Park, C., Oh, M., and Oh, E. (2004). *Comparison of phonology: Korean, English, and Japanese* [in Korean]. Seoul: Hankukmoonwhasa.

Seok, D. (2004). *Treatment of articulation and phonological disorders* [in Korean]. Daegu: Daegu University Press.

Shin, J., and Cha, J. (2003). *Korean speech sound system* [in Korean]. Seoul: Hankookmunhwasa.

Shin, M., and Kim, Y. (2002). *A practice of Korean articulation and phonology* [in Korean]. Seoul: Hakjisa.

Yoon, H , Pae, S., Kim, M , and Shin, B. (2006). Korean 1st, 2nd, 3rd graders' word recognition ability in relation with phonological awareness and language ability [in Korean]. Manuscript in preparation.

SUMMARY OF STUDIES OF TYPICAL KOREAN SPEECH ACQUISITION

Authors	Year	Country	No. of children	Age of children	Information	Sample type	Data collection
Cheon and Lee	1999	Seoul	286	2;0–7;11	PCC of /s, s*/	Single word	Cross-sectional
Hong and Pae	2002	Chuncheon	50	2;0–5;11	Acquisition of syllable-final consonant	Single word	Cross-sectional

Authors	Year	Country	No. of children	Age of children	Information	Sample type	Data collection
Hong and Sim	2002	Seoul	1	1;6–2;0	Consonant inventory and syllable types	Connected speech	Longitudinal
Hong et al.	2002	Seoul	72	4–6	Phonological awareness	Single word	Cross-sectional
Kim	In preparation	Seoul	220	2;6–6;5	Phonological processes	Single word	Cross-sectional
Kim and Pae	2000	Seoul	24	2–4	Phonological process	Single-word	Cross-sectional
Kim and Pae	2005	Seoul	220	2;6–6;5	PCC, age of consonant acquisition	Single word	Cross-sectional
Kim	1992	Seoul	48	2;0–6;5	Percentage of phonological processes	Single word	Cross-sectional
Kim	1996	Seoul and Daegu	155	2–6	PCC, ages of consonant acquisition	Single word	Cross-sectional
Kim and Shin	1992	Daegu	50	2;0–6;5	Percentage of phonological processes	Single word	Cross-sectional
Kwon	1981	Seoul	20	3;3–5;5	Development and error patterns of vowels	Connected speech	Cross-sectional
Kwon, Lee, and Son	1979		33	3;3–6;0	Development and error patterns of consonants	Connected speech and single word	Cross-sectional
Oum	1986	Seoul	150	3–5	Age of consonant acquisition	Single word	Cross-sectional
Oum	1994	Seoul	150	3–5	Developmental and error patterns of /l, s, s*/, vowel acquisition	Single word	Cross-sectional
Pae	1994	Seoul	10	1;4–3;11	Syllable structure, phonetic inventory, phonological processes	Connected speech	Cross-sectional
Pae	1995	Seoul	320	0;5–7;1	Ages of consonant acquisition	Connected speech	Cross-sectional
Pae and Kim	2005	Seoul	90	1;0–1;11	Phonetic inventory, Early development	Connected speech	Cross-sectional
Yoon et al.	2006	Chuncheon	90	1st to 3rd graders	Phonological awareness	Single word	Cross-sectional

Note. PCC = percentage of consonants correct

Chapter 47

Maltese Speech Acquisition

Helen Grech

INTRODUCTION

Maltese is the national language of the Maltese archipelago, situated in the middle of the Mediterranean Sea. It has been recognized as an official language of the European Union. The Maltese language is derived from Arabic introduced in Malta and Gozo sometime between AD 870 and 1090 during the Arab occupation. It is closely related to the North African dialect of Arabic. Maltese has developed independently and has become a unique language influenced by the Romance and Anglo-Saxon languages, particularly southern Italian and English. See the Resources section for materials pertaining to Maltese.

Where Maltese is spoken

Maltese is spoken by around 400,000 people living on the Maltese islands. However, there are more Maltese expatriates living mainly in Australia, Canada, and the USA than there are Maltese living in Malta and Gozo, and some of these still speak Maltese with their families (see accompnying map and Appendix D).

Components of Maltese

The Maltese grammar is still mainly Semitic, so that adjectives follow nouns that often inflect for pluralization and gender in accordance with Semitic rules. They may also take the definite article. The verbs can be conjugated with prefixes, suffixes, and infixes, characterizing the Semitic pattern. Two tenses are possible, namely present and perfect. In the Maltese of today, new Italian words and expressions are being observed, while English ones continue to be added and molded into the Maltese grammatical forms. For example, the verb system can include English verbs with the classical Semitic prefixes and suffixes added to them (e.g., *ixxutjajna* derived from 'to shoot'). Maltese grammar can also show a Romance or Anglo-Saxon pattern, depending on the word origin (e.g., *lingwi* for 'languages', an Italian loanword pluralized in accordance with the Romance pattern).

Maltese vocabulary is a hybrid of Arabic roots and Sicilian Italian words as well as English and French loan words. Words marking basic concepts and ideas are Semitic (e.g., *tifla*, *tifel*, *tfal*, indicating 'girl', 'boy', and 'children'). More recently adopted words such as those related to law, education, art, literature, and information technology are derived from the Romance languages and English (e.g., *teatru* from 'teatro' and *strajk* from 'strike'). Malta is experiencing linguistic change. With the increasingly apparent degree of code switching among the Maltese, loanwords are becoming commonplace, especially in child-directed speech. This may reflect the prestige that English still enjoys on the Islands. Borg (1980) refers to the Maltese English used which is really utterances containing both Maltese and English words/phrases. He claims that the amount of mixing of the two languages depends on the linguistic abilities, social context, sex, and social background of the individual.

The National Minimum Curriculum (Ministry of Education, 1999) endorses bilingualism as the basis of the educational system. Most children are taught a third language in schools. Sciriha (1999) reports that more than 80 percent of children attending church or independent schools and 10 percent of those in state schools are taught a fourth language. What we have today is children who from a very early age use Maltese with English words amalgamated into Maltese child language.

Consonants

The sound system of Maltese derived by Azzopardi (1981) and later updated in Borg and Azzopardi-Alexander (1997) includes 22 consonantal phonemes, three of which are affricates. [dz] is not usually given full phonemic status and will not be considered as a phoneme in this chapter. Table 47-1 summarizes the place and manner of articulation of each phoneme.

Vowels and diphthongs

Azzopardi (1981) distinguishes quantitatively as well as qualitatively between the 11 monophthongs, which can all exist as stressed vowels. She lists relative distances between cardinal vowels and the Maltese vowels as indicated in Figure 47-1. Vowels are longest in monosyllables. Their duration depends on the number of syllables in the word. Unstressed syllables never include long vowels. Azzopardi (1981) claims that Maltese has seven Maltese diphthongs /ɐʊ, ɐɪ, ɛʊ, ɛɪ,

TABLE 47-1   Consonants produced in Maltese

	Bilabial	Labiodental	Dental	Alveolar
Plosive	p b			t d
Nasal	m			n
Trill				
Tap or flap				
Fricative		f v		s z
Lateral fricative	███			
Affricate				ts
Approximant	w (labio velar)			ɹ
Lateral approximant	███			l

Black = articulations judged impossible

Based on the International Phonetic Alphabet. Courtesy of the International Phonetic Association (c/o Department of Linguistics, University of Victoria, Victoria, British Columbia, Canada).

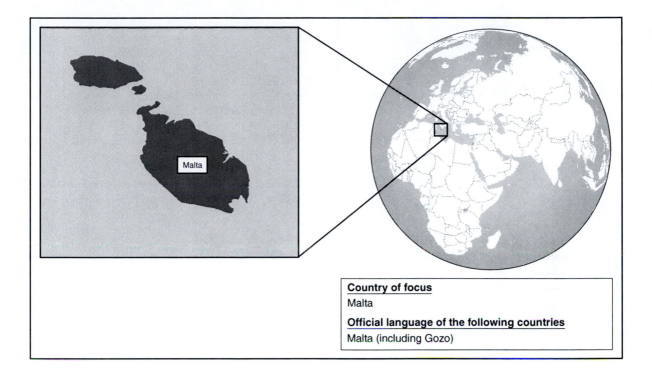

Country of focus
Malta

Official language of the following countries
Malta (including Gozo)

ɪʊ, ɔɪ, ɔʊ/. She states that the greatest degree of close-ness of such combinations is heard when the second element of the diphthong functions both as syllable final and syllable initial of the preceding and following syllable respectively.

Phonotactic restrictions

Syllables

The syllable structure of Maltese is (C)(C)(C)V(C)(C). Words can be monosyllabic in Maltese, but multisyllabic

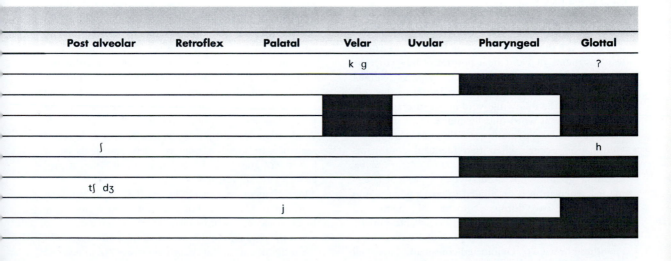

	Post alveolar	Retroflex	Palatal	Velar	Uvular	Pharyngeal	Glottal
				k g			ʔ
	ʃ						h
	tʃ dʒ						
			j				

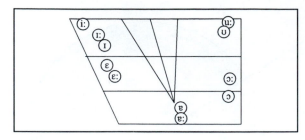

Figure 47-1 The 11 Maltese monophthongs organized according to relative distance between cardinal vowels (Note: The relative distances are only approximations as variation exists between speakers; Adapted from Azzopardi (1981); Maltese phonemic transcription as in Borg & Azzopardi-Alexander, 1997).

words are more common. These are usually composed of up to five syllables. Maltese words can be composed of one or more morphemes. There is a tendency to reduce the syllable to (C)(C)V(C) internally in multisyllabic words. Syllable division has preferences. If consonants occur between vowels the preferred pattern for occurrence is syllable-initially in the second syllable (i.e., V-CV). When two intervocalic consonants or geminated consonants occur, there is a preference for these to split up as consonant sequences to allow a closed syllable to precede a consonant-released syllable (Azzopardi, 1981, p. 74). With a three-consonant sequence intervocalically, the tendency is for the following order of preference: C-CC, CC-C, but never -CCC or CCC- . The syllable nucleus in a Maltese syllable almost always consists of a vowel. The nasals /m/, /n/, lateral /l/, and /ɹ/ may be syllabic when they occur word-initially.

Consonants and consonant clusters

- There is no opposition between voiced and voiceless obstruents in word-final position. Only voiceless obstruents occur word-finally (e.g., /kɛlp/ vs. /kɛlbɐ/ meaning 'dog' vs. 'bitch'). One exception to this rule occurs when the following word in the utterance has a voiced obstruent word-initially and the two words are not separated by a pause (e.g., /kɛlb zɐɪːɹɪ/- 'puppy').
- Gemination occurs when two identical consonants are adjacent to each other (e.g., /nɐnːɐ/ for 'nanna' meaning 'grandma'). It occurs when a particular segmental articulation is prolonged to cover what would otherwise be two distinct segments. No geminated consonant occurs word-initially or syllable-initially in Maltese, since this would be preceded with a short epenthetic vowel /ɪ/. Geminated consonants have dual syllable memberships (except word-finally) even when the first operates syllabically.

- Voicing assimilation occurs when pairs of voiced and voiceless sounds are brought together as a result of grammatical process or juxtaposition of words (usually regressive) (e.g., /hɐbɐt/ ⇨ /hɐptɐ/ 'he crashed' ⇨ 'crash').
- Complete assimilation where the modified segment takes on the complete bundle of distinctive features proper to its neighbor also occurs in Maltese. Such is the case with the definite article /l/ or /ɪl/, as in the case of Arabic. The article assimilates in words whose syllable-initial word-initial phoneme is any of the following phonemes: /t, d, n, s, z, ʃ, ts, tʃ, ɹ, l/.
- Sibilant assimilation is displayed in two ways in Maltese. One occurs by the juxtaposition of /ʃɪ/ meaning 'what' with words beginning with /s/ and /z/.
- The other kind of assimilation occurs when there is co-occurrence of the discontinuous morpheme /mɐ...ʃ/ (indicating negative) with the verb form ending in /s/ or /t/.
- Dissimilation occurs very rarely in Maltese. Borg (1975) gives one example of such occurrence where it can be observed in the replacement of /n/ by /l/: /nɔfsɪnɐːr/ ⇨ 'midday' which is often realised as /lɔfsɪnɐːɹ/.
- Metathesis is common in Maltese also where two contiguous phonemes exchange position to conform with certain phonological rules or preferences attested in the language; for example, some Maltese speakers reverse the positions of the first and second radical as in the pronunciation of certain verb forms and say /kpɛɪt/ ⇨ 'I cried' rather than /pkɛɪt/.
- All consonants can occur singly in syllable-initial word-initial position. Although CC combinations occur as clusters word-initially and word-finally (i.e., function together as onset or offset of syllable) they are dismissed from qualifying as clusters within a multisyllabic word because they are bound by syllabic division. In the circumstances they become consonantal sequences. There are only a few restrictions for CC sequence combinations across syllabic boundaries. Obstruents (plosives, fricatives, and affricates) in a cluster are either all voiced or all voiceless, depending on the last obstruent in the group. This rule does not apply to /l, m, n, ɹ/. /w, j, h, ʔ/ are not affected by other consonants in a cluster or sequence. In addition, only voiceless obstruents occur before /ʔ/ and /h/. /h/ is often voiced when it precedes a voiced obstruent.
- Three-element consonant clusters (CCC) are not very common in Maltese and they do not occur word-finally. In three-element word-initial clusters, when a choice is given the speaker may choose a simpler structure with the introduction of the epenthetic vowel /ɪ/ to separate the initial CCC cluster into two syllables: e.g., /ʃɪ/ + /flɪː ʃkɛn/ rather than /ʃflɪː ʃkɛn/.

Tones

In Maltese tone does not function at word, syllabic, or segmental level to contrast lexical meaning or to mark grammatical properties. Changes in segment duration can result from specific intonation patterns such as those marking surprise (Borg and Azzopardi-Alexander, 1997). Pitch variation functions in Maltese at sentence level only.

Stress and intonation

All long vowels are stressed in Maltese. Azzopardi (1981) claims that vowel length and stress are not clues to syllable division. Aquilina (1959) claims that there can be only one stress in the same Maltese word and that in multisyllabic words, the stress falls on the penultimate or the last syllable. Borg (1973) gives a more detailed account and claims that words bears stress on a long vowel or diphthong and in their absence stress is borne on a short vowel preceding a geminated consonant, affricate, or consonant cluster. Polysyllabic words that have none of the above bear stress on the penultimate syllable. If there is more than one long vowel, stress is borne on the last of these. Words having more than one affricate, geminated consonant, or cluster bear stress on the vowel preceding the last of these. Geminated consonants take precedence over affricates.

In Maltese any stress shift concomitant with grammatical processes such as pluralization, negativization, and so on, is often accompanied by loss or displacement of vocal length; for example, /biːp/ ⇨ /bibiːn/ 'door' ⇨ 'doors'.

Stress shift can sometimes also be accompanied by qualitative vowel changes in Maltese, for example, /kʰiːseh/ ⇨ /kɛshˈiːn/ 'cold' (singular) ⇨ 'cold' (plural).

Writing system

Maltese is the only Semitic language that is written using the Latin alphabet. The Maltese orthographic system was officially devised in the 1920s. The supremacy of English in the schools, in the past decades, reflects on the fact that nowadays many Maltese still find it easier to write English than Maltese. Apart from local newspapers, most educated people still prefer English books to the relatively few available in Maltese.

Varieties of Maltese

The varieties of Maltese are intelligible anywhere on the archipelago. Aquilina (1959) claims that a considerable number of phonetic dialectal variations occur and still exist today. Borg (1988) reports that the dialectal variations of Maltese vary widely in aspects such as phonetics, morphology, syntax, semantics, and lexis. He argues that Maltese is not homogeneous but varies geographically and socially. Maltese "dialects" are considered by some linguists as differences of "accents." They thus describe it as one language with different modes of pronunciation. Variations of Maltese are also found within the same town or village. Borg (1988) defines standard Maltese as being that which carries a privileged status. Azzopardi (1981) claims that standard Maltese is that spoken by most of the people living in the urban area centered on the capital city, Valletta. Dialectal phonetic variations include the tendency to replace /ɐ/ by /ɔ/ in certain positions as in the form /tɔːtʊ/, which in standard speech would be said as /tɐːtʊ/; and to replace /ɔ/ by /ɛ/ as in the form /triːkɛl/, where in standard speech it would be uttered as /triːkɔl/.

Variations affecting consonants are rarer (Borg, 1973). Nevertheless, it is not uncommon to hear an elderly Maltese replace the glottal stop with a slightly affricated back velar stop.

Typical acquisition of Maltese

The Summary of Studies Table at the end of the chapter contains studies of the acquisition of Maltese that have been evaluated in Grech (2006).

Acquired sounds

Consonants

Tables 47-2 and 47-3 contain age of acquisition data related to the contrastive phones for Maltese.

Consonant clusters

Table 47-4 highlights the percentage of children who used various consonantal cluster types at 3;6 years of age. Due to the vastness of such possibilities in Maltese, cluster production was recorded for types rather than describing each cluster combination. Space constraints do not permit reporting other data pertaining to consonantal cluster usage of the same children at 2;0, 2;5, and 3;0 years of age. The reader is referred to Grech (1998) for further information.

Vowels and diphthongs

The development of monophthongs and diphthongs for Maltese has not been studied to date.

TABLE 47-2 Syllable-initial adult phonemes used by the Maltese children to convey the same contrast

Age	Nasal	Plosive	Fricative	Affricate	Approximant
2;0	m	p b			l
	n	t d			
		ʔ			
2;5	m	p b	f v		w
	n	t d	s		l
		k g			ɹ
		ʔ	ʃ		j
			h		
3;0	m	p b	f v		
	n	t d	s z	tʃ	l
		k g	ʃ		ɹ
		ʔ	h		j

Note. Data from Grech (1998). Phonemes used by 75 percent or more of the children; most of the phonemes were produced with variation

Percent correct

Consonants

Percentage of consonants produced correctly has not been reported to date.

Consonant clusters

Percentage of consonantal clusters produced correctly has been studied by Grech (1998), who reported respective data at age 2;0, 2;5, 3;0, and 3;6 for syllable-initial and syllable-final position of clusters, respectively. In syllable-initial position the children's attempts at 3;6 years of age matched with the adult form between 46 and 83 percent depending on cluster type. In final position, results were even more favorable; all attempts made (irrespective of contrastive cluster type) matched with the adult ones in 75 percent or more of the cases.

Vowels

Percentage of vowels produced correctly has not been reported to date.

Phonological processes

Figure 47-2 summarizes the chronology of typical Maltese developmental processes as reported in Grech

TABLE 47-3 Syllable-final adult phonemes used by the Maltese children to convey the same contrast

Age	Nasal	Plosive	Fricative	Affricate	Approximant
2;0					w
	n				
2;5	m	p	f		w
	n	t	s		l
		k	ʃ		ɹ
					j
3;0	m	p			
	n	t	s		l
		k			ɹ
					j

Note. Data from Grech (1998). Phonemes used by 75 percent or more of the children; most of the phonemes were produced with variation

TABLE 47-4   Maltese children using consonant clusters at age 3;6

Consonant cluster type	Syllable position	percent usage at age 3;6
plosive + approximant	initial	100.00 percent
fricative + approximant	initial	100.00 percent
fricative + nasal	initial	94.74 percent
plosive + plosive	initial	80.00 percent
affricate + approximant	initial	66.67 percent
others	initial	100.00 percent
nasal + fricative	final	94.12 percent
nasal + affricate	final	100.00 percent
approximant + plosive	final	88.89 percent
approximant + approximant	final	75.00 percent
plosive +fricative	final	100.00 percent
others	final	90.00 percent

Note. Data from Grech (1998).

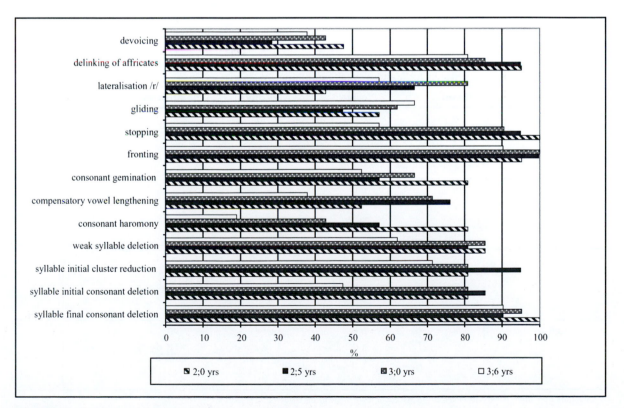

Figure 47-2   Chronology of developmental processes in Maltese

(2006). Some of the processes exhibited by the children are in line with universal trends. However, language-specific processes and preferences, such as gemination of consonants, were also identified.

Intelligibility

To date there is no study of intelligibility of Maltese children.

Phonetic inventory

Table 47-5 indicates the phone inventory of the Maltese children in Grech's (1998) study.

Common mismatches

Phoneme inventories of typical Maltese children are cited in Grech (1998). The data highlight the specific mismatches of each of the 21 informants, in syllable-initial and -final position between 2;0 and 3;6 years of age. By 3;6 years most of the children's phonemes matched respective adult ones. Some variants (other than adult allophonic variation) were still perceived, particularly for the affricates and fricatives. This indicated that the children were producing these adult phonemes customarily but full mastery had still not been achieved by this age.

Syllable structure

Table 47-6 summarizes the data about the canonical structures of the children for mono- and disyllabic structures at different developmental stages.

Prosody

To date there is no study of Maltese children's prosody.

Phonological awareness

There have been a few small-scale unpublished studies reporting typical phonological awareness skills of Maltese children. Manduca (2004) studied 24 children aged between 5;0 and 5;11 years with a gender ratio of 1:1. The children were assessed for syllable segmentation, blending, deletion, and reversal on words that included monosyllabic, disyllabic, trisyllabic, and quadrisyllabic structures. Results showed a decrease in the number of correct responses by the children as the word structure increased in complexity. Syllable blending was considered easiest, while syllable reversal seemed to be the most difficult. Pace Gellel (2004) assessed 36 children 4 years of age on various aspects of phonological awareness skills. Phoneme segmentation and rhyme awareness seemed to be difficult tasks for the Maltese children.

TABLE 47-5 Phone inventories for Maltese-speaking children

Age	Nasal	Plosive	Fricative	Affricate	Approximant
2;0	m	p b	h		w
	n	t d			l
		k			j
		ʔ			
2;5	m	p b	f		w
	n	t d	s		ʁ
		k	ʃ		ɹ
		ʔ	h		j
3;0	m	p b	f v		w
	n	t d	s	tʃ	l
		k g			ɹ
		ʔ	h		j
3;6	m	p b	f v		w
	n	t d	s z	tʃ dʒ	l
		k g	ʃ		ɹ
		ʔ	h		j

Note. Data from Grech (1998). Data indicates 75 percent or more usage by the children.

TABLE 47-6 Canonical structures of Maltese-speaking children

Syllabic structures	Age	Canonical structures	Percentage of children
Monosyllabic	2;0	CV	66.6
Monosyllabic	2;0	CVC	23.8
Monosyllabic	2;5	CVC	95.2
Monosyllabic	3;0	CVC	100
Monosyllabic	3;6	CVC	100
Disyllabic	2;0	CV,CV	61.9
Disyllabic	2;0	V,CV	19.05
Disyllabic	2;0	CVC,CV	14.29
Disyllabic	2;5	CVC,CV	33.3
Disyllabic	2;5	CV,CV	28.5
Disyllabic	2;5	V,CV	23.8
Disyllabic	3;0	CV,CV	28.57
Disyllabic	3;0	CVC,CVC	23.8
Disyllabic	3;6	CVC,CVC	38.1
Disyllabic	3;6	CV,CVC	23.8
Disyllabic	3;6	CVC,CV	9.52

Note. Data from Grech(1998). C = nonsyllabic segment; V = syllabic segment

Speech assessment for Maltese children

SLPs working in Malta use a variety of published English tests of phonology and/or articulation when assessing English-speaking children. However, the standardized norms are not relevant for the local bilingual children. The situation is more challenging when SLPs have to assess the speech of Maltese-speaking children. To date there is no speech test standardized on the local children. Clinicians use adaptations of English tests to obtain a rough idea that helps them reach a differential diagnosis. Mallia Borg (2004) adapted the *Diagnostic Evaluation of Articulation and Phonology (DEAP)* (Dodd, Hua, Crosbie, Holm, and Ozanne, 2003) for use with Maltese-speaking children. It is hoped that the new *Maltese-English Speech Assessment for Children: Mesa* (Grech and Dodd, 2006), will be standardized on Maltese children in the coming years.

Speech intervention for Maltese children

To date there are no publications of studies regarding speech intervention for Maltese children. However, clinical records are available. Maltese SLPs are familiar with most of the techniques used for speech intervention around the world. Most of them use traditional articulation and minimal pairs approaches. An increasing number of SLP graduates of the University of Malta are also applying Dodd and McCormack's (1995) model of the speech processing chain for differential diagnosis of speech disorders. Speech therapy in Malta and Gozo is relatively young and has been expanding gradually since the early 1980s. Nowadays, the service is offered in a range of settings that includes community-based clinics (health centers), acute hospitals (inpatients and outpatients), institutional settings, rehabilitation centers, day centers, school settings (special and mainstream), and the clients' homes. Therapy may take various forms, such as individual or group therapy and direct or indirect intervention.

Working in the Maltese Islands

SLPs wishing to work in Malta or Gozo need to be registered with the local Board for Professions Complementary to Medicine. The University of Malta offers a four-year undergraduate full-time degree course leading to the award of B.Sc.(Hons) in Communication Therapy. Individuals holding this qualification or its equivalence are eligible to apply for registration to practice.

PHONETICALLY SPEAKING

Pronunciation of Malta: /mɛltɪ/

Relevant words for speech assessment and intervention

Word/Phrase	Formal usage	Pronunciation	Informal usage	Pronunciation
Tongue	*ilsien*	lsɪːn	*ilsien*	lsɪːn
Teeth	*snien*	snɪːn	*snien*	snɪːn
Lips	*xuftejn*	ʃuftɛɪn	*xuftejn*	ʃuftɛɪn
Hard palate	*saqaf tal-ħalq*	seʔeftɛlhɛlʔ	*saqaf tal-ħalq*	seʔeftɛlhɛlʔ
Soft palate	*saqaf tal-ħalq (minn wara)*	seʔeftɛlhɛlʔ mɪnːaɹawɛɹɐ	*qanpiena*	ʔempɪːnɐ
Larynx	*larinġi*	leɹɪndʒɪ	*gerżuma*	gɛɹzuːme
Lungs	*pulmun*	pʊlmuːn	*pulmun*	pʊlmuːn
Nose	*imnieħer*	mnɪːhɛɹ	*imnieħer*	mnɪːhɛɹ
Sound	*ħoss*	hɔsː	*ħoss*	hɔsː
Word	*kelma*	kɛlmɐ	*kelma*	kɛlmɐ
Sentence	*sentenza*	sɛntɛntse	*sentenza*	sɛntɛntse
Paragraph	*paragrafu*	peɹegɹefʊ	*paragrafu*	peɹegɹefʊ

RESOURCES

Books

Borg, A. J., andAzzopardi-Alexander, M. (1997) *Maltese*. London: Routledge.

Grech, H. (1998) *Phonological development of normal Maltese speaking children*. Unpublished Ph.D. thesis, University of Manchester, UK.

Professional associations

Association of Speech-Language Pathologists (Malta)

Malta Federation of Professional Associations, Sliema Road, Gzira, Malta

University offering course in communication therapy

Communication Therapy Division, Institute of Health Care, University of Malta, http://www.um.edu.mt

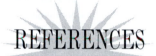

REFERENCES

Aquilina, J. (1959). *The structure of Maltese*. Malta: University of Malta.

Azzopardi, M. (1981). *The phonetics of Maltese: Some areas relevant to the deaf*. Unpublished Ph.D. thesis. Edinburgh: University of Edinburgh.

Borg, A. (1973). The segmental phonemes of Maltese. *Linguistics, 109*, 5–11.

Borg, A. (1975). Maltese morphophonemics. *Journal of Maltese Studies, 4*, 11–28.

Borg, A. J. (1980). Language and socialisation in developing Malta. *Work in Progress, 13*, 60–71. Edinburgh: Department of Linguistics, University of Edinburgh.

Borg, A. J. (1988). *Ilsienna*. Malta: Has-Sajjied.

Borg, A. J., and Azzopardi-Alexander, M. (1997). *Maltese*. London: Routledge.

Dodd, B., Hua, Z., Crosbie, S., Holm, A., and Ozanne, A. (2003). *Diagnostic evaluation of articulation and phonology (DEAP)*. London: Psychological Corporation.

Dodd, B., and McCormack, P. (1995). A model of speech processing for differential diagnosis of phonological disorders In B. Dodd, (Ed.), *Differential diagnosis and treatment of children with speech disorder* (pp. 65–90). London: Whurr.

Environment Science Research Institute. (2004). Retrieved November 2, 2004, from http://www.esri.com/.

Frendo, G. (2002). *The phonology of three-year old maltese speaking twins*. Unpublished undergraduate dissertation. Malta: University of Malta.

Grech, H. (1998) *Phonological development of normal Maltese speaking children*. Unpublished Ph.D. thesis, University of Manchester, UK.

Grech, H. (2006). Phonological development of Maltese-speaking children. In H. Zhu and B. Dodd (Ed.), *Phonological development and disorders: A multilingual perspective* (pp. 135–177). Clevedon: Multilingual Matters.

Grech H., and Dodd, B. (2006). *Maltese-English speech assessment for children (MESA)*. Unpublished, Research Version. Guardamangia, Malta: Communication Therapy Division, Institute of Health Care, University of Malta

Mallia Borg, R. (2004). *Assessment and categorisation of Maltese-speaking children presented with sub-groups of disordered speech*. Unpublished undergraduate dissertation, University of Malta.

Manduca, V. (2004). *Syllabic awareness skills of Maltese children in year one*. Unpublished undergraduate dissertation, University of Malta.

Ministry of Education. (1999). *National minimum curriculum*. St. Venera, Malta: Klabb Kotba Maltin.

Pace Gellel, C. (2004). *A phonological awareness programme for Maltese pre-school children*. Unpublished M.A. dissertation, University of Malta.

Sciriha, L. (1999). *A sociolinguistic survey of the Maltese Islands 111*. Msida, Malta: Cyclostyled, Department of English, University of Malta.

SUMMARY OF STUDIES OF TYPICAL MALTESE SPEECH ACQUISITION

Author	Year	Country	No. of children	Age of children	Information	Sample type	Data collection
Azzopardi	1997	Malta	10	4;0	Consonantal phone & phoneme inventories; phonological processes	Single word-picture naming	Cross-sectional
Frendo	2002	Malta	3 sets of twins & 3 matched singletons	3;0	Consonantal phone & phoneme inventories; phonological processes	Single word-picture naming	Cross- sectional
Grech	1998	Malta	21	2;0–3;6	Consonantal phone & phoneme inventories; phonological processes; consonantal clusters; phonotactic structures	Picture naming and spontaneous speech sampling	Longitudinal
Manduca	2004		24	5;0–5;11	Syllabification skills	Elicited	Cross-sectional
Pace Gellel	2004		36	4 years	Phonological awareness skills	Elicited	Longitudinal

Chapter 48

Norwegian Speech Acquisition

Kristian Emil Kristoffersen

INTRODUCTION

Norwegian belongs to the northern branch of the Germanic languages and is the major language spoken in Norway. It is closely related to two other North Germanic languages: Swedish, spoken in Sweden, and Danish, spoken in Denmark. Norwegian, Swedish, and Danish are mutually intelligible. Two other North Germanic languages are spoken in the region, Icelandic in Iceland, and Faroese in the Faroe Islands. See the Resources section for materials about Norwegian.

Where Norwegian is spoken

Today Norwegian is primarily spoken in Norway (see accompanying map and Appendix D), although as late as 1990 more than 80,000 persons in the USA reported that they used Norwegian as their home language. Some 4.5 million people have Norwegian as their first language. In addition to Norwegian, several minority languages are spoken in Norway; for example, Sami, Finnish, Urdu, Vietnamese, English, Spanish, Bosnian/Croatian/Serbian, Arabic, Albanian, Turkish, and Somali.

Components of Norwegian

Consonants

In what follows, components of the variety of Norwegian known as Urban East Norwegian (UEN; G. Kristoffersen, 2000) will be presented. UEN has 22 consonants,

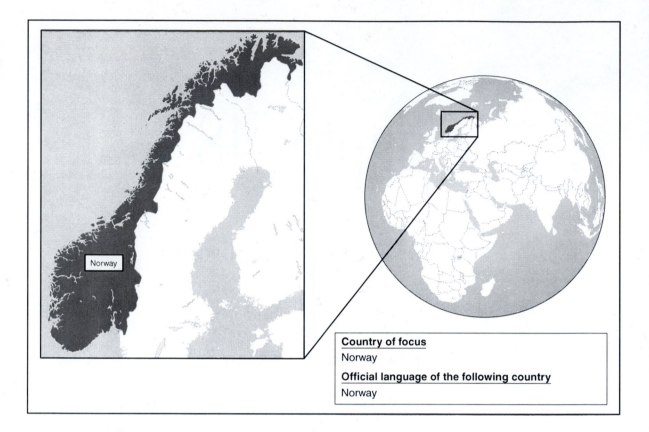

Country of focus
Norway

Official language of the following country
Norway

many of which are also part of the consonant inventory of many accents of English (see Table 48-1). Information on a selection of these consonants (laminal and apical plosives and fricatives), with recordings by UEN speakers, Electromagnetic articulography (EMA) profiles, and Electropalatography (EPG) patterns, can be found at the Web site *An electronic database of Norwegian speech sounds* (http://www.hf.uio.no/ilf/forskning/phonetics/) at the Department of Linguistics and Scandinavian Studies, University of Oslo.

UEN has two series of coronal consonants, laminal (alveolar) /t, d, n, s, l/ and apical (retroflex) /ʈ, ɖ, ɳ, ʂ, ɭ/.

TABLE 48-1   Consonants produced in Norwegian (UEN)

	Bilabial	Labio-dental	Laminal (Alveolar)
Plosive	p b		t d
Nasal	m		n
Tap or flap			ɾ
Fricative		f	s
Lateral fricative	▮▮▮▮▮		
Approximant		ʋ	
Lateral approximant	▮▮▮▮▮		l

Black = articulations judged impossible

Based on the International Phonetic Alphabet. Courtesy of the International Phonetic Association (c/o Department of Linguistics, University of Victoria, Victoria, British Columbia, Canada).

In a study of apical and laminal plosives Simonsen, Moen, and Cowen (2006) demonstrate with the help of EMA and EPG measures that there is considerable overlap in terms of the passive articulator for these two classes, varying between alveolar and post-alveolar. The main difference between these two series of consonants is that /ṭ, ḍ/ can be characterized by having the apex as the active articulator and a flat tongue middle, whereas /t, d/ lack these features.

Norwegian differs from English in having voiceless fricatives only. At the labial place of articulation, the voiceless fricative /f/ corresponds to a voiced approximant /ʋ/. Moreover, there appears to be an ongoing merger in Norwegian today between the fricatives /ç/ and /ʂ/ (Simonsen and Moen, 2004; van Dommelen, 2003). The merger started in the younger generations and is at present extending into the older generations.

UEN also has an apico-post-alveolar flap /ɽ/, which is also found in some dialects of Swedish, but not in the other Germanic languages. This consonant can occur word-medially and finally, but not word-initially.

Vowels and diphthongs

UEN has 19 vowels, 9 short and 9 long monophthongs, and 3 diphthongs, which can all occur in stressed syllables (see Table 48-2). In unstressed syllables all short vowels as well as *schwa* /ə/ can occur. The short monophthongs are somewhat lowered compared to the long ones. Moreover, /æ:/ and /æ/ have a somewhat marginal status, in that they occur only before apical consonants.

A special feature of the UEN vowel system (and the vowel systems of all other dialects of Norwegian) is the abundance of front rounded vowels: /y:, y, ø:, ø/. In addition, Norwegian has a pair of high central rounded vowels /ʉ, ʉ:/.

Phonotactic restrictions

There are some restrictions on the distribution of UEN consonants. First, the apical plosives /ṭ, ḍ/, the apical nasal /ɳ/, and the flap /ɽ/, and in addition the dorsal nasal /ŋ/, cannot occur in word-initial position. Second, /h/ and /ç/ cannot occur in word-final position. Third, the voiceless plosives have two allophones, an aspirated one, which occurs at the beginning of a stressed syllable and word-initially, and an unaspirated one, which occurs in all other positions.

Syllables

Syllables in Norwegian words can have from zero to three consonants in the onset; cf. the following words:

å	/oː/	infinitival marker		trå	/troː/	'step'
rå	/roː/	'raw'		strå	/stroː/	'straw'

In polysyllabic words up to four consonants can occur intervocalically:

ete	/'eːtə/	"eat"	ødsle	/'ødslə/	'squander'
etse	/'etsə/	'corrode'	mønstre	/'mønstrə/	'inspect'

In the syllable coda we find from zero to three consonants:

blå	/bloː/	'blue, masc./fem.'	blåst	/bloːst/	'blown'
blått	/blot/	'blue, neuter'	blomst	/blomst/	'flower'

Consonants and consonant clusters

UEN allows several different types of two-element consonant clusters in word-initial position. First, words

	Apical (Retroflex)	Dorsal	Velar	Pharyngeal	Glottal
	t ḍ		k g		
	ɳ		ŋ		
	ɽ				
	ʂ	ç			h
		j			
	l				

TABLE 48-2   Vowels produced in Norwegian (UEN) compared to General American English

American English location	American English vowels (Smit, 2004)	American English examples	Norwegian location	Norwegian vowels	Norwegian examples
High-front	i	_beat_	High-front, unrounded	iː	_bite_ /ˈbiːtə/ 'bite'
	ɪ	_bit_		i	_sitte_ /sit/ 'sit'
			High-front, rounded	yː	_syn_ /syːn/ 'vision'
				y	_synde_ /ˈsyndə/ 'sin'
			High-central, rounded	ʉː	_ku_ /kʉː/ 'cow'
				ʉ	_kutt_ /kʉt/ 'cut'
Mid-low front	e	_raid_	Mid front, unrounded	eː	_sete_ /ˈseːtə/ 'seat'
	ɛ	_bed_		e	_sette_ /ˈsetə/ 'set'
			Mid-front, rounded	øː	_søt_ /søːt/ 'sweet, masc/fem'
				ø	_søtt_ /søt/ 'sweet, neuter'
	æ	_bad_	Low–front	æː	_være_ /ˈʋæːrə/ '(to) be'
				æ	_verre_ /ˈʋærə/ 'worse'
High-back, rounded	u	_blue_	High-back, rounded	uː	_bok_ /buːk/ 'book'
	ʊ	_book_		u	_bukk_ /buk/ 'buck'
Mid-back, rounded	o	_boat_	Mid-high, back, rounded	oː	_gå_ /goː/ '(to) go'
	ɔ	_form_		o	_gått_ /got/ 'gone'
Low back	ɑ	_drop_	Low back	ɑː	_sag_ /sɑːg/ 'saw'
				ɑ	_sang_ /sɑŋ/ 'song'
Central	ə	_about, occur, upon,_	Central	ə	_bite_ /ˈbiːtə/ 'bite'
					sitte /ˈsitə/ 'sit'
Diphthongs	aɪ	_my, bike_		æi	_skei_ /ʂæi/ 'spoon'
	aʊ	_out, mouse_		øi	_øy_ /øi/ 'island'
	ɔɪ	_boy_		æʉ	_sau_ /sæʉ/ 'sheep'

can begin with a stop (voiceless or voiced) or fricative (which is always voiceless in Norwegian) followed by a sonorant (e.g., _blomst_ /blomst/ 'flower'). Second, a word-initial cluster may consist of a stop followed by a /l/, /r/, or /j/ (e.g., _slå_ /ʂloː/ 'beat'). Finally, word-initial clusters can consist of /s/ followed by a voiceless stop, for example, _stå_ /stoː/ 'stand'. These possibilities, with restrictions on particular sounds, are shown in Table 48-3.

Also, some three-element consonant clusters occur in UEN, the first member of which is always /s/ or (marginally) /ʂ/:

strå   /stroː/   'straw'   _skrive_   /ˈskriːʋə/   'write'
språk /sproːk/ 'language'   _skli_   /skli̥ː/   'skid'

Tones

Most Norwegian dialects use lexical tones to differentiate meaning. Two distinct melodies (commonly called _accents_ or _tonemes_) are found, contrasting words of more than one syllable, like the following:

Accent 1:   Accent 2:
bønder /¹bønər/ 'farmers'   _bønner_ /²bønər/ 'prayers'
tanken /¹taŋkən/ 'the tank'   _tanken_ /²taŋkən/ 'the thought'

Stress and intonation

A typical disyllabic word in Norwegian has stress on the first syllable; cf. the examples in the preceding section.

TABLE 48-3 Two-element consonant clusters in UEN

C2 → / C1 ↓	m	n	l	r	j	ʊ	p	t	k
p		x	x	x					
b		x	x	x					
t			x	(x)	x				
d			x	x	x				
k		x	x	x		x			
g		x	x	x		(x)			
f		x	x	x	x				
s	x	x				x	x	x	x
ʂ			x			(x)			
ʊ			x						
m				(x)					
n				(x)					

However, more generally both the final, the penultimate, and the antepenultimate syllable can receive stress:

Final stress: *banan* /baˈnɑːn/ 'banana'
Penultimate stress: *balanse* /baˈlɑŋsə/ 'balance'
Antepenultimate stress: *bevegelig* /beˈʋeːgəlɪ/ 'moveable'

Syllables of Norwegian words can have three different degrees of stress: primary stress, secondary stress, or no stress. The following word has primary stress (signaled by accent 1 and length) on the first syllable and secondary stress (signaled by length only) on the third syllable. The remaining syllables are unstressed:

kaffekoppen	/ˈkɑfəˌkopən/	'coffee-cup-the'

Writing system

Norwegian uses alphabetic writing. The Norwegian version of the Latin alphabet includes three letters that are not found in English: "æ, ø, å". There are two official written standards of Norwegian: *Nynorsk*, used by around 600,000, and *Bokmål*, used by 3,900,000 people. The main differences between the two standards are morphological and lexical. Both standards have equal status.

Varieties of Norwegian

There are several distinct dialects of Norwegian, of which UEN is the dialect spoken by the majority of Norwegians. An important dialect difference in Norwegian is between those dialects that have an apical *r*-sound (an apical tap: /ɾ/), and those that have a uvular *r*-sound (a uvular approximant). The latter is found along the southern and western coast north to the city of Florø, whereas the rest of the country has the apical *r*.

Another important dialectal difference concerns the number of coronal and dorsal consonants. In UEN there are three series: one apical, one laminal, and one dorsal (cf. Table 48-1), and this system is gaining ground in Norway these days. In the southern and western part of the country north to the city of Ålesund there are two series, alveolar and dorsal. In the region around Trondheim and further to the north we find four series: laminal, apical, palatoalveolar, and dorsal.

As for lexical tones, most Norwegian dialects have them, except for an area around the city of Bergen on the western coast and in scattered dialects in northern Norway. The dialects with lexical tones can be divided in two distinct groups with respect to phonetic realization (G. Kristoffersen, 2000). In southwestern, western, and northern Norway, accent 1 is realized with a high tone on the stressed syllable. In eastern Norway, accent 1 is realized with a low tone on the stressed syllable.

Typical acquisition of Norwegian

The Summary of Studies table at the end of this chapter contains studies of the acquisition of Norwegian.

Acquired sounds
Consonants

There are few studies of acquisition of Norwegian speech sounds. The first to appear was Vanvik (1971), a longitudinal diary study of the phonetic and phonological development of one girl from when she was born until she was nearly 12 years old. Fintoft, Bollingmo, Feilberg, Gjettum, and Mjaavatn (1983) was a cross-sectional study of 73 children (31 males, 42 females; mean age 4;2) from eight different regions in Norway. Simonsen (1990, 1997) was a longitudinal study of acquisition of consonants in three children (between 2;0 and 4;1). In general, Simonsen demonstrates that there is much intersubject variability in developmental patterns, as can be seen from Table 48-4.

TABLE 48-4   Age of acquisition for Norwegian (UEN) consonants

	Tomas (2;0 – 4;1)			Nora (2;3 – 3;5)			Vera (2;2 – 2;6)		
	Word-initial	Word-medial	Word-final	Word-initial	Word-medial	Word-final	Word-initial	Word-medial	Word-final
p	n.a.	2;0	2;0	n.a	2;3	2;3	n.a.	2;2	2;2
b	2;0	–	–	2;4	2;4	–	2;2	2;2	–
m	2;0	2;0	2;0	2;3	2;3	2;3	2;2	2;2	2;2
f	2;2	2;0	–	2;11	2;8	–	2;2	2;6	–
ʋ	3;3	2;0	2;0	2;4	2;4	2;8	2;2	2;2	2;2
t	2;0	2;0	2;0	2;8	2;3	2;3	2;2	2;2	2;2
d	n.a.	2;2	n.a.	2;4	2;4	–	2;6	2;2	–
n	2;0	2;5	2;0	2;3	2;3	2;3	2;2	2;2	2;2
s	4;1	4;1	n.a.	2;8	2;8	2;8	n.a.	n.a.	2;6
r	3;10	3;0	n.a.	3;5	n.a	n.a.	n.a.	n.a.	n.a.
l	0	4;1	3;10	0	2;3	–	0	2;6	n.a.
ʈ	0	–	2;0	0	2;3	2;3	0	–	2;2
ɖ	0	–	0	0	2;11	0	0	–	0
ɳ	0	–	2;0	0	2;8	2;11	0	–	2;6
ʂ	2;5	–	–	2;3	2;8	–	2;2	–	2;2
ɽ	0	–	–	0	–	–	0	–	–
ɭ	2;5	2;9	2;0	2;8	2;3	2;11	2;6	2;2	n.a.
ç	n.a.	–	0	n.a.	–	0	n.a.	–	0
j	2;9	–	4;1	3;2	3;2	n.a.	2;6	2;2	n.a.
k	3;3	2;0	2;0	2;11	2;3	2;3	2;6	2;2	2;2
g	n.a.	2;0	n.a.	2;8	2;3	–	2;6	2;2	–
ŋ	0	2;9	2;2	0	2;3	2;4	0	2;2	–
h	2;2	–	0	2;4	–	0	2;2	–	0

Note. Adapted from Simonsen (1990). Dates of acquisition are based on the criterion of 75 percent correct.

n.a. = not acquired

– = data are not sufficient to determine date of acquisition with certainty

0 = the sound does not occur in this position in the target language

However, Simonsen also found several more general trends (cf. also Simonsen, 1997). First of all, phonation in plosives was problematic for all three subjects throughout the period. In Table 48–4 this is most clearly seen in the fact that none of the three children acquired the target /p/ word-initially—the realizations for this phoneme vary from [pʰ] to [p] to [b]. Second, /r/ is acquired late—the earliest date for this consonant in Table 48–4 is 3;0 (Nora in word-medial position). Third, none of the subjects acquired /ç/ in the course of the study. And finally, all three subjects had problems with /s/.

Simonsen's (1990) results are in many respects similar to those of Vanvik (1971) and Fintoft et al. (1983). Vanvik's participant did not acquire /ç/ until she was

7;6. And Fintoft et al. reported that their children (with mean age 4;2) had two types of problems, on the one hand with /ɾ/, and on the other with the fricatives /s/ and /ç/.

Consonant clusters

Vanvik (1971) reported that the first correctly produced consonant clusters appear just after 2 years of age. However, his data indicate that clusters are not acquired properly until much later. This is confirmed by Fintoft et al. (1983), who observed that 4-year-old children still have problems with consonant clusters. Unfortunately, the exact nature of these problems is not specified.

The data from Simonsen's (1990) 3 children give us a more detailed picture of the period between 24 and 36 months. In general there was much variation in all types of clusters for all three children. Typical patterns were reductions and insertion of an epenthetic vowel.

Vowels and diphthongs

To date there is no study of acquisition of vowels and diphthongs for Norwegian. But again the few studies that exist (see the Summary of Studies table) indicate that the high front rounded vowels /y:/ and /y/ are acquired late.

Percent correct

To date there is no study of percentage correct for children acquiring Norwegian.

Phonological processes

Simonsen (1990) reports the following processes involving single segments: deletion of weak syllables, deletion of single segments, assimilation, fronting, backing, stopping, voicing and devoicing, denasalization, and substitution. Consonant clusters, on the other hand, are typically reproduced either as single consonants (e.g., [boː] for [bloː] 'blue'), or they are broken up by an epenthetic vowel (e.g., [bə'loː] for [bloː] 'blue'). The latter type is reported as sporadic in acquisition studies for other languages, but in Simonsen's participants it is common.

Intelligibility

To date there is no study of intelligibility for Norwegian.

Phonetic inventory

Simonsen (1990) reports that in children between 2;0 and 4;1 phonetic inventories vary in size depending on position. Word-initial inventories are largest, followed by word-medial inventories. Word-final inventories are small throughout the period.

Common mismatches

To date there is no study of common mismatches produced by Norwegian children.

Syllable structure

To date there is no study of syllable structure produced by Norwegian children.

Prosody

To date there is no study of Norwegian children's prosody.

Phonological awareness

To date there is no study of phonological awareness of children acquiring Norwegian.

Speech assessment for Norwegian children

The most popular tests for assessing Norwegian children's speech sounds are the following:

- *Norsk Fonemtest* [Norwegian phoneme test] (Tingleff, 2002)
- *Norsk Logopedlags Språklydprøve* [The Norwegian Association of Speech Therapist's speech sound test.] (Vidsjå, Hauglid, Kloser-Jensen, and Skei, 1983)
- *Artikulasjonsprøve B* [Articulation test B] (Backe, n.d.)
- *Artikulasjonsprøve for Registrering av Uttalefeil* [Articulation test for registration of pronunciation errors] (Johnsen, 1987)
- *Illinois Test of Psycholinguistic Abilities (ITPA)* – sound blending subtest. Norwegian version (Gjessing and Nygaard, 1975)

No analyses have been designed for analyzing Norwegian speech specifically, but Grunwell's PACS

(Grunwell, 1985) have been used in a couple of studies of Norwegian acquisition (Simonsen, 1990; Bjerkan, 1994).

Speech intervention for Norwegian children

The speech intervention techniques that have been developed for Norwegian include the following:

- *Dansk metafonboks: 726 billedkort til metafonundervisning* (in Danish) (Benn Thomsen, 1996)
- *Praxis*, an intervention method (developed for Swedish) for children with dyspraxia (Hellquist, 1996)

Working in Norway

In Norway most speech therapists work within the resource centers for special education, in schools, and in hospitals. Job vacancies for Norway are advertised in newspapers and on the Internet. The most important Web site is that of *Nav*, the Norwegian public employment service: http://www.nav.no. Aetat's site also provides important information in English for those who seek employment in Norway and other EEA countries (EEA = the countries of the European Union, Iceland, Norway, and Liechtenstein). Another Web site where vacant jobs are advertised is http://www.stillinger.no/.

PHONETICALLY SPEAKING

Pronunciation of *Norwegian*: [noʂk]

Relevant words for speech assessment and intervention

Word/Phrase	Formal usage	Pronunciation	Informal usage	Pronunciation
Tongue	*tunge*	[ˈtʰuŋə]	*tunge*	[ˈtʰuŋə]
Teeth	*tenner*	[ˈtʰenər]	*tenner*	[ˈtʰenɽ̩]
Lips	*lepper*	[²lepər]	*lepper*	[²lepɽ̩]
Hard palate	*den harde ganen*	[ˌdən ²harə ²ganən]	*den harde ganen*	[ˌdn̩ ²harə ²gann̩]
Soft palate	*den bløte ganen*	[ˌdən ²bløtə ²ganən]	*den bløte ganen*	[ˌdn̩ ²bløtə ²gann̩]
Larynx	*larynx*	[ˈlaryŋks]	*larynx*	[ˈlaryŋks]
Lungs	*lungene*	[²luŋənə]	*lungene*	[²luŋŋə]
Nose	*nese*	[²neːsə]	*nese*	[²neːsə]
Sound	*lyd*	[lyːd]	*lyd*	[lyːd]
Word	*ord*	[oːr]	*ord*	[oːr] or [oːɽ]
Sentence	*setning*	[²setniŋ]	*setning*	[²setniŋ]
Paragraph	*avsnitt*	[²aʊsnit]	*avsnitt*	[²aʊsnit]

RESOURCES

Books

Enger, H. O., and Kristoffersen, K. E. (2000). *Innføring i norsk grammatikk.* [Introduction to Norwegian grammar]. Oslo: Cappelen.

Kristoffersen, G. (2000). *The phonology of Norwegian.* Oxford, UK: Oxford University Press.

Kristoffersen, K. E., Simonsen, H. G., and Sveen, A. (2005). *Språk - en grunnbok.* [Language - an introduction]. Oslo: Universitetsforlaget.

Lind, M., Uri, H., Moen, I., and Bjerkan, K. M. (2000). *Ord som ikke vil – innføring i språkpatologi.* [Introduction to language pathology]. Oslo: Novus.

Strandskogen, A. B., Strandskogen, R., and White, B. (1995). *Norwegian: An essential grammar.* London: Routledge.

CD-ROM

Afasi og språk [Aphasia and language]. University of Oslo, Bredtvet resource center and Sunnaas hospital and school.

Journal

• *Norsk tidsskrift for logopedi.* http://www.norsk-logopedlag.no/tidsskrift.htm. *NTL* is the official journal of the Norwegian Association of Speech and Language Therapists.

Professional associations

The professional association of speech-language pathologists within Norway is *Norsk logopedlag* (Norwegian Association of Speech and Language Therapists), http://www.norsk-logopedlag.no/.

Useful Norwegian Web sites

• *Statped.* Norwegian support system for special education. http://www.statped.no/ (in Norwegian and English).
• *Bredtvet Resource Centre.* http://www.statped.no/bredtvet. BRC is a national center for special education in Norway, representing interdisciplinary expertise within the fields of speech, language, and communication disorders (in Norwegian and English).
• *Eikelund kompetansesenter* (Eikelund Resource Centre). http://www.statped.no/eikelund/. (in Norwegian only).
• *Logopedisk senter i Nordland.* (Logopaedic centre in Nordland). http://lsn.no/velkom.htm. (in Norwegian only).
• *Sørlandet kompetansesenter.* (Sørlandet Resource Centre). http://www.statped.no/sorlandet/. (in Norwegian only).
• University of Oslo, Department of Linguistics and Scandinavian Studies, Research group in clinical linguistics, http://www.hf.uio.no/iln/.

REFERENCES

Backe, L. (n.d.). *Artikulasjonsprøve B.* [Articulation Test B] Oslo: Norsk logopedlag.

Benn Thomsen, I. (1996). *Dansk metafonboks: 726 billedkort til metafonundervisning.* Herning: Special-pædagogisk forlag.

Bjerkan, K. M. (1994). *Fonologi i avvikende barnespråk. En analyse av fonologien til et barn med funksjonelt språkavvik.* [Phonology in impaired child language. An analysis of the phonology of a child with Specific Language Impairment.] Master's thesis, University of Oslo.

Fintoft, K., Bollingmo, M., Feilberg, J., Gjettum, B., and Mjaavatn, P. E. (1983). *4 år. En undersøkelse av normalspråket hos norske 4-åringer.* [4 years: A study of typical language in Norwegian four-year-olds] Unpublished manuscript. Trondheim: University of Trondheim.

Gjessing, H., and Nygaard, H. (1975). *ITPA Handbok. Norsk utgave.* [ITPA Manual. Norwegian version.] Oslo: Universitetsforlaget.

Grunwell, P. (1985). *Phonological assessment of child speech.* San Diego, CA: College-Hill Press.

Hellquist, B. (1996). *Praxis.* Malmö: Pedagogisk Design.

Johnsen, K. (1987). *Artikulasjonsprøve for registrering av uttalefeil.* [Articulation test for registration of pronunciation errors.] Jaren, Norway: Vigga forlag.

Kristoffersen, G. (2000). *The phonology of Norwegian.* Oxford, UK: Oxford University Press.

Simonsen, H. G. (1990). *Barns fonologi: System og variasjon hos tre norske og et samoisk barn.* [Children's phonology: System and variation in three Norwegian and one Samoan child] Doctoral dissertation, University of Oslo.

Simonsen, H. G. (1997). Norske barns fonologi: Universelle trekk og individuell variasjon [The phonology of Norwegian children: Universal characteristics and individual variation]. In R. Söderberg (Ed.), *Från joller til läsning och skrivning* (pp. 33–46) Kristianstad: Gleerups.

Simonsen, H. G., and Moen, I. (2004). On the distinction between Norwegian /ʂ/ and /ç/ from a phonetic perspective. *Clinical Linguistics & Phonetics, 18* (6-8), 605–620.

Simonsen, H. G., Moen, I., and Cowen, S. (2006). Retroflex consonants: Are they really? Evidence from EMA and EPG. Manuscript submitted for publication.

Smit, A. B. (2004). *Articulation and phonology: Resource guide for school-age children and adults.* Clifton Park, NY: Thomson Delmar Learning.

van Dommelen, W. A. (2003). An acoustic analysis of Norwegian /ç/ and /ʃ/ as spoken by young people. *Journal of the International Phonetic Association, 33,* 131–142.

Vanvik, A. (1971). The phonetic-phonemic development of a Norwegian child. *Norsk tidsskrift for sprogvidenskap, 24,* 269–325.

Vidsjå, I., Hauglid, J., Kloster-Jensen, M., and Skei, A. (1983). *Norsk logopedlags språklydsprøve.* Oslo: Universitetsforlaget.

SUMMARY OF STUDIES OF TYPICAL NORWEGIAN SPEECH ACQUISITION

Authors	Year	Country	No. of children	Age of children	Information	Sample type	Data collection
Fintoft et al.	1983	Norway	73	3;8 – 4;10 (mean 4;2)	Acquisition of single consonants and clusters	Connected speech	Cross-sectional
Simonsen	1990	Norway	3	2;0 – 4;1	Acquisition of single consonants and consonant clusters	Connected speech	Longitudinal
Vanvik	1971	Norway	1	0 – 7;6	Age of acquisition of vowels and consonants	Single word and connected speech	Longitudinal

Chapter 49

Portuguese Speech Acquisition

Mehmet Yavaş and Helena B. Mota

INTRODUCTION

Portuguese belongs to the Romance subfamily of Indo-European languages, which is a group of related vernaculars descended from Latin. Together with its closest relative Spanish, Portuguese forms the Ibero-Romance subgroup. The language developed in the western Iberian peninsula from the spoken Latin brought there by the Romans in the 3rd century B.C. The differentiation of Portuguese from other Romance languages begins in the 5th century after the fall of the Roman empire.

Where Portuguese is spoken

Portuguese's 215 million speakers are rather unevenly divided among 4 continents (see accompanying map and Appendix D). Brazil in South America accounts for 187 million speakers. Angola, Cape Verde, Guinea-Bissau, Mozambique, and Sao Tome and Principe in Africa total about 16 million speakers. In Europe, Portugal is the only Portuguese-speaking country with about 11 million. Finally, Portuguese is spoken in East Timor and Macao in Asia by less than half a million. In this chapter, we focus on Brazilian Portuguese, which represents 87 percent of the total number of speakers. See the Resources section in this chapter for materials about Portuguese.

Components of Brazilian Portuguese

Consonants

Brazilian Portuguese has 19 consonant phonemes (see Table 49-1).

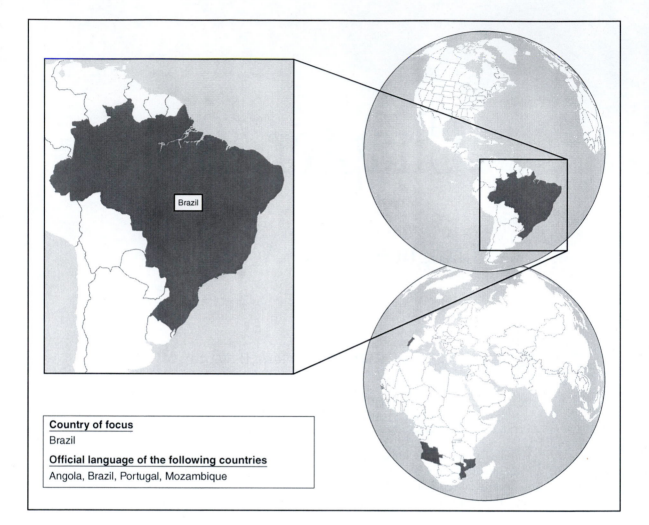

Country of focus
Brazil

Official language of the following countries
Angola, Brazil, Portugal, Mozambique

Although the two rhotics (/ɾ/ and /x/) are separate phonemes, they contrast only in intervocalic position (e.g., *caro* 'expensive' [kaɾu] – *carro* 'car' [kaxu]). In non-intervocalic onset position only /x/ can occur. The coda position is dialectally determined. While in the Southern dialect, /ɾ/ is the norm, others use /x/ (e.g., *carne* 'meat' [kaɾni] / [kaxni], *mar* 'sea' [maɾ] / [max]). Also, the alveolar lateral is highly velarized and in fact has given way to a glide [w] in coda position (e.g., *Brazil* [braziw], *caldo* 'broth' [kawdu]). In several dialects of Brazilian Portuguese, the dental stops /t/ and /d/ have palato-alveolar affricate allophones [tʃ] and [dʒ] respectively before /i/, as in *tia* 'aunt' [tʃiɐ], *dia* 'day' [dʒiɐ]. The glides [w] and [j] are marginal phonemes. In most cases, they result from the semivocalization of atonic /i, u/.

Vowels and diphthongs

Portuguese has seven oral and five nasal vowels (see Figure 49-1).

The diphthongs of Brazilian Portuguese are the following:

- Oral diphthongs: [aj, ej, ɛj, oj, ɔj uj aw, ew, ɛw]
- Nasal diphthongs: [ẽj, ẽj, õj, ũj, ẽw̃]

All seven vowels occur in stressed syllables. However, in prestressed position, the number is reduced to five (lower-mid /ɛ/ and /ɔ/ do not occur in this position). The contrasts are further reduced to three (/i/, /a/, /u/) in unstressed final position. The set of five nasal vowel phonemes is similar to the oral vowels found in the pre-stressed position. [ɐ] is an allophone of /a/ in post-tonic

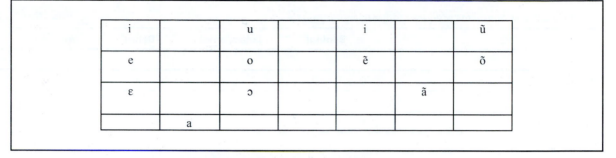

i		u		i		ũ
e		o		ẽ		õ
ε		ɔ			ã	
	a					

Figure 49-1 Portuguese vowels. Note [ɐ] is an allophone of /a/ in post-tonic and in nasal contexts.

and in nasal contexts. Glides [j] and [w] are also nasalized in nasal diphthongs, as in *mão* 'hand' [mãw̃], *viagem* 'trip' [viaʒẽj].

Phonotactic restrictions

Syllables

The Portuguese syllable structure can be described as (C)(C)V(C)(C), also written as $C_{(0-2)}VC_{(0-2)}$. The obligatory nucleus can be a simple vowel or a diphthong. Consonant clusters are basically onsets; double codas are restricted to a limited number of items only in syllable-final within-word position.

Consonants

All consonants occur word-medially as onsets, and most of them, except /ɾ/, /ʎ/, and /ɲ/, also occur word-initially. Only three consonants of Portuguese are allowed to occur in coda position. These are the alveolar liquids /l/ and /ɾ/, and the voiceless alveolar fricative /s/ (/ʃ/ in some dialects). In addition, /m/ and /n/ are allowed to occur as codas only within the word (e.g., *lembrar* 'to remember', *entrar* 'to enter').

Consonant clusters

Double onsets are formed by the combination of C1 = stop/voiceless labio-dental fricative /f/ and C2 = alveolar liquids (/l/, /ɾ/), thus giving us the following possibilities, which are valid in word-initial as well as word-medial position:

- C2 = /ɾ/: /pɾ, bɾ, tɾ, dɾ, kɾ, gɾ, fɾ/ (word-medially, /vɾ/ is also allowed; e.g., *palavra* 'word')
- C2 = /l/: /pl, bl, fl, kl, gl/ (/tl, dl/ are not allowed; very rarely /vl/, as in the name *Vladimir*)

Tones

Portuguese is not a tone language.

Stress and intonation

For the majority of nouns (and adjectives) ending in an oral vowel, stress falls on the penultimate syllable. However, the stress falls on the last syllable when nouns end in a consonant. These statements reflect the general tendencies and counter examples are easily found. The words ending in diphthongs or nasal vowels present final stress. As for verbs (simple forms), the stress falls on the final vowel of the stem, unless this vowel is word-final, when penultimate stress is the rule. Although Brazilian Portuguese has considerable reduction of atonic final vowels, it remains mainly a syllable-timed language (the stress-timed European Portuguese).

Writing system

Portuguese is written using the Latin alphabet with 26 letters (letters k, w, and y are used only for words of non-Portuguese origin). It uses ç and marks irregular stress patterns by a written accent. These accents also indicate vowel quality; the circumflex accent ˆ indicates higher vowels [ɐ, e, o], while the acute accent ´ indicates their lower counterparts [a, ε, ɔ] and is also used to mark stress on i and u. The grave accent ` has a very limited use, to indicate unreduced atonic vowels. Tilde accent ˜ is used on nasal vowels and diphthongs.

Varieties of Brazilian Portuguese

The following are commonly referenced regional varieties of Brazilian Portuguese: *Caipira* (countryside of São Paulô, *Baiano* (region of Bahia, northeast), *Fluminense* (States of Rio de Janeiro and Espirito Santo; the city of Rio de Janeiro has a particular variety of speaking), *Gaucho* (Rio Grande de Sul, the southernmost state), *Mineiro* (State of Minas Gerais), *Nordestino* (northeastern

TABLE 49-1 Consonants produced in Brazilian Portuguese

	Bilabial	Labiodental	Dental	Alveolar
Plosive	p b		t d	
Nasal	m		n	
Trill				
Tap or flap				r
Fricative		f v	s z	
Lateral fricative	███████		███████	
Affricate				
Approximant				
Lateral approximant	███████		███████	l

* The back vibrant is realized as a fricative or a frictionless continuant, the range of phonetic variants including [h, x, χ, ʁ]

Black = articulations judged impossible

Based on the International Phonetic Alphabet. Courtesy of the International Phonetic Association (c/o Department of Linguistics, University of Victoria, Victoria, British Columbia, Canadā.

states of Brazil), *Nortista* (Amazon Basin states), *Paulistano* (city of São Paulō, *Sertanejo* (States of Goias and Mato Grossō, and *Sulista* (south of Brazil, other than the state of Rio Grande de Sul).

Typical acquisition of Brazilian Portuguese

The Summary of Studies Table includes studies that have considered speech acquisition of children who speak Brazilian Portuguese.

Acquired sounds

Consonants

Similar to many other languages, stops and nasals are acquired earlier, followed by fricatives and liquids.

Stops. Along with nasals, stops are the earliest consonants acquired (before 2;0) (Hernandorena, 1990; Lamprecht, 1990; Rangel, 1998; Yavaş, 1988). Voiceless stops generally emerge earlier than their voiced counterparts. Alveolar stops /t/ and /d/, as mentioned earlier, have affricate allophones [tʃ] and [dʒ] respectively, before /i/. The typical emergence of these sounds is a little later, around 2;2 to 2;3 (Ilha, 1993).

Nasals. Two of the three-member nasal group, /m/ and /n/, emerge before 2;0; and /ɲ/ is clearly the last member in acquisition (Mota, 1996; Rangel, 1998; Yavaş, 1988).

Fricatives. Fricatives are among the later-acquired sounds. However, there are obvious differences within the group. The labio-dentals /f/ and /v/ are generally acquired before 2;0. Next in line are the alveolars /s/ and /z/, which emerge between 2;0 and 2;6. Palato-alveolars /ʃ/ and /ʒ/ are the last in this group, typically emerging between 2;6 and 3;0 (Oliveira, 2002; Savio, 2001).

Liquids. Liquids are the last acquired sounds (Azambuja, 1998; Hernandorena and Lamprecht, 1997; Rangel, 1998). As in many other languages, alveolar lateral /l/ is the earliest in this group, and is generally acquired before 3;0. Next in line is /x/ (or /χ/, /ʁ/, /h/ depending on the dialect). The typical emergence of the palatal lateral /ʎ/ is around 4;0, which is followed by the last member of this group, alveolar tap /ɾ/.

While the above generalizations are valid, the following comments about /n, s, ɾ, l/ should also be noted. These four consonants are the only ones that can occur as codas as well as single onsets. In the acquisition timetable, their emergence as single onsets is earlier than their single coda position, which is discussed in 4.6. The only exception to this is /l/, which emerges earlier as a coda (Oliveira, Mezzomo, de Freitas, and Lamprecht, 2004).

Consonant clusters

As mentioned earlier, the double onsets of Portuguese consist of C1 = stop /labial fricative and C2 = alveolar liquid (/ɾ/ or /l/). Although, as mentioned earlier, singleton /l/ emerges earlier than /ɾ/, there does not seem

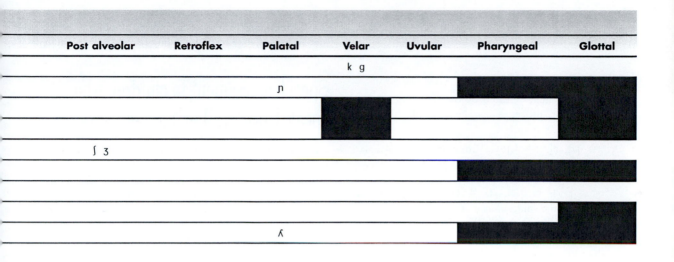

	Post alveolar	Retroflex	Palatal	Velar	Uvular	Pharyngeal	Glottal
				k g			
			ɲ				
	ʃ ʒ						
			ʎ				

to be a significant difference in the age of acquisition with respect to the changes in C2 (lateral or nonlateral) (Azambuja, 1998; Lamprecht, 1990; Ribas, 2002). As to the order of emergence in relation to the place of articulation of C1, clusters with /ɾ/ show a preference for labial stops (/pr/, /br/ earlier than others), while clusters with /l/ do not reveal any such patterns.

Vowels and diphthongs

Vowel acquisition is early and, in general, complete by 1;8 (Bonilha, 2004; Rangel, 2002). The low vowel /a/ emerges first and is followed by the two high vowels /i/ and /u/. Higher mid /e/ and /o/ follow these, leaving lower-mid /ɛ/ and /ɔ/ as the last ones.

Percent correct

There are no studies of percentage correct.

Phonological processes

Phonological processes that are prevalent in the speech of Brazilian Portuguese-speaking children can be summarized as follows. "Early processes" (generally disappearing by 3;6) are unstressed syllable deletion, final consonant deletion, stopping, fronting, initial liquid deletion, liquid substitution, liquid gliding, stopping, intervocalic voicing, and consonant harmony. "Late processes," which continue beyond 3;6, are cluster reduction, final liquid deletion, and obstruent devoicing (Yavaş, 1988).

Intelligibility

Keske-Soares (2001) suggested the following groupings with respect to phonological characteristics and intelligibility in Brazilian children.

- Speech with unusual/idiosyncratic processes. These processes include spirantization of stops, glottal replacement, deletions, and systematic sound preference, which result in highly unintelligible speech.
- Speech with persisting normal processes. These involve early simplifying processes that remain in the child's pronunciation patterns long after the age at which they would be expected to have been suppressed. Stopping, fronting of stops, devoicing, liquid gliding, and devoicing are among such processes, which result in some unintelligibility but are not as severe as the former group.
- Speech with delayed patterns. Children in this group reveal processes with delays in relation to normal acquisition. These processes include fronting of palatals, processes involving liquids, and modifying syllable structures CVC and CCV, which result in productions with little intelligibility.

Yavaş and Lamprecht (1988), analyzing in detail the speech of four children with phonological disorders, suggested that the number of words that contain more than one process may be important in determining the level of unintelligibility of the child's speech (for a similar concept, see "process density index" (Edwards, 1992).

Phonetic inventory

To date there are no studies of phonetic inventory for Portuguese-speaking children.

Common mismatches

Common mismatches created by the frequently occurring substitution processes can be exemplified in the following:

- /ʒ/ ⇨ [z], /ʃ/ ⇨ [s] via fronting (palato-alveolars become alveolars): *quiejo* 'cheese' [keʒu] ⇨ [kezu], *chapeu* 'hat' [ʃapew] ⇨ [sapew].
- /ɾ/ ⇨ [j], /l/ ⇨ [w], /ʎ/ ⇨ [j] via liquid gliding (liquids become glides): *amarela* 'yellow' [amaɾela] ⇨ [amajeja], *colo* 'lap' [kolu] ⇨ [kowu].
- /ɾ/ ⇨ [l] via liquid substitution (one liquid substitutes for the other; generally the lateral replaces the nonlateral): *passarinho* 'bird' [pasaɾiɲu] ⇨ [pasaliɲu].
- /s/ ⇨ [t] via stopping (fricatives become stops): *sopa* [sopa] ⇨ [topa].
- Cluster simplification process can reveal the elimination of C2 (liquid), as in *flor* 'flower' ⇨ [foɾ]. It also can be the source of liquid gliding (e.g., *bloco* 'block' ⇨ [bwɔku], *prego* 'nail' ⇨ [pjɛgu]) and liquid substitution (e.g., *planta* 'plant' ⇨ [pɾanta]).

Syllable structure

The order of acquisition of consonants in single onset position and of consonant clusters were given earlier. The four consonants, /l, n, s, ɾ/, that can occupy the single coda position in Portuguese, although they have different chronologies, have one pattern in common; they all individually emerge earlier in SFWF (syllable-final-word-final) position than in SFWW (syllable-final-within-word) position. The order can be given as follows (Mezzomo, 2003): /l/ SFWF (1;4), /n/ SFWF (1;7), /n/ SFWW (2;2), /s/ SFWF (2;6), /l/ SFWW (3;0), /s/ SFWW (3;0), /ɾ/ SFWF (3;10), /ɾ/ SFWW (3;10).

As for the development of the syllable structure, CV is expectedly the earliest, followed by CVC; CCV(C) is the latest acquired, around 5;0 (Ribas, 2002).

Prosody

To date we have not found any systematic study of prosody for Portuguese-speaking children.

Phonological awareness

Studies on phonological awareness generally mirror the findings in many other languages. Awareness of rhymes between 4;0 and 4;6 (Cardoso-Martins, 1994; De Freitas, 2004), phoneme awareness around 5;0 (Coimbra, 1997), and awareness at all levels including features at 6;0 (Cielo, 2000) have been reported.

Speech assessment in children who speak Brazilian Portuguese

Data collection for phonological analysis is commonly done via a spontaneous speech sample or via a formal assessment instrument. In a clinical setting, picture naming is the most commonly used procedure. This is a quick way of eliciting the desired targets in desired word and/or syllable positions. It is especially efficient in the case of unintelligible speech, as the therapist is able to easily recover the target words attempted by the child. *Avaliação Fonológica da criança* (AFC) [Phonological Assessment of Child Phonology] by Yavaş, Hernandorena, and Lamprecht (1991), which utilizes spontaneous naming, is one of the most popular assessment procedures used in Brazil. The instrument was based on five thematic pictures depicting elements, characters, and surroundings related to themes "living room," "bathroom," "kitchen," "vehicles," and "zoo." It was further expanded by another thematic picture, "circus" (Hernandorena and Lamprecht, 1997). The target words in pictures of the instrument are capable of eliciting all the consonantal phonemes of Portuguese in different positions and in different structures with multiple examples. In addition, since they are theme based, the investigator can also elicit targets in full sentences and in theme-based narrations.

Another notable assessment procedure is *ABFW— Teste de Linguagem infantile: nas áreas de fonologia, vocabulário, fluência e pragmática* [Child language examination: phonology, vocabulary, fluency, and pragmatics] by Andrade (2000), which uses "naming" and "repetition" for elicitation. Audiotaping the data is routine in Brazil, and in some cases videotaping is also used.

Contrastive assessment, distinctive feature analysis, and phonological process analysis are the methods used for phonological analysis in phonological development. Contrastive assessment is based on the principle of comparing the child's system with the ambient norm. To this end, correct productions, substitutions, and omissions for singleton targets in different positions are registered and computed. A separate inventory for consonant clusters is used. Variability of the productions is also considered.

The distinctive feature analysis aims to discover where the inadequacies are as far as the features are concerned. The changes are revealed through the substitutions observed in the inventory used from the contrastive assessment. For the model of phonological matrix for Portuguese consonants, see Mota (1996).

Phonological process analysis is probably the simplest and most economical way of describing the differences between the adult targets and the realization of these targets by children. Children's simplification patterns are examined in the following three groups. (1) syllable structure processes, (2) substitution processes, and (3) assimilatory processes. For a detailed description of these three different analyses, the reader is referred to AFC (Yavaş et al., 1991).

Speech intervention for Portuguese-speaking children

The intervention for phonological disorders is different from the purely phonetic approach of articulation disorders as such; it goes beyond motor activities and involves conceptual changes in the system. Several different models are practiced for this purpose in Brazil. Some of these models utilize processes as their base, such as the cyclical method (Hodson and Paden, 1983), modified cycles (Tyler, Edwards, and Saxman, 1987), and *Metaphon* (Dean and Howell, 1986), while others such as ABAB-withdrawal and multiple probes (Tyler and Figurski, 1994), and maximal oppositions of Gierut (1992) use features.

Although there are other differences—including number of target sounds used, techniques of the application, and the number of sessions for each target sound stimulated—these models all have the objective of generalizing treatment effects to nonspecified targets. The application of the above-mentioned models of remediation have all been proven effective for Brazilian children (Ardenghi, 2004; Bagetti, Mota, and Keske-Soares, 2005; Keske-Soares, 1996, 2001; Mota, 1990; Pereira, 1999; Ramos, 1991).

Working in Brazil

The professionals practicing speech-language therapy in Brazil are graduates of a four-year program in 'fonoaudiology' (speech pathology and audiology). Several universities have, in addition, graduate programs in the area, offering master's and doctoral degrees. Practicing speech-language therapists must be affiliated with the Federal Council of Speech Pathology and Audiology (http://www.fonoaudiologia.org.br), which regulates the profession. As for the venues of employment, private clinics, hospitals, schools, day care centers, nursing homes, various businesses, and media can be cited.

Associations that promote scientific research via meetings and publications of scientific journals include the Brazilian Association of Speech Pathology and Audiology (http://www.sbfa.org.br), which holds annual meetings and publishes *Revista da Sociedade Brasileira de Fonoaudiologia* [Journal of the Brazilian Association of Speech Pathology and Audiology], and also organizes the international speech pathology and audiology meeting. The Brazilian Audiology Association (http://www.audiologiabrasil.org.br) holds the annual meetings in audiology as well as the international audiology meeting.

For a foreign national speech-language therapist to practice in Brazil, it is mandatory that his or her degree be validated by a Brazilian university with a program in 'fonoaudiologia' (speech-language therapy).

PHONETICALLY SPEAKING

Pronunciation of Portuguese: /poɾtuges/

Relevant words for speech assessment and intervention

Word/Phrase	Formal usage	Pronunciation
Tongue	*língua*	liŋgʷa
Teeth	*dentes*	dentʃis
Lips	*labios*	labjos
Hard palate	*palato duro*	palatu duru
Soft palate	*palato mole*	palatu mɔli
Larynx	*laringe*	larindʒi
Lungs	*pulmões*	pulm jis
Nose	*nariz*	naris
Sound	*som*	s
Word	*palavra*	palavra
Sentence	*sentença*	sentensa
Paragraph	*parágrafo*	paragrafu

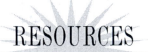

RESOURCES

Books and CD-ROMs

The following publishers and booksellers are some of the best sources:

Artmed, http://www.artmed.com.br

Revinter, http://www.revinter.com.br

Book Toy, http://www.booktoy.com.br

Pró-Fono, http://www.profono.com.br

Journals

The following are some of the several journals published in the area of communication disorders in Brazil.

- *PRO-FONO – Revista de Atualização Científica,* http://www.profono.com.br
- *Revista da Sociedade Brasileira de Fonoaudiologia,* http://www.sbfa.org.br
- *Revista Fono Atual,* http://www.fonoatual.com.br

- *Revista Distúrbios da Comunicação,* http://www.pucsp. br/educ/catalogo/periodicos
- *Revista CEFAC,* http://www.CEFAC.br
- *Revista Fonoaudiologia Brasil,* http://www.fonoaudiologia. org.br

Professional associations

Conselho Federal de Fonoaudiologia – CFFa, http://www.fonoaudiologia.org.br

Sociedade Brasileira de Fonoaudiologia – SBFa, http://www.sbfa.org.br

Academia Brasileira de Audiologia, http://www.audiologiabrasil.org.br

Universities offering degrees in speech-language pathology

For undergraduate programs, consult http://www.mec.gov.br, and http://www.educacaosuperior.inep.gov.br. For graduate programs consult http://www.capes.gov.br.

Note: Pontifícia Universidade Católica do Rio Grande do Sul (PUCRS) of Porto Alegre, although it does not have a program in speech-language pathology, is one of the most notable places for studies of phonological acquisition and disorders in Brazil. Its graduate program in linguistics and the research center in acquisition studies have produced a very significant body of resources via its projects, M.A. theses, and doctoral dissertations.

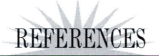

REFERENCES

Andrade, C. R. F., (2000). *ABFW – Teste de Linguagem Infantil: nas áreas de fonologia vocabulário, fluência e pragmática.* Carapicuiba, SP: Pro-Fono.

Ardenghi, L. A. (2004). *A Terapia Metaphon em casos de desvios fonológicos.* Unpublished M.A. thesis, Universidade Federal de Santa Maria, Brazil.

Azambuja, E. J. (1998). *A aquisição das líquidas laterais do português.* Unpublished M.A. thesis, Pontifícia Universidade Católica do Rio Grande do Sul, Porto Alegre.

Bagetti, T., Mota, H. B., and Keske-Soares, M. (2005). O modelo de oposições máximas modificado: Uma proposta de tratamento para o desvio fonológico. *Revista da Sociedade Brasiliera de Fonoaudiologia, 10*(1), 36–42.

Bonilha, G. F. G. (2004). Sobre a aquisição das vogais. In R. R. Lamprecht (Ed.). *Aquisição Fonológica do Português* (pp. 61–72). Porto Alegre, RS: Artmed.

Cardoso-Martins, C. (1994). Rhyme perception: Global or analytical? *Journal of Experimental Child Psychology, 57,* 26–41.

Cielo, C. A. (2000). *Habilidades em consciência fonológica em crianças de 4 a 8 anos.* Unpublished doctoral dissertation, Pontifícia Universidade Católica do Rio Grande do Sul, Porto Alegre.

Coimbra, M. (1997). *Metaphonological ability to judge phonetic and phonological acceptability in five year-old monolingual and bilingual children.* Unpublished doctoral dissertation, Pontifícia Universidade Católica do Rio Grande do Sul, Porto Alegre.

De Freitas, G. C. M. (2004). Sobre a aquisição das plosives e nasais. In R. R. Lamprecht (Ed.), *Aquisição Fonológica do Português* (pp. 73–82). Porto Alegre, RS: Artmed.

Dean, E., and Howell, J. (1986). Developing linguistic awareness: A theoretically based approach to phonological disorders. *British Journal of Disorders of Communication, 21,* 223–238.

Edwards, M. L. (1992). Clinical forum: Phonological assessment and treatment in support of phonological processes. *Language Speech and Hearing Services in Schools, 23,* 233–240.

Gierut, J. A. (1992). The conditions and course of clinically induced phonological change. *Journal of Speech and Hearing Research, 35,* 1049–1063.

Hernandorena, C. L. M. (1990). *A aquisição da fonologia do português: estabelecimento de padrões com base em traços distintivos.* Unpublished doctoral dissertation, Pontifícia Universidade Católica do Rio Grande do Sul, Porto Alegre.

Hernandorena, C. L. M., and Lamprecht, R. R. (1997). A aquisição das consoantes líquidas do português. *Letras de Hoje, 32*(4), 7–22.

Hodson, B. W., and Paden, E. P. (1983). *Targeting intelligible speech.* San Diego, CA: College-Hill Press.

Ilha, S. E. (1993). *Desenvolvimento fonológico de português em crianças com idade entre 1:8 a 2:3.* Unpublished M.A. thesis, Pontifícia Universidade Católica do Rio Grande do Sul, Porto Alegre.

Keske-Soares, M. (1996). *Aplicação de um modelo de terapia fonológica para crianças com desvios fonológicos evolutivos: a hierarquia implicacional dos traços distintivos.* Unpublished M.A. thesis,

Pontificia Universidade Católica do Rio Grande do Sul, Porto Alegre.

Keske-Soares, M. (2001). *Terapia fonoaudiológica fundamentada na çhierarquia implicacional dos traços distintivos aplicada em crianças com desvios fonológicos.* Unpublished doctoral dissertation, Pontificia Universidade Católica do Rio Grande do Sul, Porto Alegre.

Lamprecht, R. R. (1990). *Perfil da aquisição normal da fonologia do Português: Descrição longitudinal de 12 crianças 2:9 a 5:5.* Unpublished doctoral dissertation, Pontificia Universidade Católica do Rio Grande do Sul, Porto Alegre.

Lamprecht, R. R. (Ed.). (2004). *Aquisição fonológica do Português.* Porto Alegre, RS: Artmed.

Mezzomo, C. L. (2003). *Aquisição da coda no portguês brasiliero: Uma análise via teoria de Princípios e Parâmetros.* Unpublished doctoral dissertation, Pontificia Universidade Católica do Rio Grande do Sul, Porto Alegre.

Mota, H. B. (1990). *Uma abordagem terapêutica baseada nos processos fonológicos no tratamento de crianças com desvios fonológicos.* Unpublished M.A. thesis, Pontificia Universidade Católica do Rio Grande do Sul, Porto Alegre.

Mota, H. B. (1996). *Aquisição segmental do Português: Um modelo implicacional de complexidade de traços.* Unpublished doctoral disssertation, Pontificia Universidade Católica do Rio Grande do Sul, Porto Alegre.

Oliveira, C. C. (2002). *Aquisição das fricatives /f/, /v/, /ʃ/, e /ʒ/ do Português Brasiliero.* Unpublished M.A. thesis, Pontificia Universidade Católica do Rio Grande do Sul, Porto Alegre.

Oliveira, C. C., Mezzomo, C. L., de Freitas, G. C. M., and Lamprecht, R. R. (2004). Cronologia da aquisição dos segmentos e das silábicas. In R. R. Lamprecht (Ed.), *Aquisição fonológica do português* (pp. 167–176). Porto Alegre, RS: Artmed.

Pereira, L. F. (1999). *Tratamento fonológico baseado nos contrastes de oposições máximas.* Unpublished M.A. thesis, Universidade Federal de Santa Maria.

Ramos, A. P. F. (1991). *Avaliação e tratamento fonológico de crianças portadoras de fissuras do lábio e do palato reparadas na faixa etaria de 4 a 9 anos.* Unpublished M.A. thesis, Pontificia Universidade Católica do Rio Grande do Sul, Porto Alegre.

Rangel, G. A. (1998). *Uma análise auto-segmental da fonologia normal: Estudo longitudinal de 3 crianças de 1:6 a 3:0.* Unpublished M.A. thesis, Pontificia Universidade Católica do Rio Grande do Sul, Porto Alegre.

Rangel, G. A. (2002). *Aquisição do sistema vocálico do Português Brasileiro.* Unpublished doctoral dissertation, Pontificia Universidade Católica do Rio Grande do Sul, Porto Alegre.

Ribas, L. P. (2002). *Aquisição do onset complexo no Português Brasileiro.* Unpublished M.A. thesis, Pontificia Universidade Católica do Rio Grande do Sul, Porto Alegre.

Savio, C. B. (2001). *Aquisição das fricatives /s/ e /z/ do Português Brasiliero.* Unpublished M.A. thesis, Pontificia Universidade Católica do Rio Grande do Sul, Porto Alegre.

Tyler, A. A., Edwards, M. L., and Saxman, J. H. (1987). Clinical application of two phonological treatment procedures. *Journal of Speech and Hearing Disorders, 52,* 393–409.

Tyler, A. A., and Figurski, G. R. (1994). Phonetic inventory changes after treating distinctions along an implicational hierarchy. *Clinical Linguistics and Phonetics, 8*(2), 91–107.

Yavaş, M. (1988). Padrões na aquisição da fonologia do português. *Letras de Hoje, 74,* 7–30.

Yavaş, M., Hernandorena, C. L. M., and Lamprecht, R. R. (1991). *Avaliação fonológica da criança: Reeducação e terapia.* Porto Alegre, RS: Artes Medicas.

Yavaş, M., and Lamprecht, R. R. (1988). Processes and intelligibility in disordered phonology. *Clinical Linguistics and Phonetics, 2,* 329–345.

SUMMARY OF STUDIES OF TYPICAL PORTUGUESE SPEECH ACQUISITION

Authors	Year	Country	No. of children	Age of children	Information	Sample type	Data collection
Azambuja	1998	Brazil	120	2;0–4;0	Lateral liquid acq.	Single word	Cross-sectional
Cardoso-Martins	1994	Brazil	105	4;0–4;6	Phonological awareness	Single word	Cross-sectional
Cielo	2000	Brazil	85	4;0–8;0	Phonological awareness	Single word	Cross-sectional
Coimbra	1997	Brazil	55	5;0	Phonological awareness	Single word	Cross-sectional
De Freitas	2004	Brazil	33	4;0–8;0	Phonological awareness	Single word	Cross-sectional
Hernandorena	1990	Brazil	134	2;0–4;3	Distinctive feature acquisition	Single word	Cross-sectional
Hernandorena and Lamprecht	1997	Brazil	310	2;7–7;1	Liquid acquisition	Single word	Cross-sectional
Ilha	1993	Brazil	26	1;8–2;3	Phonological acquisition	Single word	Cross-sectional
Keske-Soares	2001	Brazil	35	Mean age 5;5	Disorders and treatment	Single word and connected speech	Longitudinal
Lamprecht	1990	Brazil	12	2;9–5;0	Phonological processes	Single word and connected speech	Longitudinal
Mezzomo	2003	Brazil	170	1;2–3;10	Syllable structure	Single word	Cross-sectional
Mota	1996	Brazil	25	4;0–7;0	Distinctive feature acquisition	Single word	Cross-sectional
Oliveira	2002	Brazil	103	1;0–3;8	Fricatives	Single word	Cross-sectional
Oliveira Mezzomo, de Freitas, and Lamprecht	2004	Brazil	3	1;0–4;0	General phonological acquisition	Single word and connected speech	Longitudinal
Rangel	1998	Brazil	3	1;6–3;0	Segmental acquisition	Single word and connected speech	Longitudinal
Ribas	2002	Brazil	134	1;0–5;3	Syllable structure	Single word	Cross-sectional
Savio	2001	Brazil	91	1;0–3;3	Fricative acquisition	Single word	Cross-sectional
Yavaş	1988	Brazil	72	2;4–4;4	Phonological acquisition	Single word	Cross-sectional

For the most up-to-date and comprehensive guide for references on the phonological acquisition of Brazilian Portuguese, the reader is referred to Lamprecht (2004).

Chapter 50

Putonghua (Modern Standard Chinese) Speech Acquisition

Zhu Hua

INTRODUCTION

The Chinese language is manifested in a range of varieties. As far as spoken Chinese is concerned, traditional Chinese linguists distinguish eight major varieties: *Beifang*, *Yue*, *Kejia*, *Min Bei*, *Min Nan*, *Wu*, *Xiang*, and *Gan*. Within each major variety, there are subvarieties with their own distinctive features. For example, Cantonese is a subvariety within the *Yue* variety and Hokkien in *Min Nan*. Putonghua, literally 'common speech', is a standardized language variety based on the phonological and grammatical system of *Beifang* varieties and is often referred to as Mandarin in the West. Promoted by the Mainland Chinese government since the 1950s, Putonghua is widely used in the mass media and taught in schools in China. Comprehensive descriptions and theoretical discussions of Putonghua can be found in Li and Thompson (1981), Norman (1988), and Chen (1999). See the Resources section of this chapter for materials pertaining to Putonghua.

Where Putonghua is spoken

Surveys suggest that 90 percent of the whole population in China understand Putonghua and about 50 percent of the population can communicate in Putonghua (Wu and Yin, 1984; see accompanying map and Appendix D).

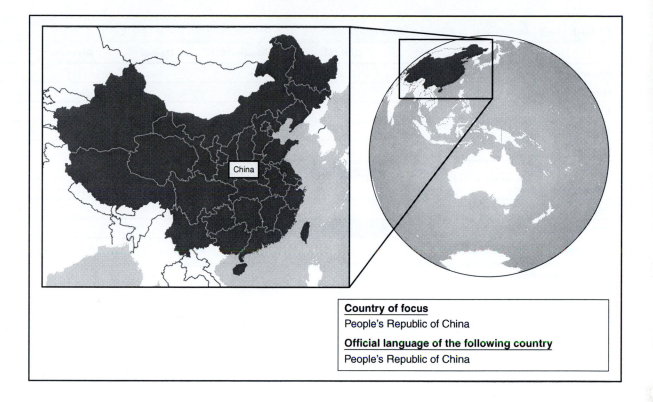

Country of focus
People's Republic of China

Official language of the following country
People's Republic of China

Components of Putonghua

Consonants

There are 22 consonants in Putonghua (the place and manner of consonants are given in Table 50-1). Aspiration serves as a distinctive feature of Putonghua consonants. There are six pairs of aspirated and unaspirated consonants, and all of them are voiceless.

Vowels

There are 22 vowels in Putonghua. They can be classified into three groups: nine simple vowels, nine diphthongs, and four triphthongs (see Figure 50-1). The nine simple vowels are /i, y, u, ɤ, o, ɑ, ə, ɛ, ɚ/ (see Putonghua vowel chart). The diphthongs can be divided further into offglides and onglides:

- /ae/, /ei/, /ɑo/, and /ou/ are offglides, the first element being longer and having more intensity
- /ia/, /iɛ/, /uɑ/, /uo/, and /yɛ/ are onglides, the second element being sonorous

In all of the four triphthongs (i.e. /iɑo/, /iou/, /uae/, /uei/), the middle element has the most intensity and is the longest.

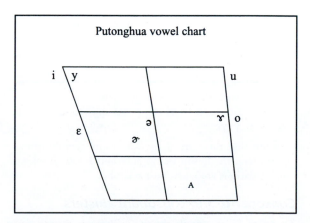

Figure 50-1 Putonghua vowel chart

TABLE 50-1 Consonants produced in Putonghua

	Bilabial	Labiodental	Dental	Alveolar
Plosive	p pʰ			t tʰ
Nasal	m			n
Trill				
Tap or flap				
Fricative		f		s
Lateral fricative	■	■	■	
Affricates				ts tsʰ
Approximant				
Lateral approximant	■	■	■	

Black = articulations judged impossible

Based on the International Phonetic Alphabet. Courtesy of the International Phonetic Association (c/o Department of Linguistics, University of Victoria, Victoria, British Columbia, Canada).

Phonotactic restrictions

Syllables

A syllable in Putonghua has the following structure: $C_{(0-1)}$ $VC_{(0-1)}$. In a Putonghua syllable, the onset and coda are optional and the vowel in the nucleus is compulsory. The onset can be one of 21 consonants and the coda can be one of only two consonants, /n/ and /ŋ/. Among the 22 consonants in Putonghua, 21 can serve as an onset with the exception of /ŋ/, which can occur only in the coda.

The great majority of syllables in Putonghua begin with a consonant. The most important phonotactic rules are the following:

- Consonants /p, pʰ, m, f/ can combine with the vowel /u/, but not with any diphthong or triphthong beginning with /u/ (i.e., /ua, uo, uae, uei/)
- Consonants /t, tʰ/ cannot occur together with the vowels /y, yɛ/
- Consonants /k, kʰ, x, s, ts, tsʰ, ɹ, ʂ, tʂ, tʂʰ/ cannot occur together with the vowels /i, ia, iɛ, iɑo, iou, y, yɛ/
- Consonants /ɕ, tɕ, tɕʰ/ can occur only with /i, ia, iɛ, iɑo, iou, y, yɛ/

Altogether there are about 420 feasible combinations of onset and rhymes in Putonghua, and 1,300 syllables if tonal variations are taken into account.

Consonants and consonant clusters

There are no consonant clusters in Putonghua.

Tones

Tones, together with vowels, are a compulsory component of syllables, and differences in tones can change the meaning of a lexical item. There are four tones in Putonghua: high level, high rising, falling-rising, and high falling, primarily characterized by voice pitch but also by length and intensity (see Table 50-2). They are referred to as tones 1, 2, 3, and 4 respectively in this chapter. *Hanyu Pinyin* (known as "Chinese phonetic writing system"), which was endorsed by the National People's Congress in 1958 in an effort to standardize pronunciation throughout China and to facilitate teaching and learning of Putonghua, uses diacritics to represent high level, rising, falling-rising, and falling tones.

Stress and intonation

Weak stress, which is often referred to as the neutral tone or weak syllable (see Norman, 1988), is an essential prosodic feature of Putonghua. It is phonologically and morphologically conditioned. Weakly stressed syllables have a very short duration and a much reduced pitch range together with other changes.

Apart from pitch variation within the domain of a morpheme (i.e., tone), Putonghua also has pitch variation within an entire utterance, that is, intonation. The main intonational patterns include falling (which is typically used to express confirmation, exclamation, etc.), rising (used in questions, calling for attention, etc.), flat (used in statements, description, and ordinary conversation), and

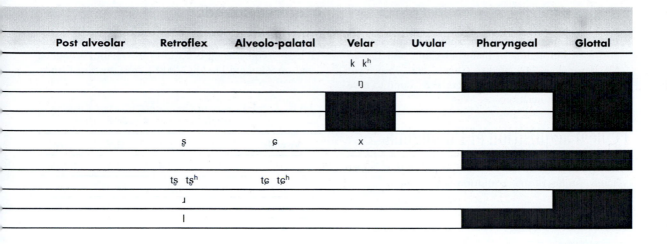

	Post alveolar	Retroflex	Alveolo-palatal	Velar	Uvular	Pharyngeal	Glottal
				k kʰ			
				ŋ			
		ʂ	ɕ	x			
		tʂ tʂʰ	tɕ tɕʰ				
		ɹ					
		l					

curve (expressing complicated emotion, exaggeration, surprise, etc.). Intonation is realized mainly on the tail, not on the head or the nucleus of an utterance.

Writing system

The Putonghua writing system is largely logographic, that is, each symbol, or character, is or originates from a logograph. Examples: 木 (wood), 林 (forest), 山 (mountain), 人 (person).

There are two writing systems: simplified and complicated characters. Simplified characters are used in the People's Republic of China and Singapore, and sentences are written horizontally from left to right. Complicated characters are used in Taiwan, Hong Kong, and overseas Chinese communities, and sentences can be written both horizontally and vertically.

Varieties of Putonghua

Though both are labeled as Mandarin in the West, there are important differences between Putonghua spoken in the People's Republic of China and Mandarin spoken in Taiwan. The latter is officially referred to as Guoyu in Taiwan (literally, 'national language'). Examples of important differences are the following:

- Rhotacization and weak stress occur less frequently in Taiwan Mandarin than in Putonghua (Chen, 1999).
- The phonological contrast between the alveolar fricative and affricates /s, ts, tsʰ/ and the retroflex fricative and affricates /ʂ, tʂ, tʂʰ/ tends to disappear in Taiwan Mandarin.
- The contrast between syllable-final consonants /n/ and /ŋ/ also tends to disappear, especially in codas /in/vs./iŋ/ and /ən/vs./əŋ/.

TABLE 50-2 The four tones of Putonghua

Tone	Syllable	Tonal indicator	Hanyu Pinyin*	English translation
High level	ba	1	bā	'eight'
Rising	ba	2	bá	'pull out'
Falling-rising	ba	3	bǎ	'target'
High falling	ba	4	bà	'Dad'

* Chinese phonetic writing system

- There are tonal differences between Putonghua and Guoyu (Yip, 1980).
- In a recent survey on pronunciation differences in the norms of Putonghua in mainland China and Taiwan Mandarin (Li, 1992, cited in Chen, 1999), 23 percent of 3,500 most common characters were found to have different pronunciations.

Typical acquisition of Putonghua

The Summary of Studies Table at the end of the chapter contains studies of the acquisition of Putonghua.

TABLE 50-3 Age of acquisition for Putonghua consonants

Consonant	75 percent group criterion	90 percent group criterion
t	2;0	2;0
t^h	2;0	3;0
m	2;0	2;0
n	2;0	2;6
x	2;0	3;0
k	2;6	3;6
tɕ	2;6	4;6
tɕ^h	2;6	4;6
ɕ	2;6	3;0
p	2;6	3;0
p^h	2;6	4;0
k^h	2;6	3;6
f	3;0	3;0
s	4;6	4;6
l	4;6	4;6
ɹ	4;6	4;6
ʂ	4;6	>4;6
tʂ	>4;6	>4;6
tʂ^h	>4;6	>4;6
ts	>4;6	>4;6
ts^h	>4;6	>4;6

Note. Data from Zhu and Dodd (2000a).

Acquired sounds
Consonants

Table 50-3 contains age of acquisition data for Putonghua based on Zhu and Dodd's (2000a) cross-sectional study.

TABLE 50-4 Age of emergence of vowels in four children in a longitudinal study

Vowels	J.J.	Z.J.	H.Y.	Z.W.
i	1;3	1;4	1;5	1;2.15
y	1;3.15	1;7	1;8.15	1;6
u	1;2.15	1;4	1;2	1;3
ɤ	1;5.15	1;9	1;2	1;2.15
o	1;7.15	1;9	no data	1;7.15
ɑ	1;2	1;4	1;2	1;2.15
ɚ	1;7.15	1;7	no data	no data
ae	1;5.15	1;8	1;4.15	1;5.15
ɑo	1;4	1;7	1;3	1;5
ei	1;2.15	1;7	1;2	1;3
oυ	1;3	1;8	1;5	1;4.15
ia	1;3.15	1;8	1;4	1;3.15
iɛ	1;3.15	1;8.15	1;2.15	1;2.15
ua	1;5.15	1;7.15	1;2.15	1;3.15
uo	1;7.15	1;9.15	1;8	1;5
yɛ	1;10	no data	no data	1;6.15
iɑo	1;3.15	1;6.15	1;6.15	1;5.15
ioυ	1;3.15	1;4.15	1;5.15	1;3.15
uae	1;6.15	1;9.15	1;5.15	1;6
uei	1;4.15	1;8	1;6	1;3.15
Mean age of emergence of simple vowels	1;4.15	1;6.9	1;3.27	1;4.2
Mean age of emergence of diphthongs	1;5	1;7.24	1;3.27	1;4.12
Mean age of emergence of triphthongs	1;4.15	1;7.3	1;5.26	1;4.18

Note. Data from Zhu (2002).

The group criteria are 90 percent and 75 percent, based on two correct realizations out of three opportunities.

Vowels and diphthongs

The acquisition of vowels takes place mainly between the ages of 1;0 and 2;0 (Zhu, 2002). Table 50-4 shows the age of acquisition of different vowels among the four children under study. Despite individual differences, some patterns were identifiable in the development of vowels in the children. Among the simple vowels, the central low vowel /ɑ/ and back high vowel /u/ were the earliest to emerge in the four children; the retroflex vowel /ɚ/ and the back vowel /o/ seemed to be the last simple vowels to emerge in the children's output. Among diphthongs, /ei/ was the first to emerge for all the children, and /yɛ/ the last. Among triphthongs, /ioʊ/ emerged first in three children's speech, while /uae/ was the last for three children.

Percent correct
Consonants

The average percentage of consonants correct in children's production in each age group is summarized in Table 50-5.

Phonological processes

According to the cross-sectional study of Zhu and Dodd (2000a), 15 error patterns were present in the speech of more than 10 percent of the children in the youngest age group (1;6 to 2;0). These could be generalized into three groups: assimilation, deletion, and systematic substitution. Five patterns (i.e., fronting of alveolar-palatals as alveolars, stopping of alveolar fricatives as alveolar stops, affrication, aspiration, and gliding) disappeared in

more than 90 percent of the children in the oldest age group (4;0 to 4;6). The chronology of these error patterns (i.e., the age of onset, persistence, and disappearance of error patterns) is given in Figure 50-2.

Intelligibility

To date there is no study of intelligibility of Putonghua-speaking children.

Phonetic inventory

Table 50-6 summarizes the phonetic inventories of four subjects in Zhu's longitudinal study (2002). The phonetic inventories consist of sounds that a child can produce in a meaningful unit irrespective of whether it is the correct target.

Common mismatches

To date there is no systematic study of common mismatches produced by Putonghua-speaking children. The following summary of common mismatches in young

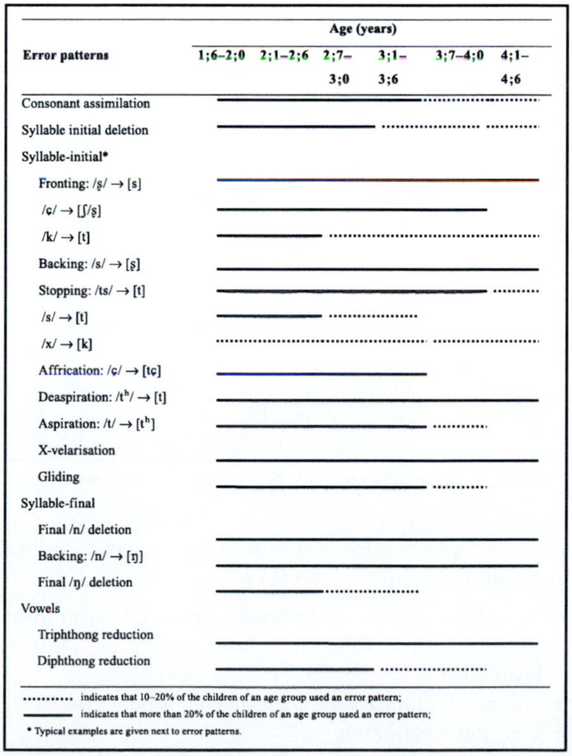

Age	Percentage of consonants correct
1;6–2;0	63.9 percent
2;1–2;6	74.4 percent
2;7–3;0	81 percent
3;1–3;6	86.4 percent
3;7–4;0	89.5 percent
4;1–4;6	92.2 percent

TABLE 50-5 Percent correct for Putonghua consonants

Note. Data from Zhu and Dodd (2000b).

Figure 50-2 Chronology of Putonghua error patterns

TABLE 50-6 Four children's phonetic inventories at different ages

Age	J.J.	Z.J.	H.Y.	Z.W.
1;2			m	m
1;2.15	k, ŋ		p	t, n-
1;3	p		t	
1;3.15	t, m			s, x
1;4		t		p
1;4.15	n-, -n	ŋ	ŋ	ŋ
1;5	tɕ	p	l	ʂ
1;5.15	tʰ, x, ɕ		n-	ɕ, tʂ, ts, -n
1;6	f			f, l
1;6.15	ts	m, n-		k, tɕ
1;7	s, tsʰ	s	k	
1;7.15	pʰ, l, ɻ			
1;8		tɕ, -n	pʰ, tʰ, s, x, tɕ, -n	
1;8.15		x, ts	ɕ	no data
1;9		k, ɻ		no data
1;9.15		l	f	no data
1;10	ʂ	tʂ	kʰ	no data
1;10.15	tʂ	f	tsʰ	no data
1;11		tʰ	ʂ, tʂ	no data
1;11.15		ɕ	ts, tɕʰ	no data
2;0	tɕʰ			no data
2;0.15				no data
Missing phonemes	kʰ, tɕʰ	pʰ, kʰ, ʂ, tɕʰ, tsʰ, tʂʰ	ɻ, tʂʰ	pʰ, tʰ, kʰ, ɻ, tɕʰ, tʂʰ, tsʰ

Note. 'n-'= syllable-initial consonant /n/; '-n' = syllable-final consonant /n/.

children's speech is based on the error patterns described above and Ha's description (1996).

- Alveolar /s, ts, tsʰ / and retroflex /ʂ, tʂ, tʂʰ/ tend to be used interchangeably, especially by people from northern China
- Aspirated sounds and unaspirated sounds tend to be used interchangeably

- /n/ tends to be pronounced as /l/ by people from southern China

Syllable structure

Zhu's (2002) longitudinal study of four Mandarin-speaking children indicates that core syllables CV and reduplicated core syllables CVCVCV are popular in children's early speech. Final consonant deletion is a very common process. V and CVC develop much later, followed by VC.

Tones

According to Zhu (2002), the acquisition of tones is completed by the age of 1;10, earlier than that of consonants and vowels. Tone is also resistant to impairment during the process of phonological acquisition. Both phonologically disordered children and hearing-impaired children are found to have very little difficulty with tones. A feature is considered to have *emerged* when it is produced correctly at least once in the speech. According to the longitudinal study conducted by Zhu (2002), the order and age of emergence of tones is as follows:

- High level/high falling tones emerge at 1;2 to 1;4
- Rising tones emerge at 1;3 to 1;4
- Falling-rising tones emerge at 1;4 to 1;7

A feature is considered to be *stabilized* when it is accurately and consistently produced on at least two of three opportunities. The order and age of stabilization of tones is as follows (Zhu, 2002):

- High level tones stabilize at 1;2.15 to 1;5.15
- High falling tones stabilize at 1;4 to 1;7
- Rising/falling-rising tones stabilize at 1;4.15 to 1;10

Table 50-7 shows the most frequent substitute(s) for each tone.

Phonological awareness

Numerous studies have been conducted on the phonological awareness of children speaking Putonghua in the People's Republic of China or Mandarin in Taiwan. The main findings are summarized below:

- Despite the fact that Chinese is not an alphabetic language, significant correlations exist between Chinese children's phonological awareness skills and readings skills, probably because phonological knowledge helps children to use the phonetic components in Chinese characters (Ho and Bryant, 1997).

TABLE 50-7 Putonghua children's most frequent substitutes for each tone

Target tones	Most frequent substitute(s)
High level	High falling
Rising	High level
Falling-rising	High level /Rising
High falling	High level

- Phonological awareness skills acquired in Chinese can be transferred to another language such as English (Chien, Kao, and Li Wei, 2004; Holm and Dodd, 1996).

Speech assessment and intervention for children who speak Putonghua

Speech disorders in Putonghua-speaking children are rarely reported in the literature. This is partly because of the lack of normative data and partly because of a lack of awareness of such a developmental phenomenon. As a result, speech therapy resources are still to be developed in China, and where resources are available, priority seems to have been given to hearing impairment. It was reported that among several speech and hearing clinics newly opened in China, almost all aimed to provide audiological services for the hearing impaired (Cheng, 2001). A lack of understanding of the nature of speech difficulties often leads to clinical misdiagnosis. Xu and Ha (1992) reported that in some clinics children with speech difficulties had been unanimously misdiagnosed as having a short frenum, and their unintelligible speech did not improve after the frenum had been cut.

The following speech assessment tools are available in Putonghua:

- *Putonghua Segmental Phonology Test* (So and Zhou, 2000)
- *Putonghua Picture-Naming and Picture-Description Tasks* (Zhu Hua, 2002)

Zhu and Dodd (2000b) describe the characteristics of disordered speech of Putonghua-speaking children.

Working in the People's Republic of China

Since speech and language therapy is underdeveloped in China, there is no professional body for speech-language pathologists. Neither is there any training program for speech-language pathologists. Researchers who carry out research on Putonghua language development or disorders are usually based in special needs centers or psychology departments affiliated with Chinese universities.

All foreign nationals wishing to work in China must apply for an employment visa before entering China or shortly thereafter. They also need to apply for a residence permit within 30 days of entering China. The Web site of the China-Britain Business Council (http://www.cbbc.org/market_intelligence/hr/working.html) contains useful information on how to apply for these documents and information on Chinese culture and living in China.

PHONETICALLY SPEAKING

Pronunciation of Putonghua: /putɔŋhua/
Relevant words for speech assessment and intervention

Word	Chinese character	Romanization (Pinyin)	Pronunciation
Tongue	舌头	/Shetou	/ʂɤ təu/
Teeth	牙齿	Yachi	/ia tʂʰi/
Lips	嘴唇	Zuichun	/tsuei tʂʰun/
Hard palate	硬腭	Yinge	/iŋɣ/
Soft palate	软腭	Ruane	/ɹuanɣ/
Larynx	喉咙	Houlong	/həu lɔŋ/
Lungs	肺	Fei	/fei/
Nose	鼻子	Bizi	/pi tsi/
Sound	声音	Shengyin	/ʂəŋ in/
Word	词	Ci	/tsʰi/
Character	字	Zi	/tsi/
Sentence	句	Ju	/tɕy/
Paragraph	段落	Duanluo	/tuaŋ luo/

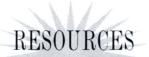

RESOURCES

Books on Chinese languages

Chen, Ping (1999). *Modern Chinese: History and sociolinguistics.* Cambridge, UK: Cambridge University Press.

DeFrancis, J. (1984). *The Chinese language: Fact and fantasy.* Honolulu: University of Hawaii Press.

Li, C. N., and Thompson, S. A. (1981). *Mandarin Chinese. A functional reference grammar.* Berkeley: University of California Press.

Norman, J. (1988). *Chinese.* Cambridge, UK: Cambridge University Press.

Information regarding Chinese acquisition norms and language tests

Li, P., Tan, L. H., Bates, E., and Tzeng, O. (Eds.) (2005). *Handbook of East Asian psycholinguistics: Chinese.* Cambridge, UK: Cambridge University Press.

So, L. K. H., and Zhou, J. (2000). *Putonghua Segmental Phonology Test.* Nanjing: Nanjing Normal University Press.

Wu, Jiang (1997). *Language, play and general development for Chinese infant-toddlers: Using adapted assessments.*

Unpublished doctoral dissertation, University of Colorado, Boulder.

Zhou, J. (2002). *Pragmatic development of Mandarin speaking children: From 14 month to 32 months*, NJ: Nanjing Normal University Press, China. (周兢: **汉语儿童语用能力发展**, 南京师范大学出版社, 2002年) 。

Zhu Hua (2002). *Phonological development in specific contexts*. Clevedon: Multilingual Matters (with norms and test).

Zhu Hua (2002). Putonghua-speaking children with developmental speech disorders. *Speech & Hearing Review, 3*, 69–90.

Zhu Hua and Dodd, B. (2000). Putonghua (Modern Standard Chinese)-speaking with speech disorder. *Clinical Linguistics and Phonetics, 14*(3), 165–191.

Zhu Hua and Dodd, B. (2000). Development and change in the phonology of Putonghua-speaking children with speech difficulties. *Clinical Linguistics and Phonetics, 14*(5), 351–368.

Zhu Hua and Dodd, B. (2000). The phonological systems of a set of Putonghua-speaking twins. *International Journal of Language and Communication Disorders, 35*(4), 487–506.

Zhu Hua and Li Wei (1999). Stylistic variations in the early lexical development of young Putonghua-speaking children. *Asia Pacific Journal of Speech, Language and Hearing, 4*, 39–51.

張仁俊，朱曼殊 (1987). 嬰兒語言的發展：一個個案的分析.《心理科學通訊》No. 5

吳天敏，許政援 (1979). 初生到三歲兒童語言發展記錄的初步分析.《心理科學通訊》No. 2

彭祖智等 (1984). 3-6 歲兒童語言發展記錄的初步分析. 中國心理學會, 1984 年學術年會論文。

李向農 (1992). 1-5 歲兒童運用方位詞及方位介詞情況的調查分析.《心理學報》1(3), 49–51

Journals

- *Speech and Hearing Review.* A bilingual annual journal published by National Kaohsiung Normal University Special Education Center, Taiwan since 2000. Editors are Li-Rong Lilly Cheng and Chin-Hsing Tseng.

Professional associations

Speech and language therapy service is underdeveloped in China. The Speech Therapy Clinic of the Division of Speech and Hearing Sciences, Hong Kong University, is a teaching and research clinic that mainly focuses on Cantonese (a dialect of Chinese).

Amity foundation, http://www.amityfoundation.org/ is a Christian organization that promotes health, education, and welfare and has established a center for hearing-impaired children in China.

Dr Caroline Bowen's Web site lists contacts regarding China, http://members.tripod.com/Caroline_Bowen/Asia.htm

Useful Dialect/Language Web sites

- *Learning Chinese online*, http://www.csulb.edu/~txie/online.htm, a resource Web site teaching visitors to speak, write, and read Chinese.
- *BBC Real Chinese*, http://www.bbc.co.uk/languages/chinese/real_chinese/

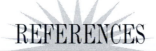

REFERENCES

Chao, Y. R. (1951/1973). The Cantian idiolect: An analysis of the Chinese spoken by a twenty-eight-month-old child. In C. A. Ferguson and D. I. Slobin (Eds.), *Studies of child language development* (pp. 13–33). New York: Holt, Rinehart and Winston.

Chen, P. (1999). *Modern Chinese: History and sociolinguistics.* Cambridge. UK: Cambridge University Press.

Cheng, L. L-R. (2001). Educating speech-language pathologists to work in multicultural populations—An Asian-Pacific perspective. *Speech and Hearing Review, 2*, 192–213.

Chien, C-N., Kao, L., and Li Wei (2004). *A preliminary study on the role of phonological awareness development in young EFL Chinese learners.* Unpublished manuscript.

Clumeck, H. (1977). *Studies in the acquisition of Mandarin phonology.* Unpublished Ph.D. thesis, University of California, Berkeley.

Clumeck, H. (1980). The acquisition of tone. In G. Yeni-Komshian, J. Kavanagh, and C. Ferguson (Eds), *Child phonology 1* (pp. 257–276). New York: Academic Press.

Ha, Ping-an (1996). *Yuyan yu yanyuzhangau lunji.* Beijing: Beijing Capital Normal University Press.

Ho, C. S., and Bryant, P. (1997). Development of phonological awareness of Chinese children in Hong Kong, *Psycholinguistics Research, 26*(1), 109–126.

Holm, A., and Dodd, B. (1996). The effect of first written language on the acquisition of English literacy. *Cognition, 59*, 119–147.

Hsu, J. (1987). *A study of the various stages of development and acquisition of Mandarin Chinese by children in Taiwan milieu.* M.A. dissertation, College of Foreign Languages, Fu Jen Catholic University.

Jeng, Heng-hsiung (1985). A developmentalist view of child phonology. *Studies in Languages and Literature* (periodical published by National Taiwan University), *1*, 1–29.

Li, C. N., and Thompson, S. A. (1977). The acquisition of tone in Mandarin-speaking children. *Journal of Child Language, 4*, 185–199.

Li, C. N., and Thompson, S. A. (1981). *Mandarin Chinese: A functional reference grammar.* Berkeley: University of California Press.

Li, Paul J.-K. (1977). Child language acquisition of Mandarin phonology. In R. Cheng, Y. C. Li, and Ting-chi Tang (Eds.), *Proceedings of the Symposium on Chinese Linguistics: 1977 Linguistic Institute of the Linguistic Society of America.* Taipei: Student Books.

Norman, J. (1988). *Chinese.* Cambridge, UK: Cambridge University Press.

Shiu, Huei-shiou (1990). *The phonological acquisition by Mandarin-speaking children: A longitudinal case study on children from 9 months through three years old.* Unpublished M.A. thesis, Taiwan Normal University.

Su, A.-T. (1985). *The acquisition of Mandarin phonology by Taiwanese children.* M.A. thesis, Fu Jen Catholic University.

Wu, Renyi, and Yin, Binyong (1984). Putonghua shehui diaocha [A survey of Putonghua]. *Wenzi Gaige*, 11, 37–38.

Xu, Fang, and Ha, Ping-An (1992). Articulation disorders among speakers of Mandarin Chinese. *American Journal of Speech-Language Pathology, 1*, 15–16.

Yip, M. (1980). *The tonal phonology of Chinese.* Unpublished Ph.D. thesis, Massachusetts Institute of Technology.

Zhu Hua and Dodd, B. (2000a). The phonological acquisition of Putonghua (Modern Standard Chinese). *Journal of Child Language, 27* (1), 3–42.

Zhu Hua and Dodd, B. (2000b). Putonghua (Modern Standard Chinese)-speaking with speech disorder. *Clinical Linguistics and Phonetics, 14*(3), 165–191.

Zhu Hua (2002). *Phonological development in specific contexts: Studies of Chinese-speaking children.* Clevedon: Multilingual Matters.

Zhu Hua (2006). The normal and disordered phonology of Putonghua [Modern Standard Chinese]-speaking children. In Zhu Hua and B. Dodd (Eds), *Phonological development and disorders: A multilingual perspective* (pp. 81–108). Clevendon: Multilingual Matters.

SUMMARY OF STUDIES OF TYPICAL MANDARIN/PUTONGHUA SPEECH ACQUISITION

Authors	Year	Country	No. of children	Age of children	Information	Data collection
Chao	1951/1973	Mandarin in USA	1 girl	2;4	Phoneme inventory, tone inventory	Longitudinal
Clumeck	1977	Mandarin in USA	1 boy	1;2–2;9	Process of tonal acquisition	Longitudinal
Clumeck	1980	Mandarin in USA	1 boy 1 girl	2;3–3;5 1;10–2;10	Order of acquisition of tones	Longitudinal
Hsu	1987	Mandarin in Taiwan	28	1;0–6;0	Age of acquisition of phoneme and tones	Longitudinal
Jeng	1985	Mandarin in Taiwan	2 boys	0;2–1;8 1;3–2;7	Order of acquisition of phonemes and tones	Longitudinal
Li	1977	Mandarin in Taiwan	1 boy 1 girl	2;0–3;0 1;1–1;8	Order of acquisition of phonemes and tones	Longitudinal

Authors	Year	Country	No. of children	Age of children	Information	Data collection
Li and Thompson	1977	Mandarin in Taiwan	17	1;6–3;0	Order of acquisition of tones & tone sandhi Error patterns	Longitudinal
Shiu	1990	Mandarin in Taiwan	1 boy 1 girl	1;0–3;0 0;7–2;4	Order of acquisition of phonemes and tones Error patterns	Longitudinal
Su	1985	Mandarin in Taiwan	1 boy 1 girl	1;5–2;4 1;2–1;11	Order of acquisition of phonemes and tones Error patterns	Longitudinal
Zhu	2002	Putonghua in Beijing	2 girls, 2 boys	1 girl 1;1–2;1 1 girl 1;2–1;8 1 boy 1;0–2;0 1 boy 0;10–2;1	Order of acquisition of tone & tone sandhi, consonants and vowels Error patterns	Longitudinal
Zhu and Dodd	2000a	Putonghua in Beijing	61 girls + 68 boys	1;6–4;6	Age of acquisition of phonemes Error patterns	Cross-sectional

Acknowledgements

This chapter is based on Zhu Hua (2006).

Chapter 51

Sesotho Speech Acquisition

Katherine Demuth

INTRODUCTION

Sesotho (also called Sotho, or Southern Sotho) is a southern Bantu language spoken in the country of Lesotho and adjacent parts of South Africa. It is one of the Sotho languages, which also include Setswana (or Tswana) and Sepedi (or Northern Sotho), spoken in Botswana and northern South Africa. Although these languages share basic vocabulary and linguistic structure, rendering them "mutually intelligible" with some effort, they also have many segmental, tonal, morphological, and syntactic differences, and are considered separate languages, having their own dictionaries and grammars. They constitute three of the 11 official languages of South Africa. Another three of South Africa's official languages come from the Nguni group of Bantu languages (including Xhosa, Zulu, and Swazi). Sotho and Nguni languages are related to other Bantu languages, such as Swahili, spoken throughout East Africa.

With the exception of Sepedi, all of the languages mentioned above, plus Isangu (Gabon), Chichewa (Malawai), and Kigiriama (Kenya), have been the subject of some language acquisition research, generally focusing on morphosyntactic acquisition (e.g., Connelly, 1984; Deen, 2002; Demuth, 1992; Kunene, 1979; Suzman, 1991; Tsonope, 1987), see Demuth (2003) for a review. Phonological studies examining the acquisition of segments have mostly focused on Xhosa and Zulu (e.g., Gxilishe, 2004; Lewis, 1994; Lewis and Roux, 1996; Mowrer and Burger, 1991; Naidoo, 2003; Tuomi, Gxilishe, and Matomela, 2001). However, the most well-studied language to date is Sesotho. This language will therefore be the focus of this chapter. The data are primarily drawn from publications based on 98 hours of longitudinal spontaneous speech samples from four children aged 2;1 to 4;7 in rural Lesotho (see the Demuth Sesotho Corpus, http://childes.psy.cmu.edu/).

The study of Bantu language acquisition is interesting for several reasons. First, there are approximately 500 Bantu languages, each with slightly different linguistic structures. This provides an ideal laboratory for understanding the nature of language development. Second, many speakers of these languages grow up with bilingual or multilingual experience (Penn, 1998), raising questions regarding the nature of children's linguistic abilities in the case of language delay (e.g., Demuth and Suzman, 1997). It is therefore imperative that information regarding normative monolingual development be available to practitioners working with such children. However, as will be seen, such work is all too often unavailable. It is hoped that this chapter may stimulate others to take this research further (Alcock, Rimba, Abubakar, and Holding, 2005; Suzman, 2002). See the Resources section for materials pertaining to Sesotho.

Where Sesotho is spoken

Sesotho is spoken in the country of Lesotho and adjacent parts of South Africa (see accompanying map and Appendix D).

Components of Sesotho

Consonants

Sesotho has a rich inventory of 40 consonants, including an extensive array of affricates, laterals, and syllabic nasals. Sesotho also exhibits phonemic use of aspiration, and has one click (see Table 51-1).

Vowels

Many Bantu languages have five or seven vowels. Sesotho has nine vowels, with three different heights of mid vowels (see Table 51-2).

Phonotactic restrictions

Syllables

As in many other Bantu languages, most Sesotho syllables exhibit basic CV structure. However, the possible Sesotho syllable structures include (C)(G)V, or a syllabic consonant (nasal or /l/). Vowel-initial syllables and words are permitted, though not common, most consisting of English or Afrikaans loanwords. Sesotho also permits syllabic liquids

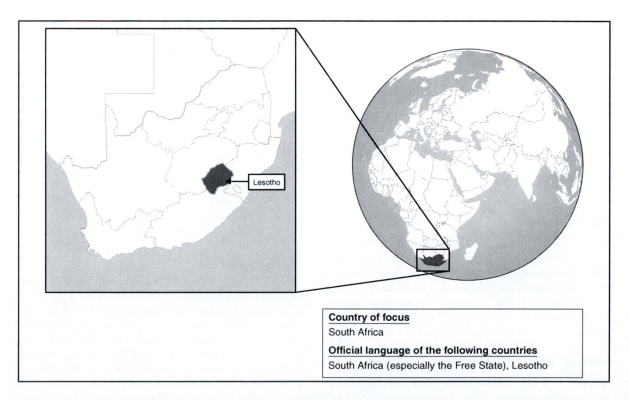

Country of focus
South Africa

Official language of the following countries
South Africa (especially the Free State), Lesotho

TABLE 51-1 Consonants produced in Sesotho

	Bilabial	Labiodental	Dental	Alveolar
Plosive	pʼ pʰ b			tʼ tʰ d
Nasal	m m̥			n n̩
Trill				r
Tap or flap				
Fricative		f [v]		s
Lateral fricative	■■■			ɬ
Affricate				tsʼ tsʰ tɬʼ tɬʰ
Approximant	(w) (labiovelar)			
Lateral approximant	■■■			l ɭ
Consonants (non-pulmonic)				
Coarticulated consonants	pʃʼ pʃʰ bʒ	fʃ		

Key. Consonants in parentheses indicate alternative place of articulation, and consonants in square brackets appear in loanwords.

Black = articulations judged impossible

Based on the International Phonetic Alphabet. Courtesy of the International Phonetic Association (c/o Department of Linguistics, University of Victoria, Victoria, British Columbia, Canada).

(e.g., *mamello* /mamɛlɔ/ 'patience') and nonmorphemic syllabic nasals, which can be found word-initially (e.g., *ntja* /n̩tja/ 'dog'), word-medially (e.g., *banna* /ban̩na/ 'men'), and word-finally (e.g., *ratang* /ratan̩/ 'love! pl.') (Doke and Mofokeng, 1985).

Consonants and consonant clusters

Glides can occur as part of a complex onset (e.g., *ngwana* /ŋwana/ 'child'). All other consonant clusters (and word-final consonants) found in English and Afrikaans words introduced into Sesotho are adapted to obey the basic CV syllable structure of the language by using vowel epenthesis (e.g., *school* ⇨ *sekolo*) (Rose and Demuth, in press).

Tones

Sesotho uses High and Low (default) tones to mark both lexical and grammatical meaning. Verbs have either High or Low basic tone, and this tone may change in the context of certain grammatical morphemes (e.g., subject markers) and the tense/mood of the sentence to produce a specific tonal pattern or tonal melody (Demuth, 1993, 1995a). These processes of tone change are called tone sandhi.

Stress and intonation

Sesotho does not have stress like English, but lengthens the penultimate syllable of a phonological phrase. Thus, the greeting for one person is *Lumela!* /dumɛːla/, and the greeting for more than one person is *Lumelang!* /dumɛlaːŋ/, where the final syllable is a syllabic nasal. Lengthening therefore shifts to the penultimate syllable. This is independent of the tone on the penultimate syllable, which may be either High or Low.

The tonal system of Sesotho exhibits gradual down drift, with sentence-initial Low tones being higher than sentence-final High tones in a declarative sentence. However, in an interrogative sentence, down drift and penultimate lengthening are both attenuated, giving the impression of a quicker, flat contour. Although shifts in word order or a choice of different lexical items are typically used for contrastive focus, this can also be achieved by employing excessive lengthening and extreme raising of the overall pitch register of the focal lexical item(s).

Writing system

Several different orthographic conventions were used by different missionaries in the 1800s and early 1900s, resulting in no marking of tone, all mid vowels being written with the graphemes 'e' and 'o', and the palatal-alveolar click written as 'q'. Today, Lesotho uses one set of orthographic conventions, and South Africa another. The major segmental difference between the two systems is that in Lesotho orthography, phonemic /l/ is used for the [d] allophonic variant before high vowels

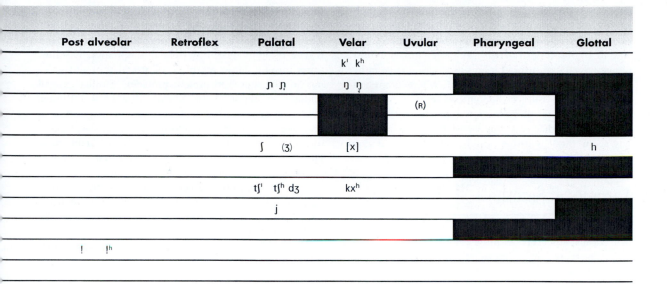

Post alveolar	Retroflex	Palatal	Velar	Uvular	Pharyngeal	Glottal
			kʼ kʰ			
		ɲ ɲ̊	ŋ ŋ̊			
				(ʀ)		
ʃ	(ʒ)		[x]			h
		tʃʼ tʃʰ dʒ	kxʰ			
		j				
ǃ ǃʰ						

TABLE 51-2 Vowels produced in Sesotho compared with General American English

American English location	American English Vowels Smit (2004)	American English examples	Sesotho location	Sesotho vowels (Doke and Mofokeng, 1985)	Sesotho examples
High-front	i	b<u>ea</u>t	High-front	i	'b<u>i</u>na' *sing*
	ɪ	b<u>i</u>t	Mid-high close	ι	'b<u>e</u>la' *boil*
	e	r<u>ai</u>d	Mid-front	e	'b<u>e</u>sa' *roast*
Mid-low front	ɛ	b<u>e</u>d	Mid-low open	ɛ	'b<u>ea</u>' *put*
	æ	b<u>a</u>d			
High-back, rounded	u	bl<u>ue</u>	High-back, rounded	u	'b<u>ua</u>' *talk*
	ʊ	b<u>oo</u>k	Mid-high back close, rounded	ω	'b<u>o</u>tsa' *ask*
Mid-back, rounded	o	b<u>oa</u>t	Mid-back, rounded	o	'b<u>o</u>nya' *flirt*
	ɔ	f<u>o</u>rm	Mid-low back, open, rounded	ɔ	'b<u>o</u>fa' *tie, bind*
Low back	ɑ	dr<u>o</u>p	Low, mid-back	ɑ	'b<u>a</u>tla' *look for*

(e.g., /li/ is pronounced [di]), and the mid vowel graphemes 'e' and 'o' are used for front and back glides /j/ and /w/, respectively. In addition, Lesotho 'ch', 'kh', 'tš', 'n', and 'm' = South African 'tjh', 'kg', 'tsh', 'nn', and 'mm', respectively. Both orthographies use a disjunctive rather than a conjunctive writing system, where grammatical morphemes (subject agreement, tense, pronominal object, verbs) are all written as separate words rather than together, that is, *ke tla li reka* vs. *ketlalireka* 'I will buy them' (lit. 'I will them buy'), as is the case in Zulu and Swahili.

Varieties of Sesotho

Sesotho is considered to be relatively homogeneous dialectically, especially within Lesotho. Even in Lesotho, however, there are some ideolectal differences with respect to tone sandhi (tonal changes). Sesotho as spoken in South Africa contains another tonal rule, shows the influence of Setswana in the tense/aspect system, and contains more loanwords from Afrikaans. 'Deep Sesotho', or *Sesotho se tebileng*, is a more formal speech register used for special purposes such as storytelling. This more ritualized use of Sesotho, as well as a more extensive vocabulary containing words for traditional foods and so forth, is generally maintained in rural areas by older generations, but it is being lost by the young and the urban. There are also an increasing number of lexical items from English, Afrikaans, Zulu, and other languages as there is more contact with these languages.

Typical acquisition of Sesotho

Due to the simple syllable structure of Sesotho, most consonants and vowels are acquired by the age of 2,

though problems with the labial glides and simplification of affricates and clicks persist until 3 (Demuth, 1992). The consonant /h/ is sometimes reduced, though this is true of adult speech as well, and aspiration is sometimes missing. However, place of articulation and voicing do not appear to present problems. Similar general findings are reported for Xhosa (Mowrer and Burger, 1991; Tuomi et al., 2001), along with late acquisition of prenasalized stops, which Sesotho does not have. Lexical tone is acquired early on Sesotho words with stable tone. However, tone sandhi processes are still being acquired at the age of 3. Like other Bantu languages, Sesotho has a rich noun class agreement system with extensive agglutinative morphology. Many of these monosyllabic morphemes are missing or reduced at 2, but are generally well formed by 3 (Demuth, 1988, 1994). The Summary of Studies table at the end of this chapter contains studies of the acquisition of Sesotho.

Acquired sounds

Consonants

Most simple consonants have been acquired by the age of 2 (Demuth, 1992); see Table 51-3. This includes syllabic nasals and voicing distinctions on labial and alveolar stops. The placement of /r/ is generally toward the back of the mouth (uvular) rather than trilled. Coarticulated sounds are typically simplified, though these are rare, and seldom appear in children's speech. The consonant [d] is an allophone of /l/ that appears only in the environment before the high vowels /i/ and /u/. Due either to its restricted (and less frequent) distribution, or to the lack of having learned the phonological rule for its use, [d] is occasionally realized as [l] until 3. Word-internally, especially after a velar nasal, /w/ may be omitted until the age of 3. The lateral

TABLE 51-3 Age of acquisition for Sesotho consonants

Consonant	Connelly (1984)	Demuth (1989)	Demuth (1992)
most consonants			2;0
/tɬ'/, /tɬʰ/			2;6
/ts'/, /tsʰ/			2;6
/w/		2;6	2;6
/r/			3;0
[d] (allophone of /l/)			3;0
/ǃ/, /ǃʰ/	3;0		3;0

affricates /tɬ/ and /ts/ are often simplified to /t/, preserving aspiration. The most problematic consonant for Sesotho-speaking children is the palatal-alveolar click /!/. Although it is spontaneously produced in isolation as early as 2;6, it is realized as /k/ within a word until around the age of 3, appropriately preserving aspiration. The later acquisition of clicks in context is probably due to the difficulty of coarticulating this consonant with a following vowel. Similar findings are reported for the three Xhosa clicks (dental 'c' /|/, palatal-alveolar 'q' /!/, and lateral /ǁ/); the palatal-alveolar and dental clicks are produced with 50–69 percent accuracy by the age of 3 (Mowrer and Burger, 1991; Tuomi et al., 2001), and all (including prenasalized clicks) are mastered by 4 (Lewis, 1994). However, the first clicks appear earlier in Xhosa (1 to 1;6) than in Sesotho, probably due to the higher frequency of clicks in that language, 15 percent of lexical items (Gxilishe, 2004).

Consonant clusters

As noted, Sesotho has no true consonant clusters. However, when /w/ is part of a complex syllable onset, it is often deleted (e.g., *ngoana* /ŋwana/ [nana] 'child') (Demuth, 1992). English loanwords with word-initial sC clusters are sometimes produced as a cluster by both adults and children, indicating possible syllable structure change due to extensive contact with English and Afrikaans (e.g., *sekolo* /sɪkolo/ [**skolo**] 'school') (Rose and Demuth, 2006).

Vowels

Little is known about the acquisition of Sesotho vowels. There is some evidence that children may have some difficulty in producing some of the finer distinctions in vowel height (e.g., *rona* /rʊna/ [runa] 'we'), but there has been no systematic study of this issue. Word-final vowels in Sesotho can also tend to be devoiced, and children sometimes omit these altogether.

Percent correct

Consonants

There are no studies with percentages of accuracy on consonant production for Sesotho. However, since Sesotho syllable structure is simple, most consonants appear to be acquired early (Connelly, 1984). The nearest estimate is presented in Table 51-4. Mowrer and Burger (1991) report similar early segmental acquisition for Xhosa: 80 percent at 3 years, compared with 40 percent for English.

TABLE 51-4 Percent correct for Sesotho consonants and vowels

Age	Consonants	Vowels
2;0	75 percent	75 percent
2;6	80 percent	80 percent
3;0	90 percent	90 percent
4;0	100 percent	100 percent

Vowels

There are no studies with percentages of accuracy on vowel production for Sesotho. However, since Sesotho does not have any diphthongs, vowel acquisition seems to be achieved relatively early. The nearest estimate, based on Demuth (1992), is presented in Table 51-4.

Phonological processes

Sesotho has several phonological processes that still cause children problems at 3 years and beyond. Labial palatalization is used in the derivation of some passives (*shapa* /ʃapa/ > *shatjoa* /ʃatʃwa/ 'lash' ⇨ 'be lashed'), and is rarely used correctly by 3. Strengthening processes take place in the environment of a nasal, such as with the first person singular object marker, where voiced plosives become voiceless ejectives (/b/ ⇨ [p'], /l/ ⇨ [t']) and fricatives become aspirated obstruents (/f/ ⇨ [pʰ], /r/ ⇨ [tʰ], /s/ ⇨ [tsʰ], etc.) (Doke and Mofokeng, 1985). Some of these forms, especially frequent imperatives like *mphe* [m̩pʰɛ] (from /ŋ + fa/) 'give me' (lit. 'me-give') are learned early as a lexical unit. However, the productivity of this phonological process is probably not complete for many children by the age of 4. Sesotho does not have the phoneme /d/; it occurs only as an allophone of /l/ after high vowels. Children between the ages of 2 and 3 years do not consistently produce the allophone [d] before high vowels, in either initial or medial position.

Sesotho also has a system of vowel harmony, where mid vowels are raised in certain phonological environments. Thus, the mid open vowel (*reka* /rɛka/ 'buy') is raised to a mid vowel when followed by a high vowel /i/ (*rekile* /rekile/ 'have bought'). Little is known about when Sesotho-speaking children acquire the rules governing vowel harmony. Like children learning many other languages, Sesotho-speaking children exhibit productive processes of consonant harmony (e.g., *Tlokoeng* /tɬokweŋ/ ⇨ [kokeŋ] 'name of a town'; *ke tla etsa*

/kʊ tɬ'a ets'a/ ⇨ [ts'a ets'a] 'I will do (it)'. These examples also show evidence of glide simplification, and a missing/ coalesced subject marker. Both are typical of Sesotho speech around 2;6 years.

Intelligibility

Despite a few problems with some complex segments, missing morphemes, and tone, Sesotho-speaking 2-year-olds are generally intelligible.

Phonetic inventory

With the exception of the trilled /r/, affricates /tɬ/ and /ts/, the click, /!/, and coarticulated consonants, Sesotho-speaking children appear to have a full phonemetic inventory by 2;6 (Demuth, 1992).

Common mismatches

The trilled /r/ is often replaced by its uvular counterpart. The affricates /tɬ/ and /ts/ are typically realized as /t/, and the click /!/ is realized as /k/, often preserving ejective or aspirated status.

Syllable structure

Glides occurring as part of the syllable onset may be deleted until 3. Word-medial and word-final syllabic nasals may be syllabified as coda consonants, though this requires further investigation.

Prosody

Sesotho-speaking 2-year-olds seem to have learned that the penultimate syllable of a phonological phrase is lengthened. However, the degree of lengthening may be shorter than that of adults, leading to a lack of falling tone on the penultimate syllable in certain contexts (Demuth, 1993, 1995a). Declarative/interrogative intonation is generally produced by 2;0 to 2;6.

Tonal development

The acquisition of fixed lexical tones (High and Low) appears to be completed by the age of 2. However, the rules governing tone sandhi (i.e., tonal change in context, such as the lowering of an underlying High tone when preceded by another underlying High tone in the same prosodic domain) are learned only by the age of 3. This especially affects the first tone of verbs, which at 2 years tends to be produced with High tone, even if the verb is lexically Low. Less is known about the acquisition of grammatical tonal melodies, which distinguish,

for example, the affirmative, negative, and subjunctive (Demuth, 1993, 1995a).

Phonological awareness

There is little research on Sesotho-speaking children's phonological awareness. However, 3-year-olds often shift to different speech registers when playing house, talking to their newborn siblings, or interacting with nonnative speakers (Demuth, 1992).

Speech assessment for Sesotho-speaking children

There is little in the way of speech assessment tools for Sesotho or any other southern Bantu language. Preliminary tests of the *MacArthur Communicative Development Inventory* (CDI) (Fenson et al., 1993) are being developed for Swahili and Kigiriama (Alcock et al., 2005). This may be adaptable to other Bantu languages, though vocabulary items will vary depending on the country and climate and on urban/rural context.

There are no standardized tests for assessing Sesotho-speaking children's speech sounds.

Speech sampling tools that have been developed for use with Sesotho-speaking children include the following:

- Spontaneous speech interactions with family members and peers (e.g., Demuth, 1989, 1990).
- Elicited production tasks focusing on specific grammatical constructions (Demuth, Machobane, and Moloi, 2003; Demuth, Machobane, Moloi, and Odato, 2005).

The following analyses have been designed for analyzing Sesotho speech:

- Quantitative analysis of morphological development in spontaneous speech (Ziesler and Demuth, 1995).
- Quantitative analysis of syntactic development using both spontaneous speech and elicited production tasks (Demuth, 1995b; Demuth et al., 2003; Demuth et al., 2005).

Speech intervention for Sesotho-speaking children

To date, no speech intervention techniques have been developed for Sesotho or any other southern Bantu language.

Working in Lesotho and South Africa

Working in Lesotho and South Africa has many challenges, but also many opportunities. Under-five clinics and preschools exist in much of Lesotho, even in rural areas, and the same is true in many parts of South Africa. Most parents are generally interested in their children's language development. Many who can afford to do so enroll their children in English-medium preschools to ensure that good English language skills are acquired early, because they are the key to later economic success. This makes documentation of normative monolingual development of Sesotho, as well as that of the other South African Bantu languages, all the more pressing.

PHONETICALLY SPEAKING

Pronunciation of Sesotho: /sɪsʊtʰʊ/

Relevant words for speech assessment and intervention

Word	Formal usage	Pronunciation
Tongue	*leleme*	/lɪlɪmɪ/
Teeth	*meno*	/mɪnɔ/
Lips	*melomo*	/mɪlomʊ/
Hard palate	*lehalapa*	/lɪhalapa/
Soft palate	*leshano*	/lɪshanʊ/
Larynx	*kolu*	/kolu/
Lungs	*matšoafo*	/matsʰwafʊ/
Nose	*nko*	/ŋ̩kɔ/
Sound	*molumo*	/mʊdumɔ/
Word	*lentsoe*	/lɪntswe/
Sentence	*polelo*	/pʊlɛlo/
Paragraph	*seratsoana*	/sɪratswana/

RESOURCES

Books

Doke, C. M., and Mofokeng, S. M. (1985). *Textbook of Southern Sotho grammar*. Cape Town, South Africa: Longman.

Paroz, R. A. (1974). *Southern Sotho-English dictionary*. Morija: Morija Printing Works.

Journals

- *South African Journal of African Languages* publishes articles on all aspects of African language research, including occasional papers on language acquisition.
- *The South African Journal of Communication Disorders* publishes articles on all aspects of communication disorders.
- *Southern African Linguistics and Applied Language Studies*, http://www.ingenta.com/, publishes articles on a wide range of linguistic and applied linguistic topics

(e.g., syntax, phonology, semantics, sociolinguistics, language teaching, language policy). Acts as a forum for research into all the languages of southern Africa, including English and Afrikaans.

Professional associations

The South African Speech-Language-Hearing Association (SASLHA), www.saslha.co.za/

Useful Sesotho Web sites

- *Sesotho Web Page*, http://www.sesotho.web.za/
- *Ethnologue*, http://www.ethnologue.com/show_language.asp?code=sot
- *National African Language Research Center*, http://lang.nalrc.wisc.edu/nalrc/prog-serv/mat-dev/mat-dev.html
- *Nation Master – Sesotho*, http://www.nationmaster.com/encyclopedia/Sesotho-language/

REFERENCES

Alcock, K. J., Rimba, K., Abubakar, A., and Holding, P. (2005). *First words, nouns, and verbs – data from two East African languages.* Paper presented at the 10th International Association for the Study of Child Language, Berlin.

Connelly, M. (1984). *Basotho children's acquisition of noun morphology.* Unpublished Ph.D. dissertation, University of Essex, UK.

Deen, K. U. (2002). *The acquisition of Nairobi Swahili: The morphosyntax of inflectional prefixes and subjects.* Unpublished doctoral dissertation, University of California at Los Angeles.

Demuth, K. (1988). Noun classes and agreement in Sesotho acquisition. In M. Barlow and C. A. Ferguson (Eds.), *Agreement in natural language: Approaches, theories, descriptions* (pp. 305–321). Stanford, CA: Stanford University Center for the Study of Language and Information.

Demuth, K. (2003). The acquisition of Bantu languages. In D. Nurse and G. Phillipson (Eds.), *The Bantu languages.* (pp. 209–222). Surrey, UK: Curzon Press.

Demuth, K., and Suzman, S. (1997). Language impairment in Zulu. In E. M. Hughes and A. Green (Eds.), *Proceedings of the 21st Annual Boston University Conference on Language Development* (Vol. 1, pp. 124–135). Somerville, MA: Cascadilla Press.

Demuth, K. (1989). Maturation and the acquisition of Sesotho passive. *Language, 65,* 56–80.

Demuth, K. (1990). Subject, topic and the Sesotho passive. *Journal of Child Language, 17,* 67–84.

Demuth, K. (1992). Acquisition of Sesotho. In D. Slobin (Ed.), *The cross-linguistic study of language acquisition* (Vol. 3, pp. 557–638), Hillsdale, NJ: Lawrence Erlbaum.

Demuth, K. (1993). Issues in the acquisition of the Sesotho tonal system. *Journal of Child Language 20,* 275–301.

Demuth, K. (1994). On the 'underspecification' of functional categories in early grammars. In B. Lust, M. Suñer, and J. Whitman (Eds.), *Syntactic theory and first language acquisition: Cross-linguistic perspectives* (pp. 119–134). Hillsdale, NJ: Lawrence Erlbaum.

Demuth, K. (1995a). Problems in the acquisition of tonal systems. In J. Archibald (Ed.), *The acquisition of non-linear phonology* (pp. 111–134). Hillsdale, NJ: Lawrence Erlbaum.

Demuth, K. (1995b). Questions, relatives, and minimal projection. *Language Acquisition, 4,* 49–71.

Demuth, K. (1996). The prosodic structure of early words. In J. Morgan and K. Demuth (Eds.), *Signal to syntax: Bootstrapping from speech to grammar in early acquisition* (pp. 171–184). Mahwah, NJ: Lawrence Erlbaum.

Demuth, K., Machobane, M., and Moloi, F. (2003). Rules and construction effects in learning the argument structure of verbs. *Journal of Child Language, 30*, 1–25.

Demuth, K., Machobane, M., Moloi, F., and Odato, C. (2005). Learning animacy hierarchy effects in Sesotho double object applicatives. *Language, 81* (2), 421–447.

Doke, C. M., and Mofokeng, S. M. (1985). *Textbook of Southern Sotho grammar*. Cape Town, South Africa: Longman.

Fenson, L., Dale, P. A., Reznick, J. S., Thal, D., Bates, E., Hartung, J., Pethick, S., and Reilly, J. S. (1993). *MacArthur Communicative Development Inventories: User's Guide and Technical Manual*. San Diego, CA: Singular.

Gxilishe, S. (2004). The acquisition of clicks by Xhosa-speaking children, *Per Linguam 20*, 1–12.

Kunene, E. (1979). *The acquisition of Swati as a first language: A morphological study with special reference to noun prefixes, noun classes and some agreement markers*. Unpublished Ph.D. dissertation, University of California at Los Angeles.

Lewis, P. W. (1994). *Aspects of the phonological acquisition of clicks in Xhosa*. Unpublished MA thesis, University of Stellenbosch, South Africa.

Lewis, P. W., and Roux, J. C. (1996). A phonological process analysis of the acquisition and loss of clicks in Xhosa, *South African Journal of African Languages, 16*, 1–7.

Mowrer, D. E., and Burger, S. (1991). A comparative analysis of phonological acquisition of consonants in the speech of 21/2–6-year-old Xhosa- and English-speaking children. *Clinical Linguistics and Phonetics, 3*, 139–164.

Naidoo, Y. (2003). *A developmental profile of speech sound and syllable in Zulu speaking children*. Unpublished master's dissertation, University of Pretoria, South Africa.

Penn, C. (1998). The study of child language in South Africa. *Folia Phoniatrica et Logopaedica 50*, 256–270.

Rose, Y., and Demuth, K. (2006). Vowel epenthesis in loanword adaptation: Representational and phonetic considerations. *Lingua, 116*, 1112–1139.

Suzman, S. (1991). *The acquisition of Zulu*. Unpublished Ph.D. dissertation, Witwatersrand University, Johannesburg, South Africa.

Suzman, S. (2002). Morphological accessibility in Zulu. In E. Fava (Ed.), *Clinical linguistics theory and applications in speech pathology and therapy* (pp. 155–174). *Current issues in linguistic theory 227*. Amsterdam: John Benjamins.

Tsonope, J. (1987). *The acquisition of Tswana noun class and agreement morphology, with special reference to demonstratives and possessives*. Unpublished Ph.D. dissertation, State University of New York, Buffalo.

Tuomi, S. K., Gxilishe, S., and Matomela, L. (2001). The acquisition of Xhosa phonemes. *Per Linguam, 17*, 14–23.

Ziesler, Y., and Demuth, K. (1995). Noun class prefixes in Sesotho child-directed speech. In E. Clark (Ed.), *Proceedings of the 26th Child Language Research Forum* (pp. 137–146). Stanford, CA: Center for the Study of Language and Information.

SUMMARY OF STUDIES OF TYPICAL SESOTHO SPEECH ACQUISITION

Authors	Year	Country	No. of children	Age of children	Information	Sample type	Data collection
Connelly	1984	UK	4	1;6–4;2	Noun class prefixes, clicks	Spontaneous speech corpora	Semi-longitudinal
Demuth	1988	USA	4	2;1–4;7	Noun class prefixes	Spontaneous speech corpora	Longitudinal
Demuth	1992	USA	4	2;1–4;7	Overall grammatical development, review of Bantu acquisition	Spontaneous speech corpora	Longitudinal
Demuth	1993	USA	1	2;1–3;2	Tonal development	Spontaneous speech corpora	Longitudinal

Authors	Year	Country	No. of children	Age of children	Information	Sample type	Data collection
Demuth	1994	USA	4	2;1–4;7	Prosodic constraints on nominal morphology	Spontaneous speech corpora	Longitudinal
Demuth	1995	USA	1	2;1–3;2	Tonal development	Spontaneous speech corpora	Longitudinal
Demuth	1996	USA	4	2;1–4;7	Prosodic constraints on word shape	Spontaneous speech corpora	Longitudinal
Demuth	2003	USA	4	2;1–4;7	Overall grammatical development, review of Bantu acquisition	Spontaneous speech corpora	Longitudinal
Demuth, Machobane, Moloi and Odato	2005	USA	100	3–12 yrs	Verb-argument structure	Experiments	Cross-sectional

Chapter 52

Spanish Speech Acquisition

Brian A. Goldstein

INTRODUCTION

Modern Spanish, as with all Romance languages, traces its roots to Latin. What we know as Spanish today diverged sharply from Latin in the thirteenth century when writers codified the vernacular pronunciation of Castilians during that time (Penny, 1991). Castile's literary, cultural, and scientific dominance of southern Spain served to spread that particular vernacular throughout all of the Iberian peninsula. Penny notes that the dialect of Seville also held considerable influence at the time due to that city's size and economic power. In the fifteenth and sixteenth centuries, Spanish was taken from the Iberian peninsula to other parts of the world by Spanish explorers, soldiers, settlers, priests, colonial administrators, and so on (Penny, 1991). Fifty years after Columbus landed in what now is the Dominican Republic, Spain was firmly established in the Americas with Castilian established as the dominant dialect of the language (Bedore, 1999). In the early nineteenth century, Spain was losing control over its territories in the Americas. By the end of that century, Spain no longer controlled Venezuela, Colombia, Ecuador, Peru, Bolivia, Florida, Mexico, and territories that eventually became part of the United States (e.g., California, Arizona, and New Mexico; Bedore, 1999). The Resources section of this chapter contains materials about Spanish.

Where Spanish is spoken

Currently, Spanish is the primary language for speakers in approximately 44 countries and is the third most commonly spoken language in the world with approximately 322 million speakers, excluding another 112 million people who speak Spanish as a second language (Grimes, 2002; see accompanying map and Appendix D).

Components of Spanish

Consonants

General Spanish has 18 phonemes (Hammond, 2001). These are presented in Table 52-1.

The three voiced stops /b, d, g/ are in complementary distribution with the spirants [β] (voiced biliabial), [ð] (voiced interdental), and [ɣ] (voiced velar), respectively. The spirant allophones most generally occur intervocalically both within and across word boundaries (e.g., /dedo/ 'finger' ⇨ [deðo]; /la boka/ 'the mouth' ⇨ [la βoka]) and in word-internal consonant clusters (e.g., /tigɾe/ 'tiger' ⇨ [tiɣɾe]).

Spanish also contains a large number of syllable-onset consonant clusters (e.g., /pl/ in /**pl**ato/) and word-internal abutting consonant pairs (e.g., /nt/ in /elefa**nt**e/). In the spoken Spanish of adults (Iglesias, Cohen, Gutierrez-Clellen, and Marcano, 1983), the most common initial consonant clusters are /pɾ/ *pronto*, /tɾ/ *tren*, /gɾ/ *grácias*, /kl/ *clavo*, /kɾ/ *cruz*, /pl/ *plato*, /fɾ/ *frío*, /bɾ/ *bruja*, /dɾ/ *dragón*, /bl/ *blanco*. The most commonly occurring abutting consonant pairs are /nt/ *elefante*, /st/ *estrella*, /nd/ *corriendo*, /ns/ *gansa*, /sp/ *después*, /ɾt/ *carta*, /ɾk/ *parque*, /ɾm/ *duermo*, /ɾs/ *universidad*, /mb/ *ambos*. Iglesias et al. (1983) found that approximately 25 percent of the words spoken by adult Spanish speakers contained either an onset cluster or an abutting consonant pair.

Vowels

Spanish has a basic five-phonemic vowel system (see Table 52-2). Vowels in Spanish have *relatively* the same tongue height and tongue placement as their counterparts in English with the exception of /a/, which in Spanish is usually described as a low, central vowel (Cotton and Sharp, 1988).

Phonotactic restrictions
Syllables

The syllable structure of Spanish is relatively noncomplex compared to languages such as English. The basic syllable structure of Spanish can be described as $C_{(0-2)}VC_{(0-2)}$. A single Spanish syllable contains, at most, five elements (e.g., [**klien**$te] *clien-te*) (Harris, 1983). Spanish syllables are composed of the following types:

1. V ([**a**] *a*)
2. VC ([**al**$go] *algo*)
3. CV ([**tu**] *tu*)
4. CVC ([**dos**] *dos*)
5. CCV ([**pla**$to] *plato*)
6. CCVC ([**plan**$ta] *planta*)
7. VCC ([**abs**$tɾak$to] *abstracto*)
8. CVCC ([**mons**$tɾuo] *monstruo*)

The most common syllable type is the CV syllable, followed by the CVC syllable (Navarro, 1968); thus open

TABLE 52-1 Consonants produced in Spanish

	Bilabial	Labiodental	Dental	Alveolar
Plosive	p b			t d
Nasal	m			n
Trill				r
Tap or flap				ɾ
Fricative		f		s
Affricate				
Lateral fricative	■			
Approximant	w (labiovelar)			
Lateral approximant	■			l

Black = articulations judged impossible

Based on the International Phonetic Alphabet. Courtesy of the International Phonetic Association (c/o Department of Linguistics, University of Victoria, Victoria, British Columbia, Canada).

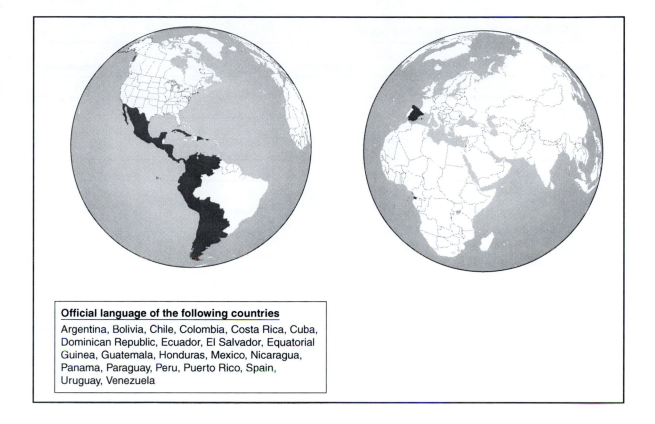

Official language of the following countries

Argentina, Bolivia, Chile, Colombia, Costa Rica, Cuba, Dominican Republic, Ecuador, El Salvador, Equatorial Guinea, Guatemala, Honduras, Mexico, Nicaragua, Panama, Paraguay, Peru, Puerto Rico, Spain, Uruguay, Venezuela

syllables are far more common than closed syllables. In terms of syllable number, multisyllabic words (e.g., *bo-ca*) are more numerous overall than monosyllabic words (e.g., *en*) (Iglesias et al., 1983). In fact, there are very few content words in Spanish that are monosyllabic (Vernon and Ferreiro, 1999).

Post alveolar	Retroflex	Palatal	Velar	Uvular	Pharyngeal	Glottal
			k g			
		ɲ				
			x			
tʃ						
		j				

TABLE 52-2   Vowel phonemic inventory of General Spanish

Description	Phoneme	Example	Spanish orthography	English translation
High-front	/i/	/hilo/	hilo	'thread'
Mid-front	/e/	/tren/	tren	'train'
Low-central	/a/	/plato/	plato	'plate'
High-back	/u/	/kutʃara/	cuchara	'spoon'
Mid-back	/o/	/sopa/	sopa	'soup'

Consonants and consonant clusters

The phonetic inventory of Spanish differs from that of English. Spanish contains some sounds that are not part of the English phonetic system. Sounds in Spanish that are not included in the phonetic inventory of English are the following:

- Voiced palatal nasal [ɲ] as in [niɲo] 'boy'
- Voiceless bilabial fricative [ɸ] as in [emɸeɾmo] 'sick'
- Voiceless velar fricative [x] as in [relox] 'watch'
- Voiced spirants [β] as in [klaβo] 'nail' and [ɣ] as in [laɣo] 'lake'
- Alveolar trill [r] as in [pero] 'dog'
- Voiced uvular trill [ʀ] as in [ʀoto] 'broken'

English also contains sounds that do not exist in Spanish. Consonant sounds not in the inventory of Spanish include:

- Aspirated stops (e.g., [pʰ] as in [pʰɛn] 'pen')
- Velar nasal (e.g., [ŋ] as in [sʌŋ] 'sung')
- Fricatives ([v] as in [vot] 'vote'; [θ] as in [mæθ] 'math'; [ʃ] as in [ʃu] 'shoe'; [ʒ] as in [mɛʒɚ] 'measure')
- Affricate (e.g., [dʒ] as in [dʒʌmp] 'jump')
- Liquid (e.g., [ɹ] as in [ɹid] 'read').

Some of the sounds listed above, [ŋ], [v], [θ], [ʃ], [ʒ], and [dʒ], do appear in the phonetic inventories of some Spanish dialects (Núñez-Cedeño and Morales-Front, 1999). It is important to consider the differences in phonetic inventories across Spanish dialects because they affect the consonant inventory more than the vowel inventory.

Tones

Spanish does not use tones to differentiate meaning.

Stress and intonation

Phonology encompasses not only segmental and syllabic features of a language (i.e., consonants, vowels, syllable types, and syllable number) but also nonsegmental aspects (i.e., stress, pitch, and intonation). Spanish is considered a syllable-timed language in which there is a recurrence of syllables, rather than stress, at regular intervals (Ladefoged, 2001). Thus, in general, there is more of a duration difference between stressed and unstressed syllables in stress-timed languages than in syllable-timed languages. In comparison to stress-timed languages (e.g., German, English), there may be an effect on syllable duration in syllable-timed languages as well. For example, stressed syllables in Spanish are 1.2 to 1.3 times longer than unstressed syllables compared with English in which stressed syllables are 1.5 times longer, on average, than unstressed syllables (Delattre, 1965). The effects of syllable length are particularly noticeable in utterance-medial, open syllables (e.g., *la persona fue a la tienda*). In those types of syllables, Spanish stressed syllables (e.g., *fue* in the example sentence) are only 1.1 times longer than unstressed syllables (e.g., *persona* in the example sentence), whereas in English, stressed syllables are 1.6 times longer than unstressed syllables (Dauer, 1983).

Stress in Spanish can occur on the final syllable (e.g., *xamón*), on the penultimate syllable (e.g., *elefante*), or on the antepenultimate syllable (e.g., *música*). The two most common patterns for stress in Spanish are penultimate stress on words ending in vowels and final stress for words ending in consonants (Hochberg, 1988). Pitch also varies as a function of the ambient language being acquired. Overall, pitch does not modulate as much in Spanish as in other languages like English (Hadlich, Holton, and Montes, 1968). Thus, the pitch range is smaller for Spanish speakers than it is for English speakers. In terms of intonation contours in Spanish, utterances begin at a relatively low pitch with the major pitch change usually taking place on the first stressed syllable (Hadlich et al., 1968). For example, in the sentence *voy a la TIENDA*, the sentence begins with a fairly low pitch that is raised on the word *tienda* (the first stressed syllable of the sentence).

Writing system

There are 24 letters in Spanish, 19 single letters (b, c, d, f, g, j, k, l, m, n, ñ, p, q, r, s, t, y, v, z), 3 digraphs or combinations of letters (ch, ll, rr), and 5 vowels (a, e, i, o, u). Spanish orthography is usually considered to be transparent because there is a basic one-to-one correspondence between phoneme and grapheme (González and Valle, 2000; Gutierrez-Clellen, 1999). For example, 'pen', in Spanish, is pronounced as [pluma] and spelled as *pluma*. Even when the form of the word is changed (e.g., from an infinitive *cerrar* to present tense, *cierro*), both pronunciation and spelling remain relatively intact (Goyen, 1989). Researchers have found that children who are acquiring languages with a more transparent orthography (e.g., Spanish) show higher decoding accuracy than children acquiring languages with a less transparent orthography (e.g., English) (Goshami, Gombert, and Fraca de Barrerra, 1998).

There are, of course, exceptions to the one-to-one concept. For example, the word 'blocks', in Spanish, is pronounced as [blokes] but spelled as *bloques*. There are also letters that correspond to more than one pronunciation. For example, the letter "c" may be produced as either [s] as in [sena] *cena* or as [k] as in [kama] *cama*. Spanish spelling also utilizes digraphs that alter the one-to-one correspondence; for example, the digraph "ch" is produced as [tʃ]. The one-to-one correspondence between production and spelling may also be impacted by the dialect of the speaker. There may be less of a one-to-one correspondence between production and spelling for speakers of radical dialects (defined in the next section) who are altering their pronunciations as part of their spoken dialect. For example, the number 'two', in Spanish, is typically pronounced as [dos] and spelled similarly as *dos*. Individuals who aspirate syllable final /s/ may pronounce the word as [doʰ] but must still learn to spell it as *dos*. The same is true for sounds that are substituted for one another. For example, the word 'letter', in Spanish, is generally pronounced as [kaɾta] and written as *carta*. Speakers who pronounce this word as [kalta] or even [katta] must learn to spell it as *carta*. Of course, all speakers must learn to spell exceptional words like those containing digraphs (e.g., *leche, arroz, llamar*).

Varieties of Spanish

The production of consonants in Spanish often varies widely according to the dialect of its speakers. Guitart (1996) distinguished two general types of dialects in Spanish: conservative (e.g., the variety of Spanish spoken in many parts of Spain) and radical (e.g., Puerto Rican Spanish). Conservative dialects are ones that preserve consonants in the rhyme (i.e., segments following the syllable nucleus; for example, [s] in /dos/) whereas radical dialects are ones in which consonants are altered in the rhyme. Guitart proposed the following characteristics of radical dialects: First, final segments (/s/, /d/, /ɾ/) are deleted (e.g., /dos/ ⇨ [do]). Second, fricatives are laryngealized (e.g., /dos/ ⇨ [doʰ]). Third, preconsonantal stops are laryngealized or velarized (e.g., [peʔsi] or [peksi] for *Pepsi*). Fourth, /n/ is produced as nasalization of preceding vowel or as velar nasal [ŋ], even before nonvelars (e.g., /xamon/ ⇨ [xamõ] or [xamoŋ]). Finally, flap /ɾ/ and liquid /l/ are neutralized. For example, /l/ may be rhotacized (e.g., /arbol/ ⇨ [aɾboɾ]), /ɾ/ may be lateralized (e.g., /kaɾta/ ⇨ [kalta]), or both are realized as a third segment that may not be either a flap or liquid (e.g., /kaɾta/ ⇨ [katta]). It should be noted that not all features listed here are used by all speakers of that particular dialect and not all speakers will utilize all features in every context (Goldstein, 2001).

Typical acquisition of Spanish

Acquisition data for two populations will be described here. First, typical acquisition of monolingual Spanish-speaking children will be recounted. Then, a short section focusing on Spanish-English bilingual children will follow. The Summary of Studies table at the end of this chapter contains studies of the acquisition of Spanish.

Acquired sounds

Consonants

Research related to consonant acquisition is somewhat difficult to characterize given the different methods researchers used in their studies (Acevedo, 1993; Anderson and Smith, 1987; de la Fuente, 1985; Fantini, 1984; Jimenez, 1987; Linares, 1981; Melgar, 1976) (see the Summary of Studies table). Thus, the acquisition data are displayed in Table 52-3 by the age at which the sound is typically mastered.

Consonant clusters

Preschool (i.e., 3- and 4-year-olds) Spanish-speaking children are able to produce consonant clusters relatively accurately (Goldstein and Iglesias, 1996) with near accuracy of 100 percent by 5 years of age (Bichotte, Dunn, Gonzalez, Orpi, and Nye, 1993).

TABLE 52-3   Age of acquisition for Spanish consonants

	Biliabial	Labio-dental	Alveolar	Alveo-palatal	Palatal	Velar
Plosive	p (by 4;0)		t (by 4;0)			k (by 4;0)
	b (by 4;0)		d (by 4;0)			g (by 5;0)
Nasal	m (by 3;0)		n (by 4;0)		ɲ (by 4;0)	
Trill			r (by 6;0)			
Tap/Flap			ɾ (by 5;0)			
Fricative		f (by 4;0)	s (by 4;6)			x (by 4;0)
Affricate				tʃ (by 4;0)		

Note. The number in ( ) indicates age by which sound is mastered.

Vowels

Given that there are only five phonemic vowels in Spanish, they are acquired early (Goldstein and Cintrón, 2001; Goldstein and Pollock, 2000; 2004; Maez, 1981), most by the age of 2 years.

Percent correct

Consonants

At 2 years of age, percentage of correct consonants for typically developing Spanish speakers is approximately 75 percent, although the range can be variable, between 55 and 86 percent (Goldstein and Cintrón, 2001).

Consonant clusters

The percentage of clusters produced correctly for 3-year-olds was 85 percent. That percentage increased to over 90 percent for 4-year-olds. By the time Spanish-speaking children are 5 years of age, consonant cluster accuracy is near 100 percent (Bichotte et al., 1993).

Vowels

In a group of 3 monolingual, Spanish-speaking children, Maez (1981) found that all 5 phonemic vowels were mastered (produced accurately greater than 75 percent of the time) by 18 months. In general, Spanish-speaking children produce few vowel errors. Goldstein and Cintrón (2001) found that percentage of correct vowels was 93 percent, on average, for a group of typically developing, monolingual Spanish-speaking 2-year-olds living in Puerto Rico. In addition, Goldstein and Pollock (2001; 2004) found that even monolingual, Spanish-speaking children with phonological disorders produced few vowel errors. Percentage of correct vowels was 98 percent, on average, for the 3- and 4-year-olds in those studies.

Phonological processes

The use of phonological processes by Spanish-speaking children has been investigated for children between the ages of 2 and 6. Anderson and Smith (1987) assessed six monolingual Puerto Rican Spanish speakers, ages 2;4 to 2;10. In that group of children only cluster reduction was exhibited in over 50 percent of the possible occurrences. Five other processes—initial, medial, and final consonant deletion, unstressed syllable deletion, and glottalization of alveolars—were exhibited in 25–50 percent of the possible occurrences. The majority of studies of phonological processes in Spanish-speaking children have focused on 3- and 4-year-olds. In children of this age, cluster reduction, final consonant deletion, and tap/trill deviations are the most commonly occurring processes (Goldstein and Iglesias, 1996; Gonzalez, 1981; Stepanof, 1990).

These children also exhibit error types other than those phonological processes listed above. In a group of 3- and 4-year-old Spanish-speaking children, Goldstein and Iglesias (1996) found that approximately 85 percent of the children's errors could be categorized by a set of 9 phonological processes. Approximately 15 percent of the errors, however, could not be categorized by one of those types. The other error types that these children exhibited included deaffrication (e.g., /letʃe/ ⇨ [leʃe]); backing (e.g., /raton/ ⇨ [rakon]); spirantization (e.g., /boka/ ⇨ [βoka]); denasalization (e.g., /mansana/ ⇨ [pasana]); addition (e.g., /plato/ ⇨ [panta]); palatalization (e.g., /sopa/ ⇨ [ʃopa]); and metathesis (e.g., /sopa/ ⇨ [posa]).

Intelligibility

To date, there is no study of intelligibility in Spanish-speaking children.

Phonetic inventory

Relatively few studies have focused on the phonetic inventory of Spanish speakers. Maez (1985) examined the consonant and vowel phonetic inventories of three female, Spanish-speaking monolingual children (although all were exposed to English, primarily through television). Results (Table 52-4) indicate that by 24 months, Spanish-speaking children produce all the segments of the inventory with the exception of the trill.

Goldstein and Cintrón (2001) examined the phonetic inventories of three male, monolingual Spanish-speaking 2-year-old boys residing in Puerto Rico. Results were commensurate with those of Maez (1985). Additionally, Goldstein and Cintrón found that there was a wide range in the percentage of consonants included in the inventory—from 52 to 91 percent (mean = 74 percent). Moreover, two of the three children produced consonant clusters. One child produced one cluster type, [pl], and another child produced five cluster types, [kl], [gl], [tɾ], [dɾ], and [gɾ]. Finally, one child did produce a trill, in contrast to the children in Maez's study.

Common mismatches

In this section, we will focus on substitution patterns in Spanish-speaking children. Goldstein (2005) examined the substitution patterns of 39 typically developing Spanish-speaking children who ranged in age from 3;2 to 4;11 and 39 Spanish-speaking children with phonological disorders who ranged in age from 3;1 to 4;9. All 78 children spoke the Puerto Rican dialect of Spanish, and those dialect features were taken into account in the analyses and not scored as errors.

Results indicated that the target, singleton sounds most commonly substituted for were somewhat different for typically developing children and children with phonological disorders. For typically developing children, the targets most commonly substituted for (in descending order) were [r], [ɾ], [t], [tʃ], and [s]. For children with phonological disorders, the targets most commonly substituted for (in descending order) were [s], [r], [tʃ], [k], and [ɾ]. Moreover, sounds most commonly used as substitutes for targets also differed between the two groups. For typically developing children, the sounds most commonly used as substitutes were (in descending order): [ɾ], [b], [l], [g], and [k]. For children with phonological disorders, the sounds most commonly used as substitutes were (in descending order): [t], [n], [b], [k], and [j]. Finally, error patterns for consonant clusters tended to differ between the two groups. Typically developing children tended to preserve the first element of the cluster and substitute for the second member (usually a glide for the target /l/ or /ɾ/). Children with phonological disorders, however, tended to simply delete the second member of the cluster and occasionally substitute a glide for it.

Barlow (2003) examined cluster production in three Spanish-speaking children: one typically developing child and two children with phonological disorders. The

TABLE 52-4 Phonetic inventory of Spanish-speaking children

	18 months*	21 months	24 months
Plosive	[p, b, t, d, k, g]	[p, b, t, d, k, g]	[p, b, t, d, k, g]
Nasal	[m, n]	[m, n]	[m, n, ɲ]
Trill	–	–	–
Tap/Flap	[ɾ]	[ɾ]	[ɾ]
Fricative	[f, v, s, h]	[f, v, s, z, h]	[f, v, s, z, h]
Spirant	[ß, ð]	[ß, ð, ɣ]	[ß, ð, ɣ]
Affricate	[tʃ]	[tʃ]	[tʃ]
Lateral Approximant	[w, j, l]	[w, j, l]	[w, j, l]
Vowels	[i, e, u, o, a]	[i, e, u, o, a]	[i, e, u, o, a]

*produced by at least 2 of 3 children at that age

children exhibited different error patterns. The typically developing child and one of the children with phonological disorders deleted the sonorant and preserved the obstruent (e.g., /plato/ 'plate' ⇨ [pato] (p. 186)). The other child with a phonological disorder, however, produced all syllable-initial clusters accurately.

Syllable structure

At 2 years of age, almost half the syllable types produced are CV syllables, and about 20 percent each are CVC and VC syllables (Goldstein and Cintrón, 2001). Finally, approximately two-thirds of the words the children produce are 2 syllables in length; 23 percent are single-syllable words; and 5 percent are 3-syllable words (Goldstein and Cintrón, 2001).

Additionallly, data on syllable structure development can be extrapolated from other research. For example, data from Anderson and Smith (1987) indicated that Spanish-speaking 2-year-olds tended to exhibit unstressed syllable deletion and cluster reduction. Thus, one can assume that the majority of productions by these children were disyllabic words with a CV syllable structure. In a group of three Spanish-speaking 2-year-olds, Goldstein and Cintrón (2001) found that the most prevalent syllable types in the children's connected speech samples were CV and V syllables. However, all three children did produce CVC, VC, and CCVC syllables. The children in that group also predominantly produced two-syllable words, followed by one-, three-, four-, and then five-syllable words. It should be noted that only two of the three children produced three-syllable words, and only one of the three children produced four- and five-syllable words.

Prosody

In Spanish, word level stress most commonly takes one of two forms: (1) stress is placed on the penultimate syllable of words ending in a vowel, /n/, or /s/ (e.g., [elefánte] 'elephant') or (2) stress is placed on the final syllable in other words (e.g., [relóx] 'watch'). There are, of course, exceptions to these general rules (Hochberg, 1987), so irregular stress is marked with an accent in the orthographic representation (e.g., [baldés] *Valdés*). Hochberg (1987) hypothesized that Spanish-speaking children are sensitive to irregular stress forms and would show this preference by regularizing stress in words with irregular stress patterns. She examined this hypothesis in 50 3-, 4-, and 5-year-old Spanish-speaking children living in California who had "various degrees of proficiency in English" (p. 58). Her results indicated the children more accurately imitated stress on words with regular stress than words with irregular stress. In addition, the children overwhelmingly regularized words with irregular stress. Finally, her results indicated that "children's stress rule learning was essentially complete by age 3" (p. 62).

In order to determine if Spanish-speaking children showed a preference for penultimate stress, Hochberg (1988) examined four Spanish-speaking children living in California. As in the previous study, these children also were dominant in Spanish but exposed to English. The results indicated that the children did not have a clear bias for penultimate stress. In fact, in the children's spontaneous productions, three of the four children were more accurate in producing words with final stress than with penultimate stress.

Acquisition in Spanish-English bilingual children

The relatively few studies on acquisition in typically developing bilingual (Spanish-English) children indicate that their phonological development is similar, although not identical, to monolingual speakers of either language. It appears that the phonological skills of younger bilingual children are less like their monolingual peers (e.g., Gildersleeve, Davis, and Stubbe, 1996; Gildersleeve-Neumann and Davis, 1998).

In two studies of bilingual 3-year-olds, Gildersleeve and colleagues found that the bilingual children exhibited an overall lower intelligibility rating, made more consonant and vowel errors, and produced more uncommon error patterns than either monolingual English or monolingual Spanish speakers. As bilingual children get older, however, skills across the two groups become commensurate (Goldstein and Washington, 2001). In examining the English and Spanish phonological skills of typically developing 4-year-old bilingual (Spanish-English) children, Goldstein and Washington (2001) found no significant differences between the two languages on percentage of correct consonants; percentage of correct consonants for sound classes; or percentages of occurrence for phonological processes. Also, their results indicated that overall phonological skills of the bilingual 4-year-olds were similar to monolingual children. However, the bilingual children were less accurate than monolingual speakers on spirants, flap, and trill in Spanish. Finally, in comparing the phonological skills of 5-year-old Spanish-English bilingual children with predominantly monolingual Spanish- and English-speaking children, Goldstein, Fabiano, and Washington (2005) found almost no significant differences between the groups on measures of consonant accuracy. Stops were the only significant difference between the Spanish of the bilingual children and the Spanish of the monolingual children.

Despite the fact that the phonological skills of bilingual children are largely similar to their monolingual peers, it should be recognized that the phonotactic structure of one language might have an effect on the phonotactic structure of the other language. Thus, bilingual children may exhibit cross-linguistic effects (e.g., /fɪʃ/ 'fish' ⇨ [fɪtʃ]). Although the frequency of such effects is generally low, they typically are bidirectional (Goldstein et al., 2003). Thus, they affect the children's production in both English and Spanish.

Phonological awareness

One of the key predictors for spelling proficiency is phonological awareness (Durgunoğlu, 1998). Phonological awareness is the "ability to reflect on and manipulate the structure of an utterance (e.g., into words, syllables or sounds) as distinct from its meaning" and also involves the ability to divide words and syllables into smaller units (Stackhouse, 1997, p. 157). Phonological awareness has been studied through a variety of tasks such as finding rhyming words, determining the first sound in a sequence, and noting the number of syllables in a word (Vernon and Ferreiro, 1999).

In two studies of language and literacy development in first graders enrolled in Spanish-English bilingual education classrooms, Durgunoğlu, Nagy, and Hancin-Bhatt (1993) and Durgunoğlu (1998) found that phonological awareness in Spanish is closely related to word recognition and spelling in Spanish. Conversely, the studies also found that schooling and learning to read and spell aided phonological awareness. In a study of segmental and syllabic segmentation in Spanish-speaking preschoolers and first graders, de Manrique and Graminga (1984) found that phonological skills were developmental. The older children exhibited greater skill than the younger children. Younger children who had training in phonological awareness, however, were able to show similar skills compared to the older children. In terms of pedagogical application of these studies, Durguno lu et al. (1993) recommended that "children need to identify the phonological subcomponents of the spoken words and understand how orthographic symbols are mapped onto those phonological subcomponents" (p. 462).

Speech assessment for Spanish-speaking children

Currently, four tests are commonly used to assess the phonological skills of Spanish-speaking children:

- *Austin Spanish Articulation Test* (Carrow, 1974)
- *Southwest Spanish Articulation Test* (Toronto, 1977)
- *Spanish Articulation Measures* (Mattes, 1995)
- *Assessment of Phonological Processes–Spanish* (Hodson, 1986)

The *Austin Spanish Articulation Test* assesses single consonant and vowel sounds, diphthongs, and consonant clusters. Normative data were collected on 29 children of Mexican American descent. The *Southwest Spanish Articulation Test* tests all the Spanish consonants in initial, medial, and final positions. The *Spanish Articulation Measures* assess the 18 consonant phonemes of Spanish in initial, medial, and word-final position and also can be used to assess phonological processes. The *Assessment of Phonological Processes–Spanish* targets 38 phonological processes. Although no normative data are reported, this assessment has been used in the research literature (e.g., Stepanof, 1990).

Because these tests largely do not have normative data associated with them, clinicians will need to use them as a criterion-referenced measure with supplemental connected speech samples. They then will have to use developmental data outlined above and in the research literature to compare the child's performance against his or her peer group.

There are three readily available computer programs that SLPs can use to transcribe and analyze Spanish:

- *Computerized Profiling* (Long, Fey, and Channell, 2004) http://www.computerizedprofiling.org/
- *Logical International Phonetic Programs* (Oller and Delgado, 2000) http://www.ihsys.com/public_html/LIPP.asp/
- *Computerized Articulation and Phonology Evaluation System* (Masterson and Bernhardt, 2001)

Speech intervention for Spanish-speaking children

Appropriate intervention begins with a least-biased assessment (Yavaş and Goldstein, 1998). Eliciting both single word and connected speech samples is necessary in helping to plan intervention for Spanish-speaking children. Once these samples are collected, SLPs should complete independent (i.e., not comparing the child's skills to the adult target) and relational analyses (i.e., comparing the child's skills to the adult target). When analyzing the results of Spanish-speaking children, it is important that SLPs take the children's dialect features into account and do not score these features as errors. Scoring these features as errors may result in the over-identification of Spanish-speaking children with phonological disorders or result in inappropriate choices for goal selection (Goldstein and Iglesias, 2001).

Once an appropriate diagnosis is made and the child's strengths and weaknesses are identified, then it is fitting to plan for intervention. There is no reason to believe that the general approaches used for English-speaking children will not be appropriate for Spanish-speaking children, although there are few efficacy studies in this area. Approaches to remediation of speech sound disorders are traditionally dichotomized into motoric and linguistic approaches (Bankson and Bernthal, 2004). Bankson and Bernthal point out, however, that it is likely that both approaches will need to be used in the intervention for phonological disorders, given the inextricable link between motoric and linguistic aspects of speech production.

In choosing specific remediation targets, Fey (1986) suggests three strategies for determining specific goals. The first strategy is the *vertical approach* in which one goal is taught in each session and taken to a prespecified criterion. The second strategy is the *horizontal approach* in which multiple goals are addressed in each session. The final strategy is a *cyclical approach* in which a number of goals are cycled although only one goal is focused on in each session. (Hodson and Paden, 1983, treat the latter approach in more detail.) It is likely that the choice of specific remediation targets might be different than for English-speaking children. For example, in English-speaking preschool children with phonological disorders, the phonological pattern of *final consonant deletion* is often an initial intervention target because of the number of final consonants in English and the impact on intelligibility of deleting them. That specific pattern is unlikely to be an initial intervention target for Spanish-speaking children because of the few final consonants in the language. Thus, deleting final consonants in Spanish will have a minimal impact on the child's intelligibility. A pattern such as *unstressed syllable deletion* will have a greater impact on intelligibility in Spanish-speaking children, given that the majority of words in Spanish are multisyllabic.

For remediating communication disorders in bilingual children, Kohnert and Derr (2004) have outlined two general approaches to remediation. The *bilingual approach* focuses on structures and/or error patterns that are similar across the two languages. The *cross-linguistic approach* focuses on structures and/or error patterns that are unique to each language. Yavaş and Goldstein (1998) have suggested a similar approach in remediating phonological disorders in bilingual children. Specifically, they suggest determining remediation targets based on the error rates of patterns in both languages. Thus, initial intervention targets would be sounds or patterns that show high error rates in both languages (e.g., /s/ or cluster reduction); that is, a bilingual approach. Then, sounds or patterns that show high error rates in the child's first language would be targeted; that is, a cross-linguistic approach. Finally, sounds or patterns that show high error rates in the child's second language would be targeted; also a cross-linguistic approach. The stimuli for these targets, of course, would be different depending on the language of intervention. For example, Spanish and English have different cluster types; Spanish has flap clusters (e.g., /tɾen/ 'train'), which English does not. Thus, in the end, intervention likely will have to take place in both languages.

PHONETICALLY SPEAKING

Pronunciation of Spanish: /spænɪʃ/

Relevant words for speech assessment and intervention

Word/Phrase	Formal usage	Pronunciation	Informal usage	Pronunciation
Tongue	*lengua*	[lɛŋua]	*lengua*	[lɛŋua]
Teeth	*dientes*	[dientes]	*dientes*	[diente]
Lips	*labios*	[laβios]	*labios*	[laβios]
Hard palate	*paladar duro*	[paladar duro]	*paladar duro*	[paladar duro]
Soft palate	*paladar blando*	[paladar blando]	*paladar blando*	[paladar blando]
Larynx	*laringe*	[larinxe]	*laringe*	[larinxe]
Lungs	*pulmones*	[pulmones]	*pulmones*	[pulmone]
Nose	*nariz*	[naris]	*nariz*	[naris]
Sound	*sonido*	[soniðo]	*sonido*	[soniðo]
Word	*palabra*	[palaβra]	*palabra*	[palaβra]
Sentence	*frase*	[frase]	*frase*	[frase]
Paragraph	*parafo*	[parafo]	*parafo*	[parafo]

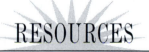

RESOURCES

Books

Alvar, M. (Ed.). *Manual de dialectología Hispánica* [Manual of Hispanic dialectology]. Barcelona, Spain: Ariel.

Carasquillo, A., and Sagan, P. (Eds.). *The teaching of reading in Spanish to the bilingual student: La enseñeza de la lectura en Español para el estudiante bilingüe.* Mahwah, NJ: Lawrence Erlbaum.

Cárdenas, D. (1960). *Introducción a una comparación fonológico del español y del inglés* [Introduction to a phonological comparison of Spanish and English]. Washington, DC: Center for Applied Linguistics.

Goldstein, B. (2000). *Cultural and linguistic diversity resource guide for speech-language pathology.* San Diego, CA: Singular.

Journal articles

Brea-Spahn, M., Masterson, J. J., Apel, K., and Goldstein, B. (2003). El deletreo en inglés y en español: desarrollo, evaluación e intervención [Spelling in English and Spanish: Development, assessment, and intervention]. *Revista Chilena de Fonoaudiologia* [Chilean Journal of Speech Pathology and Audiology], *4*, 17–30.

Goldstein, B. (1995). Spanish phonological development. In H. Kayser (Ed.), *Bilingual speech-language pathology: An Hispanic focus* (pp. 17–38). San Diego, CA: Singular.

MacDonald, M. (1989). The influence of Spanish phonology on the English spoken by United States Hispanics. In P. Bjarkman and R. Hammond (Eds.), *American Spanish pronunciation: Theoretical and applied perspectives* (pp. 215–236). Washington, DC: Georgetown University Press.

Mann, D., and Hodson, B. (1994). Spanish-speaking children's phonologies: Assessment and remediation of disorders. *Seminars in Speech and Language, 15*, 137–147.

Journals

- *Revista de Logopedia, Foniatría y Audiología* (Spain)
- *Revista Chilena de Fonoaudiologia* (Chile)
- *La Revista Fonoaudiológica* (Argentina)

Professional associations

International Association of Logopedics and Phoniatrics, http//www.ialp.info/index2.html

Associación Argentina de Logopedia Foniatría y Audiología (Argentina), http//www.asalfa.org/

Sociedad Médica Española de Foniatría (SOMEF) (Spain)

Asociación Española de Logopedia Foniatria y Audiologia (AELFA) (Spain), http//www.aelfa.org/

Colegio de Fonoaudiólogos de Chile

Asociación Colombiana de Fonoaudiología y Terapia del lenguaje, http://www.linemed.com/colombia/asofono/

Asociación de Fonoaudiologos en Costa Rica, http//espanol.geocities.com/fonoaudiologoscr

La Sociedad Ecuatoriana de Foniatría, Audiología y Logopedia–SEFAL (Ecuador)

El Colegio Nacional de Fonoaudiòlogos de Panamà, http//conadefo.0catch.com/espanol

Useful Web sites

- *Spanish phonology* (from Answers.com), http://www.answers.com/topic/spanish-phonology
- *fənɛtɪks The sounds of spoken language,* http://www.uiowa.edu/~acadtech/phonetics/#
- *Fonética española,* http//liceu.uab.es/~maria/bibliografia.html
- *History & Dialectology of Spanish,* http//people.cas.sc.edu/deholt01/links/Historyofspanishlinks.html
- *Real Academia Española,* http//www.rae.es/
- *Estudios de Lingüística del Español,* http//elies.rediris.es/
- *Fundación Verbum para el Lenguaje y la Comunicación,* http//www.fundacionverbum.org/

REFERENCES

Acevedo, M. A. (1993). Development of Spanish consonants in pre-school children. *Journal of Childhood Communication Disorders, 15,* 9–15.

Anderson, R., and Smith, B. (1987). Phonological development of two-year-old monolingual Puerto Rican Spanish-speaking children. *Journal of Child Language, 14,* 57–78.

Bankson, N., and Bernthal, J. (2004). Treatment approaches. In J. Bernthal and N. Bankson (Eds.), *Articulation and phonological disorders* (5ᵗʰ ed.) (pp. 292–347). Boston: Allyn & Bacon.

Barlow, J. (2003). Asymmetries in the acquisition of consonant clusters in Spanish. *Canadian Journal of Linguistics, 48,* 179–210.

Bedore, L. (1999). The acquisition of Spanish. In O. Taylor and L. Leonard (Eds.), *Language acquisition across North America: Cross-cultural and cross-linguistic perspectives* (pp. 157–208). San Diego, CA: Singular.

Bichotte, M., Dunn, B., Gonzalez, L., Orpi, J., and Nye, C. (1993, November). *Assessing phonological performance of bilingual school-age Puerto Rican children.* Paper presented at the annual convention of the American Speech-Language-Hearing Association, Anaheim, CA.

Carrow, E. (1974). *Austin Spanish Articulation Test.* Austin, TX: Learning Concepts.

Cotton, E., and Sharp, J. (1988). *Spanish in the Americas.* Washington, DC: Georgetown University Press.

Dauer, R. (1983). Stress-timing and syllable-timing re-analyzed. *Journal of Phonetics, 11*, 51 –62.

de la Fuente, M. T. (1985). *The order of acquisition of Spanish consonant phonemes by monolingual Spanish speaking children between the ages of 2.0 and 6.5.* Unpublished doctoral dissertation, Georgetown University, Washington, DC.

de Manrique, A. M. B., and Gramigna, S. (1984). La segmentación fonológica y silábica en niños de preescolar y primer grado [Phonological and syllabic segmentation in children in preschool and first grade]. *Lectura y vida: Revista latinoamericana de lectura, 5*, 4–14.

Delattre, P. (1965). *Comparing the phonetic features of English, French, German and Spanish: An interim report.* Heidelberg: Julius Verlag.

Durguno lu, A. (1998). Acquiring literacy in English and Spanish in the United States. In A. Durgunog lu and L. Verhoeven (Eds.), *Literacy development in a multilingual context: Cross-cultural perspectives* (pp. 135–145). Mahwah, NJ: Erlbaum.

Durguno lu, A., Nagy, W., and Hancin-Bhatt, B. (1993). Cross-language transfer of phonological awareness. *Journal of Educational Psychology, 85*, 453–465.

Eblen, R. (1982). A study of the fricatives by three-year-old children learning Mexican Spanish. *Language and Speech, 25*, 201–220.

Fantini, A. (1978). *Language acquisition of a bilingual child: A sociolinguistic perspective (to age 10).* San Diego, CA: College Hill Press.

Fey, M. (1986). *Language intervention in young children.* San Diego, CA: College Hill Press.

Gildersleeve, C., Davis, B., and Stubbe, E. (1996, November). *When monolingual rules don't apply: Speech development in a bilingual environment.* Paper presented at the annual convention of the American Speech-Language-Hearing Association, Seattle, WA.

Gildersleeve-Neumann, C., and Davis, B. (1998, November). *Learning English in a bilingual preschool environment: Change over time.* Paper presented at the annual convention of the American Speech-Language-Hearing Association, San Antonio, TX.

Goldstein, B., and Iglesias, A. (1996). Phonological patterns in normally developing Spanish-speaking 3- and 4-year-olds of Puerto Rican descent. *Language, Speech, and Hearing Services in Schools, 27*, 82–90.

Goldstein, B., and Washington, P. (2001). An initial investigation of phonological patterns in 4-year-old typically developing Spanish-English bilingual children. *Language, Speech, and Hearing Services in Schools, 32*, 153–164.

Goldstein, B. (2001). Transcription of Spanish and Spanish-influenced English. *Communication Disorders Quarterly, 23*, 5460.

Goldstein, B. (2005). Substitution patterns in the phonology of Spanish-speaking children. *Journal of Multilingual Communication Disorders, 3*, 56–63.

Goldstein, B., and Cintron, P. (2001). An investigation of phonological skills in Puerto Rican Spanish-speaking 2-year-olds. *Clinical Linguistics and Phonetics, 15*, 343–361.

Goldstein, B., and Iglesias, A. (2001). The effect of dialect on phonological analysis: Evidence from Spanish-speaking children. *American Journal of Speech-Language Pathology, 10*, 394–406.

Goldstein, B., and Pollock, K. (2000). Vowel errors in Spanish-speaking children with phonological disorders: A retrospective, comparative study. *Clinical Linguistics and Phonetics, 14*, 217–234.

Goldstein, B., and Pollock, K. (2004). Vowel production in Spanish-speaking children with phonological disorders: Dialect and sampling issues. *Journal of Multilingual Communication Disorders, 2*, 147–160.

Goldstein, B., Fabiano, L., and Iglesias, A. (2003, April). *The representation of phonology in sequential Spanish-English bilingual children.* Poster session presented at the 4th Annual International Symposium on Bilingualism, Tempe, AZ.

Goldstein, B., Fabiano, L., and Washington, P. (2005). Phonological skills in predominantly English, predominantly Spanish, and Spanish-English bilingual children. *Language, Speech, and Hearing Services in Schools, 36*, 201–218.

Gonzalez, A. (1981). *A descriptive study of phonological development in normal speaking Puerto Rican preschoolers.* Unpublished doctoral dissertation, Pennsylvania State University, State College, PA.

González, J., and Valle, I. (2000). Word identification and reading disorders in the Spanish language. *Journal of Reading Disabilities, 33*, 44–60.

Goshami, U., Gombert, J., and Fraca de Barrerra, L. (1998). Children orthographicrepresentations and linguistic transparency: Nonsense word reading in English, French, and Spanish. *Applied Psycholinguistics, 19*, 19–52.

Goyen, J. (1989). Reading methods in Spain: The effect of a regular orthography. *The Reading Teacher, 42*, 370–373.

Grimes, B. (Ed., 2002). *Ethnologue* (14th ed.). Dallas, TX: Summer Institute of Linguistics, Inc. [http://www.ethnologue.com]

Guitart, J. (1996). Spanish in contact with itself and the phonological characterization of conservative and radical styles. In A. Roca and J. Jensen (Eds.), *Spanish in contact: Issues in bilingualism* (pp. 151–157). Somerville, MA: Cascadilla Press.

Gutierrez-Clellen, V. (1999). Mediating literacy skills in Spanish-speaking children with special needs. *Language, Speech, and Hearing Services in Schools, 30*, 285–292.

Hadlich, R., Holton, J., and Montes, M. (1968). *A drillbook of Spanish pronunciation.* New York: Harper & Row.

Hammond, R. (2001). *The sounds of Spanish: Analysis and application (with special reference to American English).* Somerville, MA: Cascadilla Press.

Harris, J. (1983). *Syllable structure and stress in Spanish: A nonlinear analysis.* Cambridge, MA: MIT Press.

Hochberg, J. (1987). The acquisition of word stress rules in Spanish. *Papers and Reports in Child Language Development, 26*, 56–63.

Hochberg, J. (1988). First steps in the acquisition of Spanish stress. *Journal of Child Language, 15*, 273–292.

Hodson, B. (1986). *Assessment of phonological processes–Spanish.* San Diego, CA: Los Amigos Research Associates.

Hodson, B., and Paden, E. (1983). *Targeting intelligible speech.* San Diego, CA: College Hill Press.

Iglesias, A., Cohen, L., Gutierrez-Clellen, V., and Marcano, M. (1983). *Permitted complexity of spoken Spanish.* Seminar presented at the convention of the American Speech-Language-Hearing Association, Washington, DC.

Jimenez, B. C. (1987). Acquisition of Spanish consonants in children aged 3–5 years, 7 months. *Language, Speech, and Hearing Services in Schools, 18*, 357–363.

Kohnert, K., and Derr, A. (2004). Language intervention with bilingual children. In B. Goldstein (Ed.), *Bilingual language development and disorders in Spanish-English speakers* (pp. 311–342). Baltimore: Brookes Publishing.

Ladefoged, P. (2001). *A course in phonetics* (4th ed). Fort Worth, TX: Harcourt College Publishers.

Linares, T. A. (1981) Articulation skills in Spanish-speaking children. In R. Padilla (Ed.), *Ethnoperspectives in bilingual education research: Bilingual education technology* (pp. 363–367). Ypsilanti: Eastern Michigan University Press.

Long, S., Fey, M., and Channell R. (2004). *Computerized profiling* (MS-DOS version 9.6) [computer software]. Milwaukee, WI: Marquette University.

Macken, M., and Barton, D. (1980). The acquisition of the voicing contrast in Spanish A phonetic and phonological study of word-initial stop consonants. *Journal of Child Language, 7*, 433–458.

Macken, M. (1975). The acquisition of intervocalic consonants in Mexican Spanish: A cross sectional study based on imitation data. *Papers and reports on child language development, 29–45*.

Maez, L. (1981). *Spanish as a first language.* Unpublished doctoral dissertation, University of California, Santa Barbara.

Maez, L. (1985). The acquisition of the Spanish sound system by native Spanish-speaking children. In E. Garcia and R. Padilla (Eds.), *Advances in bilingual education research* (pp.3–26). Tucson, AZ: University of Arizona Press.

Masterson, J., and Bernhardt, B. (2001). *Computerized articulation and phonology evaluation System.* Austin, TX: Pro-Ed.

Mattes, L. J. (1995). *Spanish articulation measures* (Rev. ed.). Oceanside, CA: Academic Communication Associates.

Melgar de Gonzalez, M. (1976). *Como detectar al niño con problemas del habla* [Identifying the child with speech problems]. Mexico City: Trillas.

Navarro, T. (1968). *Studies in Spanish phonology.* Coral Gables, FL: University of Miami Press.

Núñez-Cedeño, R., and Morales-Front, A. (1999). *Fonología generativa contemporánea de la lengua española* [Contemporary generative phonology of the Spanish language]. Washington, DC: Georgetown University Press.

Oller, D. K., and Delgado, R. (2000). *Logical International Phonetic Programs* (v. 2.02). Miami, FL: Intelligent Hearing Systems.

Penny, R. (1991). *A history of the Spanish language.* Cambridge, UK: Cambridge University Press.

Stackhouse, J. (1997). Phonological awareness: Connecting speech and literacy problems. In B. Hodson and M. L. Edwards (Eds.), *Perspectives in applied phonology* (pp. 157–196). Gaithersburg, MD: Aspen Publishers.

Stepanof, E. R. (1990). Procesos phonologicos de niños Puertorriqueños de 3 y 4 años evidenciado en la prueba APP-Spanish [Phonological processes evidenced on the APP-Spanish by 3- and 4-year-old Puerto Rican children]. *Opphla, 8*(2), 15–20.

Stoel, C. (1973). Note on the acquisition of sonorants in Spanish. *Papers and Reports on Child Language, 6*, 107–115. [ERIC document ED101562].

Toronto, A. (1977). *Southwestern Spanish Articulation Test.* Austin, TX: National Education Laboratory Publishers, Inc.

Vernon, S., and Ferreiro, E. (1999). Writing development: A neglected variable in the consideration of phonological awareness. *Harvard Educational Review, 69*, 395–415.

Yavaş, M., and Goldstein, B. (1998). Phonological assessment and treatment of bilingual speakers. *American Journal of Speech-Language Pathology, 7*, 49–60.

SUMMARY OF STUDIES OF TYPICAL
SPANISH SPEECH ACQUISITION

Authors	Year	Dialect	Language status	No. of children	Age of children	Information	Sample type	Data collection
Acevedo	1993	Mexican	Spanish as primary language	120	3;0–5;11	Consonants	Single word	Cross-sectional
Anderson and Smith	1987	Puerto Rican	Monolingual Spanish	6	2;4–2;10	Consonants; phonological processes		Cross-sectional
Eblen	1982	Mexican	Monolingual Spanish	6	3;0	Fricatives	Single word; sentences	Cross-sectional
Goldstein and Cintron	2001	Puerto Rican	Monolingual Spanish	3	1;10, 2;4, 2;5	Consonants; vowels; phonological processes	Connected speech	Cross-sectional
Goldstein, Fabiano, and Washington	2005	Puerto Rican	Bilingual Spanish-English	15	5;0–5;5	Consonants; vowels; phonological processes	Single word	Cross-sectional
Goldstein and Iglesias	1996	Puerto Rican	Spanish as primary language	54	3;2–4;11	Phonological processes	Single word	Cross-sectional
Goldstein and Washington	2001	Puerto Rican	Bilingual Spanish-English	12	4;0	Consonants; vowels; phonological processes	Single word	Cross-sectional
Jimenez	1987	Mexican	Monolingual Spanish	120	3;0–5;7	Consonants	Single word	Cross-sectional
Macken	1975	Mexican	Monolingual Spanish	(1) 6 from California (2) 6 from Mexico	(1) 2;4–3;3 (2) 1;6–6;1	Intervocalic consonants	CVC syllables	Cross-sectional
Macken and Barton	1980	Mexican	Monolingual Spanish	4	(1) 1;7–1;9 (2) 3;6–4;0	Word initial stops	Single words	Longitudinal
Maez	1985	No information	Monolingual Spanish (but exposed to English)	3	18, 21, 24 months	Consonants and vowels	Connected speech	Longitudinal
Stoel	1973	No information	Monolingual Spanish	6	2;4–3;3	Nasals and liquids	Nonsense syllables	Longitudinal

*This chart represents published studies. Research based on theses and dissertations, for example, was not included, given that those sources are difficult for clinicians to obtain. In addition, this list of studies is not meant to be exhaustive but merely representative.

Chapter 53

Thai Speech Acquisition

Preeya Lorwatanapongsa and Sumalai Maroonroge

INTRODUCTION

Thai, the official or national language of Thailand, is from the Chinese-Thai branch of the Sino-Tibetan family. The Thai language in use today is the result of a centuries-long maturation and is still growing as more words from other languages are fused into the language. Many of the polysyllabic words within the Thai language are borrowed from Khmer, Pali or Sanskrit, European languages, and English. Thai is predominantly a monosyllabic, uninflected tonal language (Kingkam, 2004). The Thai language has its own alphabet, which traces back to a script of India. This chapter focuses on Central Thai, the official dialect of the majority of Thai people. The Resources section of this chapter contains materials about Thai.

Where Thai is spoken

According to the 2000 census, 65–66 million people live in Thailand. An estimated 80 percent of the people speak Thai, while the rest use over 60 different languages that are not related to Thai (see accompanying map and Appendix D). The latter are ethnic minorities scattered in various parts of the country.

Four major dialects are accepted as variations of the Thai language; however, due to a lack of commonalities in speech/language structures, most listeners require special training to understand them. Central Thai or Standard Thai is taught in all schools and is widely understood by Thai people in all regions. All educated Thai are bidialectal due to the success of the central government's literacy programs (Hinds, 1988). However, strong regional identity has kept the local dialects alive (Kingkam, 2004). Outside Bangkok and the central plains, other dialects coexist with the Standard Thai. Northern Thai is spoken in the north and Southern Thai is used in the south and the northern part of Malaysia. Northeastern Thai, or Isan, resembles the dialect of the Lao language, mainly used in the northeast of Thailand. There are small ethnic minority groups, composed of natives from hill tribes, Indians, Chinese, Indo-Chinese, and Europeans who live in Thailand. They speak over 60 different languages that are not related to Standard Thai.

Components of Thai

The Thai language is representative of a class of complex languages whose characters are composed of a number of symbols. Thai belongs to the Sino-Tibetan family of languages (Chaichana, 1963). Thai is a monosyllabic tone language with many structures similar to Chinese, with further influences from the Indian languages Pali and Sanskrit.

Standard Thai is composed of at least three distinct forms of social contexts. Social appropriateness or "linguistic etiquette" is essential in Thai. Based on the speech patterns, most listeners familiar with the language will be able to separate speakers of Standard Thai from the non-Standard Thai. Speech patterns reveal regional, social, or ethnic background, and possibly values, behaviors, and intentions (Smalley, 1994). The classifications and descriptions of variations in Central Thai are Street Thai, an informal Thai used between relatives and friends (ภาษาพู); Elegant Thai, the official and spoken/written version used by news media (ภาษาเขียน); and Royal Thai, which is rarely used except among the royal families (ราชาศัพท์).

This chapter will focus on Street and Elegant Thais, the common forms of Central Thai dialect. The Thai language has various pronunciation rules, tonal rules, and structure rules. The spoken Thai language has a pleasing rhythmic pattern that is very poetic; it uses tones to distinguish meanings of the words.

The grammar of the Thai language is simple. Most significantly, there are no tenses, suffixes, plurals, genders,

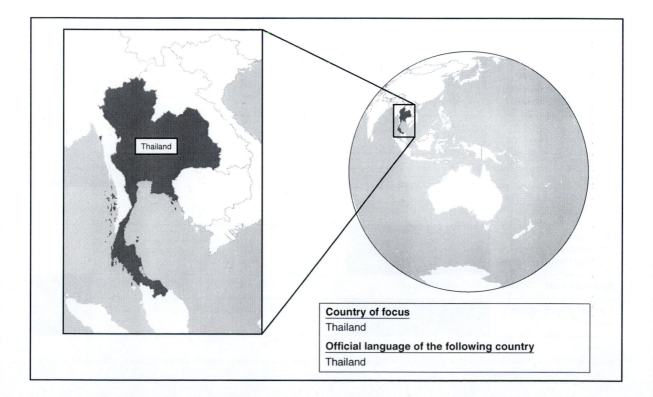

Country of focus
Thailand

Official language of the following country
Thailand

subject-verb agreement, or articles such *as a, an,* or *the.* The basic structure of Thai sentences is subject/verb/object with adjectives following nouns (the National Language from http://www.mahidol.ac.th). For example, "this is a white cat" is English, but in Thai, it would be "this is a cat white." In many cases, verbs can be changed into nouns with the use of a prefix. Time is indicated by standard auxiliaries, and marked by adverbs and time expressions or context within the sentence. Mood, questions, and other parts of speech are constructed by adding certain words to the sentences.

Consonants

The 44 consonant forms in Thai represent 21 consonant sounds. The following consonants are pronounced like the sounds of English consonant counterparts: /b, d, m, n, l, r, w, y, f, s, h/, while the remaining consonants are pronounced a bit differently from English. The 44 consonants are grouped into three classes, high, mid, and low, based on the tone of a syllable. The /kʰ/ ฅ, ฅ consonants are obsolete and not commonly found in everyday speech.

In English, consonants are voiced/unaspirated or unvoiced/aspirated. Thai consonants have an additional group of unvoiced/unaspirated consonants, similar to the English allophone. The sample of this will be /p/ as in 'spin'. The unvoiced/unaspirated consonants are observed in alveolar /t/, /tʰ/, /d/, post-alveolar /tɕ/, /tɕʰ/, and the velar /k/, /kʰ/.

Table 53-1 shows the 44 Thai consonant forms and 21 consonant sounds. Several consonant sounds have multiple consonant forms. Originally the forms represented separate sounds, but over the years the distinction between those sounds was lost; the consonant forms are dictated by the tones. The six main consonants /m, ʔp, n, ʔt, ŋ, ʔk/ can be in either initial or in final positions. The rest of the consonants in Table 53-1 can be only in the initial position; if they appear in the final positions, they carry the pronunciation of one of the six main consonants (Thai Language Page from Thammasat University, http://thaiarc.tu.ac.th/). For each cell, International Phonetic Alphabet (IPA) is shown with the Thai consonant forms. Consonants within the same cell have identical pronunciation but different written forms.

TABLE 53-1 Consonants produced in Thai

	Bilabial	Labio-dental	Alveolar	Alveolar-palatal	Palatal	Velar	Glottal
Plosive							
voiceless aspirated	pʰ		tʰ			kʰ	ʔ
voiceless unaspirated	ʔp		ʔt			ʔk	
voiced unaspirated	b		d				
Nasal							
voiced	m		n			ŋ	
Flap							
voiced			r				
Fricative							
voiceless		f	s				h
Affricate							
voiceless aspirated				tɕʰ			
voiceless unaspirated				tɕ			
Approximant	w (labiovelar)				j		
Lateral approximant							
voiced			l				

Black = articulations judged impossible

Based on the International Phonetic Alphabet. Courtesy of the International Phonetic Association (c/o Department of Linguistics, University of Victoria, Victoria, British Columbia, Canada).

Vowels and diphthongs

The vowels are by far the most difficult part of the Thai language. There are 18 vowel forms, and many of the vowels do not have equivalent sounds in English. Depending on the form, they can be placed above, below, before, and after the consonants. Some vowels have complex forms that are composed of multiple parts that embrace the consonants. Thai diphthongs and triphthongs are created by a combination of single vowels. All diphthongs and triphthongs have longer duration compared to the single vowels (Wikipedia, 2005).

Vowels

The Thai vowels associated with consonants are nonsequential: they can be located before, after, above, or below their associated consonant. In terms of articulation, the basic Thai vowels are formed from front to back and from close to open. Table 53-2 displays the basic Thai vowels. In column 1, the vowels are shown with the place of articulation and

duration. Long versus short duration creates distinct phonemes representing unrelated words in Thai. For example, the short vowel /khao/ (เขา) means 'he or she' or 'mountain' in Thai. The long vowel /khao/ (ขาว) means 'white' in Thai. The equivalent English pronunciation in IPA is in column 3. The Thai vowel forms are displayed in column 4. The dash (–) indicates the position of the initial consonant in which the vowel is pronounced.

Diphthongs

The basic vowels can be combined into diphthongs as shown in Table 53-3. Although some minor disagreements appear over the number of diphthongs, it is reasonable to conclude that there are 15 diphthongs and 3 triphthongs. The Thai diphthongs are very different from the English diphthongs, and it is difficult to find the equivalent English sounds to describe them. The diphthongs have short and long forms as described in Table 53-3. Some may not be true diphthongs but are influenced by the glide consonant.

TABLE 53-2 Thai vowels with International Phonetic Alphabet (IPA), sound equivalent, and vowel forms

Location	Pronunciation (IPA)	English equivalent	Vowel form
High front (short)	i	pin, sin	◌ิ
High front (long)	iː	see, me, we	◌ี
High central (short)	ɯ	–	◌ึ
High central (long)	ɯː	–	◌ื
High back (short)	ui	book, look	◌ุ
High back (long)	uː	zoo, blue,	◌ู
Mid-high front (short)	e	set, let, met	เ–ะ
Mid-high front (long)	eː	same, name	เ–
Mid-high central (short)	ɤ	–	เ–อะ
Mid-high central (long)	ɤː	earn, burn	เ–อ
Mid-high back (short)	o	–	โ–ะ
Mid-high back (long)	oː	sew, soul	โ–
Mid-low front (short)	ɛ	bat, sat, mat	แ–ะ
Mid-low front (long)	ɛː	am, ham, jam	แ–
Mid-low back (short)	ɔ	–	เ–าะ
Mid-low back (long)	ɔː	saw, law	–อ
Low-front (short)	a	hut, nut, just	–ะ
Low-front (long)	aː	Father, jar	–า

TABLE 53-3 Diphthongs in Thai (/:/ indicates a long vowel)

Short vowels		Long vowels	
ai	ไ- ใ- ไ-ย	aːi	-าย
ɑu	เ-า	ɑːu	-าว
eu	เ-ึ่ว	eːu	เ-ว
ʊɪ	-ุย		
iu	-ึว		
		iːa	เ-ีย
		uːa	-ัว
		ɯːa	เ-ือ
		ɛːu	แ-ว
		ɤːi	เ-ย
		oːi	โ-ย
		ɔːi	-อย

Triphthongs

Triphthongs are the combination of three different vowels. The Thai triphthongs are pronounced differently from English sounds. The closest pronunciation of Thai triphthongs is shown in Table 53-4. Column 1 represents the pronunciation using the International Phonetic Alphabet (IPA) and column 2 shows the Thai triphthongs.

Phonotactic restrictions

The Thai syllable has very complex rules on how consonants are pronounced. Multiple consonants often have the same pronunciation (sound) due to the phonological changes in the Thai language in the past few hundred years. The pronunciation of many Thai consonants can be altered by their position within the syllable. Among the 44 consonants, there are only six main consonants,

TABLE 53-4 Thai triphthongs with their IPA pronunciation

Pronunciation (IPA)	Thai triphthongs
iau	เ-ียว
ɯai	เ-ือย
uai	-วย

namely /m, ʔp, n, ʔt, ŋ, ʔk/, that are used to end syllables. Other consonants can be used to end the syllable, but they must be pronounced as one of the six main consonants.

Syllables

The Thai sound system is best described in relationship to the syllable, the tone-bearing unit. A Thai syllable has the maximum shape CV, VC, CVV, or CVC (Anchaleenukul, 2004; Thongkam, 2003). The sounds represented by selective consonants can change when they are used to end or begin a syllable.

Consonants and consonant clusters

A consonant cluster is a group of consonants that have no intervening vowel. There are at least 12 consonant clusters in Thai in which two consonants are paired and pronounced as a blend unit. Six initial consonants (/kʰ, ʔk, pʰ, ʔp, tʰ, ʔt/) can be paired with three specific consonants (/w, r, l/) to form the clusters. Examples are listed in Table 53-5. The first column shows the prounciation in the International Phonetic Alphabet. Thai clusters are displayed in the second column and the sample words for these clusters are shown in the third column. The meanings of the Thai clusters are listed in the last column.

Tones

The Thai language uses tones to differentiate meaning. There are four tone markers but five tone sounds: middle, low, high, falling, and rising. Tone marks are placed above the initial consonant of the syllable. Tone can be placed on top of the vowel if the vowel is placed above the consonant. Figure 53-1 demonstrates the average fundamental frequency contours for tones, modified from Gandour (1976).

There are five distinctive pitches in Standard Thai. The tonal symbols are placed above the initial consonant of the syllable. Not all consonant forms will have all five tones. Table 53-6 shows graphics of Thai tone with the description.

Stress and intonation

There is no stress in Thai speech, as the majority of Thai words are single units unless they are loanwords from other languages, but most Thai will ignore the stress in the loanwords. The intonation is at suprasegmental or compound words/sentences levels. The syllables with tones are considered at the segmental level.

TABLE 53-5 Thai consonant clusters

IPA	Thai	Example words	Meaning
kʰw	คว ขว	ควาย ขวาน ควัน	'buffalo', 'axe', 'smoke'
ʔkw	กว	กวาง กวาด	'deer', 'sweep'
kʰr	คร ขร	ครู ครัว	'teacher', 'kitchen'
ʔkr	กร	กรง กรุง	'cage', 'city'
kʰl	คล ขล	คลาน เคลื่อน	'crawl', 'move'
ʔkl	กล	กลับ เกลือ	'back', 'salt'
ʔtr	ทร	ทรา(จันทรา)	'the moon'
pʰr	ดร	ตรวจ ตรง	'check', 'straight'
tʰr	พร ผร	พระ พริก	'monk', 'pepper'
pʰl	พล ผล	ผลัก พลิก	'push', 'turn over'
ʔpr	ปร	แปรง ปรับปรุง	'brush', 'improve'
ʔpl	ปล	เปลี่ยนแปลง ปลา	'change', 'fish'

Writing system

One of the most striking features of the modern Thai writing system is the absence of the spaces between words. Words, consisting of consonants or vowels, generally flow uninterruptedly through a sentence. When spaces occur, they often correspond to some form of punctuation mark in English, similar to periods or commas. There are no question marks or capital letters in the Thai script.

The writing and reading of words in sentences are from left to right. From a linguistic or phonetic point of view, the Thai writing system is very complex due to the

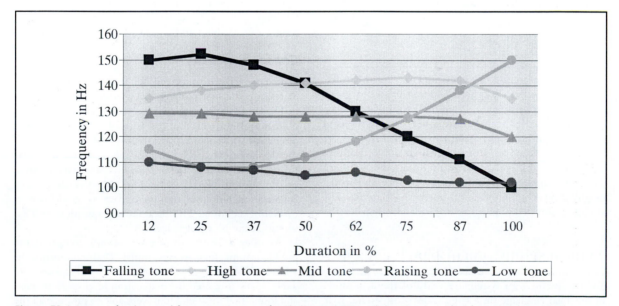

Figure 53-1 Average fundamental frequency contours for Thai tones in Hz and duration (modified from Gandour, 1976)

TABLE 53-6 The five pitches of Standard Thai

Thai symbols	Tonal description
No tone mark	mid level tone
่	low tone
้	falling tone
๊	high tone
๋	rising tone

different locations of the vowels, consonants, and tones. Thai scripts are written into four parallel lines. The following description provides some insight into the complexity of Thai script (http://thaiarc.tu.ac.th):

- The base line is where the consonants and some vowels are written, for example: **นก** /nok/ 'bird,' **ชาม** /tɕʰam/ 'bowl'.
- The line above the base line is used for writing upper vowels and upper diacritics, for example: **กิน** /ʔkin/ 'eat', **จันทร์** /tɕan/ 'moon'.
- The line above the upper vowel line is used for writing tone marks and upper diacritics, for example: **เพื่อน** /pʰɯːan/ with the falling tone 'friend'.
- The line below the base line is used for writing lower vowels and lower diacritics, for example: ถุง /tʰuŋ/ 'bag', ลุง /luŋ/ 'uncle', สูง /suːŋ/ 'tall'.

Varieties of Thai

Thai language consists of Standard Thai and three dialects of the northern, southern, and northeastern regions. Official or Standard Thai is based on the idealized speech of the educated elite of Bangkok and large portions of the Central Plain. The other main regional dialects are Northern Thai, spoken around Chiangmai; Northeastern Thai (Isan), spoken to the east of Korat; and Southern Thai, spoken south of Chumporn province and in the neighboring communities of northern Malaysia. The younger, educated population of Thailand is bidialectal.

Typical acquisition of Thai language

To date there is no systematic study of the acquisition of the Thai language on a large scale. Most studies have involved smaller research samples based on master's theses from the Department of Communicative Disorders at Mahidol University in Bangkok, Thailand. Since most studies have small samples, it is difficult to make generalizations. This chapter is based on clinical observation combined with a few smaller studies in Thai speech acquisition. The Summary of Studies table at the end of this chapter contains studies of Thai speech acquisition.

Acquired sounds

Thai children produce gurgling, cooing, or babbling before developing intelligible sounds. The early common sounds are bilabial and nasal, such as /ma ma/ for mother, /pa pa/ for father; basic vowel sounds such as /a, e, i, o, u/ and glottal sounds emerge by the age of 9 months. First utterances of meaningful words (first words) are assumed to be produced, as in English, at the approximate age of 11 months. Complex consonants and consonant clusters are not developed before 2 years of age. The later development of complex sounds may be related to physiological and motor functions of the child. Children are able to produce complex vowels and consonant clusters to a degree similar to adults by the age of 5. Many children will exhibit normal dysfluency and less than perfect articulatory production when they first acquire these sounds. No systematic research confirms the above assumptions, but the guidelines are used by many Thai speech-language pathologists in the assessment of delayed speech and language. Most of the Thai normative information is based on the English standard. Children are considered delayed when they are unable to produce or comprehend words by age 2.

Consonants

Dardarananda, who received her training in the United States, was the first pioneer speech-language pathologist in Thailand. She is the driving force in the development of many assessment tools as part of students' research projects. Dardarananda (1993) provided a summary of the development of Thai consonants in children similar to the one shown in Table 53-7. Her summary is based on Boonyathitisuk's (1982) studies. Many Thai speech-language pathologists use these data as guidelines in evaluating children. The data show acquisition of Thai sounds at the 80 percent level.

Another study by Muknguen (1980) compared the production of final versus initial Thai consonants in school children aged 3 to 8 years in Bangkok (see Table 53-8). She used the acquisition level of 75 percent and found that most children were able to produce all the final consonants by age 3.5. Most initial consonants were

TABLE 53-7 Age of acquisition for Thai consonants

Age in years and month	Intelligible consonants
2;1–2;6	ม [m] , ณ,น [n], ห,ฮ [h], ญ,ย [j], ค[kʰ], _[ʔ]
2;8–3;0	ว [w], บ [b], ก [k], ป [p]
3;1–3;6	ท [tʰ], ฏ,ต [t], ล [l], จ [tɕ], ย [j] พ [pʰ]
3;7–4;0	ง [ŋ], ค [kʰ]
4;1–4;6	ฟ [f]
5;1–5;6	ส [s], ซ [s]
>7	ร [r] and the rest of the unlisted consonants

Note. Data from Boonyathitisuk (1982) and Dardarananda (1993).

acquired by age 5 except /s/ and /r/. It is interesting that the final consonants were developed earlier than some initial consonants. It may be due to the limited numbers of final consonants in Thai (n = 8) compared to the 44 initial consonants.

Consonant clusters

Muknguen (1989) and Boonyathitisuk (1982) found that only two Thai consonant clusters /kʰw/ and /ʔkw/ are pronounced correctly by 5 years. They concluded that it is common for children to delete the second consonant in consonant clusters, so /ʔk lai/ will be pronounced as [ʔk ai], /ʔplao/ as [ʔpao], and /kʰrap/ as /kʰap/.

Vowels and diphthongs

To date there is no systematic study of vowels and diphthongs. Many of the practicing speech and language pathologists modify normative data from research on the English language except when addressing diphthongs and triphthongs.

TABLE 53-8 Percent correct for Thai consonants

Age	Consonants
3;0–3;5	6 final Thai sounds were acquired at 75 percent correct.
4;6–4;11	42 initial Thai sounds, except /s/ and /r/, were acquired at 75 percent correct.

Note. Data from Muknguen (1980).

Percent correct

To date there is no study of the percentage of correct consonants, vowels, or consonant clusters produced by Thai-speaking children at different ages.

Phonological processes

As children become more mature, phonological errors decrease. The ability to master complex sounds is related to the maturation of motor functions. Although there is no formal study on the phonological processes in Thai, the following generalizations can be made:

- Backing: Substitution of the final consonants with the initial consonants, for example, /-ŋ/ for /-n/ and /-ʔk/ for /-ʔt/.
- Cluster reduction: Reduction of a cluster to a single consonant, for example, /ʔpa:/ for /ʔpla:/ (means fish).
- Deletion of final consonants: Final consonants are not as essential as in English.
- Fronting: Substitution of anterior phonemes.
- Initial consonant deletion: Deletion of the initial consonant sound, substitution of initial consonants with /ʔ/.
- Labialization: Substitution of labial phonemes for other consonants.
- Stopping: Substitution of a stop for a fricative or affricate.
- Nonaspirated: Substitution of a nonaspirated phoneme for an aspirated phoneme.
- Stridency deletion: Omission of a strident or the substitution of a nonstrident consonant.

Intelligibility

Intelligibility of speech depends on dialect and language background as well as socioeconomic status of the child. Based on clinical experience and observations reported by speech–language pathologists, the intelligibility of speech depends on the area where the children live; children who speak variations of dialects from smaller cities tend to be less intelligible when they speak the Central dialect. Speech intelligibility may be related to the socioeconomic structures of the child.

According to Dardarananda (1993), basic simple consonants and vowels were well developed by age 3 (80 percent accuracy). The production of consonants, complex vowels, and consonant clusters continues to develop and approximates adultlike speech by age 7. For the production of loanwords from other languages and complex sentences, most children will show some difficulties in the complex sound sequences.

Phonetic inventory

There are no large-scale studies on establishing norms for speech acquisition in young Thai children. Dardarananda (1993) reported that children produce babbling below 12 months of age. Table 53-7 indicates the phonological inventory for Thai children from age 2 to 7 years. The increase in phonetic inventory is correlated with the rapid increase in vocabulary.

Common mismatches

Dardarananda (1993) reported the following observations based on her clinical experiences working with young Thai children from the Division of Communicative Disorders at Ramathibodi Hospital:

- Although Thai syllables or words can end only with /m, ʔp, n, ʔt, ŋ, ʔk/, the endings of most Thai consonants in the final position are usually half-pronounced. There is a tendency for final consonant deletion.
- The *l* and *r* sounds are often used almost interchangeably in Thai, though they are separate sounds. /r/ is difficult to pronounce, even for many Thai adults.
- Cluster reduction is common in Thai. For cluster consonant blends, it is common for Thai speakers to omit the second consonant of the cluster.
- Initial consonant deletion or substitution of /ʔ/ for other phonemes is also found.

Syllable structure

Thai syllable structures consist of CV, VC, CVC, CCV, and the tone-bearing unit. Acquisition of Thai syllables progresses from simple CV or VC to complex clusters of CCV. Although Thai is a monosyllabic language, many of the nouns are formed by compound words made up of multiple syllables. They may consist of two to four syllables; each syllable has a unique meaning and can stand alone.

Prosody

To date there is no large-scale study on how children acquire prosody.

Phonological awareness

Wei (2005) investigated the relationship between phonological awareness and reading ability. The subjects were a group of children from the primary schools in Thailand. Thai phonological awareness was found to be related to the ability to read syllables. Since Thai has no word boundaries, it is essential for the children to segment each syllable from a long string of syllables. They must develop the ability to detect initial and final sounds, in addition to rhyming, before they can develop the skills to read.

Speech assessment for Thai children

Most speech-language pathologists have developed their own tests to assess speech impairment in their work settings. Some have developed the assessment tools based on their master's thesis. At present no Thai language standardized test has been published.

Most of the speech evaluation information is obtained from the following sources:

- Case history
- Informal observation during parent interview. The examiner will stimulate the child with toys to obtain appropriate speech samples for later analysis. Behavior observation, delayed speech, articulation problems, and fluency are noted.
- Informal assessment with locally developed speech picture cards. Each set of cards is designed to cover all the speech sounds in Thai.

Speech intervention for Thai children

There are two or more groups of professionals who provide speech and language services to Thai children: speech-language pathologists and special education teachers. Therapy techniques vary depending on the educational background and the nature of speech problems. The special education teachers tend to follow the traditional methods, which include articulation drill and placement methods. The SLP group tends to use newer methods, which include sensorimotor techniques and cognitive-linguistic approaches. Auditory verbal therapy techniques are used with hearing-impaired children. Computer software such as IBM Speech Viewer and other biofeedback techniques are popular among modern SLPs.

Working in Thailand

The population of Thailand is 65 million. There is only one training program for master's level speech-language pathologists, at Mahidol University, which commenced around 1975. Currently there are about 65 SLPs with graduate degrees in Thailand.

Thaisha is a national organization of speech-language pathology and audiology in Thailand (http://www.thaisha.org). However, membership is limited to speech-language pathologists and audiologists, and some qualified technicians. There is an attempt to develop licensure, but it is difficult because there are insufficient trained personnel to serve individuals with communicative disorders. The license is from the Ministry of Public Health to work as SLP/Audiologists. Licenses are issued to individuals with graduate degrees in communication disorders. Thaisha organizes an annual conference for the members to obtain continuing education units (CEU) and network opportunities.

PHONETICALLY SPEAKING

Pronunciation of Thai: /pʰaː saː tʰai/

Relevant words for speech assessment and intervention

Word	Thai script	Pronunciation
tongue	ลิ้น	/lin/
teeth	ฟัน	/fan/
lips	ริมฝีปาก	/rimfiː?paː?k/
hard palate	เพดานปาก	/pʰe daːn ?paː?k/
soft palate	เพดานอ่อน	/pʰe daːn ?ɔːn/
larynx	กล่องเสียง	/?kɔːŋ siaːŋ/
lung	ปอด	/?pɔːd/
nose	จมูก	/tɕa muː?k/
sound	เสียง	/siaːŋ/
word	คำ	/kʰam/
sentence	ประโยค	/?pra joː?k/
paragraph	ย่อหน้า	/jɔː naː/

Note.   symbol /ː/ = long vowel

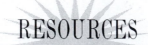

RESOURCES

Journal articles, books, and dissertations

- Manochiopinig, S., Pracharitpukdee, N., and Lertsarunyapong, S. (1998). The articulation characteristics of normal Thai children aged 3-10 years, *Siriraj Hospital Gazette, 50*(8), 763–769.
- Pattamadilok, K. (1977). *The history of the Thai language.* Chiangmai, Thailand: Chiangmai University Press.
- Tiencharoen, S. (1987). *A comparative study of spoken and written Thai: Linguistic and sociolinguistic perspectives.* Unpublished doctoral dissertation, Georgetown University.
- Tuaychareon, P. (1990). *Phonetics.* Bangkok, Thailand: Thammasat University Press.

Journals

There is no journal related to communication disorders published in Thailand.

Professional associations

Thaisha is the profession association of speech-language pathology and audiology in Thailand.

Useful Web sites

- Official Web site for Thai Speech-language Pathology and Audiology: http://www.thaisha.org/.
- Official Web site of Chiengrai Rajabhat University in Thailand: http://www.lib.ricr.ac.th/.
- Thai Language Audio Resource Center, Thammasat University in Thailand: http://thaiarc.tu.ac.th/.
- Thai Language Learning Framework and Forum by John Hartmann, Northern Illinois University: http://www.seasite.niu.edu/thai/LLF/profile.htm.
- ScienceDaily, an online magazine about science, technology, and medicine http://www.sciencedaily.com/encyclopedia/thai_alphabet.

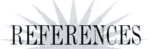

REFERENCES

Anchaleenukul, S. (2004). *Thai word system.* Bangkok, Thailand: Chulalongkorn University Press.

Boonyathitisuk, P. (1982). *Articulatory characteristics of kindergarten children aged three to four years eleven months in Bangkok.* Unpublished master's thesis, Mahidol University, Bangkok, Thailand.

Chaichana, C. (1963). *History of Thailand.* Bangkok, Thailand: Kasembanakit Press.

Dardarananda, R. (1993). *The life and work of Professor Dardarananda: Collection of articles from Ramathibodi Hospital.* Division of Communicative Disorders, Mahidol University, Bangkok, Thailand.

Gandour, J. (1976). Aspects of Thai tone (Doctoral dissertation, University of California at Los Angeles, 1976). *Dissertation Abstracts International, 37,* 1516-A (University Microfilms No. 76-21, 348).

Hinds, J. (1988). Conversational interaction in Central Thai. In C. Bamroongrak, G. Williams et al. (Eds.), *International symposium on language and linguistics* (pp. 150–163). Bangkok, Thailand: Thammasat University Press.

Kingkam, W. (2004). *Thai dialects.* Bangkok, Thailand: Kasetsart University Press.

Muknguen, S. (1980). *Articulatory characteristics of school children aged three to eight years in Phaya-Thai area.* Unpublished master's thesis, Mahidol University, Bangkok, Thailand.

Smalley, W. A. (1994). *Linguistic diversity and national unity: Language ecology in Thailand.* Chicago: University of Chicago Press.

Thongkam, L. (2003). *Thai accent. Laryngectomees.* Bangkok, Thailand: Chulalongkorn University Press.

Wei, Y. F. (2005). *The relationship between phonological awareness and reading ability of Thai students in English and Thai in primary schools of Thailand.* Unpublished doctoral dissertation, University of Maryland.

Wikipedia (2005). Thai Language. http://en.wikipedia.org/wiki/Thai_language#Vowels.

SUMMARY OF STUDIES OF TYPICAL THAI SPEECH ACQUISITION

Authors	Year	Country	No. of children	Age of children	Information	Sample type	Data collection
Boonyathitisuk	1982	Thailand	1032	3–8 yrs	Articulation characteristics	Picture naming	Cross-sectional
Muknguen	1980	Thailand	400	3;0–4;11	Articulation characteristics	Picture naming	Cross-sectional
Manochiopinig et al.	1998	Thailand	560	3;0–10;0	Articulation characteristics	Picture naming	Cross-sectional

Chapter 54

Turkish Speech Acquisition

Seyhun Topbaş

INTRODUCTION

Turkish is accepted within the southwest group of Turkic languages belonging to the Oghuz branch. It is still controversial whether or not it is a branch of the Ural-Altai linguistic family (Göksel & Kerslake, 2005; Lewis, 2000). Turkish is an agglutinating language, that is, a large number of affixes may be added to the root, each of which has only one meaning or grammatical function. In strings of morphemes, each element retains its phonological and semantic identity as well as its relative position (Comrie, 1997; Erguvanlı-Taylan, 1984). The neutral word order is subject-object-verb (SOV). Please see the Resources at the end of this chapter.

Where Turkish is spoken

Modern Standard Turkish is the official and the native language of the Republic of Turkey and is spoken by over 67 million people (see accompanying map and Appendix D). About 20 percent of residents are linguistic minorities who have grown up as bilinguals. They speak Kurdish (forming the largest linguistic population of about 8 to 10 percent), Jewish, Modern Greek and Armenian (Comrie, 1992; Kornfilt, 1997; Göksel and Kerslake, 2005) as their first language. Modern Standard Turkish is used as the medium of instruction in kindergarten, school, and university all over Turkey. More than 3 million people of Turkish descent live abroad. Over a million speakers of Turkish are found in Bulgaria, Romania, Serbia, Greece and Cyprus. Thus, Turkish is also a co-official language in North Cyprus, and in some municipalities of Republic of Macedonia and Kosovo. Over 3.0 million immigrants live in Germany and other European countries,

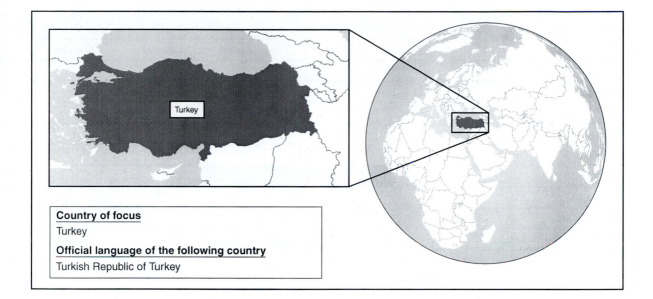

Country of focus
Turkey

Official language of the following country
Turkish Republic of Turkey

including Austria, Belgium, France, Denmark, the Netherlands, Switzerland, and the United Kingdom (Schaufeli, 1991; Göksel and Kerslake, 2005), and about 100,000 Turkish speakers live in Australia, Canada and the United States (Grimes, 1992; Yağmur, 1997; Turkish Ministry of Affairs, 2003).

Components of Turkish

Consonants

Turkish contains 21 consonant phonemes /p, b, t, d, k, g, ɣ, f, v, s, z, ʃ, ʒ, h, m, n, ɾ, l, j, tʃ, dʒ/ (see Table 54-1). The voiceless noncontinuant obstruents /p, t, k, tʃ/ are aspirated in all positions and may be released in codas unless followed by a homorganic consonant. The voiced noncontinuants /b, d, g, dʒ/ cannot occur in final position. The velar stops /k, g/ have palatal allophones [c] and [ɟ], which are conditioned by the neighboring vowels. Palatal [c] and [ɟ] occur in syllables with front vowels /i, ɛ, y, œ/ and the velar [k] and [g] occur in syllables with back vowels /ɯ, a, o, u/. The continuant obstruent /v/ has two allophones as well: it is a fricative in initial position (e.g., [vazo] 'vase'), but in medial or final position it becomes a frictionless continuant, [ʋ], (e.g., [haʋa] 'weather', [haʋlu] 'towel', [eʋ] 'house'). The orthographically preserved (soft-g) voiced velar fricative, [ɣ], indicates lengthening of the previous vowel (e.g., *oğlan* [oːɫan] 'boy', *dağ* [daː] 'mountain') in syllable-final position. When it occurs after front vowels (e.g., *iğne* [iynɛ] 'injection'), it is replaced by the palatal glide, and it

does not occur post-vocalically, in syllable-initial position (e.g., *soğan* [soan] 'onion', *doğu* [dou] 'east') (Kornfilt, 1997; Topbaş and Yavaş, in press). /h/ in final position may be realized as a voiceless velar fricative. The sonorant alveolar flap /ɾ/ has a voiceless allophone in final position, which is produced with friction (e.g., [kaɾ̥]). The alveolar lateral approximant /l/ has two allophones in native words: (a) velarized or "dark-l," [ɫ], when it occurs with a tautosyllabic back vowel (e.g., [haɫa] 'aunt'), and (b) palatalized or "clear-l" when it occurs with a tautosyllabic front vowel (e.g., [cilim] 'carpet'). All laterals in word-initial position are borrowings, which are predictably palatalized; laterals are also predictably palatalized when either the immediately preceding or following vowel is front, even if that vowel is not tautosyllabic (e.g., [sɛ.lam] 'greeting'). Almost all laterals in other positions of borrowed words are of the "clear" or palatalized version regardless of their vocalic environment. There is a dispute over whether the above-mentioned allophonic variations of obstruents [k, g] and the allophonic variation of lateral [l] should be fully recognized as phonemically distinct. As in the acquisition studies of Turkish, for ease of presentation in this chapter they are treated separately (Topbaş and Yavaş, in press; Zimmer and Orgun, 1999).

Vowels and diphthongs

The vowel system of Turkish contains 8 vowels (see Table 54-2). Phonetically three degrees of height (high, mid, low) are considered; phonologically /i, y, ɯ, u/ are considered as high and /ɛ, ø, a, o/ are considered as

TABLE 54-1 Consonants produced in Turkish

	Bilabial	Labiodental	Dental	Alveolar
Plosive	p b			t d
Nasal	m			n
Trill				
Tap or flap				ɾ
Fricative		f v		s z
Lateral fricative	■		■	
Affricate				
Approximant				
Lateral approximant	■		■	ɫ l

Black = articulations judged impossible

Based on the International Phonetic Alphabet. Courtesy of the International Phonetic Association (c/o Department of Linguistics, University of Victoria, Victoria, British Columbia, Canada).

nonhigh. All vowels in Turkish are are accepted as being short. Currently, objective acoustic studies are ongoing in this respect (Turk et al., 2004; Kılıc, 2003). Long vowels may occur through the above-mentioned deletion of "soft-g," or in borrowed vocabulary. /a/ may have allophones: [a] speaker-dependent as in *para* [paɾa] 'money'; and [ʌ] elsewhere (Kopkallı-Yavuz, 2000); [ø] also has an allophone, [œ]. Turkish does not have diphthongs but the vowels followed by /j/ may create diphthong-like sounds; *ay* /aj/ 'moon'. However, the /j/ becomes the onset consonant if it is followed by a vowel (e.g., *ayı* [ajɯ] 'bear').

Phonotactic restrictions

Syllables

The canonical syllable type is CV, allowing syllable structures as (C)V(C)(C), in that the vowel nucleus is the only obligatory element. Morphological structure, applying freely across morpheme boundaries, allows syllabification with the requirements of phonological constraints. The maximum *Onset First Principle* (Clements and Keyser, 1983) is a major assignment for clusters and sequences of two consonants that are not tautosyllabic. Thus, the final consonant clusters are syllabified; the first consonant in

TABLE 54-2 Vowels produced in Turkish

Turkish location	Standard-Turkish vowels	Example words	English translation
High-front	i	*inek* [inɛc]	'cow'
High-front rounded	y	*üzüm* [yzym]	'grapes'
Mid-front	ɛ	*ekmek* [ɛcmɛc]	'bread'
Mid-front rounded	ø or œ	*ördek* [ørdɛc]	'duck'
		göl [ɟœl]	'lake'
Mid-back	ɯ	*ışık* [ɯʃɯk]	'light'
Mid-back rounded	o	*oda* [odʌ]	'room'
High-back rounded	u	*uçak* [utʃʌk]	'airplane'
Central-low	a or ʌ	*aslan* [asɫʌn]	'lion'

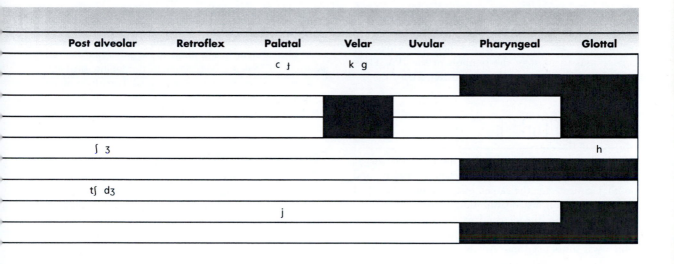

	Post alveolar	Retroflex	Palatal	Velar	Uvular	Pharyngeal	Glottal
			c ɟ	k g			
	ʃ ʒ						h
	tʃ dʒ						
			j				

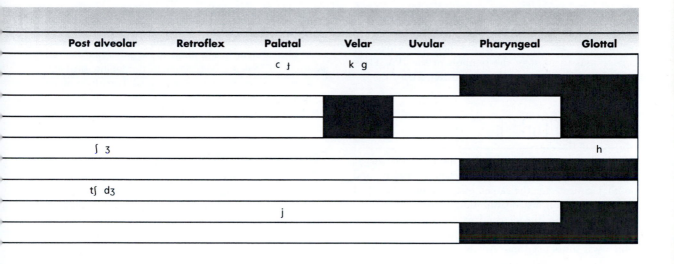

the sequence with the preceding vowel and the last one with the following vowel (e.g., *Türk* [tyɾc] 'Turkish' ⇨ *türk+üm* [tyɾ.cym] 'I'm Turkish'). Intervocalic consonants are also assigned to the following syllable and ambisyllabicity is not allowed (e.g., *çimen* [tʃi.mɛn] 'grass', *kalem* [ka.lɛm] 'pencil'). Since Turkish is an agglutinating language, words can be derived by inflections that may contain successive long strings of syllables.

Consonants and consonant clusters

There are no onset clusters, syllable-initial or word-initial. Only certain cluster codas, consisting of not more than two consonants, are permitted and can be mainly described as:

- C1= sonorant + C2= obstruent (e.g., [faɾk] 'difference', [tyɾc] 'Turkish', [ʃort] 'short pant', [tuɾp] 'radish', [ɾenk] 'color', [vintʃ] 'crane')
- C1= fricative + C2= stop (e.g., [tʃift] 'couple', [aʃk] 'love'

Loanwords or borrowed words may have a sequence of C1= /k/ + C2= /s/ (e.g., [boks] 'boxing', [ɾaks] 'dancing'). Some Western borrowed words may contain initial clusters, but these are broken up via vowel epenthesis (e.g., *kral* [kɯ.ɾʌl] 'king', *traktör* [tɯ.ɾʌk.tœr] 'tractor/caterpillar').

Phonological processes

Vowel harmony. All vowels in native words are subject to vowel harmony. Neighboring vowels in a word agree in backness (i.e., all "front" or all "back" sounds); and in addition, high vowels agree in rounding with the preceding vowel (e.g., *köy* [cœj] 'village', *köyler* [cœj.lɛr] 'villages', *köyüm* [cœj.ym] 'my village').

Final devoicing. /b, d, g/ and affricate /dʒ/ becomes voiceless in word- or syllable-final position. Words with these consonants may have different underlying representations of alternating and nonalternating roots (Kopkallı-Yavuz, 1993).

Assimilation. Place of articulation assimilation, which may affect nasals respectively, is generally regressive (e.g., *penbe* [pembe] 'pink'), and voicing assimilation, which may affect stop-initial and affricate-initial suffixes, is generally progressive in Turkish (e.g., [kap] *cup* +suffix −*de* [kap.ta] 'in the cup').

Tones

Turkish does not use tones to differentiate meaning.

Stress and intonation

Stress, in Turkish, generally falls on the last syllable, having phonetic correlates of loudness and higher pitch (e.g., [a.ɾa.bá] 'car', [a.ɾa.ba.já] 'to the car', [a.ɾa.ba.mɯ.zá] 'to our car', [a.ɾa.ba.ta.ɾɯ.mɯz] 'our cars', [a.ɾa.ba.taɾɯ.mɯ.zá] 'to our cars'). Exceptions to the final syllable rule are:

- place names in which the addition of affixes does not change the position of the stress (e.g., [a ´n.ka.ɾa], [án.ka.ɾa.ja] 'to Ankara')
- many adverbs (e.g., [kɯ́.ʃɯn] 'in winter', [hé.mɛn] 'right now', [ó.ɾa.da] 'there')
- interjections and vocatives (e.g., [háj.di] 'let's, come on')

In Turkish, a syllable-timed language, all syllables, stressed and unstressed, have more or less equal duration (Kornfilt, 1997; Topbaş & Yavaş, in press).

Writing system

Turkish uses the modern Latin alphabet. The standard orthography assigns one symbol per phoneme that corresponds to most of the symbols of the IPA. Thus, Turkish assigns 29 symbols: 8 for vowels, 21 for consonant phonemes.

Varieties of Turkish

While Modern Standard Turkish is the official language, several dialects are reported; Rumelian, Anatolian, and South Crimean are the larger ones. Modern Standard Turkish represents a standardization of the Istanbul dialect of Anatolian, the descendant of Ottoman Turkish and its predecessor, the so-called Old Anatolian Turkish, which was introduced into Anatolia by the Seljuk Turks in the late eleventh century AD (Kornfilt, 1997). There are regional accents or variations that affect the pronunciation of some consonants.

Typical acquisition of Turkish

The Summary of Studies Table at the end of this chapter contains studies of the acquisition of Turkish. They have been summarized in Topbaş and Yavaş (in press).

Acquired sounds
Consonants

Table 54-3 contains age of phoneme acquisition data from the study by Topbaş (2004/2005). In this longitudinal and cross-sectional study 665 monolingual Turkish-speaking children aged 1;6 to 8;0 were assessed for their speech abilities. No differences between boys and girls were observed (for details refer to Topbaş and Yavas, 2006)

Consonant clusters

Topbaş (2004/2005; Topbaş, Kopkallı-Yavuz, 2006) investigated the acquisition of word-final clusters of Turkish (see Table 54-4). Among the clusters the nasal + stop /ntS, nk/ clusters started to be acquired by the age of 3;0 to 3;6. Fricative + stop /ft, st/ and liquid + stop /lp, lk/ clusters were observed to be produced correctly at 3;6 and stabilizing at around 4;0; and flap + stop /ɾt, ɾk/ clusters were acquired last, around the age of 4;6 to 5;0. Although the liquids seemed to occur in children's speech much earlier, they were subject to deletion when they occurred in clusters (Topbaş and Kopkallı-Yavuz, 2006).

Vowels and diphthongs

To date no study has investigated vowel acquisition in detail.

TABLE 54-3   Age of acquisition for Turkish consonants

Age group	75 percent of children who produced phoneme at least 68 percent correct				90 percent of children who produced phoneme at least 68 percent correct			
	SIWI	SIWW	SFWW	SFWF	SIWI	SIWW	SFWW	SFWF
1;6–1;11	b, d, k, t, m, n, p, j	b, d, t, m, p, k, g, n	m, n, j, p, k, l	p, k, c, t, m, n, j	b, d, k, t, m	b, d, t, m	m, n, j	p, k, t, m, n, j
2;0–2;5	g , ɟ, tʃ, dʒ, l, s, ʃ	tʃ, dʒ, ɟ, l, ɫ, s, ʃ	ʊ, tʃ, ʃ	tʃ, ʊ, s, ʃ, l	p, g, t, n, ɟ, tʃ, dʒ, j, l	p, k, g, n, tʃ, dʒ, j	p, k, l, ʊ	c, tʃ, ʊ
2;6–2;11	f, v, z, ʒ, h	ʊ	s, ɫ	f, ʒ	s, ʃ	s, ʃ, l, ɫ	s, ʃ, tʃ, ɫ	s, ʃ, l
3;0–3,5	ɾ	f, z, h	z, f, h	z, h, ɾ̥	f, v, z, ʒ, h	f, ʒ, z, v	z, f	f, ʒ, z, h
3;6–3;11	All	ɾ	ɾ	clusters	ɾ	h	h,	ɾ̥
4;0–4;5	All	ɣ	All	ɣ	All	r, ɣ	r	ɣ, clusters
4;6–4;11	All	All	All	All	All	All	All	clusters
5;0–5;11	All	All	All	All	All	All	All	All

KeyNote. Data from Topbaş (2004/2005). SIWI = syllable initial, word initial; SIWW = syllable initial within word; SFWW = syllable final, within word; SFWF = syllable final, word final.

TABLE 54-4 Age of acquisition of consonant clusters by Turkish-speaking children

Consonant cluster	Age of acquisition
-ntʃ	3;0–3;6
-nk	3;0–3;6
-ft	3;6–4;0
-st	3;6–4;0
-lp	3;6–4;0
-lk	3;6–4;0
-rt	4;6–5;0
-rk	4;6–5;0

Note. Data from Topbaş (2004/2005); Topbaş et al. (2006).

Percent correct

Consonants

Percentage of consonants produced correctly has been studied by Topbaş (2004/2005) and Topbaş and Yavas (2006). The overall correct (PCC) and error (PCE) rate of phonemes with standard deviation values for each age group is given in Table 54-5. There were no differences for gender among the groups on the PCC.

Consonant clusters

The above study by Topbaş included the percentage of consonant clusters produced correctly (Topbaş, 2006).

Vowels

To date no study has yet investigated percentage of vowel production in detail. However, Aksu-Koç and Slobin (1985) reported that children acquire the vowel system at an early age and make few vowel errors.

Phonological processes

The most detailed studies of developmental phonological processes in Turkish were conducted by Topbaş and colleagues (1992, reanalyzed 1996; 1997; 2005; Topbaş and Konrot, 1998; Kopkallı-Yavuz and Topbaş, 1998; Topbaş and Yavas, 2006) covering longitudinal and cross-sectional data (see Table 54-6).

Topbaş and Kopkallı-Yavuz (1998) have also analyzed the phonological process of word-final devoicing (FD) concerning the /b, d, c, g/ sounds in Turkish in 30 typical children aged 16 to 30 months in a longitudinal and cross-sectional study. At 16 months children began using inflected forms, which gives evidence for the presence of the FD rule. By 18 months inflected forms became increasingly frequent. Alternations between the voiced and voiceless set of noncontinuant obstruents were examined. At 22 months, alternating forms were pretty well established, although there were a few cases of substitution of nonalternating forms for alternating ones. At 26 months the rule was completely acquired.

Intelligibility

No study has yet assessed in detail the intelligibility of typical Turkish-speaking children. There is only one small group study on speech-impaired children (aged between 5;0 and 8;0) that has assessed intelligibility. The following listener judgments were made: correlation of average words per utterance, intended words, PCC, and such suprasegmental aspects as voice (pitch, loudness, quality) and rhythm (phrasing, stress, and rate) were calculated based on Shriberg and Kwiatkowski (1982). This small group study found significant correlation between suprasegmentals and PCC. It is reported that low performance on PCC may affect a child's performance on suprasegmentals (Topbaş, 1996).

Phonetic inventory

The study by Topbaş and Yavaş (in press) analyzed the phonetic inventory of Turkish-speaking children.

Common mismatches

A few studies (Topbaş, 1997; Topbaş and Konrot (1998), Yavaş and Topbaş (2004), Topbaş and Dinçer (2002), Topbaş (2006) and Yavas and Topbaş (2006) have analyzed the error patterns by typically developing and speech-impaired children. The most common error patterns observed were liquid deviation, word-final cluster reduction, fronting, and stopping processes.

Syllable structure

Kopkallı-Yavuz and Topbaş (2000) have analyzed children's preferences for syllable and word forms in phonological acquisition in 30 typically developing children in a longitudinal and cross-sectional study when children

TABLE 54-5 Percent phonemes/consonants correct (PCC) by age group

		Age							
		1;3–2;0 (n=41)		2;1–3;0 (n=47)		3;1–4;0 (n=41)		4;1–5;0 (n=57)	
		mean	SD	mean	SD	mean	SD	mean	SD
PCC	Boys	41.10	13.21	68.50	12.76	94.88	4.29	98.72	2.26
	Girls	44.27	11.80	74.00	8.77	94.78	4.87	97.78	2.53
	Total	42.80	12.42	71.42	11.05	94.85	4.44	98.19	2.44

Note. Data from Topbaş & Yavas (in press).

reached the 15-word stage, 50-word stage, and 75-word stage. They reported that Turkish children attempted disyllabic words more frequently than monosyllabic words. In production, disyllabic words usually were not reduced to monosyllables. As for open/closed syllables, the children did not avoid closed syllables either in monosyllabic or disyllabic words. When closed syllables were reduced to open syllables, the closing consonants were /l/, /r/, /j/.

Prosody

There is as yet no study on the acquisition of prosody by typical Turkish-speaking children.

TABLE 54-6 Percentage of phonological processes used by 665 Turkish children (Topbaş, 2004/2005)

	1;6	2;0	2;6	3;0	3;6	4;0	4;6	5;0	6;0>
Structural simplifications									
Reduplication	41	9	1						
Syllable deletion (stressed/non-stressed)	37	30	22	13	2				
Consonant deletion (SI, SF)	19	21	111	6	2				
Word-final cluster reduction	56	98	71	48	30	4	3	1	
Assimilation/consonant harmony	15	22	17	3	1				
Systemic simplifications									
Liquid deviation	76	90	55	42	24	8	3	1	1
Fronting of velars	28	46	10	2					
Stopping of fricatives/affricates	44	58	36	16	5	1			
Deaffrication	7	13	5	0.5					
Affrication	8	19	6	1					
Voicing (SIWI & SIWW)	38	11	3						
Word-final devoicing /z/	21	45	17	1					
Metathesis	9	11	2						
Backing to palatals & velars	3	6	2						

Note. Data from Topbaş (2004/2005). SI = syllable-initial; SF = syllable-final; SIWI = syllable-initial, word-initial; SIWW = syllable-initial, within word.

5;1–6;0 (n=63)		6;1–7;0 (n=159)		7;1–8;0 (n=128)		8 > (n=129)		Phonologically disordered (n=70)		Total (n=735)	
mean	SD	mean	SD	mean	SD	mean	SD	mean	SD	mean	SD
97.54	3.21	98.52	2.53	99.56	1.31	99.40	1.13	60.02	18.56	90.15	18.69
98.33	2.39	98.80	2.18	99.22	1.76	99.54	1.37	65.96	18.04	90.55	17.52
97.92	2.85	98.66	2.35	99.42	1.51	99.47	1.25	62.74	18.43	90.34	18.13

Phonological awareness

No study has yet adequately investigated the acquisition of phonological awareness in typical Turkish-speaking children.

Speech assessment for Turkish-speaking children

To date a nonstandardized articulation tool developed by Özsoy (1982), and informal materials designed by clinicians, have been used to assess the speech of Turkish children. The reliability and validity of these instruments has not been evaluated. Recently two standardized tests have been developed (see Table 54-7). One of these tests, *Ankara Articulation Test*, is segment-oriented, based on a picture–naming task that targets one phoneme, and only the realization of that one phoneme is noted (Ege, Acarlar, and Turan, 2004). The second test, *Turkish Articulation-Phonology Test-SST*, was developed by Topbaş (2004/2005) in collaboration with the Ministry of Education to be used in formal assessments. *SST* is linguistically balanced, has naming reliability, validity, and

norms, and covers all aspects of speech development. It has three subtests:

- Articulation subtest: segment-oriented, based on a picture-naming task
- Auditory discrimination subtest: assesses phoneme discrimination in minimal pairs
- Phonological analysis subtest: based on continuous speech sampling by picture descriptions

The results were interpreted by phonological process analysis, severity measures, and inconsistency.

Speech intervention for Turkish-speaking children

In Turkey, speech-language pathology is a new profession and is not as well established as in the United States or European countries and, as a result, is not supported in law and through certification. Until recently, in the entire country only seven or eight persons held advanced (master's and doctoral level) degrees in speech-language pathology. They were trained overseas, mainly in England and the United States (Topbaş, 2006, b). By the efforts

TABLE 54-7   Most popular tests for assessing children's speech sounds

Tool	Author/s	SO	PO	IT	Norms
Eskisehir Speech Assessment Test	Ozsoy (1982)	+	–	–	–
Ankara Articulation Test	Ege, Acarlar, and Turan (2004)	+	–	–	+
Turkish Articulation-Phonology Test	Topbaş (2004/5)	+	+	+	+

Key. SO = Segment-orientated; PO = Process-orientated; IT = Inconsistency Test

of these SLPs, a postgraduate program offering training in speech-language pathology at the master's and Ph.D. level was initiated at Anadolu University in Turkey in 2000, and license requirements are just beginning to be established. The graduates of this program (38 graduates in 2006) have begun practicing in the field very recently. These SLPs are expected to treat people with all kinds of communication impairments. There are currently a number of additional different professionals (such as audiologists, special education teachers, and psychologists) working in the field of SLP in Turkey. Audiologists and special education teachers mostly work on the speech and language development of hearing-impaired children and mentally retarded children, and work in private and/or national special education schools and centers. In a few university hospitals some medical ear-nose-throat specialists work on voice disorders, and some neurologists work on aphasia and related neurogenic disorders. The cost of speech therapy for nonorganic or functional disorders was covered by national insurances after new legislation was enacted in late 2005.

The dominant intervention approach used in Turkey is still articulation therapy (van Riper, 1963). In the late 1990s, a change from articulation to psycholinguistically oriented phonological intervention has been introduced by the efforts of Topbaş (1994; 1997; 1998; Topbaş and Konrot, 1998; Kopkallı-Yavuz and Topbaş, 1998) based on Grunwell (1985), Ingram (1981), and Dodd (1995).

The following phonological approaches are now in the process of being adopted: Metaphon (Howell and Dean, 1995); Minimal Pair Therapy (Saben and Ingham, 1991). Single-subject efficacy methodologies in articulation and phonological therapy have also been introduced to the field (Kıran-Gerçek and Topbaş, 2005).

Working in Turkey

In order to work in Turkey as an SLP, it is not necessary to apply for a certificate that proves one's qualification as an SLP; however, foreigners need working permission from the Ministry of Foreign Affairs and Ministry of Internal Affairs. An SLP who wishes to work at or be a visiting professor at a university center can also apply to Fulbright (http://www.cies.org/us_scholars) in accordance with the contact university. Similarly, if the SLP has a contact or fellowship at a university in Turkey, that university may apply to TUBITAK [The Scientific and Technological Research Council of Turkey] (http://www.tubitak.gov.tr) for a visiting scholar supportive grant. Currently, there is no institution that is responsible for issuing certificates for SLP as in the US, and membership in a professional body is not compulsory. However, to practice as an SLP a Masters degree diploma with 400 hours of clinical practicum is compulsory. An annual conference is held by the co-efforts of DILKOM and DKBUD (listed in the Resources section).

PHONETICALLY SPEAKING

Pronunciation of Turkish: Türkçe: [tyrɛtʃɛ] Turk: Türk [tyrɛ]

Relevant words for speech assessment and intervention

Word	Formal usage	Pronunciation	Informal usage	Pronunciation
Tongue	dil	/dil/	dil	/dil/
Teeth	diş	/diʃ/	diş	/diʃ/
Lips	dudak	/dudʌk/	dudak	/dudʌk/
Hard palate	palat sert damak	/patʌt sɛrt dʌmʌk/	sert damak	/sɛrt dʌmʌk/
Soft palate	yumuşak damak	/jumuʃʌk dʌmʌk/	yumuşak damak	/jumuʃʌk dʌmʌk/
Larynx	larenks	/lʌrɛncs/	gırtlak	/gɯrttʌk/
Lungs	akciğer	/akdʒijeɾ̃/	akciğer	/akdʒijeɾ̃/
Nose	burun	/burun/	burun	/burun/
Sound	ses	/sɛs/	ses	/sɛs/
Word	sözcük	/sœzdʒyc/	sözcük	/sœzdʒyc/
Sentence	tümce	/tymdʒɛ/	tümce	/tymdʒɛ/
Paragraph	paragraf	/parʌgrʌf/	paragraf	/parʌgrʌf/

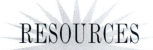

RESOURCES

Books

Topbaş, S. (2005). *Dil ve kavram gelişimi.* [Language and concept development] Ankara: Kok Pub.

Topbaş, S., and Mavis, İ. (2004). *Dil ve konuşma bozuklukları terimler sözlüğü.* [Turkish dictionary of speech and language disorders]. Ankara: Karatepe Pub.

Topbaş, S. (1998). *Konuşma sorunlu çocukların sesbilgisel çözümleme yöntemi ile değerlendirilmesi.* [Assessment of speech disordered children by phonological analysis] Eskişehir: Anadolu University Press.

Topbaş, S. (2004). The frequency effect and the acquisition of /k/, /t/, /tʃ/ sounds in Turkish. (revised M.Sc. Dissertation, City University of London, 1988). Eskişehir: Ongar Basımevi.

Kornfilt, J. (1997). *Turkish.* London: Routledge.

Balpınar, Z. (2003). *Turkish phonology, morphology and syntax.* Eskişehir: Anadolu University Press.

Demircan, Ö. (1982). *Türkçe'nin Sesdizimi.* İstanbul: İstanbul University Press.

Journals

- There are yet no journals published specifically by SLPs and/or for SLP.

Professional associations

The professional association of speech and language pathologists (DKBUD) http://www.dkbud.org was formed only recently (23 December, 2004) and the formal processes are still evolving.

Universities offering courses in Speech-Language Pathology / Logopedi in Turkey

There is no SLP program at the undergraduate university level and only one offering SLP at the postgraduate master of science/health and doctorate level under the Institute of Health Sciences at Anadolu University, Eskişehir. The course and clinical practicum requirements of this program are designed according to

ASHA and IALP regulations and are similar to those programs in the USA. Although certification is not yet supported through law, for future requirements of licensure the program offers 450 hours of clinical practicum that is required for graduation. Apart from this program, four universities offer post-graduate programs in audiology as a major and speech pathology courses as a minor.

Useful Turkish Web sites

- Education, Research, and Training Centre for Speech and Language Disorders.
  http://www.dilkom.anadolu.edu.tr
- Ministry of International Affairs.
  http://www.disisleri.gov.tr
- Ministry of Education.
  http://www.meb.gov.tr
- Council of Higher Education of Turkey.
  http://www.yok.gov.tr
- The Scientific and Technological Research Council of Turkey.
  http://www.tubitak.gov.tr

REFERENCES

Acarlar, F. (1995). *Normal ve fonolojik bozukluğu olan çocukların karşılaştırılması* [Comparative study on normally developing and phonologically disordered children]. Unpublished doctoral dissertation, Hacettepe University, Ankara, Turkey.

Acarlar, F., and Ege, P. (1996). *Türkçe kazanımda kullanılan fonolojik süreçlerin incelenmesi.* [Phonological processes in the acquisition of Turkish] *Türk Psikoloji Dergisi,* 38, 35–43.

Aksu-Koç A. A., and Slobin D. I. (1985). The acquisition of Turkish. In D. I. Slobin, (Ed.). *The crosslinguistic study of language acquisition.* (The Data Vol. 1) (pp. 839–876). Hillsdale, NJ: Lawrence Erlbaum.

Barlow, J. A. (1996). Variability and phonological knowledge. In T. W. Powell (Ed), *Pathologies of speech and language: Contributions of clinical phonetics and linguistics* (pp. 125–134). New Orleans, LA: ICPLA.

Clements, G. N., and Keyser, S. J. (1983). *CV phonology: A generative theory of the syllable.* Linguistic Inquiry Monograph 9. Cambridge, MA: MIT Press.

Comrie, B. (1992). Turkic languages. In W. Bright, (Ed.), *International encyclopedia of linguistics* (Vol. 4, pp. 187–190). New York: Oxford University Press.

Dinnsen, D., and Chin, S. (1994). Independent and relational accounts of phonological disorders. In M. Yavaş (Ed.), *First

and second language phonology* (pp. 135–148). San Diego, CA: Singular.

Dodd, B. (1995). *Differential diagnosis and treatment of children with speech disorder.* London: Whurr.

Ege, P., Acarlar, F., and Güleryüz, F. (2004). *Ankara artikülasyon testi* [Ankara articulation test] Ankara: Key Tasarım.

Erguvanli-Taylan, E. (1984). *The function of word order in Turkish grammar* (Vol 106). Berkeley and Los Angeles: University of California Press.

Göskel, A. and Kerslake, C. (2005). Turkish: A comprehensive grammar. London: Rutledge.

Grimes, B. F. (1992). *Ethnologue: Languages of the world.* Dallas, TX: Summer Institute of Linguistics.

Grunwell, P. (1985). *PACS. Phonological analysis of child speech.* Windsor: NFER-NELSON.

Grunwell, P. (1987). *Clinical phonology.* London: Croom Helm.

Howell, J., and Dean, E. (1995). *Treating phonological disorders in children—Metaphon—theory to practice* (2nd ed.). London: Whurr.

Ingram, D. (1981). *Procedures for the phonological analysis of children's language.* Baltimore: University Park Press.

Ingram, D. (1989). *Phonological disability in children* (2nd ed). London: Whurr.

Kılıç, M.A. (2003). Türkiye Türkçesi'ndeki ünlülerin sesbilgisel özellikleri. [Vowel characteristics of Turkish]. In S. Özsoy; D.Akar; M. Nakipoglu-Demiralp; E. Erguvanlı-Taylan, and A. Aksu-Koç (Eds.), *Proceedings of the 10th International Conference on Turkish Linguistics* (pp. 19–27). Istanbul: Bogaziçi University Press.

Kıran-Gerçek, E., and Topbaş, S. (2005). Serebral-Palsili çocuklarda çiğneme becerisinin geliştirilmesinde oral-motor terapinin etkililiği. [Speech therapy in the development of oral skills of cerebral-palsied children] *Abstracts of 3rd Congress of Speech and Language Disorders*. Ankara: DKUBD.

Ketrez, F. N. (1997, May). Bir çocuğun dil edinimi sürecinde ses aktarımı. [The process of metathesis in the phonology of a child acquiring Turkish] *11th Linguistics Symposium*, METU Ankara.

Kopkallı-Yavuz, H. (1993). *A phonetic and phonological analysis of final devoicing in Turkish*. Unpublished doctoral dissertation, University of Michigan, Ann Arbor.

Kopkallı-Yavuz, H. (2000). Interaction between syllable structure and vowel length: Example from Turkish /a/.In S. Özsoy; D.Akar; M. Nakipoglu-Demiralp; E. Erguvanlı-Taylan, and A. Aksu-Koç (Eds.), *Proceedings of the 10th International Conference on Turkish Linguistics* (pp. 19–27). Istanbul: Bogaziçi University Press.

Kopkallı-Yavuz, H., and Topbaş, S. (1998). Phonological processes of Turkish phonologically disordered children: Language specific or universal? In W. Ziegler and K. Deger (Eds.), *Clinical Phonetics and Linguistics* (pp. 88–97). London: Whurr.

Kopkallı-Yavuz, H., and Topbaş, S. (2000). Children's preferences in early phonological acquisition: How does it reflect sensitivity to the ambient language? In A. Göksel and C. Kerslake (Eds.) *Studies on Turkish and Turkic Languages. Turcologica* (pp. 291–299). Harrassowitz Verlag, Wiesbaden: Oxford University.

Kornfilt J. (1997). *Descriptive grammars: Turkish*. London: Routledge.

Özsoy Y. (1982). *Eskişehir Konuşma Değerlendirme Test Takımı* [Eskisehir assessment of speech test]. Eskişehir, Turkey: Anadolu University Press.

Saben, C. B., and Ingham, J. C. (1991). The effects of minimal pairs treatment on the speech sound production of two children with phonologic disorders. *Journal of Speech and Hearing Research*, 34, 1023–1040.

Schaufeli, A. J. (1991). *Turkish in an immigrant setting. A comparative study of the first language of monolingual and bilingual Turkish children*. Universiteit van Amsterdam: Academisch Poefschrift.

Shriberg, L. D., and Kwiatkowski, J. (1982). Phonological disorders I: A diagnostic classification system. *Journal of Speech and Hearing Disorders*, 4, 226–241.

Stoel-Gammon, C. (1985). Phonetic inventories, 15–24 months: A longitudinal study. *Journal of Speech and Hearing Research*, 28, 505–512.

Topbaş, S. (1994). *Konuşma sorunlu çocukların sesbilgisel çözümleme yöntemi ile değerlendirilmesi*. [Phonological analysis of speech disordered children] (pp. 150–250). Published doctoral thesis (1998). Eskişehir: Anadolu Üniversitesi Press.

Topbaş, S. (1996). Phonological analysis of speech disordered children: A supra-segmental study. *Abstracts of VII International Congress for the Study of Child Language (IASCL)*. Boğaziçi University, Istanbul.

Topbaş, S. (1997). Turkish children's phonological acquisition: Implications for phonological disorders. *European Journal of Disorders of Communication*, 32, 377–397.

Topbaş, S. (1998). *Konuşma sorunlu çocukların sesbilgisel çözümleme yöntemi ile değerlendirilmesi*. [Assessment of speech disordered children by phonological analysis] Eskişehir: Anadolu University Press.

Topbaş, S. (2004). *The frequency effect and the acquisition of /k/, /t/, /tʃ/ sounds in Turkish*. (Revised M.Sc. Dissertation, City University of London, 1988). Eskişehir: Ongar Basımevi.

Topbaş, S. (2004/2005). *Türkçe Sesletim-Sesbilgisi Testi* [Turkish Articulation and Phonology Test]. Ankara: Milli Eğitim Yayınevi 4. Akşam Sanat Okulu

Topbaş, S. (2005). *Dil ve kavram gelişimi*. [Language and concept development] Ankara: Kok Pub.

Topbaş, S. (in press-a). Does the phonology of Turkish-speaking children differ from children learning other languages? *Clinical Linguistics and Phonetics*.

Topbaş, S. (in press-b) A Turkish perspective on communication disorders. *Logopedics, Phoniatrics and Vocology*.

Topbaş, S., and Bleile, K. (2004, May). Early phoneme acquisition in Turkish and English. *Abstract Proceedings of the 2nd National Congress in Speech and Language Disorders*, Anadolu University, Eskişehir, Turkey.

Topbaş, S., and Dinçer, B. (2002, July). Universal and language specific aspects of variability in phonological patterns. *Abstract Proceedings of IASCL-SRCLD Conference*, University of Wisconsin, Madison, WI.

Topbaş, S., and Konrot, A. (1998). Variability in phonological disorders: Can we search for systematicity? Evidence from Turkish-speaking children. In W. Ziegler and K. Deger (Eds), *Clinical Phonetics and Linguistics* (pp. 79–87). London: Whurr.

Topbaş, S., and KopkallI-Yavuz, H. (1998). The onset of a linguistic system: Is there evidence from the acquisition of final devoicing in Turkish? In A. Sorace, C. Heycock, and R. Shillcock (Eds), *Proceedings of the GALA (Generative Approaches to Language Acquisition) Conference* (pp. 284–290). Edinburgh: Edinburgh University Human Communication Centre Press.

Topbaş, S., Kopkallı-Yavuz, H., and Unal, O. (2006, May). *Reviewing sonority for word-final consonant cluster simplifications in Turkish*. Paper presented at 11th ICPLA Congress, Dubrovnik, Croatia.

Topbaş, S., and Yavaş, M. (in press). Phonological acquisition and disorders in Turkish. In Zhu Hua and B. Dodd, (Eds), *Phonological development and disorders in children: A multilingual perspective* (pp. 233–265). Clevedon, UK: Multilingual Matters.

Turkish Ministry of Foreign Affairs (2003). *Turkish*. Retrieved October 24, 2003, from http://www.disisleri.gov.tr/.

Türk, O., Şayli, Ö., Özsoy, A. S., Arslan, L. Türkçede Ünlülerin Formant Frekans İncelemesi.[Formant frequency analysis of Turkish vowels.] *18. Türk Dilbilim Kurultayı*, Ankara Univ., 2004.

Van Riper, C. (1963). *Speech correction: Principles and methods* (4th ed.). Englewood Cliffs, NJ: Prentice Hall.

Yağmur, K. (1997). Sociolinguistic aspects of first language attrition among Turkish migrants in Sydney. *Proceedings of the 8th International Conference on Turkish Linguistics*. (pp. 231–241). Ankara, Turkey: Ankara University Press.

Yavaş, M., and Topbaş, S. (2004). Liquid development in Turkish: Salience vs. frequency. *Journal of Multilingual Communication Disorders*, 2, 110–123.

Zimmer, K., and Orgun, O. (1999). Turkish. In International Phonetic Association (Ed.). *Handbook of the International Phonetic Association: A guide to the use of the International Phonetic Alphabet*. (pp. 154–156). Cambridge, UK: Cambridge University Press.

SUMMARY OF STUDIES OF TYPICAL TURKISH SPEECH ACQUISITION

Authors	Year	No. of children	Age of children	Information	Sample type	Data collection	Focus
Acarlar	1995	20 20 PD	2.1–5;0	Phonological Processes	Single-word	Cross-sectional	Comparison of typical and impaired children
Acarlar and Ege	1996	20	2;1–5;0	Consonants Phonological Processes	Single word	Cross-sectional	Phonological process usage in typical children
Ketrez	1997	1	1;3–2;0	Metathesis process	Spontaneous speech	Longitudinal	A typical case study of metathesis phonological process
Kopkallı-Yavuz and Topbaş	1998	10	5;2–6;3	Phonological processes	Picture-naming	Cross-sectional	Phonological processes are discussed in comparison to seven languages from the literature: Qualitative analysis of phonological processes
Kopkallı-Yavuz and Topbaş	2000	30	3;0–6;11	Syllable structure	Connected speech	Longitudinal Cross-sectional	Children's preferences for syllable /word forms in phonological acquisition
Topbaş	1988	20	1;3–2;11	Acquisition of /k, t, tʃ/	Connected speech	Cross-sectional Longitudinal	The frequency effect-Analysis: PCC, substitution errors
Topbaş	1996	10 PD	4;0–8;0	Consonants Suprasegmentals voice (pitch, loudness, quality) and rhythm (phrasing, stress and rate)	Connected speech	Cross-sectional	Intelligibility of the speech of PD children by listener judgments: correlation of average words per utterance, intended words, PCC and suprasegmental aspects based on Shriberg and Kwiatkowski (1982)

Authors	Year	No. of children	Age of children	Information	Sample type	Data collection	Focus
Topbaş	in press	70 PD	4;0–8;0	Consonants Clusters Phonological processes Severity	Connected speech, Single-word picture naming	Longitudinal Cross-sectional	Comparison of classification with other languages
Topbaş	1997	22 1 PD	1;3–2;11	Consonants, Phonological processes	Connected speech	Cross-sectional longitudinal	Age of phoneme acquisition and phonological processes are compared with the PD system of a single child.
Topbaş and Bleile	2004	30	0;9–2;0	Consonants, Clusters	Connected speech	Longitudinal	Comparison of phoneme emergence in Turkish and English based on Stoel-Gammon (1982)
Topbaş and Dinçer	2002	40 PD	4;0–8;0	Consonants, Phonological processes: Universal and language specific aspects of variability	Picture naming	Cross-sectional	The correct underlying representations (CUR) and substitution errors to verify incorrect underlying representations (IUR) were analyzed according to Dinsen and Chin (1994), Barlow (1996).
Topbaş and Konrot	1998	10	5;2–6;3	Phonological processes	Picture-naming	Cross-sectional	Variability in phonological impairment and the sub-classification of phonological disorders
Topbaş and Kopkallı-Yavuz	1998	30	1;3–2;6	Word-final devoicing rule	Connected speech	Longitudinal Cross-sectional	Phonological process of word final devoicing (FD) concerning the /b, d, dʒ, g/ sounds in Turkish
Topbaş and Yavaş	in press	665 70 PD	1:3–8;0	Consonants, Clusters, Phonological processes	Connected speech, Single-word Pic-naming	Longitudinal Cross sectional	Normative study

Note. PD = phonologically disordered/speech impaired

Chapter 55

Vietnamese Speech Acquisition

Deborah A. Hwa-Froelich

INTRODUCTION

Vietnamese is the national language of Vietnam. The Vietnamese language comes from the Austro-Asiatic languages. Within the Austro-Asiatic languages are three branches: (a) Munda, including Santali and Mundari languages of India, (b) Mon-Khmer, containing Mon (languages of Burma and Thailand) and Khmer (Cambodian and Kampuchea languages), and (c) the branch of Viet-Muong, consisting of Vietnamese and Muong (Grimes, 1996; Ruhlen, 1987). Some authors, however, would place the Vietnamese language within the Mon-Khmer branch (Grimes, 1996).

Several other languages such as Chinese, English, French, and Malay have influenced the Vietnamese language. Some examples of Vietnamese words from other languages include *mit-tinh* for the English word 'meeting'; *xa-rông* for the Malay word 'sa-rong' (a type of clothing); and *xà-bông* for the French word 'savon' (soap) (Cheng, 1991). The Chinese language, however, has had the greatest influence on the Vietnamese language. Vietnam was ruled by China for a thousand years from 111 BC to AD 938; consequently, over one-third of the Vietnamese vocabulary consists of Chinese words (McWhorter, 2000). Other linguistic similarities between Chinese and Vietnamese include the syllabic nature of the languages and the use of tones for semantic meaning. See the Resources section of this chapter for materials pertaining to Vietnamese.

Where Vietnamese is spoken

Vietnamese is spoken primarily in Vietnam and the surrounding countries of Cambodia, Laos, and Thailand as well as in parts of Myanmar and the Indo-Chinese peninsula (see accompanying map and Appendix D). A significant number of Vietnamese speakers also migrated to or were relocated to Australia, Canada, Cote d'Ivoire, Japan, Senegal, the United States, and parts of Europe (Grimes, 1996).

Components of Vietnamese

Consonants

Vietnamese has 24 consonants (see Table 55-1) and is most closely related to Cantonese (see Chapter 36). The Vietnamese alphabet is phonemic, that is, one letter or a specific combination of letters corresponds to one phoneme. The final consonants are limited to either a voiceless stop or a nasal. Final consonants include /p/, /t/, /k/, /m/, /n/, and /ŋ/. The Vietnamese language does not have consonant clusters (Cheng, 1991; Thompson, 1965).

The 24 consonants include nine plosives /p, b, t̪, t̪ʰ, t̪, d, c, k, ʔ/, one affricate /tʃ/, five fricatives /f, z, ɣ, x, h/, four nasals /m, n, ɲ, ŋʔ/, two glides /j, w/, and three liquids /l, r, ɽ/. Not all dialects include the same phonemes. Some phonemes /dʒ, z/ were observed in the speech of a central dialect speaker and some /v, ʒ/ in the speech of a northern dialect speaker but not in the speech of a southern dialect speaker (Hwa-Froelich, Hodson, and Edwards, 2002). Tang and Barlow (2006) reported that the glottal stop /ʔ/ in the initial position is noncontrastive (does not change word meaning). Thus, the glottal stop adds meaning only in medial or final word positions. Different authors have reported varying perceptions of speaker productions in response to the grapheme "r". Thompson (1965), Cheng (1991), and Campbell (1998) reported that the "r" grapheme was produced as an alveolar voiced fricative /z/ by northern dialect speakers. Hwa-Froelich and colleagues (2002) reported that the northern and southern dialect speakers produced /ɽ/ but the central dialect speaker produced /ɹ/. According to other authors, there are different opinions regarding /r/ productions by southern dialect speakers. Cheng (1991) reported that southern dialect speakers produced a post-alveolar fricative /ʒ/ and a trilled /r/. Tang and Barlow (2006) reported that the "r" grapheme is represented as the retroflex voiced fricative /ʐ/ with a regional variant of /ɽ/ in the Vietnamese linguistic literature.

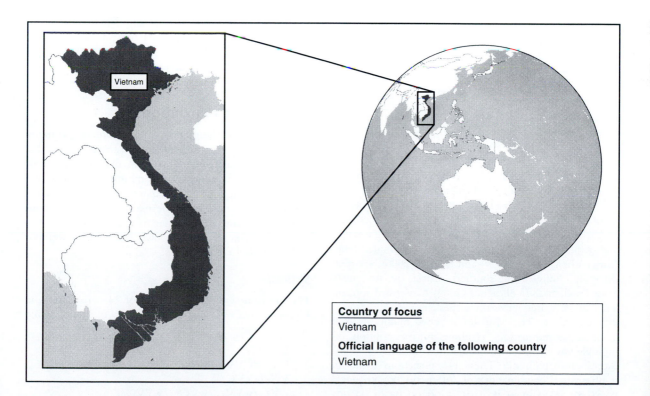

Country of focus
Vietnam

Official language of the following country
Vietnam

TABLE 55-1 Consonants produced in Vietnamese

	Bilabial	Labiodental	Dental	Alveolar
Plosive	p b		t̪	t̪ˀ d
Nasal	m			n
Trill				
Tap or flap				
Fricative		f v		s zᴺ
Affricate				
Lateral fricative	███████			
Approximant	w (labiovelar)	ʋ		l

Note. ᶜcentral dialect, ᴺnorthern dialect, and ˢsouthern dialect. Not all sounds are represented in each dialect.

Black = articulations judged impossible

Based on the International Phonetic Alphabet. Courtesy of the International Phonetic Association (c/o Department of Linguistics, University of Victoria, Victoria, British Columbia, Canada).

Vowels and diphthongs

Vietnamese speakers produce 11 different single vowels (see Table 55-2). Vowel productions vary across the three major dialects and are influenced by other vowels in the word; vowels are also influenced by semivowels following another vowel (Hwa-Froelich et al., 2002; Tang and Barlow, 2006). Due to these variations, different authors have reported different vowel inventories. For example, Cheng (1991) reported /i, ɛ, e, a, ɐ, ʌ, u, ɯ, ɔ, o, ɤ/ Hwa-Froelich et al. (2002) reported /æ, ɛ, e, i, ʌ, ɒ, u, ɯ, o, ɤ/ (ɤ was reported as œ in Hwa-Froelich et al., 2002) across three dialect speakers of Vietnamese. In an analysis of the southern dialect, Tang and Barlow (2006) listed the following 11 vowel singletons: /i, e, ɛ, ɯ, ɤ, ɤ̆, a, ʌ, u, o, ɔ/. These differences may also be due to the differences in native vs. nonnative speech perception of Vietnamese. For example, Cheng and Hwa-Froelich and colleagues are nonnative listeners of Vietnamese, whereas Tang is a native Vietnamese speaker.

Variations in listener identification of diphthongs and triphthongs may also exist. For example, Tang (native Vietnamese speaker) and Barlow (2006) reported three diphthongs in the southern dialect, /ie, ɯɤ, uo/. Hwa-Froelich and colleagues (2002) transcribed spoken Vietnamese words across three speakers, each speaking a different dialect. The word list included multiple vowel grapheme combinations resulting in transcription of multiple vowel combinations that may not be true diphthongs or triphthongs. These pronunciations included double vowel combinations of /ɑɪ, ai, ɑʊ, ɒo, ɒʊ, ei, ɛɪ, ɛo, ɛʊ, ɛu, iʌ, iə, io, iʊ, iɛ, iu, iɪ, ɪə, oɑ, oʊ, ʊɛ, ʊi, ʊə, ʊɑ, ʊɛ, ʊi, ui, uə/ and triple vowel combinations of /ɛʊi, iɛʊ, oɑi, uiə, uei, ʊɑi, ʊia, ʊiʊ, ʊeə, ʔʊi, ʊiə, ʊiʔ/.

Tang and Barlow (2006) cite Dinh and Nguyen (1998), authors of a Vietnamese phonetics text, who report semivowels that occur in the word-final position. These semivowels include /-u/ and /-i/. According to Tang and Barlow, "the semivowel /-i/ only appears after nonfront vowels such as in /ai, ɤi, ɯi, oi, ɔi, ui/. The semivowel /-u/ appears after unrounded vowels: /iu, eu, ɛu, ɯu, au, āu/" (Tang and Barlow, 2006).

Phonotactic restrictions

The phonotactic constraints in Vietnamese primarily involve syllable structure rules. Vietnamese is a syllabic language that allows consonants in the initial or final position with multiple vowel combinations. Other languages have phonotactic constraints for consonant clusters, but Vietnamese has none except for combinations with the semivowel /w/. There may be other constraints not yet documented that involve consonant-vowel and multiple vowel combinations.

Syllables

The Vietnamese alphabet consists of 24 consonants and 11 vowels that can be combined in any of the following possible ways:

/V/, /VV/
/CV/, /CVV/, /CVC/, /CVVC/
/VC/, /VVC/
/wV/, /wVV/, /wVC/, /wVVC/

Post-alveolar	Retroflex	Palatal	Velar	Uvular	Pharyngeal	Glottal
	ʈ	c	k g			ʔ
		ɲ	ŋ			
		r				
ʃ^{c,s} ʒ	ʐ	ß j^s	ɣ x			h
tʃ dʒ^c						
	ɽ^{N,S}	ɹ j^{c,s}				

TABLE 55-2 Vowels produced in Vietnamese compared to General American English

American English location	American English Vowels Smit (2004)	American English examples	Vietnamese location	Vietnamese vowels	Vietnamese examples
High-front	ɪ	*beat*		ɪ	va-li 'suitcase'
	i	*bit*	i		
	e	*raid*		e	pɤ̆m 'night'
Mid-low front	ɛ	*bed*	æ	ɛ	pem 'to take'
	æ	*bad*	ɛ, a	æ	ba 'three'
High-back rounded	u	*blue*		u	thu 'autumn'
				unrounded	su' 'monk'
				ɯ,ɤ	mo· 'dream'
	ʊ	*book*	u, ʌ		
Mid-back rounded	o	*boat*		o	tố 'big bowl'
	ɔ	*form*		ɔ	to 'big'
Low-back [r]-colored	ɑʳ	*drop*			
	ɚ				
	ɛʳ	*never, color*			
Central	ʌ	*up*		ʌ	cấn 'to weigh'
				low ɒ	cho 'to give'
	ə	*about, occur, upon*			

Table 55-2 continued

Diphthongs*	aɪ	*my, bike*	ău,ie	sầu riêng 'a fruit'
	ou	<u>out</u>, m<u>ou</u>se	ei,eu,uɑ	ấ y 'that'
				kếu 'to order food'
				quăn 'to be curled'
	ɔɪ	b<u>oy</u>	ɯɤ	Gửo,ng 'mirror'

*Diphthongs may vary across dialect, therefore, only a few are listed here (Cheng, 1991; Hwa-Froelich et al., 2002; Tang and Barlow, 2006).

/CwV/, /CwVV/, /CwVC/, /CwVVC/, where /w/ is a semivowel that sometimes may follow the initial consonant (Nguyen, 1987). Thus, the possible syllables of Vietnamese can be summarized as $C_{(0-1)}w_{(0-1)}V_{(1-2)}C_{(0-1)}$.

As new words are created in the language, more polysyllabic forms have been reported. Borrowed terms from other languages and names of technological advances have produced multisyllabic Vietnamese words. For example, *máy bay* is a single word meaning 'aeroplane' and *vali* means 'suitcase'.

Consonants and consonant clusters

There are no consonant clusters in the Vietnamese language. Consonants may be combined with /w/, but this is the only multiconsonant combination. A Vietnamese word example is *quốc ngữ* the name for the written Vietnamese language. In addition Thompson (1965) states, "the Vietnamese speaker insists on a two-syllable expression of some sort—a phrase, compound, pseudo-compound or derivative" (p. 310). Thus, it is likely that multisyllabic combinations of phonemes are produced across syllable boundaries.

Tones

The Vietnamese language is a tonal language developed before the twelfth century (Thompson, 1965; Thuy, 1975). Most often six tones are identified in the Vietnamese language (Cheng, 1991; Hwa-Froelich et al., 2002; McWhorter, 2000; Thompson, 1965). Represented graphically by small markings over or under the vowel of a syllable, the six tones include the following:

- High-rising or *sắc* [á]
- Emphasized high-rising or dipping-rising labeled as *hỏi* [ả]
- Mid-level or *không dấu* [a]
- Mid-rising or creaky called *ngã* [ã]
- Low-falling or *huyền* [à]
- Low-rising or constricted identified as *nặng* [ạ]

Cheng (1991) described the six tones using different adjectives, which include (a) level, (b) breathing rising, (c) breathing falling, (d) falling rising, (e) creaky rising (low rising), and (f) low falling (low constricted).

Differences in the reported number of tones for Vietnamese can be explained by dialectal differences. Some authors have specified five tones (Language and Orientation Resource Center, 1981). Thuy (1975) explained that two of the tones are so similar that some linguists consider them to be the same. Dialect differences in tone production may help to explain differences in tone perception. In the southern dialect, speakers produce five tones, eliminating the *ngã* mid-rising or creaky tone [ã], which is produced the same as emphasized h\i high-rising or dipping-rising tone [ả] (Tang and Barlow, 2006). In the central dialect the emphasized h\i high-rising or dipping-rising tone [ả] is produced like *huyền* low-falling [à]. All six tones are produced differently, however, in the northern dialect (Hwa-Froelich et al., 2002). Thus, dependent on the dialect of the speakers being studied, the speakers may express five or six tones.

It is important to note the tonal differences between speaker pronunciation and a listener's auditory perception of tones. In addition, writing a clear description of the tone differences is difficult. (Please refer to Hwa-Froelich et al., 2002, for a chart pictographically representing tone production across three Vietnamese dialects.) The practitioner should listen to a group of native speakers demonstrating tonal use to develop a regional baseline for tone production. The rising and falling aspect of tonal languages is dynamic during the production of the vowel and difficult to detect in each vowel or syllable during a conversation. Because the tone changes word meaning, producing the correct tonal pattern is essential for successful communication in this language.

Stress and intonation

Three stress levels that vary in loudness are used in the Vietnamese language: (a) loud syllables, (b) medium syllables, and (c) weakly stressed syllables (Thompson, 1965).

According to Thompson (1965, p. 17) most syllables are produced with medium stress, but at least one in each phrase or "pause group" has heavy stress and an occasional weakly stressed syllable. The heavier stress is used to denote new or important information (Thompson, 1965).

Writing system

During the time of Chinese rule, from 111 BC to AD 938, the official written language was Chinese until approximately the tenth century AD. At this time, a new script called *Chữ' Nôm* was created. This writing system was used until the seventeenth century, and was replaced when Western missionaries influenced the creation of a writing system, *Chữ' Quốc Ngữ'*. This new and current writing system is based on the Latin alphabet (*Chinese, Japanese and Vietnamese writing systems*, 2005).

The consonant graphemes used in Vietnamese writing include the following: A a, Ă ă, Â â, B b, C c, CH ch, D d, Đ đ, E e, Ê ê, G g, GI gi, H h, I i, K k, KH kh, L l, M m, N n, NG ng, NH nh, O o, Ô ô, O'o', PH ph, QU qu, R r, S s, T t, TH th, TR tr, U u, U' u', V v, X x, and Y y (Thompson, 1965; Thuy, 1975). When written with tonal markings, multiple diacritics are used.

Varieties of Vietnamese

As described previously, there are three major regional dialects of Vietnamese. These include

- The northern dialect associated with the region surrounding Ha Noi,
- The central dialect related to Hue, and
- The southern, Ho Chi Minh City or Saigon dialect (Cheng, 1991; Hwa-Froelich et al., 2002; Thompson, 1965).

Pronunciation of some of the sounds varies from one dialect to another (central, northern, and southern), but in Vietnamese dialects, one sound typically corresponds to the same symbol or combination of symbols (Hwa-Froelich et al., 2002). Although there are differences in tonal use, as well as pronunciation of consonants, vowels, and different lexical items, these three regional Vietnamese dialects are mutually intelligible to all speakers. In addition to these three major dialects, Vietnam also has many minority ethnic groups and languages. Grimes (1996) reported 54 ethnic groups and 86 spoken languages.

Typical Acquisition of Vietnamese

At present no studies have been published in English regarding acquisition of Vietnamese speech. Only one study on phonological assessment of Vietnamese children could be found. Tang and Barlow (2006) recently conducted a study with four monolingual Vietnamese children (two were 4;4 and two were 5;5 at the time of the study). All children's parents and teachers reported poor speech intelligibility. Each child was exposed to both northern and southern Vietnamese dialects. Based on their assessment data, the authors concluded that these children may have had phonological impairments. Because typically developing children have acquired adultlike speech patterns by the age of 4;6 to 5;0 (Grunwell, 1997; Hodson and Paden, 1991), the 4- and 5-year-olds in this study may have been exhibiting phonological delay. Acquisition of Vietnamese will be discussed in light of the error patterns these four children exhibited.

Acquired sounds

It is important to note that all of the four children in the Tang and Barlow (2006) study had previously acquired correct tonal production. Acquisition of tones has been reported in the literature to occur by 1;8 for children speaking Cantonese and Putonghua (Campbell, 1998; Hua, 2002).

Consonants

Generally, the four children with speech impairment from Tang and Barlow (2006) acquired most of the stops, nasals, and glides. A southern dialect adult phonemic inventory for the syllable-initial position includes /b, ʈ, ʈʰ, d, ʃ, c, k, m, n, ɲ, ŋ, f, s, ʂ, z, x, ɣ, h, w, l, j/ and syllable-final position includes /pˀ, tˀ, kˀ, m, n, ŋ/. When compared to the adult southern dialect speaker consonant inventory, the four children expressively produced these phonemes: /b, tʃ, d, k, m, ɲ, h, w, j/. The 4;4-year-old children had acquired the following word-initial consonant sounds: /b, ʈ, d, k, m, ɲ, h, w, j/. One of the 4;4-year-old children also had acquired /ʈʰ, c, n, ŋ, ɣ, g/ and the other had acquired /f, θ, s, ʂ, x, l/. The two children who were 5;5 exhibited these correctly produced phonemes: /b, tʃ, d, ʈ, c, k, m, n, ɲ, ŋ, f, ɣ, h, w, j/. One 5-year-old child also produced /s, ʂ/ and the other produced /g, kʰ, x, l/.

For word-final consonants, the four children correctly produced: /pˀ, kˀ, m, ŋ/. Three of the children also produced /tˀ/ correctly and two children, a 4-year-old and a 5-year-old, produced /n/ correctly.

Consonant clusters

There are no consonant clusters in the Vietnamese language.

Vowels and diphthongs

All four participants with speech impairment in the Tang and Barlow (2006) study correctly produced all vowels. Only participant 2, who was 4;4 years old at the time of the study, reduced seven diphthongs /ɤɪ, ao, ɛo, ɔɪ, ɔa, ɯa, ɑɪ/ to a single vowel. These findings are similar for other studies on Cantonese and Putonghua (Hua, 2002) in that most of the children acquired the vowels and tones of their native language. Tones and vowels may be acquired before acquiring consonants in tonal languages.

Percent correct

There are no studies to date that describe percentage of correct consonant (PCC) productions for typically developing Vietnamese children. The Tang and Barlow study (2006), however, provides PCC measures for four children with phonological delays: Child 1 (4;4 years) PCC = 57.3 percent; Child 2 (4;4 years) PCC = 76.6 percent; Child 3 (5;5 years) PCC = 84.1 percent; and Child 4 (5;5 years) PCC = 71.8 percent. PCC severity levels described in Bauman-Waengler (2004) listed PCCs >90 percent as mild; 65–85 percent as mild-moderate; 50–65 percent as moderate-severe; and <50 percent as severe. Therefore, according to these guidelines, only one of these children would have been considered moderate-severe and the others were at the mild-moderate level of severity.

Phonological processes

Seven phonological processes were demonstrated by at least two children with speech impairment in the Tang and Barlow study (2006). These included gliding, fronting, glottal replacement, backing, velar assimilation, stopping, and final consonant deletion. The processes of stopping, fronting, final consonant deletion, and assimilation are also documented in speakers of other languages (Goldstein and Iglesias, 1996; Hua, 2002; So and Dodd, 1994, 1995).

Uncommon processes documented in the Tang and Barlow (2006) study include gliding, glottal replacement, and backing. These processes were also documented in Cantonese children with phonological impairment (So and Dodd, 1994). In contrast, backing and gliding were considered typical phonological processes for Putonghua-speaking children during early development and glottal replacement was not observed in children with or without phonological impairment (Hua, 2002). If gliding and backing persisted past 4;6, however, these processes would be considered atypical.

Cross-linguistic similarities in error patterns for the production of velar stops and retroflex consonants exist among Vietnamese, Cantonese, and Putonghua speakers. The Vietnamese children in the Tang and Barlow (2006) study exhibited velar assimilation and incorrect retroflex /ʐ/ productions. Both So and Dodd (1994) and Hua et al. (2002) reported that Cantonese- and Putonghua-speaking children made errors with velar sounds, demonstrating either velar assimilation or velar omissions. Putonghua-speaking children also exhibited errors with more complex sounds such as retroflexes and affricates. Thus gliding, glottal replacement, velar assimilation processes, and incorrect productions of retroflex consonants may be an indication of impairment in Vietnamese children. More research specifically focusing on typical and atypical phonological processes in Vietnamese language acquisition is needed.

Tang and Barlow (2006) contend that some processes may occur more or less frequently based on structural differences among languages. In other words, Vietnamese children may acquire final consonants earlier due to the restricted number of possible final consonant sounds allowed in the Vietnamese language. Therefore, final consonant deletion may occur less often in languages that have few word-final consonants, such as Vietnamese and Chinese, and final consonant deletion processes may also be an indication of phonological impairment.

Backing as a typical process may also be explained by the number and frequency of velars in the Vietnamese language. Children may acquire velars earlier because of frequency of occurrence and consequently substitute velars for sounds they have not yet acquired. Thus backing may be a reflection of the frequency of velar occurrence in the Vietnamese language and may not indicate a phonological impairment (Hua, 2002; Tang and Barlow, 2006).

Intelligibility

To date there is no study of the intelligibility of children who speak Vietnamese.

Phonetic inventory

To date there is no study of the phonetic inventories produced at different ages by children who speak Vietnamese.

Common mismatches

Dialectal differences may occur for the graphemes "p, s, x, v, r, z". Southern dialect speakers may produce /pˀ/ only in borrowed words. In addition, southern dialect speakers produce /ʂ/ for "s", /s/ for "x", and /ʐ/ or /ʈ/ for "r". For the grapheme "v", southern dialect speakers may produce /j/ or /βj/. In contrast, northern dialect speakers may express /v/ for "v", /s/ for "s, x" and /ʈ/ for "r" (Hwa-Froelich et al., 2002; Tang and Barlow, 2006).

Hwa-Froelich and colleagues (2002) listed the possible mismatches of Vietnamese productions of English phonemes. These phonemes include /θ, ð, p, g, dʒ, ʒ, s, ʈɪ, v, ɪ, ɛ, æ, ʊ/. Because the Vietnamese language has fewer syllable-final phonemes, Vietnamese speakers may have difficulty with the following English final consonants: /b, d, f, v, s, ʃ, z, θ, l/. Table 55-3 provides possible mismatches for Vietnamese speakers' production of English sounds.

Syllable Structure

To date, there are no studies published in English on the acquisition patterns of Vietnamese syllable structure. One study by Sato (1984) found first language interference in second language learning. She studied two Vietnamese males aged 10 and 12 years, learning English as a second language. The performance of both favored the Vietnamese CVC syllable structure when learning English words. In addition, Vietnamese speakers of English have more difficulty learning syllable-final English clusters as compared to syllable-initial English clusters (Osburne, 1996; Sato, 1984).

These findings may indicate that learners of Vietnamese may acquire CVCs before CVVCs or double and triple vowel combinations.

Prosody

Currently there are no studies of Vietnamese prosodic characteristics.

Phonological Awareness

No studies on phonological awareness of Vietnamese speakers could be found.

Speech assessment for Vietnamese children

The World Health Organization's (WHO, 2001) *International Classification of Functioning, Disability, and Health* (ICF) provides a framework to evaluate the communication of children from all cultures (see Chapter 1). A comprehensive evaluation includes assessment of Body Structure, Body Function, Activity/Participation, Environmental factors, and Personal Factors as discussed in Part I of this text (McLeod and Bleile, 2004). To examine the Body Structure and Function components

TABLE 55-3   Possible mismatches for Vietnamese speakers of English

Word-initial phonemes	Confused with	Word-final phonemes	Confused with
/θ/	/t, s/	/b/	/p/
/ð/	/d, z/	/d/	/t/
/p/	/b/	/f/	/p/
/g/	/k/	/v/	/b, p/
/dʒ/	/z/	/s/	Omitted or /ʃ/
/ʒ/	/z, dʒ/	/ʃ/	Omitted
/s/	/ʃ/	/z/	/ʃ, s/
/ʈɪ/	/dʒ, tʃ, t/	/l/	/ʃ/
/v/	/j/		/n/
/ɪ/	/i/		
/ɛ/	/æ/		
/æ/	/ɛ, a/		
/ʊ/	/u, ʌ/		

Note: Adapted from Hwa-Froelich et al. (2002).

of the ICF associated with speech production, the speech assessment should include an oral muscular examination and audiological assessment, if possible. Any medical records indicating neurological dysfunction would also be included in looking at Body Structure support for communication. The Body Function areas of the ICF relevant to speech sound production concern overall ability to communicate with others. Thus, intelligibility of speech (including articulation and phonological development), voice production and quality, and fluency would be the main Body Function areas that would need to be evaluated. Qualitative measures of the participant's intelligibility in the environments in which he or she participates could be gathered. It is also important to assess receptive and expressive language skills and, because phonological processing affects reading and writing, it is necessary to explore the individual's reading and writing skills.

Three publications include word lists that can be used to assess Vietnamese speakers:

- *Articulation Test: Vietnamese* (Cheng, 1991)
- *Vietnamese consonant word list and Vietnamese vowel word list* (Hwa-Froelich et al., 2002)
- *Southern dialect Vietnamese phonological probe* (Tang and Barlow, 2006)

Cheng (1991) published an articulation test that can be administered by asking the participant to imitate an adult model. Hwa-Froelich and colleagues (2002) published word lists to test consonant and vowel productions related to Vietnamese graphemes. Pictures, objects, and/or printed words can be used to elicit spontaneous productions of these phonemes. Finally, Tang and Barlow (2006) created a word list for young southern dialect speakers. Pictures and/or objects can be used to elicit the words on the Tang and Barlow list. A conversational language sample will provide a means for the examiner to evaluate fluency, resonance, voice, intelligibility, and general language discourse. An educational assessment of reading and writing skills can be provided by the participant's teacher, place of employment, or family member.

There may be a mismatch between expectations of children's performance on standardized assessments and the children's expectations of the examiner's behavior. Hwa-Froelich (2000) found American standardized tests were based on the expectation that children would guess when they did not know the correct answer. Vietnamese children, however, preferred not to respond when they did not know the answer. In addition, Vietnamese parents socialized their children to follow and practice an adult model to learn new tasks. When an adult model was not provided, the Vietnamese children looked for the adult to provide clues to indicate the expected behavior or choice (Hwa-Froelich, 2000).

The Activity/Participation and Environmental Factors components of the ICF are particularly crucial in the evaluation of the speech of Vietnamese children because of the likelihood that the speech therapists will be of a different culture than the child. How children interact with their environment will be influenced by the regional variations of their Vietnamese culture. It would thus be important to gather information regarding the participant's view of how the communication impairment affects his or her participation in daily activities as well as the attitudes and expectations of family members, schoolteachers, or business associates, and other social participants. In addition, the examiner should investigate the resources available to the individual for continued treatment.

Speech intervention for Vietnamese children

In addition to the child's immediate environment of family and friends, another important environmental factor is the overall society's view of disability, specifically speech disability. Not all cultures or governments identify speech differences as impairments or disabilities (Hwa-Froelich and Westby, 2003). These viewpoints may affect the amount of support provided for assessment and treatment services. Hwa-Froelich and Westby (2003) found that Vietnamese parents defined disability as loss of appendages or senses. Speech impairment was not considered a form of learning disability. Children with such learning differences were included in regular education and no special services were available. However, these children may experience difficulty in school, such as the child with phonological disorders who has difficulty learning to read. If this speech difficulty is not recognized as a disability, then it is possible that the child could be viewed as simply not trying or as intellectually limited. Children who had overt physical anomalies causing their speech difficulty, such as children with cleft palates or cerebral palsy, were often teased at school, and if these children did not perform well at school, they stayed at home or tried to find other work in their communities (Hwa-Froelich, 2000; Hwa-Froelich and Westby, 2003).

Working in Vietnam

There are few trained speech-language pathologists in Vietnam (Ducote, 2001; Tang and Barlow, 2006). In addition, there are few studies regarding typical or atypical speech development of Vietnamese children. Only one publication (Tang and Barlow, 2006, discussed earlier in this chapter) studied speech impairment in Vietnamese children.

In 1996, Dr. Charlotte Ducote, a speech-language pathologist, volunteered to work with Operation Smile, a nonprofit organization based in Norfolk, Virginia, that provides surgery and related services to persons in other countries as well as the United States (Ducote, 2001). She wrote,

Of the 80 million Vietnamese individuals in the country, fewer than 10 have held the title of "speech therapist,"

and none of them have a degree in speech therapy. Their degrees are in medicine, physical therapy, dentistry, linguistics, psychology, nursing, or other areas. None have attended a formal university course in speech therapy as this has not been available in Vietnam, and no interested individuals have had sufficient foreign language skills to be admitted to a speech therapy program in another country (p. 3).

From this initial experience in 1996, Dr. Ducote with Ann Marie Juul initiated the Speech-Therapy Vietnam Project in 1998. This project sponsors seminars and presentations at hospitals and universities in Vietnam. They have also recruited individual and corporate donors who contributed equipment, supplies, and textbooks.

PHONETICALLY SPEAKING

Pronunciation of Vietnamese: Tiếng Việt /ʈɪŋ viɛtˀ/
Relevant words for speech assessment and intervention

Word	Formal usage	Pronunciation	Informal usage	Pronunciation
Tongue	*lưỡi*	/luwi/		
Teeth	*răng*	/ʈæŋ/		
Lips	*môi*	/moi/		
Hard palate				
Soft palate				
Larynx	*(giải phẫu) thanh quản*			
Lungs	*phổi*	/foi/		
Nose	*mũi*	/mui/	*lỗ mũi*	/lo mui/
Sound	*tiếng*	/ʈɪŋ/		
Word	*từ*	/tu/		
Sentence	*nguyên câu*	/hwɪn gau/		
Paragraph	*đoạn văn*	/dwætˀ væn/		

RESOURCES

Books

Nguyễn, D. L. (1970). A contrastive phonological analysis of English and Vietnamese. In D. L. Nguyen (Ed.), *A contrastive analysis of English and Vietnamese* (Vol. 4). Sydney: Pacific Linguistics.

Thompson, L. C. (1965). *A Vietnamese grammar.* Seattle: University of Washington Press.

Thuy, V. G. (1975). *Vietnamese in a nutshell.* New York: Funk and Wagnalls.

Professional associations

There is currently no professional association in Vietnam. The chapter author can be e-mailed for a list of contacts in the United States and Vietnam.

Useful Vietnamese Web sites

Language

• UCLA Language Materials Vietnamese Language Profile, http://www.lmp.ucla.edu/prfiles/profv01.htm
• Vietic Languages, http://www.anu.edu.au/~u9907217/languages/AAlecture6.html.
• Sound system in Vietnamese, http://www.de-han.org/vietnam/chuliau/lunsoat/sound; http://www.geocities.com/CollegePark/Campus/6336/pronunciation.html.
• Vietnamese culture and language *Adopt Vietnam,* http://www.adoptvietnam.org/vietnamese/.
• *Journey into the Vietnamese culture,* http://www.viet-spring.org/.
• *Vietnamese language and culture,* http://www.seasite.niu.edu/vietnamese/VNMainpage/vietsite/vietsite.htm.
• *Omniglot: The guide to written language,* http://www.omniglot.com/writing/vietnamese.htm.
• *Vietnamese Language, Culture, Van-Hoa, History,* http://www.saigon.com/~nguyent/language.html.

Vietnamese dialects

• *Vietnamese dialects,* http://www.glossika.com/en/dict/dialectv.php.

Vietnamese online dictionaries

• *Vietnamese=English=French Dictionary,* http://www.yourdictionary.com/languages/austasia.html.
• *Vietnamese - English - French Dictionary,* http://vdict.com/.
• *Free English-Vietnamese-French-German On-Line Dictionary,* http://www.saigon.com:8081/~vietdict/.
• *English-Vietnamese,* http://www.ksvn.com/anhviet.htm.

REFERENCES

Bauman-Waengler, J. (2004). *Articulatory and phonological impairments.* Boston: Pearson.

Campbell, G. L. (1998). *Concise compendium of the world's languages.* New York: Routledge.

Cheng, L. L. (1991). *Assessing Asian language performance* (2nd ed.). Oceanside, CA: Academic Communication Associates.

Chinese, Japanese, and Vietnamese Languages writing systems. (2005) Retrieved June 2, 2005, from http://www.cjvlang.com/writing/writviet.html.

Ducote, C. (2001). *A speech-language pathologist in Vietnam.* Retrieved January 1, 2005, from http://www.asha.org/about/publications/leader-online/archives/2001/vietnam.htm?.

Goldstein, B., & Iglesias., A. (1996). Phonological patterns in normally developing Spanish-speaking 3- and 4-year-olds of Puerto Rican descent. *Language, Speech, and Hearing Services in Schools, 27,* 82–90.

Grimes, B. F. E. (1996). *Ethnologue: Languages of the world,* Retrieved from http://www.sil.org/ethnologue/ethnologue.html.

Grunwell, P. (1997). Developmental phonological disability: Order in disorder. In B. W. Hodson & M. L. Edwards (Eds.), *Perspectives in applied phonology* (pp. 61–84). Gaithersburg, MD: Aspen.

Hodson, B. W., & Paden, E. P. (1991). *Targeting intelligible speech* (2nd ed.). Austin, TX: Pro-Ed.

Hua, Z. (2002). *Phonological development in specific contexts: Studies of Chinese-speaking children.* Clevedon, England: Multilingual Matters.

Hwa-Froelich, D. A. (2000). *Frameworks of education: Perspectives of Asian parents and Head Start staff.* Unpublished dissertation, Wichita State University, Wichita, KS.

Hwa-Froelich, D. A., Hodson, B. H., & Edwards, H. T. (2002). Vietnamese phonology: A tutorial. *American Journal of Speech-Language Pathology, 11,* 264–273.

Hwa-Froelich, D. A., & Westby, C. E. (2003). Frameworks of education: Perspectives of Southeast Asian parents and Head Start staff, *Language, Speech, and Hearing Services in Schools, 34,* 299–319.

McLeod, S., & Bleile, K. (2004). The ICF: A framework for setting goals for children with speech impairment. *Child Language Teaching and Therapy, 20*(3), 199–219.

McWhorter, J. (2000). *Spreading the word: Language & dialect in America.* Portsmouth, NH: Heinemann.

Nguyen, D. H. (1987). Vietnamese. In B. Comrie (Ed.), *The world's major languages* (pp. 777–796). New York: Oxford University Press.

Osburne, A. G. (1996). Final cluster reduction in English L2 speech: A case study of a Vietnamese speaker. *Applied Linguistics, 17*(2), 164–181.

Ruhlen, M. (1987). *A guide to the world's language, Vol. 1: Classification.* Stanford, CA: Stanford University Press.

Sato, C. (1984). Phonological processes in second language acquisition: Another look at interlanguage syllable structure. *Language Learning, 34*(4), 43–57.

Smit, A. B. (2004). *Articulation and phonology: Resource guide for school-age children and adults.* Clifton Park, NY: Thomson Delmar Learning.

So, L., & Dodd, B. (1995). The acquisition of phonology by Cantonese-speaking children. *Journal of Child Language, 22,* 473–495.

So, L., & Dodd, B. (1994). Phonologically disordered Cantonese-speaking children. *Clinical Linguistics and Phonetics, 8,* 235–255.

Tang, G., & Barlow, J. (2006). Characteristics of the sound system of monolingual Vietnamese-speaking children with phonological impairment. *Clinical Linguistics and Phonetics, 20*(6), 423–445.

Thompson, L. C. (1965). *A Vietnamese grammar.* Seattle: University of Washington Press.

Thuy, V. G. (1975). *Vietnamese in a nutshell.* NY: Funk and Wagnalls.

World Health Organization (2001). *ICF: International classification of functioning, disability, and health.* Geneva, Switzerland: WHO.

SUMMARY OF STUDIES OF TYPICAL VIETNAMESE SPEECH ACQUISITION

As mentioned previously, to date no studies have been published in English describing typical speech acquisition for Vietnamese children.

Acknowledgements

The author would like to thank Giang Tang, Jessica Barlow, and Lilly Cheng for their help with this manuscript and their generosity in sharing their charts and word lists. Travis Threats offered insightful comments and suggestions on the ICF, which helped make this manuscript easier to read and understand. Julie Hoffman helped with the transcription and clarification of phonetic symbols and explanations. I am indebted to them for both their time and their patience.

Chapter 56

Welsh Speech Acquisition

Siân M. Munro, Martin J. Ball, and Nicole Müller

INTRODUCTION

Welsh (*Cymraeg* in Welsh) is a Celtic language, belonging to the Brythonic group along with Cornish, and Breton (spoken in Brittany). Census figures (see National Statistics Online, 2003) confirm that Welsh is the liveliest of the modern Celtic languages, both in terms of actual numbers of speakers (575,168), and in terms of percentage of speakers within the political boundaries of the country (20.5 percent). Full linguistic descriptions of Welsh can be found in Williams (1980) and Thomas (1996); with shorter accounts in Thomas (1992), Watkins (1993), and Ball (2007). Ball and Jones (1984) and Ball and Williams (2001) are devoted to Welsh phonology and phonetics respectively. Ball, Müller, and Munro (2006) looks at Welsh-English bilingualism in the clinical context. See the Resources section of this chapter for materials pertaining to Welsh.

Where Welsh is spoken

Welsh is spoken in Wales (*Cymru* in Welsh), with a small Welsh-speaking community still extant in Patagonia (Argentina), the result of emigrants establishing a Welsh-speaking 'colony' (*Y Wladfa* in Welsh) in the nineteenth century (Jones, 1998). The percentage of the population speaking Welsh differs across the country (see accompanying map and Appendix D).

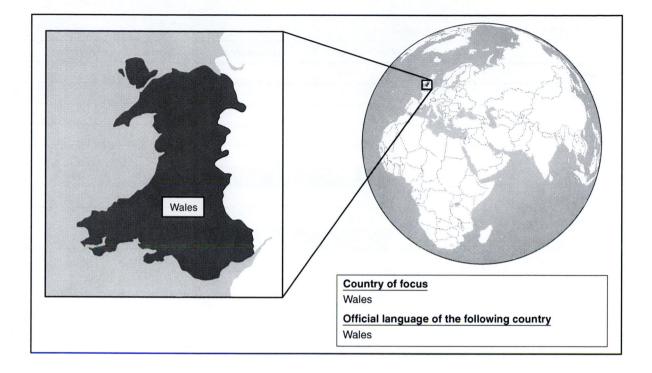

Country of focus
Wales

Official language of the following country
Wales

Components of Welsh

Northern standard pronunciation of Welsh will form the basis of this section as the phonological system is larger than in southern varieties; differences between northern and southern standards are pointed out in the relevant sections following.

Consonants

Welsh has 25 consonant phonemes (see Table 56-1).

Vowels and diphthongs

The vowel system is large in northern varieties, with 13 monophthongs and 13 diphthongs. Southern varieties have smaller systems, however, with a formal register probably distinguishing 11 monophthongs and 8 diphthongs (see Table 56-2). Monophthongs are normally paired in descriptions of the language into phonologically long and short vowels; northern varieties have smaller qualitative differences between the members of each pair than southern. Different transcribers of Welsh,

therefore, have used length-based or quality-based transcriptions of the vowel system (see Ball and Williams 2001). In the following transcriptions we will not show vowel length, adopting instead a different symbol for each vowel to show the kind of quality distinctions that are heard; readers are asked to bear in mind, though, the differences between northern and southern accents referred to above.

Mutations

Mutations are phonological changes to word-initial consonants that are triggered by a range of morpho-syntactic contexts. Initial consonant mutations are common to all the Celtic languages and are historical remnants of processes once triggered by phonological contexts, which have subsequently been lost during various sound changes. A full account of mutations and the environments that trigger them is given in Ball and Müller (1992), but we can give a brief description of them here. There are three main sets of consonants changes: soft mutation (SM) or lenition, nasal mutation (NM) or nasalization, and aspirate mutations (AM) or

TABLE 56-1 Welsh consonant phonemes

	Bilabial	Labiodental	Dental	Alveolar
Plosive	p b		t̪ d̪	
Nasal	m		n̪	
Trill				r̥ʰ r
Tap or flap				
Fricative		f v	θ ð	s
Lateral fricative	■			ɬ
Affricate				
Approximant	w (labiovelar)			
Lateral approximant	■			l

Note. /x/ may also be realized as [χ]; dental plosives and nasal are alveolar in southern varieties; /r̥ʰ/ is often merged with /r/ in southern varieties and /h/ deleted; southern varieties may use /z/ in loanwords; /tʃ/ and /dʒ/ occur in loanwords and through coalescence.

Black = articulations judged impossible

Based on the International Phonetic Alphabet. Courtesy of the International Phonetic Association (c/o Department of Linguistics, University of Victoria, Victoria, British Columbia, Canada).

spirantization. Table 56-3 shows the changes in orthography and phonology.

Common triggering environments for these mutations are as follows:

- SM: feminine singular noun after the article, after the numeral *un*; adjective following feminine singular noun; word following *ei* 'his', *dy* 'your' (singular); words following a range of common prepositions; verbs following a range of preverbal particles (e.g., marking questions, statements, negatives); items following a range of numeral forms (e.g., *dau/dwy* 'two', *ail* 'second'); adjectives following the complementizer *yn* (but not verbs); direct object of an inflected verb (but not of a periphrastic construction), and adverbials of time, among numerous others.
- NM: words following *fy* 'my'; nouns following the preposition *yn* 'in'; various set expressions with numerals and time expressions.
- AM: words following *ei* 'her'; words following a range of prepositions (*â, gyda* 'with', *tua* 'towards'); words following various negative particles; words following the numerals *tri* 'three' masc., *chew* 'six', and the adverb *tra* 'very'.

A feature called prevocalic aspiration by Ball and Müller (1992) can also occur in some contexts, and here an /h/ is added to vowel-initial words, for example, following *ei, ein, eu* 'her, our, their'.

Phonotactic restrictions
Syllables

The syllable structure of Welsh allows V, VC, CV, and CVC types. The Welsh syllable can be $C_{0-3}VC_{0-2}$; consonant clusters are allowed at both C positions (see the following section).

Consonants and consonant clusters

Phonotactic restrictions for consonants and consonant clusters are illustrated in Table 56-4.

Tones

Welsh does not use tones to differentiate meaning.

Stress and intonation

Suprasegmental aspects of Welsh phonology have not been studied to the same extent as segmental (though see Ball and Williams, 2001, and references cited within). Word stress in Welsh is regularly on the penult with a very small number of exceptions (mostly borrowings, or the result of syllabic contraction). Interestingly, however, major pitch movements of the intonation system take place on the final syllable of accented words, and so pitch and stress are separated. Nuclear tones (or major pitches) have been

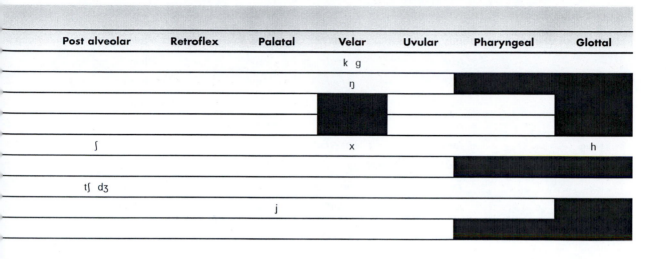

Post alveolar	Retroflex	Palatal	Velar	Uvular	Pharyngeal	Glottal
			k g			
			ŋ			
ʃ			x			h
tʃ dʒ						
		j				

TABLE 56-2 Welsh vowel phonemes

Location	Northern Welsh vowel phonemes	Southern Welsh vowel phoneme equivalents	Example words	English translation
High-front	/i/	/i/	pîn	'pines'
	/ɪ/	/ɪ/	pin	'pen'
Mid front	/e/	/e/	pêr	'sweet'
	/ɛ/	/ɛ/	pen	'head'
Low-front	/a/	/a/	pan	'when'
Low back	/ɑ/	/ɑ/	pân	'fulled cloth'
High-back, rounded	/u/	/u/	pŵl	'stupid'
	/ʊ/	/ʊ/	pwl	'fit, attack'
Mid-back, rounded	/o/	/o/	pôr	'lord'
	/ɔ/	/ɔ/	pont	'bridge'
Central	/ɨ/	/i/	p'un	'which one'
	/ɪ̵/	/ɪ/	pum	'five'
	/ə/	/ə/	pyrs	'purse'
Diphthongs				
Fronting	/aɪ/	/aɪ/	llais	'voice'
	/ɔɪ/	/ɔɪ/	rhoi	'give'
	/əɪ/	/ɪe/	lleidr	'thief'

Table 55-2 continued

backing	/ɪʊ/	/ɪʊ/	lliw	'colour'
	/ɛʊ/	/ɛʊ/	llew	'lion'
	/aʊ/	/aʊ/	llaw	'hand'
	/əʊ/	/əʊ/	llywiau	'helms'
	/iʊ/	/ɪʊ/	llyw	'helm, rudder'
centering	/aɨ/	/aɪ/ ~ /ɔɪ/	llau	'lice'
	/ɑɨ/	/aɪ/ ~ /ɑ/	llaes	'loose'
	/ɔɨ/	/ɔɪ/ ~ /ɔ/	lloer	'moon'
	/ʊɨ/	/ʊɪ/	llwy	'spoon'
	/əɨ/	/əɪ/	lleu	'to light'

described by several authors (Ball and Williams, 2001; Pilch, 1975; Rhys, 1984; Thomas, 1967). The consensus view is that the language has four broad categories of pitch movement: fall, rise, rise-fall, and level, but that high and low versions of these exist, at least at the level of phonetic difference. Thomas (1967) posits a variety of prenuclear patterns in intonation (both "preheads" and "heads"), and Williams (1985) found some support for these. They are normal, high rising, high level, and low level preheads, and saw-toothed, rising, and level heads.

Writing system

The grapheme-phoneme correspondence in Welsh is fairly close, especially for the northern accents. Generally, each phoneme described above has only one written form, and each grapheme only one pronunciation. There is some departure from this ideal, but often this is predictable. We give in Tables 56-5, 56-6, and 56-7 below the grapheme-phoneme correspondences for consonants and vowels, and the order of the alphabet in Welsh and the pronunciation of the letters.

The order of the alphabet in Welsh is: a, b, c, ch, d, dd, e, f, ff, g, ng, h, i, l, ll, m, n, o, p, ph, r, rh, s, t, th, u, w, y. The pronunciation (standard northern) of these letters is: /ɑ, bi, ɛk, ɛx, di, ɛð, e, ɛv, ɛf, ɛg, ɛŋ, aɪtʃ, i, ɛl, ɛɬ, ɛm, ɛn, o, pi, fi, ɛr, r̥ʰi/r̥ʰo, ɛs, ti, ɛθ, i/ɨ bɛdɔl, u, ə/. The name *u-bedol* means 'horseshoe-u' and is used in southern pronunciations to distinguish the letter name from that of *i*. "j" is not considered part of the traditional alphabet but is used for borrowings. It is placed in dictionaries after "i"

TABLE 56-3   Initial Welsh consonant mutations

	Radical	Soft mutation		Nasal mutation		Aspirate mutation	
p	p	b	b	mh	mʰ	ph	f
t	t	d	d	nh	nʰ	th	θ
c	k	g	g	ngh	ŋʰ	ch	x
b	b	f	v	m	m		
d	d	dd	ð	n	n		
g	g	deleted	–	ng	ŋ		
m	m	f	v				
ll	ɬ	l	l				
rh	r̥ʰ	r	r				

Note. Unfilled boxes mean that the mutation does not change the radical in these cases

TABLE 56-4 Phonotactic constraints with Welsh consonants

Syllable type	Consonant type	Examples
CV*	obstruents	p t k b d g f v θ s ʃ x ɬ tʃ dʒ
	sonorants	m n l r̥ʰ j w h
VCV	obstruents	p t k b d g f v θ ð s ʃ x ɬ tʃ dʒ
	sonorants	m n ŋ l r̥ʰ r j w h
VC	obstruents	p t k b d g f v θ ð s ʃ x ɬ tʃ dʒ
	sonorants	m n ŋ l r
CCV*	obstruents+obstruent	sb, sd, sg
	obstruent+sonorant	kn, tr, dr, tl, fr, gl
VCCV	obstruents+obstruent	gv, xg, ɬd
	sonorant+sonorant	rm, rl, mn
	sonorant+obstruent	ŋg, mð, rd, rθ
	obstruent+sonorant	dn, br, vn, vl
VCC	obstruents+obstruent	sg, ɬd
	sonorant+sonorant	rn, rm
	sonorant+obstruent	mp, rd, rð, lx
	obstruent+sonorant†	dr, br, vn
CCCV	/s/+stop+liquid	sdr, sgl
VCCCV	/s/+stop+liquid	sgr, sbr
	nasal+stop+liquid	ndl, ntr

* Excluding mutation reflexes (see above)

† Except in very formal speech these clusters are normally separated by a copy epenthetic vowel in southern varieties.

and pronounced as in English. "k", "q", "v", and "z" are pronounced as in British English when referred to.

Varieties of Welsh

Welsh has a strong differentiation between the literary language and various regionally differentiated colloquial forms (see also Ball, 1988; Jones, 1993). These differences range over phonology, morphology, syntax, and lexis to an extent almost reminiscent of the diglossic situations described for languages such as Arabic (Ferguson, 1959).

Traditionally, Welsh was divided into four broad dialect areas: Venedotian (northwest Wales), Powysian (northeast and mid Wales), Demetian (southwest Wales), and Gwentian (southeast Wales) (see Morris Jones, 1913). However, due to disproportionate percentage decline of Welsh speakers in different areas over the last 150 years, these dialect zones have to large extent been fragmented, and the Gwentian dialect has been severely reduced. Thomas (1973) proposes a major division between southern varieties, midland

varieties, and northern varieties, with each of these areas subdivided into east and west. Further, he suggests that midland and northern varieties share certain features that allow an overarching grouping and division between south and north (as we use in this chapter).

Typical acquisition of Welsh

The Summary of Studies Table at the end of this chapter contains studies of the acquisition of Welsh.

Acquired sounds

Most of the studies included below have approached Welsh within the context of Welsh-English bilingualism, as the majority of Welsh-speaking children also speak English.

Consonants

Discussion of Welsh consonant acquisition is primarily based on Munro, Ball, Müller, Duckworth, and Lyddy

TABLE 56-5 Grapheme-phoneme correspondences for Welsh consonants

Grapheme	Phoneme	Comments
p	/p/	
t	/t/	
c	/k/	"k" and "c" in early texts
b	/b/	
d	/d/	
g	/g/	
j	/dʒ/	Not considered part of the alphabet
ff	/f/	
ph	/f/	Only in mutation reflexes of "p"
th	/θ/	
s	/s/	
ch	/x/	
h	/h/	
f	/v/	"v" and "u" in early texts
dd	/ð/	
z	/z/	Only in southern accents. Not counted as part of the alphabet; usually replaced by "s"
m	/m/	
n	/n/	
ng	/ŋ/	Occasionally /ŋg/
l	/l/	
ll	/ɬ/	
r	/r/	
rh	/r̥ʰ/	In southern accents often /r/
i	/j/	See also vowels
w	/w/	See also vowels

Note. /ʃ/ is written 'si' initially, "s" or "sh" finally (e.g., *siarad* 'talk', *brws/brwsh* 'brush')

/tʃ/ is written "tsi" or "tsh" initially, and "ts" or "tsh" finally (e.g., *Tsiechof* 'Chekhov', *mats/matsh* 'match')

TABLE 56-6 Grapheme-phoneme correspondences for Welsh monophthongs

Grapheme	Phoneme	Comments
i	/i/, /ɪ/	See note on circumflex below
e	/e/, /ɛ/	See note on circumflex below
a	/ɑ/, /a/	See note on circumflex below
o	/o/, /ɔ/	See note on circumflex below
w	/u/, /ʊ/	See note on circumflex below
u	N - /i/, /ɪ/ S - /i/, /ɪ/	See note on circumflex below
y	N - /i/, /ɪ/, /ə/ S - /i/, /ɪ/, /ə/	See note on circumflex below

Note. N stands for northern accents, S for southern.

A circumflex can be added to show a long vowel in those syllable types where minimal pairs are possible (e.g., *ton* 'wave' ~ *tôn* 'tune'); but not all such instances have the diacritic.

"y" is not schwa when in monosyllables (except for a few function words and borrowings), in the final syllable of polysyllabic words, in the penult or antepenult if preceding a vowel or following "w"; elsewhere it is schwa.

which consonants the children used contrastively. The formula used was that a consonant was acquired for each age cohort if at least 75 percent of the children in each cohort achieved at least 75 percent accuracy for that consonant. Simultaneous and successive Welsh/English bilinguals were included in the study, the subjects being organized into 6-monthly age bands from 2;6 to 5;0.

The study by Munro et al. (2005) classified the children according to language dominance before analysis began. The limitations of such *a priori* classification and the methods used are contained in the 2005 publication. Language dominance was considered essential because children in Wales learn Welsh within diverse linguistic, educational, and familial contexts. A simple Welsh dominant vs. English dominant distinction went at least some way to recognizing this diversity.

Table 56-8 contains age of acquisition data for Welsh. In this table, single entries denote a lack of difference between Welsh dominant and English dominant subjects in terms of age of acquisition. Where there are differences, details for Welsh dominant children are provided first, with English dominant information in brackets. "Uneven" refers to a pattern where there is apparent acquisition by younger children that is not maintained by older children.

(2005), as this is the only detailed study available. In that study acquisition was defined as the developmental sequence of phonological contrasts, though crude, frequency definitions were adopted as a means of reflecting

TABLE 56-7 Grapheme-phoneme correspondences for Welsh diphthongs

Grapheme	Northern phoneme	Southern Phoneme
ai	/aɪ/	/aɪ/
ae	/ɑɨ/	/aɪ/ ~ /ɑ/
au	/aɨ/	/aɪ/ ~ /ɔɪ/
aw	/aʊ/	/aʊ/
ei	/əɪ/	/əɪ/
eu	/əɨ/	/əɪ/
ew	/ɛʊ/	/ɛʊ/
iw	/ɪʊ/	/ɪʊ/
oi	/ɔɪ/	/ɔɪ/
oe	/ɔɨ/	/ɔɪ/ ~ /ɔ/
uw	/ɨʊ/	/ɪʊ/
wy	/ʊɨ/, /wɨ/, /wə/	/ʊɪ/, /wɪ/, /wə/
yw	/ɨʊ/, /əʊ/	/ɪʊ/, /əʊ/

Note. "ey" sometimes occurs for "ei" and "ou" for "oe". "ow" can be found for /aʊ/, and for a marginal diphthong /oʊ/ derived from inflections. Finally "ow" can represent /ɔu/.

"yw" is generally /ɨʊ/ ~ /ɪʊ/ in monosyllables and final syllables. "wy" is generally /wɨ/ ~ /wɪ/ following /g/ or /x/ in monosyllables, but /wɪ/ after /g/ in polysyllables. Elsewhere it is /ʊɨ/ ~ /ʊɪ/.

With reference to the data in the first column of Table 56-8, /ð/ appeared to be acquired by 3;6, regardless of dominance, but in the Welsh dominant children there was a later period of instability (the "uneven" category) with acquisition not being re-established until 4;6. A similar pattern presented across targets /g/, /w/, and /v/, with Welsh dominant children reaching the acquisition criterion before 3;6 but the English dominant not until 3;6, followed by a period of instability until 4;6 or later.

Although Welsh dominant children seemed to acquire /ʃ/ before 3;6 and the English dominant children by 3;6, both then demonstrated instability until 4;6. However, in the case of /tʃ/, Welsh dominant subjects demonstrated acquisition by 3;6 followed by instability until 4;6 whereas the English dominant presented with firm acquisition patterns before 3;6.

Returning to Table 56-8, the ages cited by Donohue, Holding, and Jones (1983) are contained in the *Dyfed Screening Test of Articulation and Language* (see later). The acquisition ages are broadly similar to those in the first column in about 70 percent of cases, and it is interesting to note that the relatively late acquisition quoted by Donohue et al. for targets /v/, /ð/, and /ʃ/ are mirrored by some unevenness of development in the Munro et al. study. What is not clear are the reasons for the differences in age of acquisition with regard to /l/, /j/, /s/, and /x/, as the articulation test manual does not give details of methodology such as subject selection and the working definition of acquisition.

TABLE 56-8 Age of acquisition for Welsh consonants

Consonant	Munro et al. (2005)	Donohue, Holding, and Jones. (1983)
p	before 3;6	by 3;0
b	before 3;6	by 3;0
t	before 3;6	by 4;0
d	before 3;6	by 4;0
k	before 3;6	by 4;0
g	before 3;6 (uneven)	by 4;0
m	before 3;6	by 3;0
n	before 3;6	by 3;0
ŋ	by 4;6 (not by 5;0)	–
l	before 3;6	by 6;0
r/r̥ʰ	not by 5;0	by 6;0
w	before 3;6 (uneven)	by 3;0

Table 56-8 continued

j	before 3;6 (by 3;6)	by 7;0
f	before 3;6	by 4;0
v	before 3;6 (uneven)	by 7;0
θ	by 4;6 (not by 5;0)	by 7;0
ð	uneven (by 3;6)	by 7;0
s	before 3;6	by 6;0
z	–	by 7;0
ʃ	uneven	by 7;0
x	before 3;6	by 6;0
ɫ	by 4;6 (not by 5;0)	by 6;0
h	before 3;6	by 3;0
tʃ	uneven (before 3;6)	–
dʒ	by 3;6 (before 3;6)	–

Consonant clusters

The data obtained by Munro et al. (2005) have not yet been analyzed with regard to consonant clusters. However, some information is available from earlier sources and is described under Phonological Processes.

Vowels and diphthongs

To date there has been no study of the acquisition of vocalic segments in Welsh.

Percent correct

Percentage correct scores can be reported for the speakers in the Munro et al. (2005) study, for five different age ranges. These scores are available for consonants only, and are presented for the male and female speakers separately in Table 56-9.

Phonological processes

Munro (1985) gave an account of simplifying phonological processes in normal Welsh-English simultaneous bilingual children, the data being drawn mostly from Harrison and Thomas (1975). It should be noted that the summarized information below is based on only three children, Lowri, Nia, and Roderic (the English data are excluded from this chapter). Examples are confined

to the earliest and latest ages at which the processes appeared, and are shown in Table 56-10.

Intelligibility

No work to date has been reported on intelligibility issues in Welsh acquisition or phonological disorder.

Phonetic inventory

The work of Munro et al. (2005) reported earlier points to typical phonetic inventories at different ages.

Common mismatches

The phonological process section above reports many common realizations of target sounds in disordered speech. In typical acquisition, Munro et al. (2005) describe the use of similar patterns, including velar fronting (but not for /x/, which is acquired early), fricative simplification, and some liquid gliding. Of most interest were the realizations of the trills and the lateral fricative (see Ball, Müller, and Munro, 2001a, b). With the lateral fricative, a large number of substitutions were used, though the tendency among English-dominant subjects was to use a voiceless velar fricative, or that fricative together with the voiced alveolar lateral approximant ([x], [xl]). With the Welsh dominant subjects the lateral fricative was less often substituted, and patterns of [s] and [x] usage were noted.

The Welsh trill was the sound that showed the most varied substitution patterns of all, though many of these occurred only once or twice. A common substitution for all speakers was the approximant-r ([ɹ]), as found in English. Interestingly, there was also a considerable use of voiced fricatives (especially [ð]) by all subjects. This may be due to the acoustic similarity between this fricative and the target trill.

Syllable structure

See the section on phonological processes.

Prosody

No work to date has been reported on prosody in Welsh acquisition or phonological disorder.

Phonological awareness

No work to date has been reported on phonological awareness in Welsh acquisition or phonological disorder.

Speech assessment for Welsh-speaking children

There are very few published speech assessments for Welsh speaking-children. The *Dyfed Test* was developed by speech and language therapists in Mid Wales and contains both Welsh and English sections (Donohue, Holding, and Jones, 1983). The assessment is not standardized; rather, it is a means of recording a child's realizations and comparing them with the acquisition guidelines supplied. The assessment is presented in sets of three pictures per consonant, one each in word-initial, medial and final positions. The score sheet is organized into developmental levels as is the administration of the test. It is intended as a screening device for therapists, teachers, and medical officers.

CWLWM (Rees and Trythall, 1995) is also published as a phonological screening test; the manual recommends that it is a starting point for the gathering of data rather than an analytical tool. Devised by Rees and Trythall, speech and language therapists in North West Wales, *CWLWM* consists of black and white line drawings with which to elicit phonemes in various word positions. The type:token ratios vary across consonants and across word

positions. Data from the recording sheet can be mapped on to grids allocated to each phoneme. No acquisition guidelines are provided.

Given the paucity in number of Welsh speech assessments and the absence of standardized tests, popularity is not a useful concept as choice is so restricted. Therapists use one of the above assessments or their own, unpublished methods of collecting and analyzing data (see below).

Additional speech sampling tools have been developed for use with Welsh-speaking children. The Munro et al. (2005) study incorporated word lists for the sampling of consonants. Criteria by which phonological data should be collected were stipulated and the target words used in the study were selected on the basis of the given criteria, the lists being included in the 2005 publication. This was a development of earlier work by Ball and Munro (1981).

Analyses of Welsh phonological data are often based on clinical tools developed for English. Speech and language therapists analyze a child's phonetic inventory along with the correspondence between target phonemes and a child's realizations. Many also describe the phonological processes in a set of data, although consideration of the clinical significance of the processes (in terms of delay or deviance) is limited because of the absence of a robust Welsh developmental yardstick.

Nevertheless, the analysis of processes remains useful because of their effects on a child's contrastive system. Therapists are more likely to adopt the *Phonological Assessment of Child Speech* (PACS)(Grunwell, 1985) to analyze contrastivity where a child presents with a complex phonological problem. The focus of PACS is on the child's own system, based on universal principles underlying the organization of phonological systems. Thus it can, to an extent, be used for Welsh data, although other studies are required in order to make quantitative and qualitative comparisons with normal children from the same linguistic background. (The further usefulness of this approach in dealing with Welsh-English bilingual phonological data is discussed in Ball et al., 2006.)

There has been an increase in the analysis of phonological disorders within a psycholinguistic framework, particularly that developed by Stackhouse and Wells (1997). Individual therapists or groups of therapists have adapted the framework to Welsh but the information is not published. A further, interesting perspective is the potential use of such a framework for analyzing bilingual data (Munro, Murray, and Pandeli, 2006).

TABLE 56-9   Percent correct for Welsh consonants

Age	2;6–3;0		3;0–3;6				3;6–4;0	
Dominance	Welsh		Welsh		English		Welsh	
Sex	male	female	male	female	male	female	male	female
tʃ	44.4	66.7	33.3	60	80	100	100	85.7
dʒ	100	100	61.1	60	93.3	83	100	85.7
l	95.4	100	78.8	93.1	96.1	100	98.1	100
r/r̥ʰ	0	0	0	10.9	1.82	5.2	17.4	4.2
w	100	100	100	89.7	80	66.7	88.9	95.2
j	95.2	100	100	100	70	66.7	100	100
f	75	91.7	100	100	100	100	100	100
v	97.7	90.7	88	95	81.2	69.7	83.3	96.9
θ	22.2	53	28.7	23.6	5.8	16.7	96.3	72.4
ð	40	100	0	93.5	50	100	88.9	89.6
s	97.7	98.3	100	100	96.6	100	100	97.6
z	0	100	100	0	0	0	100	100
ʃ	80	69.3	40.2	58.5	63.7	100	100	97.6
ʒ	0	0	0	0	0	0	0	0
x	76.7	91.7	93.65	70	94.2	61.9	100	100
ɬ	60.4	74.1	17.2	56.3	11.4	49.9	74.7	68.4
h	97.2	97	91.7	100	100	100	91.7	100
m	100	100	100	99.4	98	100	100	100
n	98.5	91	94.8	96.4	94.4	98.7	95.7	94.4
ŋ	27.7	63	55.7	33.2	58	25	50	38.3
p	100	94.3	94.3	100	100	96.3	100	94.9
b	93.7	100	100	98.4	97	93.7	96.3	99.1
t	97.7	97.3	90.7	100	100	100	100	98.9
d	92	95.8	96.7	98.2	88.2	78.3	95.3	97.1
k	71.3	91.5	97.3	97.6	97	90.3	100	99.3
g	78	94	90.5	89.1	85.5	76.2	90.7	93.4

Auditory discrimination assessment is included in the Stackhouse and Wells framework, but analysis of children's responses on auditory discrimination tasks has been common in clinical practice for many years. It is not surprising, therefore, that Welsh versions exist, though these are resources designed by individuals or groups and shared on a relatively informal basis.

Speech intervention for Welsh-speaking children

Again, approaches for speech intervention for Welsh-speaking children are based on those originating in

| 3;6–4;0 | | | | 4;0–4;5 | | | | 4;5–5;0 | |
| English | | Welsh | | English | | Welsh | | English | |
male	female	male	female	male	female	male	female	male	female
100	100	60	80	100	75	100	100	100	83.3
91.7	100	100	80	100	93.8	100	100	80	100
98.1	88	93.6	97.5	98.4	91.2	100	100	100	94.45
4.7	14	42.1	45.7	6.7	23.5	49.4	44.8	39.3	23.1
80.1	94.4	93.3	100	92.9	66.7	100	100	87	87.5
100	66.7	80	100	100	87.5	100	100	100	100
100	89	100	100	100	95.8	100	100	100	100
74.7	88.7	97.8	96	72.8	53.6	93.4	87.5	77	74.9
45.1	60	74.2	53.4	31	83.3	93.4	100	63.4	83.7
66.7	0	25	100	0	100	100	100	83.3	100
100	93.3	100	100	100	100	100	100	100	94.5
100	0	0	0	0	0	0	0	0	0
95.8	93.3	68	71.4	88	91.7	100	100	95	94.45
0	0	0	0	0	0	0	0	0	0
93.5	77.4	93	94.3	98	73.8	100	95.8	100	100
31.8	57.5	34.6	100	48.7	66.9	100	100	58	77.8
100	100	100	100	100	100	100	100	100	100
97.2	100	100	100	100	98.3	97.2	100	100	97.67
92.9	95	91.7	97.6	95.5	98	97	92.5	96.2	91.5
34.7	33	79.2	75.4	22.3	38.5	100	100	30	41.7
97	100	100	100	100	100	100	100	100	100
87	100	98.6	100	95	98.5	100	100	98.2	93.7
96.7	91.7	100	100	100	100	100	100	100	90.3
95.3	95	95	97.4	91.9	81.8	100	100	86.6	98.5
97.7	100	99.2	100	88.1	100	100	100	93.8	97.9
81	87	96.6	93.6	70.4	88.4	100	98.25	100	93.5

English. Therapists select from a range of approaches such as metaphonological, discrimination, and articulatory placement therapies, depending on their personal preferences and the needs of each child. Materials have been adapted into Welsh. The largest percentage of Welsh-speaking therapists is in North West Wales and so it is not surprising that most of the Welsh materials have emanated from that area. Some of those materials have, relatively recently, been made available to other therapists in Wales as a result of Welsh Assembly Government grants.

TABLE 56-10   Phonological processes in Welsh

Process	Example	Ages	Comment
Weak syllable deletion	R: *awyren* 'aeroplane' /aˈwərɛn/ ⇨ [ˈjavja]	1;8	Not a major process for any of the children
	N: *mamgu* 'grandmother' /mamˈgi/ ⇨ [gi]	1;6	
	N: *Eleri* [personal name] /ɛˈleri/ ⇨ [ˈleji]	1;10	
	L: *oren* 'orange' /ˈorɛn/ ⇨ [on]	1;10–1;11	
Fronting	No instances for Nia and only a very few for the other 2 children		
Stopping	Hardly any instances in Roderic's data and none for Nia and Lowri		
Final consonant deletion	R: *ieir* 'chickens' /jeɪr/ ⇨ [jeɪ]	1;8–2;0 (few 2;3)	
	N: *diolch* 'thanks' /ˈdiɔlx/ ⇨ [dja]	1;7–2;8	
	L: *dŵr* 'water' /dur/ ⇨ [du]	1;10–2;2	
Metathesis	Of little relevance as there were only 2 instances for each child		
Cluster reduction	R: *drws* 'door' /drus/ ⇨ [du];	2;2	A common process for all 3 children in all word positions. More evidence was available for word-initial Cluster Reduction than for other word positions. With reference to these initial clusters, where targets involved stop+liquid, it was the stop that all children retained. Where targets involved /s/ + stop/ nasal, Nia and Roderic dropped the /s/ but in Lowri's case it was the /s/ that was retained.
	Cymraeg 'Welsh [language]' /kəmˈraːg/ ⇨ [gəˈmaːg]	3;3	
		1;10; 2;1	
	N: *cloc* 'clock' /klɔk/ ⇨ [kɔk]; *drws* /drus/ ⇨ [dus]	1;10; 2;8	
	L: *bwlch* 'gap' /bulx/ ⇨ [bux]; *llofft* 'upstairs' /ɬɔft/ ⇨ [ɬɔf]		
Gliding	R: *Eleri* /ɛˈleri/ ⇨ [ɛiˈejei]	1;10	Most commonly the realization of target /l/ and /r/ by the glides [w, j].
	Gareth [personal name] /ˈgarɛθ/ ⇨ [ˈgawɛθ]	2;7	
	N: rare		
	L: nonexistent		
Voicing	R: *pen* 'head' /pɛn/ ⇨ [bɛw]	1;8	
	castell 'castle' /ˈkastɛɬ/ ⇨ [ˈdasdɛ]	2;10	
	N: *ci* 'dog' /ki/ ⇨ [gi]; *ti* 'you [sing]' /ti/ ⇨ [di]	1;4; 1;8	
	L: *coch* 'red' /kox/ ⇨ [gox]	1;10	
	pedwar 'four [masc]' /ˈpɛdwar/ ⇨ [ˈbɛdwah]	3;5	
Reduplication and assimilation	R: *dyna* 'there is/are' /ˈdəna/ ⇨ [ˈwəwə]	1;8	
	llaeth 'milk' /ɬaɪθ/ ⇨ [ɬaɪɬ]	2;5	
	N: *helo* 'hello' /ˈhɛlo/ ⇨ [ˈlala]	1;3–1;10	
	L: *dere* 'come!' [sing] /ˈderɛ/ ⇨ [ˈdɛdɛ]	1;9	
	cregyn 'shell' /ˈkrɛgɪn/ ⇨ [ˈdɛdɪn]		
	trowsus 'trousers' /ˈtrousɪs/ ⇨ [ˈsɪsɪs]; *Eleri* /ɛˈleri/ ⇨ [aˈlɛli]	1;11	

Note. From Munro (1985).

R: Roderic; N: Nia; L: Lowri

Additionally, a Welsh version of the POPAT phoneme awareness program (Popat, 1991) is being developed in Pembrokeshire (South West Wales).

In conclusion, it should be pointed out that there are very few Welsh-speaking speech and language therapists, and only some of these work with children. This has had an effect on the time available to develop Welsh clinical resources.

Working in Wales

The required qualifications for working within Wales are the same as those for the United Kingdom as a whole (see Royal College of Speech and Language Therapists, http://www.rcslt.org.uk). Clearly, if one wishes to work in a strongly Welsh-speaking part of the country, a knowledge of Welsh would be extremely helpful.

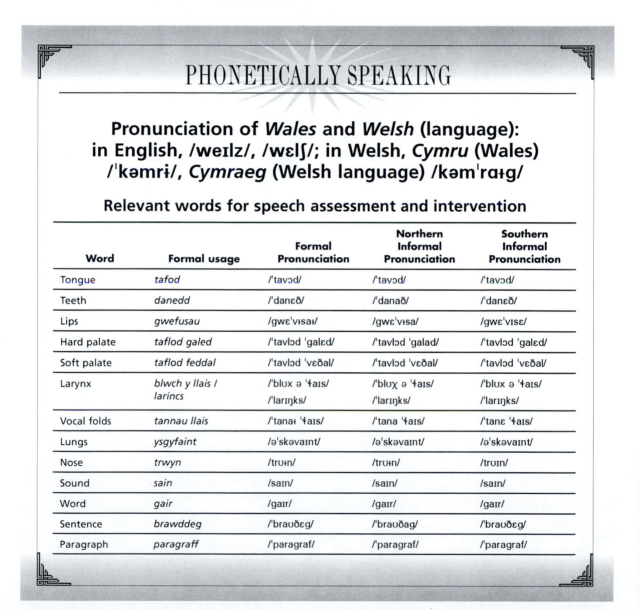

PHONETICALLY SPEAKING

Pronunciation of *Wales* and *Welsh* (language): in English, /weɪlz/, /wɛlʃ/; in Welsh, *Cymru* (Wales) /ˈkəmrɨ/, *Cymraeg* (Welsh language) /kəmˈraɨg/

Relevant words for speech assessment and intervention

Word	Formal usage	Formal Pronunciation	Northern Informal Pronunciation	Southern Informal Pronunciation
Tongue	*tafod*	/ˈtavɔd/	/ˈtavɒd/	/ˈtavɒd/
Teeth	*danedd*	/ˈdanɛð/	/ˈdanað/	/ˈdanɛð/
Lips	*gwefusau*	/gwɛˈvɪsaɨ/	/gwɛˈvɪsa/	/gwɛˈvɪsɛ/
Hard palate	*taflod galed*	/ˈtavlɔd ˈgalɛd/	/ˈtavlɔd ˈgalad/	/ˈtavlɔd ˈgalɛd/
Soft palate	*taflod feddal*	/ˈtavlɔd ˈvɛðal/	/ˈtavlɔd ˈvɛðal/	/ˈtavlɔd ˈvɛðal/
Larynx	*blwch y llais / larincs*	/ˈblʊx ə ˈɬaɪs/ /ˈlarɪŋks/	/ˈblʊχ ə ˈɬaɪs/ /ˈlarɪŋks/	/ˈblʊx ə ˈɬaɪs/ /ˈlarɪŋks/
Vocal folds	*tannau llais*	/ˈtanaɨ ˈɬaɪs/	/ˈtana ˈɬaɪs/	/ˈtanɛ ˈɬaɪs/
Lungs	*ysgyfaint*	/əˈskəvaɪnt/	/əˈskəvaɪnt/	/əˈskəvaɪnt/
Nose	*trwyn*	/trʊɨn/	/trʊɨn/	/trʊɪn/
Sound	*sain*	/saɪn/	/saɪn/	/saɪn/
Word	*gair*	/gaɪr/	/gaɪr/	/gaɪr/
Sentence	*brawddeg*	/ˈbrauðɛg/	/ˈbrauðag/	/ˈbrauðɛg/
Paragraph	*paragraff*	/ˈparagraf/	/ˈparagraf/	/ˈparagraf/

RESOURCES

Books

King, G. (2005). *Colloquial Welsh: A complete language course.* London: Routledge.

Brake, P. (1998). *Welsh in three months.* Woodbridge: Hugo's Language Books.

Gruneberg, M. M. (1996). *Linkword Welsh.* Llandysul: Gomer.

Rhys Jones, T. J. (1992). *Welsh.* Sevenoaks: Teach Yourself.

O'Riain, F. (1991). *Lazy way to Welsh.* Talybont: Y Lolfa.

CD-ROMs and CDs

See selection available on the Acen Web site. Online course in Welsh available at University of Wales, Lampeter (see Web site below).

Journals

* *Journal of Celtic Linguistics,* http://www.uwp.co.uk
  Linguistics
* *Studia Celtica,* http://www.uwp.co.uk
  Language, history, and archaeology
* *Acen,* http://www.acen.co.uk
  Learners' magazine

Professional associations

The professional association of speech-language pathologists within Wales is the Royal College of Speech and Language Therapists (London).

Useful Welsh Web sites

* Acen: Welsh learners' site, http://www.acen.co.uk/
* Welsh language board site, http://www.bwrdd-yr-iaith.org.uk/
* BBC Welsh learners' site, http://www.bbc.co.uk/wales/learnwelsh/
* BBC learners' course, http://www.bbc.co.uk/wales/catchphrase/
* Welsh department, University of Cardiff, http://www.cardiff.ac.uk/cymraeg/
* Welsh department, University of Wales, Aberystwyth, http://www.aber.ac.uk/cymraeg-welsh/
* Welsh department, University of Wales, Bangor http://www.bangor.ac.uk/adran_cymraeg/indecs.htm
* Welsh department, University of Wales, Swansea, http://www.swan.ac.uk/cymraeg/
* Welsh department, University of Wales, Lampeter, http://welsh.lamp.ac.uk/Department/Cymraeg/

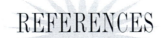

REFERENCES

Ball, M. J. (Ed.) (1988). *The use of Welsh.* Clevedon: Multilingual Matters.

Ball, M. J. (2007). Welsh. In D. Britain, (Ed.), *Language in the British Isles* (2nd ed.). Cambridge, UK: Cambridge University Press.

Ball, M. J., and Jones, G. E. (Eds.) (1984). *Welsh phonology. Selected readings.* Cardiff: University of Wales Press.

Ball, M. J., and Müller, N. (1992). *Mutation in Welsh.* London: Routledge.

Ball, M. J., Müller, N., and Munro, S. (2001a). The acquisition of the lateral fricative in Welsh-English bilinguals. *Multilingua, 20,* 269–284.

Ball, M. J., Müller, N., and Munro, S. (2001b). The acquisition of the rhotic consonants by Welsh-English bilingual children. *International Journal of Bilingualism, 5,* 71–86.

Ball, M. J., Müller, N., and Munro, S. (2006). Welsh/English-speaking bilingual children. In Zhu Hua and B. Dodd, (Eds.), *Phonological development and disorders from a cross-linguistic perspective* (pp. 346–382). Clevedon: Multilingual Matters.

Ball, M., and Munro, S. (1981). Language assessment procedures for linguistic minorities: An example. *Journal of Multilingual and Multicultural Development, 2,* 231–241.

Ball, M. J., and Williams, B. (2001). *Welsh phonetics.* Lewiston, NY: Edwin Mellen Press.

Bellin, W. (1984). Welsh phonology in acquisition. In M. J. Ball and G. E. Jones (Eds.). *Welsh Phonology* (pp. 156–175). Cardiff: University of Wales Press.

Donohue, A., Holding, J., and Jones, V. (1983). *Dyfed Screening Test of Articulation and Language.* Swansea: East Dyfed Health Authority.

Ferguson, C. (1959). Diglossia. *Word, 15*, 325–340.

Grunwell, P. (1985). *Phonological assessment of child speech*. Windsor: NFER-Nelson.

Harrison, G., and Thomas, C. (1975). *The acquisition of bilingual speech by infants*. Final Report on SSRC Grant HR2104/1. [Social Science Research Council, U.K.].

Jones, R. O. (1993). The sociolinguistics of Welsh. In M. J. Ball (Ed), *The Celtic languages* (pp. 536–605). London: Routledge.

Jones, R. O. (1998). Yr iaith Gymraeg yn y Wladfa. In G. H. Jenkins (Ed.), *Iaith carreg fy aelwyd: Iaith a Chymuned yn y Bedwaredd Ganrif ar Bymtheg* (pp. 281–305). Caerdydd: Gwasg Prifysgol Cymru.

Morris Jones, J. (1913). *A Welsh grammar: Historical and comparative*. Oxford, UK: Clarendon Press.

Munro, S. (1985). *An empirical study of specific communication disorders in bilingual children*. Unpublished Ph.D. thesis, University of Wales.

Munro, S., Ball, M. J., Müller, N., Duckworth, M., and Lyddy, F. (2005). The acquisition of Welsh and English phonology in bilingual Welsh-English children. *Journal of Multilingual Communication Disorders, 3*, 24–49.

Munro, S., Murray, A., and Pandeli, H. (2006). Psycholinguistics assessment of a Welsh-English bilingual child. Manuscript in preparation.

National Statistics Online (2003). Retrieved March 12, 2003, from http://tables.neighbourhood.statistics.gov.uk/tables/eng/TableViewer/wdsview/print.asp.

Pilch, H. (1975). Advanced Welsh phonemics. *Zeitschrift für Celtische Philologie, 34*, 60–102.

Popat, P. (1991) A phoneme awareness programme. London: College of Speech Therapists Bulletin Numbers, 467–468.

Rees, O., and Trythall, M. (1995). *CWLWM*. Edinburgh: Langlearn Communications.

Rhys, M. (1984). Intonation and the discourse. In M. J. Ball and G. E. Jones (Eds.). *Welsh Phonology* (pp. 125–155). Cardiff: University of Wales Press.

Stackhouse, J., and Wells, B. (1997). *Children's speech and literacy difficulties*. London: Whurr

Thomas, A. R. (1973). *The linguistic geography of Wales*. Cardiff: University of Wales Press.

Thomas, A. R. (1992). The Welsh Language. In D. MacAulay (Ed), *The Celtic languages* (pp. 251–345). Cambridge, UK: Cambridge University Press.

Thomas, C. H. (1967). Welsh intonation – a preliminary study. *Studia Celtica*, 2, 8–28.

Thomas, P. W. (1996). *Gramadeg y Gymraeg*. Caerdydd: Gwasg Prifysgol Cymru.

Watkins, T. A. (1993). Welsh. In M. J. Ball (Ed), *The Celtic languages* (pp. 289–348). London: Routledge.

Williams, B. (1985). Pitch and duration in Welsh stress perception: The implications for intonation. *Journal of Phonetics*, 13, 381–406.

Williams, S. (1980). *A Welsh grammar*. Cardiff: University of Wales Press.

SUMMARY OF STUDIES OF TYPICAL WELSH SPEECH ACQUISITION

Authors	Year	Country	No. of children	Age of children	Information	Sample type	Data collection
Bellin	1984	UK	3	1;0–4;6	Variety	Single word and connected speech	Longitudinal
Donohue, Holding, and Jones	1983	Wales	300	3;0–8;0	Age of acquisition	Single word	Cross-sectional
Harrison and Thomas	1975	Wales	3	1;6–3;6	Variety	Single word and connected speech	Longitudinal
Munro et al.	2005	Wales	83	2;6–5;0	Variety	Single word and connected speech	Cross-sectional

Chapter 57

San Lucas Quiaviní Zapotec
Speech Acquisition

Joseph Paul Stemberger and Felicia Lee

INTRODUCTION

San Lucas Quiaviní Zapotec is an indigenous language of southern Mexico, spoken primarily in the state of Oaxaca. It is one of roughly 50 mutually unintelligible languages in the Zapotec language family. The Zapotec languages belong to the Otomanguean stock, which also includes Amuzgoan, Chinantecan, Mixtecan, Otopamean, Popolocan, and Tlapanecan languages. Zapotec is not an official language of government, though it is used in bilingual or trilingual signage in some locations (e.g., archeological sites). Although the basic characteristics of the grammars of many Zapotecan languages have been worked out, there is still much research remaining to be done before we have as full a picture of these languages as we do for intensively studied languages such as English. There has been only a little research on the acquisition of Zapotec by typically developing children, and little is known about children with language impairments. While Zapotec is still healthy in many respects, encroachment by Spanish and English leads us to classify it as threatened. This chapter reports on the specific variant of Zapotec spoken in the village of San Lucas Quiaviní. See the Resources section for materials pertaining to San Lucas Quiaviní Zapotec.

Where San Lucas Quiaviní Zapotec is spoken

San Lucas Quiaviní Zapotec and related variants of Zapotec are spoken in the Tlacolula Valley, southeast of the city of Oaxaca in the state of Oaxaca in southern Mexico (see accompying map and Appendix D).

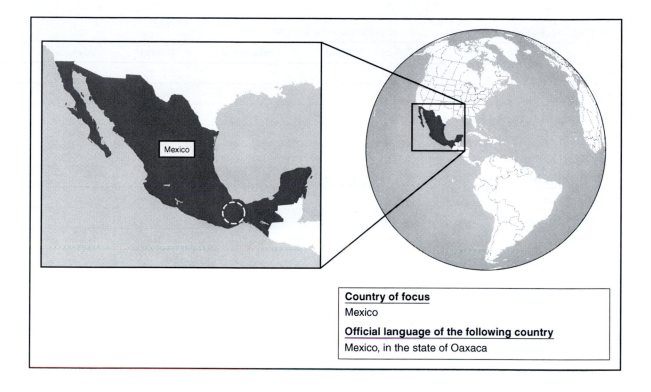

Country of focus
Mexico
Official language of the following country
Mexico, in the state of Oaxaca

Components of San Lucas Quiaviní Zapotec

Consonants

San Lucas Quiaviní Zapotec has 28 consonants (see Table 57-1). There is no true distinction of voicing, but rather a contrast that is described as "fortis vs. lenis"; in Table 57-1, the fortis consonant (marked with separate symbols for voiceless obstruents and with a length mark for sonorants) is listed first in a cell. For obstruents, lenis consonants are shorter, are sometimes lightly fricated, and are often voiced; for sonorants, lenis consonants are shorter and possibly of lower intensity. The affricates and two of the fricatives have no lenis counterparts. Trilled /r/ is found primarily in Spanish loan words, but that includes many words learned early. The approximant /w/ has the bilabial-fricative allophone [β]. The language has both a dental and a post-alveolar affricate.

Vowels and diphthongs

There are six basic vowels in San Lucas Quiaviní Zapotec, each of which can appear long or short, with one of four voice qualities: modal (as in English), breathy, creaky, and checked. (Checked vowels resemble a glottal stop after, or in the middle of, a vowel, but this is not treated as a separate consonant.) Two or three voice qualities can be combined in sequence on a single vowel within a single syllable nucleus; note that the vowel is written orthographically as a double or triple vowel, but this does not lead to the degree of extra duration that this orthographic convention might suggest. Early-learned words sample from the full range of vowels and voice qualities in the language. Note that all of the words in Table 57-2 are monosyllabic.

Phonotactic restrictions
Syllables

The syllable structure of San Lucas Quiaviní Zapotec is quite complex, with consonant sequences that are unusual cross-linguistically. The minimal syllable is a single short vowel. The maximal syllable is CCGVVVCG (where "G" refers to a glide /j, w/).

Consonants and consonant clusters

Many syllables lack codas. If a coda is present, it consists of either a single consonant (which can be any consonant

TABLE 57-1 Consonants produced in San Lucas Quiaviní Zapotec

	Bilabial	Labiodental	Dental	Alveolar
Plosive	p b		t d	
Nasal	m: m		n: n	
Trill				r
Tap or flap				ɾ
Fricative		f	s z	
Lateral fricative	■■■			
Approximant	w (labiovelar)			
Lateral approximant	■■■		l: l	
Affricate			ts	

Black = articulations judged impossible

Based on the International Phonetic Alphabet. Courtesy of the International Phonetic Association (c/o Department of Linguistics, University of Victoria, Victoria, British Columbia, Canada).

in the language) or a sequence of a consonant followed by a glide (e.g., *bèe'cw* /beẽʔkw/ 'dog'); the latter sequence is odd cross-linguistically (counter to the "sonority sequencing principle") because high-sonority glides tend to precede lower-sonority true consonants in codas, not follow them (e.g., Greenberg, 1965). Onsets are not obligatory, but most words begin with an onset, and sequences of two vowels within a word are uncommon. Vowel-initial words are most often loanwords from Spanish (though there are a few high-frequency indigenous function words, such as the question marker *èee* /eẽː/). Onsets can consist of one or two consonants, plus a glide in second/third position (e.g., CC, CG, and CCG). CC onsets can contain two obstruents, two sonorants, an obstruent followed by a sonorant, or a sonorant followed by an obstruent. Onsets that violate the sonority sequencing principle (unusual cross-linguistically) are not uncommon (e.g., *Wsee* [wseː] 'Joseph', *rsìiilly* [rsịiːlj] 'morning'), and are common in inflected verb forms (e.g., *rdùu'b* [rduụʔb] 'sweeps'). Whether the vowel nucleus is V, VV, or VVV does not interact in any way with the size of the coda or of the onset.

Tones

San Lucas Quiaviní Zapotec has four tones (High, Low, Falling, and Rising), though their use in differentiating the meaning of words in unclear. Vowels with breathy and creaky phonation tend to have low tones, and tone is in general predictable from the voice quality and complexity of the vowel. So far, no minimal pairs have been discovered where only tone distinguishes the

two words; but descriptions of the correlation between tones and voice quality are complex and not easy to make sense of.

Stress and intonation

San Lucas Quiaviní Zapotec also has stress. The root-final syllable (which tends to be fairly complex segmentally) is termed the "key" syllable by Munro and Lopez (1999), and is generally perceived as stressed. There are a few prefixes and suffixes, which may never contain a key syllable. Words are commonly S (Strong), Sw (Strong weak, with a suffix), or wS (with or without a prefix), but longer feet also occur. All stress patterns occur among the early-learned words.

Writing system

Zapotec has no surviving traditional writing system (though a hieroglyphic system existed in pre-Columbian times), and few speakers are literate in Zapotec. Early texts were written in an adaptation of Spanish orthography. Writing systems have been established for many variants of Valley and Southern Zapotec over the past several decades. Munro and Lopez (1999) present a Latin-based orthography for San Lucas Quiaviní Zapotec in which the phonemic representation of the word is always unambiguously derivable from the spelling. However, this led to such visual complexity that they have since proposed a simplification that omits the marking of vowel length,

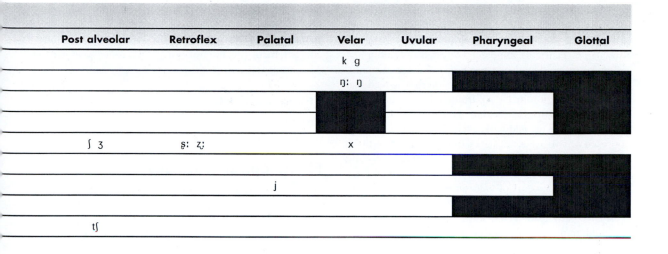

Post alveolar	Retroflex	Palatal	Velar	Uvular	Pharyngeal	Glottal
			k g			
			ŋː ŋ			
ʃ ʒ	ʂː ʐː		x			
		j				
tʃ						

TABLE 57-2	Vowels produced in San Lucas Quiaviní Zapotec

San Lucas Quiaviní Zapotec Location	San Lucas Quiaviní Zapotec vowels	San Lucas Quiaviní Zapotec examples
High-front	i	*zhi'iilly* 'sheep'
Mid front	e	*bèe'cw* 'dog'
High-central, unrounded	ɨ	*dëëzh* 'roof tile'
Low central, unrounded	a	*xniaa* 'red'
High-back, rounded	u	*cu'uch* 'pig'
Mid-back, rounded	o	*wròo'oh* 'big'
Diphthongs	ai	*rài'* 'gets cooked'
	au	*Ca'au* 'Claudia'
	ei	*Gye'eihlly* 'Mike'
	ia	*gyìa'* 'flower'
	ie	*nyieeny* 'is audible'
	iu	*byiuh* 'ground up'
	ua	*bua'rr* 'donkey'
	ue	*rrueed* 'wheel'
	ɨi	*ncwëiby* 'new

tone, and voice quality (Munro, Lillehaugen, and Lopez, 2006). Orthography is partially based on Spanish (e.g., "c" for /k/ before central and back vowels, "qu" for /k/ before front vowels).

Varieties of San Lucas Quiaviní Zapotec

San Lucas Quiaviní Zapotec is a variant of Zapotec spoken only in San Lucas Quiaviní, with a population of about 2,000 people. The variants of Zapotec spoken in other nearby towns differ substantially and are only partially mutually intelligible. Lillehaugen (2003) groups all of the variants of Zapotec spoken in the Tlacolula Valley southeast of Oaxaca City as "Valley Zapotec." Zapotec speakers from nearby towns teach in the bilingual preschool in the village and report that this is generally successful, albeit with occasional communication failures. Many other variants, which are not mutually intelligible, are grouped as "Southern Zapotec" and "Sierra Zapotec."

Typical acquisition of San Lucas Quiaviní Zapotec

The Summary of Studies table at the end of this chapter contains studies of the acquisition of San Lucas Quiaviní Zapotec.

There have been only a few studies of the acquisition of any variant of Valley Zapotec. The first two studies (Lillehaugen, 2003; Jensen de López, 1999, 2002, on San Marcos Tlapazola Zapotec) addressed only nonphonological issues (locative expressions). We are currently engaged in a long-term project to gather cross-sectional and coarse-longitudinal data from a large number of children. At the time of writing, we have just completed a second season of fieldwork; each fieldwork season has consisted of two weeks of data gathering, resulting in 32 (first season) and 29 (second season) recording sessions, which lasted between 10 minutes and 60 minutes, for a total of about 45 hours of videotaped material involving 25 different children aged 1;2 to 6;8. Each year, 18 children have participated, constituting perhaps 5 percent of the children in the target age range. Analysis of this material is as yet incomplete. Information about average age of acquisition will not be considered reliable until after several more years of data collection. For this reason, we will not state our observations in table form. All observations must be considered preliminary.

Acquired sounds

Consonants

Even the youngest children have nasals ([m, n]) and "lenis" labial and dental stops ([b, d], as well as glides [j, w]. Word-initial [ʔ] may be present, even though it is not present in the adult language. Velars and other manners of articulation are often absent initially. Obstruents appear initially to be "lenis," though the phonetics of this is unclear even for adult speech. Affricates such as [tʃ] appear early, being present for most children by 2;1. It is common for children to have one liquid by 2;1 (either /r/ or /l/), but generally not both until later.

Consonant clusters

Consonant clusters are absent in the speech of the younger children, and are often not fully established even for 5-year-olds. We have not established statistical tendencies regarding which types of cluster develop first, whether there is a difference between onset and coda cluster development, and whether the markedness of the sonority sequences matters.

Vowels and diphthongs

Vowels are accurate early. Before 2;6, there are errors on some vowels. All voice qualities seem to appear in the speech of children by 1;11, but voice quality errors are observed even after 5;0; the acoustic qualities characteristic of creaky or breathy voice in adult speech may be absent, but we do not yet know whether more subtle effects remain (on intensity or pitch). Tones have yet to be investigated.

Percent correct

There is no information available about percentage correct at any age.

Phonological processes

We have observed many processes similar to those found in other languages, such as velar fronting (e.g., *cu'uch* 'pig' /kuʔutʃ/ ⇨ [dutʃ], which also illustrates initial lenition/voicing), stopping of fricatives, gliding of /l/ and /r/ (e.g., *pelo't* 'ball' /peˈloʔt/ ⇨ [teˈjot]), reduplication (see section on prosody below), cluster simplification (e.g., *bx:àady* 'edible grasshopper' /bʃaadj/ ⇨ [ʃæd]; *bèe'cw* 'dog' /beɛʔkw/ ⇨ [βak]), and weak syllable deletion (see below). We have observed some labial backing in several children (see 'ball' in previous sentence). When one liquid is present, it can substitute for the other; we have observed [r] for /l/ and [l] for /r/, in different children. Coronal fricatives can be subject to affrication (e.g., the /ʒ/ in *zhi'iilly* 'sheep' as [dʒ]), because affricates are sometimes acquired earlier than fricatives. Glottal replacement (e.g., *pelo't* 'ball' /peˈloʔt/ ⇨ [ʔot]) and initial consonant deletion (e.g., *bèe'cw* 'dog' /beɛʔkw/ ⇨ [aʊkw]) are unusual across children, and when present generally occur only for particular target consonants (such as /l/) or are restricted to initial unstressed syllables. Coda deletion is possible, but generally affects only specific consonants (e.g., the final /g/ in *gyahg* 'tree' /gjag/ ⇨ [giˈja]). Coalescence is sometimes observed for consonant clusters in both onsets (e.g., the /bz/ of *bzihny* as [f]) and codas (e.g., *bèe'cw* 'dog' /beɛʔkw/ ⇨[bɛp]). Marked voice qualities are sometimes replaced with modal (noncreaky, nonbreathy) voice quality (see 'dog' in previous sentence). Some backing and lowering of vowels has been observed (e.g., for target mid front vowels, as in *bèe'cw* 'dog' /beɛʔkw/ ⇨ [βak]).

Intelligibility

As with all languages, children as old as 4;0 are not always fully intelligible to adults. As expected, intelligibility is often higher for members of the child's family than for adults unfamiliar with the child; when our assistant could not understand what the child had said, the mother often (but not always) was able to.

Phonetic inventory

Phonetic inventories begin highly reduced, as in other languages, and become more elaborated over time.

Common mismatches

See discussion of processes above and of syllable structure and prosody below.

Syllable structure

Codas have been present in the speech of all children in the study, though it must be borne in mind that all but one child was 1;11 or older. The one younger child had codas at 1;2, as in [daˈdat] (glossed by the mother as 'Daddy is coming': some closed-class lexical item followed by *da'ad* 'father' /daʔad/). Complex nuclei (diphthongs) may be present early. Complex onsets and codas develop later, and may not be fully established even at 5;0. Deletion (or glottal replacement) of specific consonants is observed in both onsets and codas.

Prosody

Sentence prosody has yet to be studied. We have preliminary observations about the role of stress in bisyllabic and multisyllabic words. In the acquisition of stress languages, unstressed syllables often show effects different from those of stressed syllables in the same location in the word. We observe reduction in the independent content of unstressed syllables, ranging from (1) full deletion, (2) exact reduplication of the following syllable; or, with an accurate vowel, (3) deletion of the word-initial consonant, (4) reduplication of just the word-initial consonant, to (5) use of default/unmarked features in the initial consonant, vs. more adultlike realization of the same phonemes in stressed syllables. We find examples of all of these effects in Zapotec, quite unlike in tone/pitch-accent languages. For *kaba'i* 'horse' /kaˈbaʔi/, we find [βai], [aˈβai], [βaˈβai]. For *pelo't* /peˈloʔt/ 'ball', we find [ʔot] and, from two children, at 1;11 and at 3;0, [teˈjot], the latter with default [Coronal] in place of [Labial] (where other words suggest that this is not coronal harmony). Additionally there is denasalization in *mannsaan* 'apple' /manˈsaːn/ [daˈsan]. Reduction in wwS words such as *elefann* /eleˈfan̩ː/ 'elephant' has been observed even at 5;6: [nfan], [ʔliˈfan].

Phonological awareness

There is no information available about Zapotec-speaking children's phonological awareness.

Speech assessment for San Lucas Quiaviní Zapotec children

There are no tools available for speech assessment of children speaking any variant of Zapotec. In our studies, we use pictures and toys to elicit nouns and adjectives, video clips to elicit verbs (with the use of questions to manipulate the verbal aspect that the child uses), and wordless picture books to elicit narratives (the *Frog* books by Mayer, 1967, 1969; and *Anno's Journey* by Anno, 1977). These materials have not been balanced or normed for clinical use. There are no standard analyses for clinical applications that have been applied to the collected data. One of the goals of the current research program is to develop a rough set of norms for acquisition of sounds and syllable structures that can be used as a guide by teachers in the preschool.

Speech intervention for San Lucas Quiaviní Zapotec children

To our knowledge, no speech intervention has taken place with any variant of Zapotec; certainly none has occurred in San Lucas Quiaviní. A few children have been identified as having language difficulties. Many children (but not all) enter the bilingual preschool at age 4 and continue at age 5, before entering the monolingual-Spanish primary school at age 6. There are approximately 80 children in the preschool at the time of writing, of whom 2 (2.5 percent) have been identified as having language problems, on the basis of social isolation; no details were available about their speech or language, and school officials had no clear idea what would constitute a delayed or disordered phonological system. It is unclear whether intervention would be available even in Spanish, and children at this age are in any event monolingual speakers of Zapotec. We hope in the future to obtain more information about the speech of such children, and ultimately to supply the preschool with information about identification of speech-language problems and intervention in Zapotec.

Additional information

There is a bilingual Zapotec-Spanish preschool (which is officially for three years, for 3-year-olds through

5-year-olds, but not all children attend, and enrollments are low enough that only the second and third years are offered), a Spanish-only primary school (attended by all children), and a Spanish-only distance-education secondary school (*tele-secondario*). The village has electricity, and has recently gained access to mobile telephones and a community Internet cafe, and most families have radios, TVs, video players, and often DVD players. The language of the media is monolingual Spanish. While there are still monolingual speakers of Zapotec older than 50 and younger than 6, most people become bilingual in Spanish after entering school, and fluent within a few years. In other villages (such as Santa Ana del Valle), only half of the children are learning Zapotec at all, and all of those are being raised as bilinguals in Spanish from the beginning. In the largest nearby town (Tlacolula), there are few native speakers of Zapotec below the age of 50. It is likely that San Lucas Quiaviní will follow a similar path. In addition, there is a large amount of emigration to California, where children are often being raised as English-Spanish bilinguals with little exposure to Zapotec. This variant of Zapotec, and probably all variants of Valley Zapotec, should be considered threatened.

There is a critical need to study first language acquisition by monolingual children in indigenous communities here and throughout the world, before they disappear, and to help local authorities develop strategies for language maintenance.

Working in the state of Oaxaca

Working in rural areas of the state of Oaxaca is challenging, as there is no reliable supply of clean water except in bottles, and sanitary facilities are minimal; it is necessary to be very careful about eating and drinking. Only the larger towns (such as Tlacolula) have hotels, though houses are often available for rental in smaller towns and villages. Most of the streets of San Lucas Quiaviní are unpaved and steep, and they become very muddy in the rain. Most families have farm animals, and there are few places where animal sounds cannot be heard. There are a few public buildings, but most of our research takes place in the children's homes, often in outbuildings or even in open courtyards. Rain on the tin roof of an outbuilding shuts down a recording session.

PHONETICALLY SPEAKING

Pronunciation of Zapotec: [ˈzapəˌtʰɛk] ~ [ˈzæpəˌtʰɛk]
Relevant words for speech assessment and intervention

Word	Formal usage	Pronunciation
Tongue	*lùuzh*	/lu̱u̱ʒ/
Teeth	*la'aih*	/laʔai̱/
Lips	*gui'dy ru'uh*	/giʔdj ruʔu̱/
Hard palate	*(no term known)*	
Soft palate	*dehs ru'uh*	/de̱s ruʔu/
Larynx	*(no term known)*	
Lungs	*lastòo' quìizh*	/laˈsto̱o̱ʔ ki̱iʒ/
Nose	*zhi'ih*	/ʒiʔi̱/
Sound	*(no term known)*	
Word	*dìi'zh*	/di̱i̱ʔʒ/
Sentence	*orasyonny*	/oraˈsjonːj/
Paragraph	*parrafo*	/paˈrafo/

Note. Blanks indicate gaps in the dictionary which a native speaker identified as unfamiliar concepts.

RESOURCES

Books

Lee, F. (2006). *Remnant raising and VSO clausal architecture: A case study from San Lucas Quiaviní Zapotec.* Heidelberg: Springer.

Munro, P., and Lopez, F. H. (1999). *Di'csyonaary X:tèe'n Dìi'zh Sah Sann Lu'uc.* Los Angeles, CA: UCLA Chicano Studies Research Center Publications.

Munro, P., Lillehaugen, B. D., and Lopez, F. H. (2006). *Cali Chiu? A course in Valley Zapotec.* Manuscript in preparation.

Journals

There are no journals dedicated to this language, but articles on Zapotec may often be found in the *International Journal of American Linguistics (IJAL)*, University of Chicago Press, www.journals.uchicago.edu/IJAL/home.html.

Professional associations

The professional association of speech-language pathologists within Mexico is Sociedad Mexicana de Audiologia y Foniatria.

Useful San Lucas Quiaviní Zapotec Web sites

- *A Selected Bibliography on Tlacolula Valley Zapotec*, http://www.linguistics.ucla.edu/people/grads/lillehaugen/BiblioTVZ.htm

- *Zapotec (Zapoteco)*, http://www.native-languages.org/zapotec.htm
- *Zapotecan family*, http://www.sil.org/mexico/zapoteca/00i-zapoteca.htm

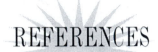

REFERENCES

Anno, M. (1977). *Anno's journey*. New York: Philomel Books.

Greenberg, J. H. (1965). Some generalizations concerning initial and final consonant sequences. *Linguistics*, *18*, 5–34.

Jensen de López, K. (1999, June). The acquisition of Zapotec body part locatives: A longitudinal case study. Paper presented at the *International Congress for the Study of Child Language*. San Sebastian, Spain.

Jensen de López, K. (2002). *Baskets and body-parts: A cross-cultural and crosslinguistic investigation of children's development of spatial cognition and language*. Unpublished Ph.D. dissertation, University of Aarhus, Denmark.

Lillehaugen, B. D. (2003). *The categorical status of body part prepositions in Valley Zapotec languages*. Unpublished M.A. thesis, Department of Linguistics, University of California, Los Angeles.

Mayer, M. (1967). *A boy, a dog, and a frog*. New York: Dial Books for Young Readers (Penguin).

Mayer, M. (1969). *Frog, where are you?* New York: Dial Books for Young Readers (Penguin).

Munro, P., and Lopez, F. H. (1999). *Di'csyonaary X:tèe'n Dìi'zh Sah Sann Lu'uc*. Los Angeles, CA: UCLA Chicano Studies Research Center Publications.

Munro, P., Lillehaugen, B. D., and Lopez, F. H. (2006). *Cali Chiu? A course in Valley Zapotec*. Manuscript in preparation.

SUMMARY OF STUDIES OF TYPICAL SAN LUCAS QUIAVINÍ ZAPOTEC SPEECH ACQUISITION

Authors	Year	Country	No. of children	Age of children	Information	Sample type	Data collection
Jensen de López	2002	Mexico	33	1;5– 3;10	Locative information	Comprehension task	Cross-sectional
Jensen de López	2002	Mexico	1	1;3–2;9	Locative information	Comprehension task	Longitudinal for one child
Lillehaugen	2003	Mexico	4	1;6–7;11	Locative information	Comprehension task	Cross-sectional
Stemberger, and Lee	in progress	Mexico	25 (so far)	1;2–6;8	Entire language	Various production and comprehension tasks	Cross-sectional; coarse longitudinal

Appendix

APPENDIX A

THE INTERNATIONAL PHONETIC ALPHABET (revised to 1993, updated 1996)

CONSONANTS (PULMONIC)

	Bilabial	Labiodental	Dental	Alveolar	Postalveolar	Retroflex	Palatal	Velar	Uvular	Pharyngeal	Glottal
Plosive	p b			t d		ʈ ɖ	c ɟ	k ɡ	q ɢ		ʔ
Nasal	m	ɱ		n		ɳ	ɲ	ŋ	ɴ		
Trill	ʙ			r					ʀ		
Tap or Flap				ɾ		ɽ					
Fricative	ɸ β	f v	θ ð	s z	ʃ ʒ	ʂ ʐ	ç ʝ	x ɣ	χ ʁ	ħ ʕ	h ɦ
Lateral fricative				ɬ ɮ							
Approximant		ʋ		ɹ		ɻ	j	ɰ			
Lateral approximant				l		ɭ	ʎ	ʟ			

Where symbols appear in pairs, the one to the right represents a voiced consonant. Shaded areas denote articulations judged impossible.

CONSONANTS (NON-PULMONIC)

Clicks	Voiced implosives	Ejectives
⊙ Bilabial	ɓ Bilabial	ʼ Examples:
ǀ Dental	ɗ Dental/alveolar	pʼ Bilabial
ǃ (Post)alveolar	ʄ Palatal	tʼ Dental/alveolar
ǂ Palatoalveolar	ɠ Velar	kʼ Velar
ǁ Alveolar lateral	ʛ Uvular	sʼ Alveolar fricative

VOWELS

Where symbols appear in pairs, the one to the right represents a rounded vowel.

OTHER SYMBOLS

ʍ Voiceless labial-velar fricative
w Voiced labial-velar approximant
ɥ Voiced labial-palatal approximant
ʜ Voiceless epiglottal fricative
ʢ Voiced epiglottal fricative
ʡ Epiglottal plosive

ɕ ʑ Alveolo-palatal fricatives
ɺ Alveolar lateral flap
ɧ Simultaneous ʃ and x

Affricates and double articulations can be represented by two symbols joined by a tie bar if necessary.
k͡p t͡s

SUPRASEGMENTALS

ˈ	Primary stress	ˌfoʊnəˈtɪʃən
ˌ	Secondary stress	
ː	Long	eː
ˑ	Half-long	eˑ
˘	Extra-short	ĕ
ǀ	Minor (foot) group	
ǁ	Major (intonation) group	
.	Syllable break	ɹi.ækt
‿	Linking (absence of a break)	

DIACRITICS
Diacritics may be placed above a symbol with a descender, e.g. ŋ̊

̥	Voiceless	n̥ d̥	̤	Breathy voiced	b̤ a̤	̪	Dental	t̪ d̪
̬	Voiced	s̬ t̬	̰	Creaky voiced	b̰ a̰	̺	Apical	t̺ d̺
ʰ	Aspirated	tʰ dʰ	̼	Linguolabial	t̼ d̼	̻	Laminal	t̻ d̻
̹	More rounded	ɔ̹	ʷ	Labialized	tʷ dʷ	̃	Nasalized	ẽ
̜	Less rounded	ɔ̜	ʲ	Palatalized	tʲ dʲ	ⁿ	Nasal release	dⁿ
̟	Advanced	u̟	ˠ	Velarized	tˠ dˠ	ˡ	Lateral release	dˡ
̠	Retracted	e̠	ˤ	Pharyngealized	tˤ dˤ	̚	No audible release	d̚
̈	Centralized	ë	̴	Velarized or pharyngealized	ɫ			
̽	Mid-centralized	e̽	̝	Raised	e̝	(ɹ̝ = voiced alveolar fricative)		
̩	Syllabic	n̩	̞	Lowered	e̞	(β̞ = voiced bilabial approximant)		
̯	Non-syllabic	e̯	̘	Advanced Tongue Root	e̘			
˞	Rhoticity	ɚ a˞	̙	Retracted Tongue Root	e̙			

TONES AND WORD ACCENTS

LEVEL			CONTOUR		
e̋ or ˥	Extra high	ě or ˩˥	Rising
é ˦	High	ê ˥˩	Falling
ē ˧	Mid	e᷄ ˧˥	High rising
è ˨	Low	e᷅ ˩˧	Low rising
ȅ ˩	Extra low	e᷈ ˧˩˧	Rising-falling
ꜜ	Downstep	↗	Global rise
ꜛ	Upstep	↘	Global fall

Reproduced with the permission of the International Phonetic Association.

APPENDIX B

extIPA SYMBOLS FOR DISORDERED SPEECH

(Revised to 2002)

CONSONANTS (other than on the IPA Chart)

	bilabial	labiodental	dentolabial	labioalv.	linguolabial	interdental	bidental	alveolar	velar	velophar.
Plosive		p̪ b̪	p͆ b͆	p͇ b͇	t̼ d̼	t̪͆ d̪͆				
Nasal			m͆	m͇	n̼	n̪͆				
Trill					r̼	r̪͆				
Fricative median			f͆ v͆	f͇ v͇	θ̼ ð̼	θ̪͆ ð̪͆	h̪͆ ɦ̪͆			ʩ
Fricative lateral+median								ʪ ʫ		
Fricative nareal	m͋							n͋	ŋ͋	
Percussive	ʬ						ʭ			
Approximant lateral					l̼	l̪͆				

Where symbols appear in pairs, the one to the right represents a voiced consonant. Shaded areas denote articulations judged impossible.

DIACRITICS

͍	labial spreading	s͍	͈	strong articulation	f͈	͊	denasal	m͊
͆	dentolabial	v͆	͉	weak articulation	v͉	͋	nasal escape	v͋
̪͆	interdental/bidental	n̪͆	\	reiterated articulation	p\p\p	͌	velopharyngeal friction	s͌
͇	alveolar	t͇	͎	whistled articulation	s͎	↓	ingressive airflow	p↓
̼	linguolabial	d̼	͢	sliding articulation	θ͢s	↑	egressive airflow	!↑

CONNECTED SPEECH

(.)	short pause
(..)	medium pause
(...)	long pause
f	loud speech [{$_f$ laʊd $_f$}]
ff	louder speech [{$_{ff}$ laʊdɚ $_{ff}$}]
p	quiet speech [{$_p$ kwaɪət $_p$}]
pp	quieter speech [{$_{pp}$ kwaɪətɚ $_{pp}$}]
allegro	fast speech [{$_{allegro}$ fast $_{allegro}$}]
lento	slow speech [{$_{lento}$ sloʊ $_{lento}$}]
crescendo, ralentando, etc. may also be used	

VOICING

ˬ	pre-voicing	ˬz
ˬ	post-voicing	zˬ
₍̥₎	partial devoicing	₍z̥₎
₍̥	initial partial devoicing	₍z̥
̥₎	final partial devoicing	z̥₎
₍̬₎	partial voicing	₍s̬₎
₍̬	initial partial voicing	₍s̬
̬₎	final partial voicing	s̬₎
=	unaspirated	$p^{=}$
h	pre-aspiration	ʰp

OTHERS

(̲), (C̲)	indeterminate sound, consonant	(( ))	extraneous noise ((2 sylls))
(V̲), (P̲l̲.v̲l̲s̲)	indeterminate vowel, voiceless plosive, etc.	¡	sublaminal lower alveolar percussive click
(N̲), (v̲)	indeterminate nasal, probably [v], etc.	!¡	alveolar and sublaminal clicks (cluck-click)
( )	silent articulation (ʃ), (m)	*	sound with no available symbol

APPENDIX C

VoQS: Voice Quality Symbols

Airstream Types

Œ	œsophageal speech	И	electrolarynx speech
Ю	tracheo-œsophageal speech	↓	pulmonic ingressive speech

Phonation types

V	modal voice	F	falsetto
W	whisper	C	creak
V̰	whispery voice (murmur)	V̰	creaky voice
Vʰ	breathy voice	C̡	whispery creak
V!	harsh voice	V!!	ventricular phonation
V̬!!	diplophonia	V̰!!	whispery ventricular phonation
V̨	anterior or pressed phonation	W̲	posterior whisper

Supralaryngeal Settings

L̝	raised larynx	L̞	lowered larynx
Vᵅ	labialized voice (open round)	Vʷ	labialized voice (close round)
V̫	spread-lip voice	Vᵛ	labio-dentalized voice
V̺	linguo-apicalized voice	V̻	linguo-laminalized voice
V˞	retroflex voice	V̪	dentalized voice
V̱	alveolarized voice	V̲	palatoalveolarized voice
Vʲ	palatalized voice	Vˠ	velarized voice
Vˣ	uvularized voice	Vˤ	pharyngealized voice
V̰ˤ	laryngo-pharyngealized voice	Vˮ	faucalized voice
Ṽ	nasalized voice	Ṽ	denasalized voice
J̞	open jaw voice	J̝	close jaw voice
J̬	right offset jaw voice	J̫	left offset jaw voice
J̟	protruded jaw voice	Θ	protruded tongue voice

USE OF LABELED BRACES & NUMERALS TO MARK STRETCHES OF SPEECH
AND DEGREES AND COMBINATIONS OF VOICE QUALITY:

[ˈðɪs ɪz ˈnɔɹməl ˈvɔɪs {₃V! ˈðɪs ɪz ˈvɛɹi ˈhɑɹʃ ˈvɔɪs ₃V} ˈðɪs ɪz ˈnɔɹməl ˈvɔɪs wʌns
ˈmɔɹ {L̝ ₁V! ˈðɪs ɪz ˈlɛs ˈhɑɹʃ ˈvɔɪs wɪð ˈloʊɚd ˈlæɹɪŋks ₁V!L̝}]

© 1994 Martin J. Ball, John Esling, Craig Dickson

Reproduced with the permission of Dr. Martin J. Ball.

APPENDIX D

Countries of Focus Where a Specific Dialect/Language is Spoken by a Significant Portion of the Population and Immigrants

Chapter no.	Dialect/ Language	Country of focus	Official language	Spoken by a significant portion of the population	Spoken by a significant portion of immigrants
22	General American English	United States of America	United States of America	–	–
23	African American English	United States of America	United States of America	United States of America (southern states and the states with particularly large cities where African Americans are populated, including Philadelphia, New York, Detroit, Los Angeles, and Chicago)	–
24	Appalachian English	United States of America	–	United States of America (Appalachian mountain range, specifically those living in eastern Kentucky, West Virginia, southwest Virginia, western North Carolina and eastern Tennessee)	–
25	Cajun English	United States of America	–	United States of America (Louisiana – the Acadian triangle)	–
26	Canadian English	Canada	Canada (Ontario, the Western Provinces [Manitoba, Saskatchewan, Alberta, British Columbia] and the North [Yukon, the Northwest Territories and Nunavut])	Canada (Quebec, Newfoundland, the Maritime Provinces [New Brunswick, Nova Scotia, Prince Edward Island])	–
27	English	United Kingdom	Akrotiri, Anguilla, Antigua, Australia, Bahamas, Barbados, Bermuda, Belize, Botswana, British Virgin Islands, Cameroon, Canada, Cayman Islands, Christmas Island, Cocos (Keeling) Islands, Cook Islands, Dhekelia, Dominica, European Union, Falkland Islands, Fiji, Gambia, Ghana, Gibraltar, Grenada, Guam, Guernsey, Guyana, Hong Kong, India, Isle of Man, Jamaica, Jersey, Kenya, Kiribati, Lesotho, Liberia, Malta, Mauritius, Marshall Islands, Federated States of Micronesia, Montserrat, Namibia, New Zealand, Nigeria, Norfolk Island,	Belize, Canada, Cayman Islands, India, Ireland, Israel, Montserrat, American Samoa, Singapore, South Africa, Surinam, Virgin Islands	–

Chapter no.	Dialect/ Language	Country of focus	Official language	Spoken by a significant portion of the population	Spoken by a significant portion of immigrants
27 (cont.)			Northern Ireland, Pakistan, Palau, Papua New Guinea, Philippines, Pitcairn Islands, Republic of Ireland, Rwanda, Samoa, Seychelles, Sierra Leone, Singapore, Solomon Islands, South Africa, St Helena, St Kitts and Nevis, St Lucia, St Vincent and the Grenadines, Swaziland, Tanzania, Trinidad and Tobago, Tokelau, Tonga, Turks and Caicos Islands , Tuvalu, Uganda, United Kingdom, United States of America, Virgin Islands, Zambia, Zimbabwe		
28	Irish English	Northern Ireland, Republic of Ireland	Northern Ireland, Republic of Ireland	–	–
29	Scottish English	Scotland	Scotland	–	–
30	Australian English	Australia	Australia	–	–
31	New Zealand English	New Zealand	New Zealand (including the Chatham Islands and Stewart Island), Cook Islands	–	–
32	Cantonese English	Australia	–	Hong Kong	Australia, Canada, the Netherlands, New Zealand, Singapore, United Kingdom, United States of America
33	Spanish English	United States of America	Andorra, Belize, United States of America	–	–
34	Jordanian Arabic	Jordan	Algeria, Bahrain, Chad, Comoros, Djibouti, Egypt, Eritrea, Iraq, Israel, Jordan, Kuwait, Lebanon, Libya, Mauritania, Morocco, Oman, Palestine, Qatar, Saudi Arabia, Sudan, Syria, Tunisia, United Arab Emirates, Yemen	–	India, Indonesia, Pakistan
35	Lebanese Arabic	Lebanon	Algeria, Bahrain, Chad, Comoros, Djibouti, Egypt, Eritrea, Iraq, Israel, Jordan, Kuwait, Lebanon, Libya, Mauritania, Morocco, Oman, Palestine, Qatar, Saudi Arabia, Sudan, Syria, Tunisia, United Arab Emirates, Yemen	–	India, Indonesia, Pakistan
36	Cantonese	China (Guangdong and Guangxi provinces)	China (Guangdong and Guangxi provinces, including Hong Kong)	–	

Chapter no.	Dialect/ Language	Country of focus	Official language	Spoken by a significant portion of the population	Spoken by a significant portion of immigrants
37	Dutch	Netherlands	Netherlands, Belgium, Suriname, Aruba, and the Dutch Antilles	Belgium (specifically, in the northern part of Belgium, in the provinces of West-Vlaanderen and Oost-Vlaanderen, Antwerpen, Limburg, and Brabant), Dutch Antilles, Surinam	Indonesia, South Africa
38	Filipino	Philippines	Philippines	Philippines (Manila, most of Luzon, and Mindoro)	Bahrain, Brunei, Canada, Guam, Italy, Japan, Jordan, Kuwait, Malaysia, Qatar, Saudi Arabia, Singapore, United Arab Emirates, United Kingdom, United States of America
39	Finnish	Finland	Finland	–	–
40	French	France	Belgium, Benin, Burkina Faso, Burundi, Cameroon, Canada (Quebec), Central African Republic, Chad, Comoros, Democratic Republic of the Congo, Congo, Republic of the Congo, Cote d'Ivoire, Djibouti, Equatorial Guinea, European Union, France, French Guiana, French Polynesia, Gabon, Guadeloupe, Guinea, Haiti, Madagascar, Mali, Martinique, Mauritius, Mayotte, Monaco, New Caledonia, Niger, Reunion, Rwanda, Saint Pierre and Miquelon, Senegal, Switzerland, Togo, Vatican City	Algiers, Brazil, Cambodia, Canada (Northern Ontario, Northern and Eastern New Brunswick), Dominica, Egypt, Greece, Grenada, Guernsey, Italy, Laos, Lebanon, Luxembourg, Mauritania, Morocco, Saint Lucia, Saint Vincent and the Grenadines, Syria, Trinidad and Tobago, Tunisia, Vanuatu, Vietnam, Virgin Islands, Wallis and Futuna	–
41	German	Germany	Austria, Germany, Lichtenstein, Luxemburg, Southern Tirol, Switzerland (eastern)	–	–
42	Greek	Greece	Greece, Cyprus	Albania (Southern), Egypt (Alexandria), Italy (Southern, east of Reggio; Salento [Colimera, Sternatía, Zollino] and Aspromonte [Bova, Condofuri, Palizzi, Roccoforte, Roghudi]), Romania (Karakatchan, Romanian nomadic shepherds), Turkey (Istanbul city), and Ukraine (Donetsk oblast, Mariupol)	–

Chapter no.	Dialect/ Language	Country of focus	Official language	Spoken by a significant portion of the population	Spoken by a significant portion of immigrants
43	Hungary	Hungary	Hungary, Serbia, Slovenia	Austria, Serbia (Vojvodina region), Slovenia	Argentina, Australia, Austria, Belgium, Brazil, Canada, Croatia, Czech Republic, Finland, France, Germany, Israel, Italy, Montenegro, the Netherlands, Romania, Serbia, Slovakia, Slovenia, South Africa, Switzerland Ukraine, United Kingdom, United States of America, Venezuela
44	Israeli Hebrew	Israel	Israel	–	–
45	Japanese	Japan	Japan	–	–
46	Korean	South Korea	North Korea, South Korea	–	–
47	Maltese	Malta	Malta (including Gozo)	–	Australia, Canada United State of America
48	Norwegian	Norway	Norway	–	–
49	Portuguese	Brazil	Angola, Brazil, Portugal, Mozambique	Cape Verde islands, Guine-Bissau, San Tome-Principe	East Timor, Goa, Malaysia, Macao
50	Putonghua	People's Republic of China	People's Republic of China	–	–
51	Sesotho	South Africa	South Africa (specifically Lesotho, and adjacent parts of the Orange Free State to the north of Lesotho)	–	–
52	Spanish	–	Argentina, Bolivia, Chile, Colombia, Costa Rica, Cuba, Dominican Republic, Ecuador, El Salvador, Equatorial Guinea, Guatemala, Honduras, Mexico, Nicaragua, Panama, Paraguay, Peru, Puerto Rico, Spain, Uruguay, Venezuela	Aruba, Belize, Brazil, European Union, Gibraltar, Netherlands Antilles, Trinidad and Tobago, Virgin Islands	Switzerland, United States of America
53	Thai	Thailand	Thailand	–	–
54	Turkish	Turkey	Turkish Republic of Turkey	–	–
55	Vietnamese	Vietnam	Vietnam	Cambodia, Laos, Myanmar, Thailand	Australia, Canada, Cote d'Ivoire, France, Japan, Philippines, Indonesia, Senegal, United States of America
56	Welsh	Wales	Wales	–	–
57	Zapotec	Mexico	Mexico, in the state of Oaxaca	–	–

Index

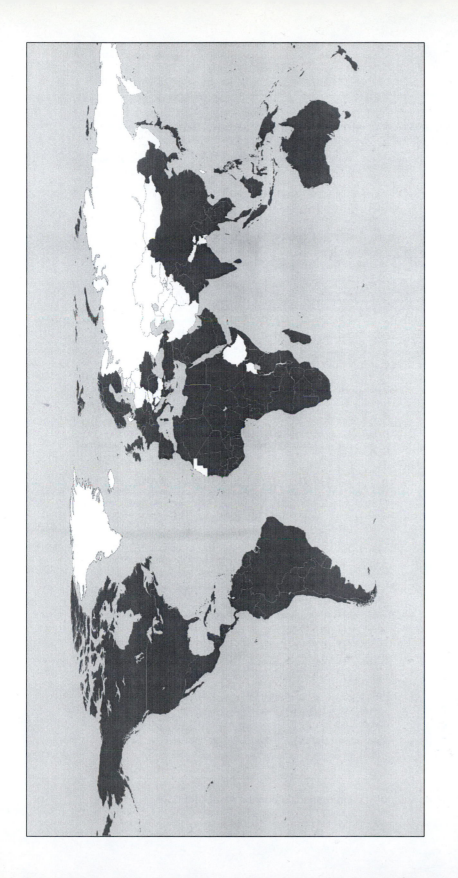

Areas Covered in International Guide to Speech Acquisition

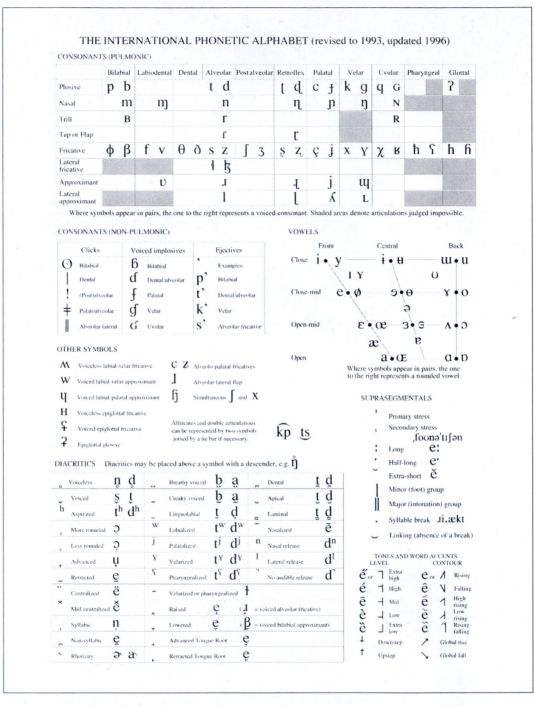

THE INTERNATIONAL PHONETIC ALPHABET (revised to 1993, updated 1996)

Reproduced with the permission of the International Phonetic Association.

CPSIA information can be obtained
at www.ICGtesting.com
Printed in the USA
FFOW03n1835020215
10763FF